Insulin Resistance and Insulin Resistance Syndrome

Insulin Resistance and Insulin Resistance Syndrome

Editor: Frank Cohen

FOSTER ACADEMICS

www.fosteracademics.com

www.fosteracademics.com

FOSTER ACADEMICS

Cataloging-in-Publication Data

Insulin resistance and insulin resistance syndrome / edited by Frank Cohen.
p. cm.
Includes bibliographical references and index.
ISBN 978-1-63242-953-7
1. Insulin resistance. 2. Metabolic syndrome. 3. Insulin antibodies.
4. Diabetes--Complications. I. Cohen, Frank.
RC662.4 .I57 2020
616.46--dc23

Foster Academics,
118-35 Queens Blvd., Suite 400,
Forest Hills, NY 11375, USA

ISBN 978-1-63242-953-7 (Hardback)

Contents

Preface

This book has been a concerted effort by a group of academicians, researchers and scientists, who have contributed their research works for the realization of the book. This book has materialized in the wake of emerging advancements and innovations in this field. Therefore, the need of the hour was to compile all the required researches and disseminate the knowledge to a broad spectrum of people comprising of students, researchers and specialists of the field.

Insulin resistance is a set of signs and symptoms that occur due to inhibited insulin activity. It is a subset of a larger group of symptoms called the insulin resistance syndrome. The condition leads to high circulating levels of insulin, and stimulates the formation of new fatty tissues, thus accelerating weight gain and leading to obesity. Insulin resistance is also associated with insulin resistance syndrome or metabolic syndrome. Insulin resistance syndrome refers to an aggregate of five known medical conditions- high blood sugar, central obesity, high blood pressure, high serum triglycerides and low serum high-density lipoprotein. It is generally considered a risk factor for type 2 diabetes and cardiovascular disease. The nature of the development of this syndrome is still an area of active medical research. It often affects older obese adults having a degree of insulin resistance and leading a sedentary life. Whether insulin resistance or obesity triggers metabolic syndrome or if they are consequences of a complex metabolic derangement is a subject of study. Each disorder manifested in metabolic syndrome is treated separately. Hypertension is treated using ACE inhibitors and diuretics, and cholesterol drugs are prescribed to manage abnormal levels of triglycerides and LDL/HDL cholesterol. Restricting the intake of carbohydrate in food is recommended for the management of both insulin resistance and insulin resistance syndrome. The topics included in this book on insulin resistance and insulin resistance syndrome are of utmost significance and bound to provide incredible insights to readers. It presents researches and studies performed by experts across the globe. It will prove to be immensely beneficial to students and researchers.

At the end of the preface, I would like to thank the authors for their brilliant chapters and the publisher for guiding us all-through the making of the book till its final stage. Also, I would like to thank my family for providing the support and encouragement throughout my academic career and research projects.

Editor

1

Effects of *Lactobacillus paracasei* CNCM I-4034, *Bifidobacterium breve* CNCM I-4035 and *Lactobacillus rhamnosus* CNCM I-4036 on Hepatic Steatosis in Zucker Rats

Julio Plaza-Diaz[1,2], Carolina Gomez-Llorente[1,2], Francisco Abadia-Molina[3], Maria Jose Saez-Lara[4], Laura Campaña-Martin[2], Sergio Muñoz-Quezada[1,2¤], Fernando Romero[5], Angel Gil[1,2], Luis Fontana[1,2*]

1 Department of Biochemistry & Molecular Biology II, School of Pharmacy, University of Granada, Granada, Spain, **2** Institute of Nutrition & Food Technology "José Mataix", Biomedical Research Center, University of Granada, Granada, Spain, **3** Department of Cell Biology, School of Sciences, University of Granada, Granada, Spain, **4** Department of Biochemistry & Molecular Biology I, School of Sciences, University of Granada, Granada, Spain, **5** Hero Global Technology Center, Hero Spain, S.A., Alcantarilla, Murcia, Spain

Abstract

We have previously described the safety and immunomodulatory effects of *Lactobacillus paracasei* CNCM I-4034, *Bifidobacterium breve* CNCM I-4035 and *Lactobacillus rhamnosus* CNCM I-4036 in healthy volunteers. The scope of this work was to evaluate the effects of these probiotic strains on the hepatic steatosis of obese rats. We used the Zucker rat as a genetic model of obesity. Zucker-Lepr$^{fa/fa}$ rats received one of three probiotic strains, a mixture of *L. paracasei* CNCM I-4034 and *B. breve* CNCM I-4035, or a placebo for 30 days. An additional group of Zucker-lean$^{+/fa}$ rats received a placebo for 30 days. No alterations in intestinal histology, in the epithelial, lamina propria, muscular layers of the ileal or colonic mucosa, or the submucosae, were observed in any of the experimental groups. Triacylglycerol content decreased in the liver of Zucker-Lepr$^{fa/fa}$ rats that were fed *L. rhamnosus*, *B. breve*, or the mixture of *B. breve* and *L. paracasei*. Likewise, the area corresponding to neutral lipids was significantly smaller in the liver of all four groups of Zucker-Lepr$^{fa/fa}$ rats that received probiotics than in rats fed the placebo. Zucker-Lepr$^{fa/fa}$ rats exhibited significantly greater serum LPS levels than Zucker-lean$^{+/fa}$ rats upon administration of placebo for 30 days. In contrast, all four groups of obese Zucker-Lepr$^{fa/fa}$ rats that received LAB strains exhibited serum LPS concentrations similar to those of Zucker-lean$^{+/fa}$ rats. Serum TNF-α levels decreased in the Zucker-Lepr$^{fa/fa}$ rats that received *B. breve*, *L. rhamnosus*, or the mixture, whereas *L. paracasei* feeding decreased IL-6 levels in the serum of Zucker-Lepr$^{fa/fa}$ rats. In conclusion, the probiotic strains reduced hepatic steatosis in part by lowering serum LPS, and had an anti-inflammatory effect in obese Zucker rats.

Editor: Jose Luis Balcazar, Catalan Institute for Water Research (ICRA), Spain

Funding: Part of the research currently in progress in the authors' laboratory is funded by the company Hero Spain, S. A. through the grant #3545 managed by the Fundacion General Empresa-Universidad de Granada. No additional external funding was received for this study. The funders played a role in the study design, but had no role in the decision to publish or preparation of the manuscript.

Competing Interests: Part of the research currently in progress in the authors' laboratory is funded by the company Hero Spain, S. A. through the grant #3545 managed by the Fundacion General Empresa-Universidad de Granada. Fernando Romero is employed by Hero Global Technology Center, Hero Spain, S.A. This center is part of the food company HERO, headquartered in Switzerland. There are no patents, products in development or marketed products to declare.

* E-mail: fontana@ugr.es

¤ Current address: National Agency for Medicines (ANAMED), Public Health Institute, Santiago, Chile

Introduction

Obesity has reached pandemic levels and is becoming a serious health problem worldwide. In developing countries, the prevalence of obesity has tripled over the last 20 years owing to the adoption of a Western lifestyle (i.e., low physical activity levels, sedentariness, and excessive eating) [1,2].

The increasing prevalence of type 2 diabetes (T2D), cardiovascular disease, and certain types of cancer is linked to obesity. Thus, approximately 90% of T2D cases are attributable to excess body weight, and 200 million people worldwide are estimated to have glucose intolerance and insulin resistance syndrome (IRS), a figure that is expected to rise to 420 million by the year 2025 [3].

Recent evidence indicates that the intestinal microbiota plays a crucial role in body weight and fat mass [4–6], and, accordingly, suggests an association between the gut microbiota and T2D [7–9]. Probiotics are live microorganisms that confer a health benefit on the host when administered in adequate amounts [10], although dead bacteria and bacterial molecular components may also exhibit probiotic properties. Strains belonging to *Bifidobacter-*

ium and *Lactobacillus* are the most widely used probiotic bacteria and are included in many functional foods and dietary supplements [11–13]. Probiotics can modulate the gut microbiota and the mucosal immune system [14–16].

For probiotics to be successful, they must exhibit certain characteristics: i.e., tolerance to gastrointestinal conditions (gastric acid and bile), ability to adhere to the gastrointestinal mucosa, and competitive exclusion of pathogens [17,18]. We have previously described the isolation of three lactic acid bacterial (LAB) strains from the feces of exclusively breast-fed newborn infants. These strains were selected based on their probiotic properties, such as adhesion to intestinal mucus, sensitivity to antibiotics and resistance to biliary salts and low pH. We identified these strains as *Lactobacillus paracasei* CNCM I-4034, *Bifidobacterium breve* CNCM I-4035, and *Lactobacillus rhamnosus* CNCM I-4036 [19].

Recently, we demonstrated the tolerance and safety of these three strains in a multi-centre, randomized, double-blind, placebo-controlled trial with healthy volunteers [20]. Oral administration of these LAB strains modified the bacterial populations in the feces of the volunteers, and all three strains exerted varying degrees of immunomodulatory effects [20]. Thus, administration of *B. breve* CNCM I-4035 resulted in a significant increase in fecal secretory IgA content. In addition, IL-4 and IL-10 was increased, whereas IL-12 was decreased, in the serum of volunteers treated with any of the three strains.

A large body of evidence has highlighted the concept that putative intestinal bacteria–derived compounds may affect liver metabolism and, therefore, cause systemic diseases [6,21,22]. Serum LPS levels have been proposed to increase upon obesity and steatosis, leading to a metabolic endotoxemia capable of modulating proinflammatory cytokines, as well as glucose and lipid metabolism in the liver or in the adipose tissue [23–26]. Endotoxemia is considered a major risk for inducing liver inflammation in nonalcoholic steatohepatitis (NASH) and nonalcoholic fatty liver disease (NAFLD) in humans [27–30]. NASH and NAFLD have been shown to be associated with increased gut permeability in humans [31,32]. Cani et al. have demonstrated the alteration of gut-barrier function in genetic models of obesity [33]. Overall, these studies strongly suggest a direct link between the gut microbiota, the gut barrier, and hepatic changes.

In the present study, we used the Zucker rat as a genetic model of obesity to test the probiotic properties of our three LAB strains. We chose the Zucker rat model because it has been exhaustively characterized and exhibits symptoms of IRS that are usually found in obese humans, including hyperglycemia, glucose intolerance, hyperinsulinemia, insulin resistance, hyperlipidemia, and hepatic steatosis [34–38]. We focused on evaluating the effects of the LAB strains on hepatic steatosis in lean and obese Zucker rats.

Materials and Methods

Ethical Statement

This study was carried out in strict accordance with the recommendations in the guidelines for animal research of the University of Granada (Spain). All animals received humane care. The protocol was approved by the Committee on the Ethics of Animal Experiments of the University of Granada (Permit Number. CEEA: 2011–377).

Microorganisms

The LAB strains *Lactobacillus paracasei* CNCM I-4034, *Bifidobacterium breve* CNCM I-4035, and *Lactobacillus rhamnosus* CNCM I-4036 have been characterized and are described elsewhere [19]. These strains were assayed for enzymatic activity and carbohydrate utilization, and they were deposited in the Collection Nationale de Cultures de Microorganismes (CNCM) of the Institute Pasteur [19].

Experimental design

Forty-eight Zucker-Lepr$^{fa/fa}$ and 16 Zucker-lean$^{+/fa}$ male rats weighing 168–180 g were purchased from Harlan Laboratories (Charles River, Barcelona, Spain). The rats were housed in metabolic cages with a 12-h light-dark cycle and had free access to water and food. After 5 days of adaptation, 8 Zucker-lean$^{+/fa}$ and 8 Zucker-Lepr$^{fa/fa}$ rats were euthanized as a reference (baseline). The remaining 40 Zucker-Lepr$^{fa/fa}$ rats were then randomly assigned to receive 10^{10} CFUs of one of the three probiotic strains, a mixture of *Lactobacillus paracasei* CNCM I-4034 and *Bifidobacterium breve* CNCM I-4035, or a placebo by oral administration each day for 30 days. An additional group of 8 Zucker-lean$^{+/fa}$ rats received placebo for 30 days. The placebo contained 67% cow's milk powder, 32.5% sucrose, and 0.56% vitamin C. The goal of this study was to examine the differences between obese rats treated with probiotics and placebo.

After the intervention, the animals were anesthetized and sedated with ketamine and xylazine. Blood was drawn from the aorta and centrifuged for 10 min at $1000\times g$ and 4°C to separate the serum from cells. Samples of intestinal mucosa and liver were also taken.

Intestinal histology

Ileum and colon samples were fixed with 4% paraformaldehyde for 4 h at room temperature and embedded in paraffin. Three pieces of each ileum and colon were respectively embedded in the same paraffin block. Five-µm-thick sections were obtained and routinely stained with haematoxylin-eosin for their microscopic examination. Two rats per group and 8 sections per rat were stained and examined.

Hepatic triacylglycerol (TG) assay

Hepatic TG content was determined using a commercial kit according to the manufacturer's instructions (SpinReact, Gerona, Spain). The TG values were normalized to liver weight.

Oil red O staining

Liver samples were fixed with 4% paraformaldehyde, cryopreserved in 30% phosphate-buffered saline (PBS)-sucrose, frozen in an isopentane liquid nitrogen bath, and embedded in OCT™ compound. Three pieces of liver from each animal were fixed and embedded in the same block. Seven µm-thick cryostat sections were obtained and stained with a solution of 0.3% Oil Red O in 60% isopropanol. Four to 8 sections per block were stained, micrographs were taken and the percentage of the micrograph area corresponding to the lipid staining was calculated using ImageJ software (National Institutes of Health, USA). Two rats per group were used for this study.

Serum biochemistry

Concentrations of glucose, insulin, phospholipids, triacylglycerols, HDL-cholesterol, LDL-cholesterol, and non-esterified fatty acids (NEFA), as well as the activities of AST and ALT were determined in the serum of the rats using commercial kits. Relative insulin sensitivity was determined by the homeostasis model assessment of insulin resistance (HOMA-IR) as described [39].

Serum lipopolysaccharide (LPS) concentration

Serum LPS was measured with an enzyme-linked immunosorbent assay kit from Cloud-Clone Corp., Houston, USA, following the manufacturer's directions.

Adipokine and cytokine quantification in serum

Serum concentrations of leptin, adiponectin, TNF-α, and IL-6 were measured using MILLIplex^{TM} immunoassays (Merck-Millipore, MA, USA) and the Luminex 200 system according to the manufacturer's instructions.

Statistical analysis

All results are expressed as the mean ± SEM unless otherwise indicated. Statistical analyses between Zucker-Lepr$^{fa/fa}$ and Zucker-lean$^{+/fa}$ male rats were performed using the t test at the baseline and after the intervention (placebo groups). Significant differences between obese rats that received placebo and any group of obese rats that received a specific strain after intervention were analyzed using one-factor ANOVA, which was corrected by an *a posteriori* Bonferroni test ($P<0.05$). All analyses were performed using the statistical package IBM SPSS (Statistical Package for the Social Sciences) Statistics 20 (Somers, NY).

Results

Zucker-Lepr$^{fa/fa}$ rats exhibited severe signs of insulin resistance syndrome (IRS) at the end of the intervention period

Although the body weights of Zucker-Lepr$^{fa/fa}$ (n = 8) and Zucker-lean$^{+/fa}$ rats (n = 8) were initially similar (179.9 g±2.2 g vs. 168.9 g±4.9 g, respectively, $P>0.3$), the Zucker-Lepr$^{fa/fa}$ rats were clearly obese after 30 days of feeding with the placebo (Zucker-Lepr$^{fa/fa}$ (n = 8) 294.4 g±5.7 g vs. Zucker-lean$^{+/fa}$ (n = 8) 241.5 g±5.6 g, $P<0.001$). No adverse events occurred during or after treatment.

We measured parameters related to carbohydrate and lipid metabolism, as well as hepatic function in the serum of the rats (n = 8 per group, Table 1). At baseline, the glucose, insulin, HOMA-IR, phospholipid, TG, total cholesterol, and HDL cholesterol concentrations were significantly greater in the Zucker-Lepr$^{fa/fa}$ rats than in the Zucker-lean$^{+/fa}$ rats ($P<0.05$). With the exceptions of phospholipids and HDL cholesterol, all of these parameters were worse in obese rats that were fed the placebo for 30 days compared to the lean controls ($P<0.05$) (Table 1).

The LDL cholesterol and NEFA concentrations were similar in both groups of rats at baseline but were significantly higher in Zucker-Lepr$^{fa/fa}$ rats that were fed the placebo for 30 days compared to Zucker-lean$^{+/fa}$ rats ($P<0.05$) (Table 1). At baseline, the AST and ALT activities differed between the Zucker-Lepr$^{fa/fa}$ rats and the Zucker-lean$^{+/fa}$ rats and remained significantly elevated in the Zucker-Lepr$^{fa/fa}$ rats after the intervention (t = 30) with the placebo ($P<0.05$) (Table 1). The concentrations of TG, total cholesterol and NEFA, as well as the ALT activity, of Zucker-Lepr$^{fa/fa}$ rats worsened after 30 days of intervention ($P<0.05$).

The TG content was also measured in the livers of the rats (Figure 1). Hepatic TG content was similar in Zucker-Lepr$^{fa/fa}$ rats and Zucker-lean$^{+/fa}$ rats at baseline. However, the liver TG content was 2.5-fold greater in the Zucker-Lepr$^{fa/fa}$ rats at the end of the intervention with the placebo ($P<0.05$) (Figure 1). Together, these results indicated that Zucker-Lepr$^{fa/fa}$ rats showed clear signs of IRS.

Table 1. Serum biochemical parameters of Zucker-lean$^{+/fa}$ and Zucker-Lepr$^{fa/fa}$ rats fed either a placebo or LAB strains.

	Baseline		Placebo		Intervention with LAB strains			
	ZL	ZO	ZL	ZO	*L. rhamnosus*	*L. paracasei*	*B. breve*	Mixture
Glucose (mg/dL)	165.2±11.1	257.4±38.7#	191.1±4.9	290.1±33.2†	267.2±14.7	243.2±38.9	229.7±19.6	272.7±15.7
Insulin (µg/L)	0.8±0.1	3.1±1.1#	1.1±0.1	3.4±0.5†	3.8±0.6	3.9±1.0	3.5±0.4	2.6±0.4
HOMA-IR	3.1±0.5	8.0±1.1#	4.2±0.2	18.2±3.9†	13.8±2.3	9.7±2.3	13.2±1.6	11.6±2.1
Phospholipids (mg/dL)	185.4±7.6	271.9±20.8#	144.4±7.8	242.9±43.2†	283.7±14.7	239.9±49.2	318.2±16.2	323.9±23.1
Triacylglycerols (mg/dL)	54.3±4.5	152.7±23.2#	46.2±1.8	256.4±25.1†*	242.5±26.9	364±12.1	269.1±51.3	297.7±46.9
Total Cholesterol (mg/dL)	123.6±6.5	143.5±4.7#	99.6±3.7	174.5±13.1†*	191±10.9	208.8±22.8	211.3±5.4	191±10.9
HDL Cholesterol (mg/dL)	32.1±0.9	40.7±2.3#	18.9±2.1	23.8±7.1	39.7±5.5	28.4±8	33.7±3.4	37.3±1.8
LDL Cholesterol (mg/dL)	80.5±5.3	77.2±8.3	70.3±3.3	99.3±11.9†	93.9±14.2	126.6±20	108.8±7.9	111.6±12.3
NEFA (mmol/L)	0.3±0.03	0.3±0.01	0.3±0.04	0.5±0.05†*	0.4±0.04	0.6±0.1	0.6±0.08	0.6±0.08
AST (U/L)	110±13.5	216.1±19.9#	97.2±10.8	356±69.3†	309.7±52.6	378.7±61.6	424.3±70.9	363.6±58.5
ALT (U/L)	39.4±2.5	130.8±19.9#	35.8±6.1	275±52.6†*	235±31.4	316.8±46.3	347.9±60.3	296±61.9

Values are the means ± SEM, n = 8 per group. #$P<0.05$ (ZL baseline vs. ZO baseline), †$P<0.05$ (ZL + placebo vs. ZO + placebo), *$P<0.05$ (ZO baseline vs. ZO + placebo). ALT, alanine aminotransferase; AST, aspartate aminotransferase; NEFA, non-esterified fatty acids. HOMA-IR, homeostasis model assessment of insulin resistance. ZL, Zucker-lean$^{+/fa}$ rats; ZO, Zucker-Lepr$^{fa/fa}$ rats.

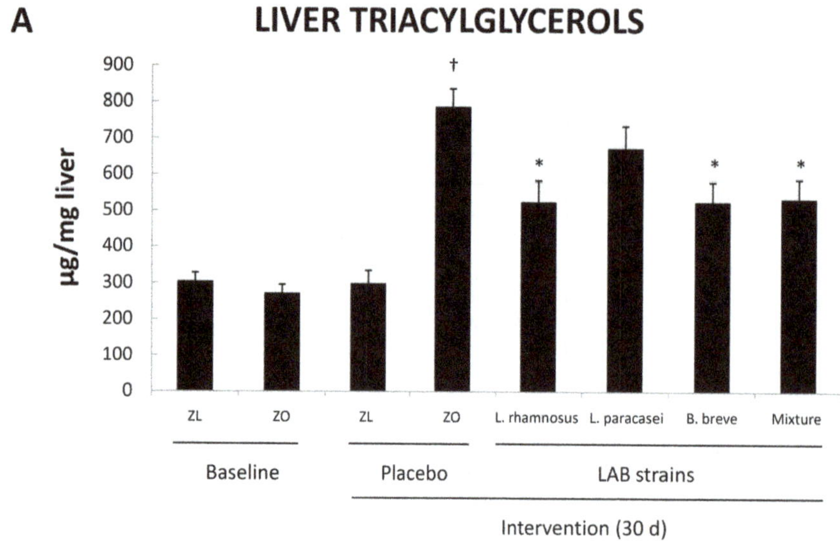

Figure 1. Liver triacylglycerol content of Zucker-lean$^{+/fa}$ and Zucker-Lepr$^{fa/fa}$ rats that were fed either a placebo or LAB strains for 30 days. Values are the means ± SEM, n = 8 per group. †*P*<0.05 (ZL + placebo vs. ZO + placebo), and **P*<0.05 (ZO + placebo vs. ZO + LAB strains). ZL, Zucker-lean$^{+/fa}$ rats; ZO, Zucker-Lepr$^{fa/fa}$ rats.

LAB strains did not exert any effect, beneficial or detrimental, on intestinal histology

No alterations in intestinal histology, of the epithelial, lamina propria, or muscular layers of the ileal or colonic mucosa, or in the submucosae, were observed in any of the experimental groups (Figure 2). The remaining intestinal layers also appeared normal in all of the experimental groups. These results suggested that the probiotics did not alter the morphology of this organ, reinforcing the safety of all three LAB strains.

Steatosis was decreased in Zucker-Lepr$^{fa/fa}$ rats that were fed LAB strains

To investigate whether the bacterial strains affected hepatic steatosis, we measured the TG content in the liver of rats fed these strains (Figure 1). Strikingly, the TG content was significantly lower in the liver of Zucker-Lepr$^{fa/fa}$ rats that were fed *L. rhamnosus* CNCM I-4036, *B. breve* CNCM I-4035, or the mixture of *B. breve* CNCM I-4035 and *L. paracasei* CNCM I-4034 for 30 days ($P<0.05$) than in the liver of Zucker-Lepr$^{fa/fa}$ rats that were fed the placebo (Figure 1).

These results were confirmed by Oil red O staining of liver sections (Figure 3). All four groups of Zucker-Lepr$^{fa/fa}$ rats that received probiotic bacteria exhibited significantly lower percentages of neutral lipids in the liver compared with Zucker-Lepr$^{fa/fa}$ rats fed the placebo (Figure 3).

LAB strains did not affect serum biochemistry

No significant differences in HOMA-IR values or any of the biochemical parameters that were analyzed in the serum were found among the various groups of Zucker-Lepr$^{fa/fa}$ rats that received LAB strains after an intervention of 30 days (Table 1),

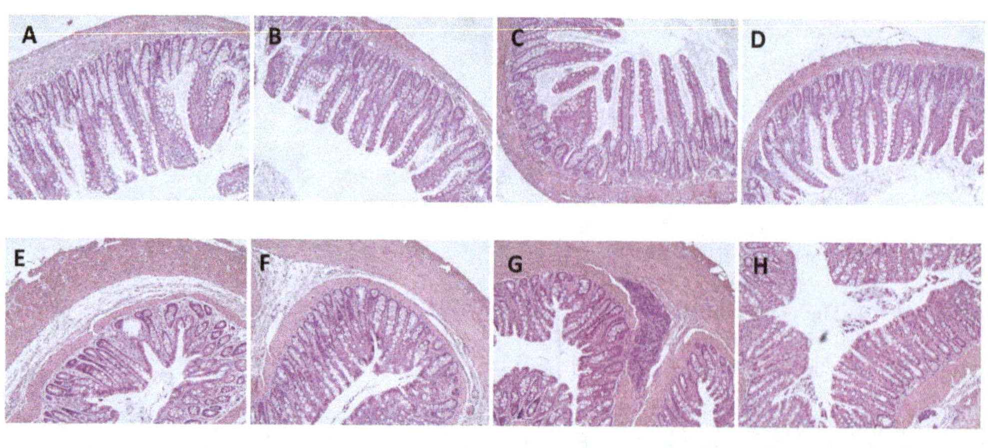

Figure 2. Haematoxylin-eosin stained, 5-µm-thick sections of ileal (top panels, A–D) and colonic (bottom panels, E–H) mucosa of Zucker-lean$^{+/fa}$ and Zucker-Lepr$^{fa/fa}$ rats that were fed either a placebo or LAB strains for 30 days. Two rats per group were used for this staining. Three pieces of tissue from each animal were fixed and embedded in the same paraffin block. Four to 8 sections per block were cut, stained and analyzed. Representative micrographs from various groups are shown. A and E: Zucker-lean$^{+/fa}$ rats at baseline; B and F: Zucker-Lepr$^{fa/fa}$ rats + placebo; C and G: Zucker-Lepr$^{fa/fa}$ rats +*L. rhamnosus*; and D and H: Zucker-Lepr$^{fa/fa}$ rats + LAB mixture.

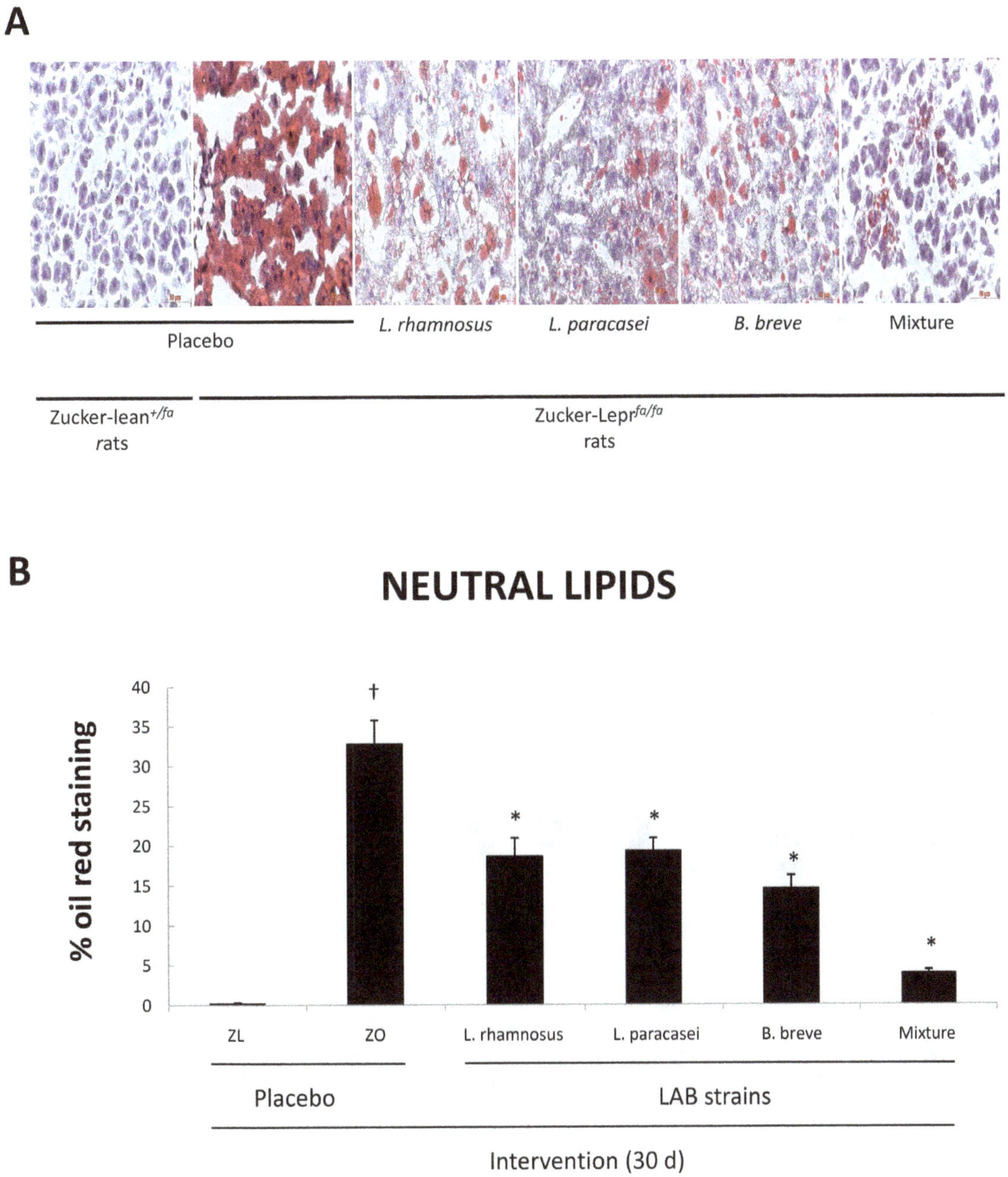

Figure 3. Representative micrographs of 7-μm-thick liver sections stained with 0.3% Oil red O in 60% isopropanol of Zucker-lean$^{+/fa}$ and Zucker-Lepr$^{fa/fa}$ rats that were fed either a placebo or LAB strains for 30 days (A). Percentage of the micrograph area corresponding to the lipid staining of liver sections described in panel A was calculated (B). Values are the means ± SEM, n = 2 per group. $^{†}P<0.05$ (ZL + placebo vs. ZO + placebo), and $^{*}P<0.05$ (ZO + placebo vs. ZO + LAB strains). ZL, Zucker-lean$^{+/fa}$ rats; ZO, Zucker-Lepr$^{fa/fa}$ rats.

suggesting that the bacterial strains did not affect serum markers of IRS.

LAB strains modified the profile of serum cytokines but not serum adipokines

We determined the serum concentrations of leptin, adiponectin, TNF-α, and IL-6. At baseline, the concentrations of leptin and adiponectin (Figure 4) were significantly greater in Zucker-Lepr$^{fa/fa}$ rats than in Zucker-lean$^{+/fa}$ rats ($P<0.05$). These results further supported the above serum biochemistry measurements that indicated that Zucker-Lepr$^{fa/fa}$ rats suffered from IRS. At the end of the intervention with the placebo, leptin concentration remained higher in the obese rats than in the lean controls ($P<0.05$) (Figure 4A). Probiotics exerted no effect on the levels of any of the adipokines that were analyzed (Figure 4).

At baseline, the serum TNF-α and IL-6 concentrations were similar in Zucker-Lepr$^{fa/fa}$ and Zucker-lean$^{+/fa}$ rats (Figure 5), but the TNF-α concentration was significantly increased (Figure 5A) in obese rats after 30 days of intervention with the placebo ($P<0.05$). Intervention with *L. rhamnosus* CNCM I-4036, *B. breve* CNCM I-4035, or the mixture of *L. paracasei* CNCM I-4034 and *B. breve* CNCM I-4035 decreased serum TNF-α concentrations in Zucker-

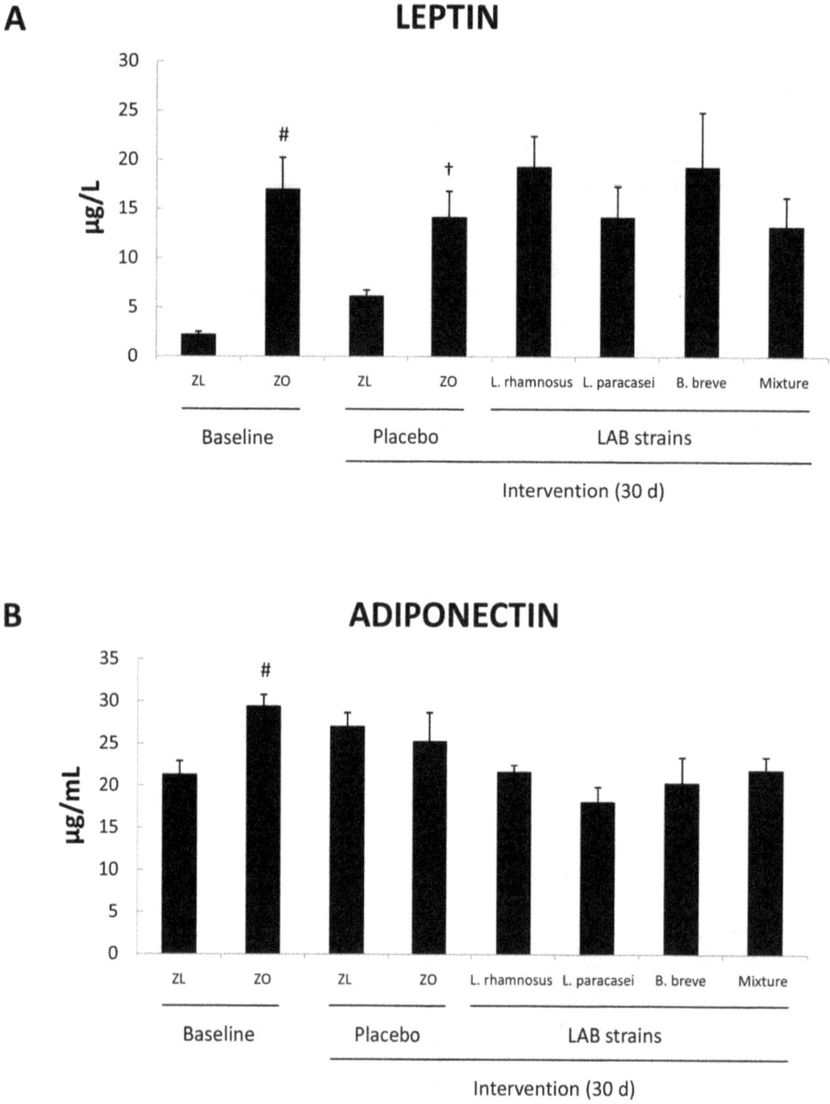

Figure 4. Serum leptin (A) and adiponectin (B) concentrations of Zucker-lean$^{+/fa}$ and Zucker-Lepr$^{fa/fa}$ rats that were fed either a placebo or LAB strains for 30 days. Values are the means ± SEM, n = 8 per group. $^{\#}P<0.05$ (ZL baseline vs. ZO baseline), and $^{\dagger}P<0.05$ (ZL + placebo vs. ZO + placebo). ZL, Zucker-lean$^{+/fa}$ rats; ZO, Zucker-Lepr$^{fa/fa}$ rats.

Lepr$^{fa/fa}$ rats ($P<0.05$) (Figure 5A). The serum IL-6 levels decreased upon *L. paracasei* CNCM I-4034 administration ($P<0.05$) (Figure 5B).

Administration of LAB strains to obese rats decreased serum LPS concentrations

To shed light on the potential mechanism of action of the probiotic strains we measured LPS concentrations in serum samples. These results appear in Figure 6. Zucker-Lepr$^{fa/fa}$ rats exhibited significantly greater LPS levels than Zucker-lean$^{+/fa}$ rats upon administration of placebo for 30 days. In contrast, all four groups of obese Zucker-Lepr$^{fa/fa}$ rats that received LAB strains exhibited serum LPS concentrations similar to those of Zucker-lean$^{+/fa}$ rats. These results matched those obtained for liver TG content (Figure 1) and clearly demonstrate the impact of probiotic administration on serum LPS.

Discussion

Metabolic syndrome, which is better termed insulin resistance syndrome (IRS), was originally defined as concomitant hyperlipidemia, hypertension, insulin resistance and obesity [40,41]. IRS often precedes the onset of type 2 diabetes and increases the risk of cardiovascular disease [42,43]; therefore, IRS has become a major public health concern. The Zucker rat shows many of the features of IRS; therefore, it is one of the most commonly used genetic models of this syndrome [43]. Under our experimental conditions, Zucker-Lepr$^{fa/fa}$ rats exhibited obesity, hyperglycemia, insulin resistance, hypercholesterolemia, hypertriglyceridemia, and elevated serum free fatty acid concentrations after 30 days of intervention with the placebo in contrast to Zucker-lean$^{+/fa}$ rats. In addition, Zucker-Lepr$^{fa/fa}$ rats had hepatic steatosis, as well as elevated serum AST and ALT activities, indicating that the liver component of IRS was also present in this model.

As we have previously described in human subjects [20], the administration of our three LAB strains was safe, as determined by

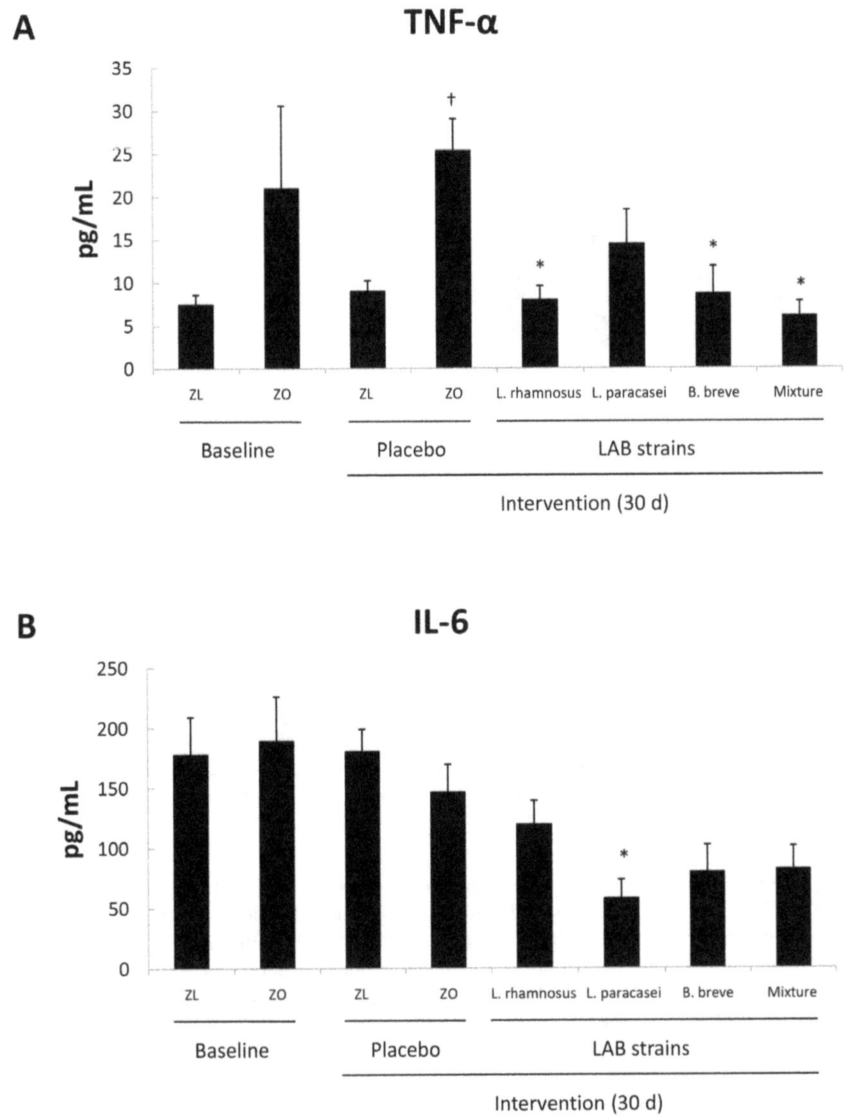

Figure 5. Concentrations of serum TNF-α (A) and IL-6 (B) of Zucker-lean$^{+/fa}$ and Zucker-Lepr$^{fa/fa}$ rats that were fed either a placebo or LAB strains for 30 days. Values are the means ± SEM, n = 8 per group. $^{\dagger}P<0.05$ (ZL + placebo vs. ZO + placebo), and $^{*}P<0.05$ (ZO + placebo vs. ZO + probiotic strains). ZL, Zucker-lean$^{+/fa}$ rats; ZO, Zucker-Lepr$^{fa/fa}$ rats.

intestinal histology, which showed no difference between LAB strain-fed rats and placebo-fed rats.

We took advantage of the Zucker rat model to investigate the effects of three probiotic strains on IRS features and inflammation. Administration of the probiotic strains did not affect serum biochemical parameters, insulin resistance, or the adipokine profile. These findings were in accordance with results recently reported in human volunteers who were fed these same three LAB strains [20].

The main finding of this study was the reduction in liver steatosis observed in obese rats fed probiotics. Zucker-Lepr$^{fa/fa}$ rats that received *L. rhamnosus* CNCM I-4036, *B. breve* CNCM I-4035, or a mixture of *B. breve* CNCM I-4035 and *L. paracasei* CNCM I-4034 had a liver TG content lower than rats fed the placebo. This drop in liver TG content may not be attributable to a decrease in serum insulin concentration because insulinemia was similar in Zucker-Lepr$^{fa/fa}$ rats fed placebo and those fed LAB strains. Additionally, given that the administration of *L. paracasei* CNCM I-4034 alone did not lower liver TG content in the obese rats, the effect observed by mixing the two probiotics might be attributable to *B. breve* CNCM I-4035. Oil red O staining of liver neutral lipids confirmed this finding in probiotic-fed obese rats.

The administration of probiotics has been reported to lower the hepatic TG and cholesterol content in mice and rats with high fat diet-induced obesity [33,44–47]. To our knowledge, however, this is the first study describing the effect of probiotics on lowering the liver TG content in genetically obese Zucker rats. This anti-steatotic effect seemed to be mediated, at least in part, by the lowering of serum LPS observed in the probiotic-fed groups of obese rats. Overall our results support the current evidence that intestinal bacteria may affect liver metabolism [6,21,43].

Clear anti-inflammatory effects of probiotics were found in this study: i) the lower serum TNF-α concentrations found in Zucker-Lepr$^{fa/fa}$ rats that received *L. rhamnosus* CNCM I-4036, *B. breve* CNCM I-4035, or a mixture of *B. breve* CNCM I-4035 and *L. paracasei* CNCM I-4034 than in Zucker-Lepr$^{fa/fa}$ rats fed the

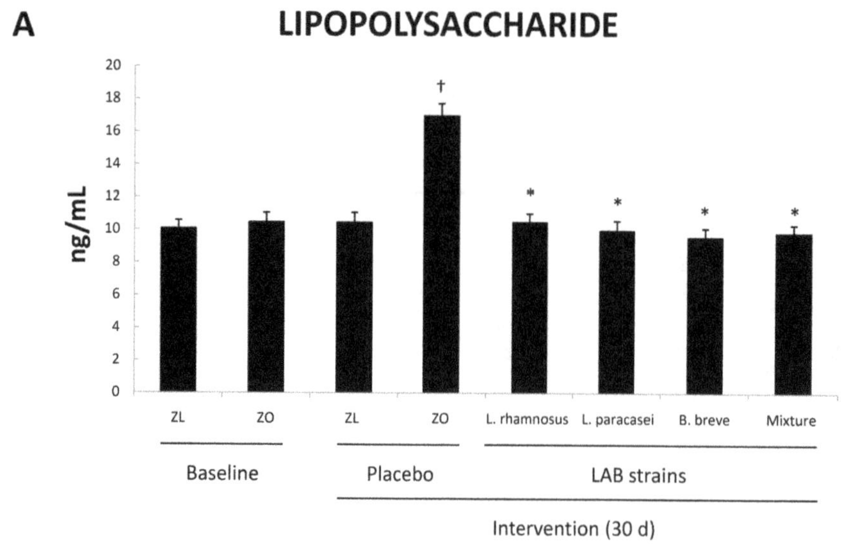

Figure 6. LPS concentration in serum of Zucker-lean$^{+/fa}$ and Zucker-Lepr$^{fa/fa}$ rats that were fed either a placebo or LAB strains for 30 days. Values are the means ± SEM, n = 8 per group. †$P<0.05$ (ZL + placebo vs. ZO + placebo), and *$P<0.05$ (ZO + placebo vs. ZO + LAB strains). ZL, Zucker-lean$^{+/fa}$ rats; ZO, Zucker-Lepr$^{fa/fa}$ rats.

placebo; and ii) the lower serum IL-6 concentrations in obese rats fed *L. paracasei* CNCM I-4034 than in obese rats fed the placebo. Two previous studies by our group have reported the effects of *L. paracasei* CNCM I-4034 and *B. breve* CNCM I-4035 on the production of cytokines and chemokines by cultured human intestinal dendritic cells challenged with *Salmonella typhi* [48,49]. *L. paracasei* CNCM I-4034 decreased the amounts of proinflammatory cytokines and chemokines in these cells [48], whereas *B. breve* CNCM I-4035 was a potent inducer of pro-inflammatory factors (TNF-α, IL-8 and RANTES (Regulated on Activation, Normal T Cell Expressed and Secreted) and anti-inflammatory factors (IL-10) [49]. In the present study, the administration of *L. paracasei* CNCM I-4034 decreased the concentrations of proinflammatory cytokines such as IL-6.

Other authors have described the anti-inflammatory effects of probiotic administration. Probiotics have been reported to significantly suppress the high-fat-diet-induced activation of nuclear factor κ-B signaling that is involved in the development of high-fat-diet-induced insulin resistance [50]. In addition, the administration of lactobacilli to rats developing alcohol-induced metabolic endotoxemia and liver disease reduced plasma endotoxin levels and the liver pathology score [51]. A mixture of bifidobacteria, lactobacilli, and *Streptococcus thermophilus* has been shown to decrease liver inflammation in genetically obese mice [52] and high-fat-diet-induced hepatic inflammation in young rats [53].

Taken together, the results suggested that our probiotic strains ameliorated hepatic steatosis through a decrease in serum LPS and diminished the serum profile of proinflammatory cytokines of obese Zucker rats. These findings, along with those previously obtained by our group using these probiotic strains in *in vivo* and human studies, warrant further study to investigate the potential use of these bacterial strains as coadjuvants in the treatment of human disease.

Author Contributions

Conceived and designed the experiments: CGLL FR AG LF. Performed the experiments: JPD FAM MJSL SMQ. Analyzed the data: JPD CGL FAM LCM AG LF. Contributed reagents/materials/analysis tools: FR. Contributed to the writing of the manuscript: JPD FAM AG LF.

References

1. Haslam DW, James WPT (2005) Obesity Lancet 366: 1197–1209.
2. Hossain P, Katar B, El Vahas M (2007) Obesity and diabetes in the developing world. A growing challenge. N Engl J Med 356: 213–215.
3. Wang Y, Lobstein T (2006) Worldwide trends in childhood overweight and obesity. Int J Pediatr Obes 1: 11–25.
4. Turnbaugh PJ, Ley RE, Mahowald MA, Magrini V, Mardis ER, et al. (2006) An obesity-associated gut microbiome with increased capacity for energy harvest. Nature 444: 1027–1031.
5. Knaapen M, Kootte RS, Zoetendal EG, de Vos WM, Dallingha-Thie GM, et al. (2013) Obesity, nonalcoholic fatty liver disease, and atherothrombosis: a role for the intestinal microbiota? Clin Microbiol Infect 19: 331–337.
6. Delzenne NM, Cani PD (2011) Interaction between obesity and the gut microbiota: relevance in nutrition. Annu Rev Nutr 31: 15–31.
7. Ley RE, Backhed F, Turnbaugh P, Lozupone CA, Knight RD, et al. (2005) Obesity alters gut microbial ecology. Proc Natl Acad Sci USA 102: 11070–11075.
8. Ley RE, Turnbaugh PJ, Klein S, Gordon JI (2006) Microbial ecology: human gut microbes associated with obesity. Nature 444: 1022–1023.
9. Backhed F, Ley RE, Sonnenburg JL, Peterson DA, Gordon JI (2005) Host-bacterial mutualism in the human intestine. Science 307: 1915–1920.
10. World Health Organization and Food & Agriculture Organization (2002) Guidelines for the Evaluation of Probiotics in Food. Report of a joint FAO/WHO working group on drafting guidelines for the evaluation of probiotics in food. London, Ontario, Canada. ftp://ftp.fao.org/es/esn/food/wgreport2.pdf
11. Gourbeyre P, Denery S, Bodinier M (2011) Probiotics, prebiotics, and synbiotics: impact on the gut immune system and allergic reactions. J Leukoc Biol 89: 685–695.
12. Macpherson AJ, Harris NL (2004) Interactions between commensal intestinal bacteria and the immune system. Nat Rev Immunol 4: 478–485.
13. Frick JS, Schenk K, Quitadamo M, Kahl F, Köberle M, et al. (2007) *Lactobacillus fermentum* attenuates the proinflammatory effect of *Yersinia enterocolitica* on human epithelial cells. Inflamm Bowel Dis 13: 83–90.
14. Yadav H, Jain S, Sinha PR (2008) Oral administration of dahi containing probiotic *Lactobacillus acidophilus* and *Lactobacillus casei* delayed the progression of streptozotocin-induced diabetes in rats. J Dairy Res 75: 189–195.

15. Power SE, O'Toole PW, Stanton C, Ross RP (2014) Intestinal microbiota, diet and health. Br J Nutr 111: 387–402.
16. Smith PM, Howitt MR, Panikov N, Michaud M, Gallini CA, et al. (2013) The microbial metabolites, short-chain fatty acids, regulate colonic Treg cell homeostasis. Science 341: 569–573.
17. Collins JK, Thornton G, Sullivan GO (1998) Selection of probiotic strains for human application. Int Dairy J 8: 487–490.
18. Ouwehand AC, Salminen S, Isolauri E (2002) Probiotics: an overview of beneficial effects. Antonie van Leeuwenhoek 82: 279–289.
19. Muñoz-Quezada S, Chenoll E, Vieites JM, Genovés S, Maldonado J, et al. (2013) Isolation, identification and characterisation of three novel probiotic strains (*Lactobacillus paracasei* CNCM I-4034, *Bifidobacterium breve* CNCM I-4035 and *Lactobacillus rhamnosus* CNCM I-4036) from the faeces of exclusively breast-fed infants. Br J Nutr 109: S51–S62.
20. Plaza-Diaz J, Gomez-Llorente C, Campaña-Martin L, Matencio E, Ortuño I, et al. (2013) Safety and immunomodulatory effects of three probiotic strains isolated from the feces of breast-fed infants in healthy adults: Setoprob study. PLoS ONE 8: e78111.
21. Nolan JP (1979) The contribution of gut-derived endotoxins to liver injury. Yale J Biol Med 52: 127–133.
22. Nolan JP, Leibowitz AI (1978) The contribution of gut-derived endotoxins to liver injury. Gastroenterology 75: 765–766.
23. Cani PD, Delzenne NM (2009) Interplay between obesity and associated metabolic disorders: new insights into the gut microbiota. Curr Opin Pharmacol 9: 737–743.
24. Cani PD, Delzenne NM (2009) The role of the gut microbiota in energy metabolism and metabolic disease. Curr Opin Pharmacol 15: 1546–1558.
25. Lanthier N, Molendi-Coste O, Horsmans Y, van RN, Cani PD, et al. (2009) Kupffer cell activation is a causal factor for hepatic insulin resistance. Am J Physiol Gastrointest Liver Physiol 298: 107–116.
26. Neyrinck AM, Cani PD, Dewulf EM, De BF, Bindels LB, et al. (2009) Critical role of Kupffer cells in the management of diet-induced diabetes and obesity. Biochem Biophys Res Commun 385: 351–356.
27. Adachi Y, Moore LE, Bradford BU, Gao W, Thurman RG (1995) Antibiotics prevent liver injury in rats following long-term exposure to ethanol. Gastroenterology 108: 218–224.
28. Verdam FJ, Rensen SS, Driessen A, Greve JW, Buurman WA (2010) Novel evidence for chronic exposure to endotoxin in human nonalcoholic steatohepatitis. J Clin Gastroenterol 5: 149–152.
29. Harte AL, da Silva NF, Creely SJ, McGee KC, Billyard T, et al. (2010) Elevated endotoxin levels in nonalcoholic fatty liver disease. J Inflamm (Lond.) 7: 15.
30. Thuy S, Ladurner R, Volynets V, Wagner S, Strahl S, et al. (2008) Nonalcoholic fatty liver disease in humans is associated with increased plasma endotoxin and plasminogen activator inhibitor 1 concentrations and with fructose intake. J Nutr 138: 1452–1455.
31. Farhadi A, Gundlapalli S, Shaikh M, Frantzides C, Harrell L, et al. (2008) Susceptibility to gut leakiness: a possible mechanism for endotoxaemia in nonalcoholic steatohepatitis. Liver Int 28: 1026–1033.
32. Miele L, Valenza V, La TG, Montalto M, Cammarota G, et al. (2009) Increased intestinal permeability and tight junction alterations in nonalcoholic fatty liver disease. Hepatology 49: 1877–1887.
33. Cani PD, Possemiers S, Van de WT, Guiot Y, Everard A, et al. (2009) Changes in gut microbiota control inflammation in obese mice through a mechanism involving GLP-2-driven improvement of gut permeability. Gut 58: 1091–1103.
34. Serkova NJ, Jackman M, Brown JL, Liu T, Hirose R, et al. (2006) Metabolic profiling of livers and blood from obese Zucker rats. J Hepatol 44: 956–962.
35. Obeid OA, Powell-Tuck J, Emery PW (2000) The postprandial rates of glycogen and lipid synthesis of lean and obese female Zucker rats. Int J Obes Relat Metab Disord 24: 508–513.
36. Erdös B, Snipes JA, Miller AW, Busija DW (2004) Cerebrovascular dysfunction in Zucker obese rats is mediated by oxidative stress and protein kinase C. Diabetes 53: 1352–1359.
37. Dokken BB, Henriksen EJ (2006) Chronic selective glucogen synthase kinase-3 inhibition enhances glucose disposal and muscle insulin action in prediabetic obese Zucker rats. Am J Physiol Endocrinol Metab 291: 207–213.
38. D'Angelo G, Mintz JD, Tidwell JE, Schreihofer AM, Pollock DM, et al. (2006) Exaggerated cardiovascular stress responses and impaired β-adrenergic-mediated pressor recovery in obese Zucker rats. Hypertension 48: 1109–1115.
39. Singh R, Wang Y, Xiang Y, Tanaka KE, Gaarde WA, et al. Differential effects of JNK1 and JNK2 inhibition on murine steatohepatitis and insulin resistance. Hepatology 2009; 49: 87–96.
40. Reaven GM (1988) Role of insulin resistance in human disease. Diabetes 37: 1595–1607.
41. Reaven GM (2004) The metabolic syndrome or the insulin resistance syndrome? Different names, different concepts, and different goals. Endocrinol Metab Clin North Am 33: 283–303.
42. Lakka HM, Laaksonen DE, Lakka TA, Niskanen LK, Kumpusalo E, et al. (2002) The metabolic syndrome and total and cardiovascular disease mortality in middle-aged men. JAMA 288: 2709–2716.
43. Kahn R, Buse J, Ferrannini E, Stern M (2005) The metabolic syndrome: time for a critical appraisal: joint statement from the American Diabetes Association and the European Association for the Study of Diabetes. Diabetes Care 28: 2289–2304.
44. Paik HD, Park JS, Park E (2005) Effects of *Bacillus polyfermenticus* SCD on lipid and antioxidant metabolisms in rats fed a high-fat and high-cholesterol diet. Biol Pharm Bull 28: 1270–1274.
45. Xie N, Cui Y, Yin YN, Zhao X, Yang JW, et al. (2011) Effects of two *Lactobacillus* strains on lipid metabolism and intestinal microflora in rats fed a high-cholesterol diet. BMC Complement Altern Med 11: 53.
46. Awaisheh SS, Khalifeh MS, Al-Ruwaili MA, Khalil OM, Al-Ameri OH, et al. (2013) Effect of supplementation of probiotics and phytosterols alone or in combination on serum and hepatic lipid profiles and thyroid hormones of hypercholesterolemic rats. J Dairy Sci 96: 9–15.
47. Yoo SR, Kim YJ, Park DY, Jung UJ, Jeon SM, et al. (2013) Probiotics *L. plantarum* and *L. curvatus* in combination alter hepatic lipid metabolism and suppress diet-induced obesity. Obesity (Silver Spring) 21: 2571–2578.
48. Bermudez-Brito M, Muñoz-Quezada S, Gomez-Llorente C, Matencio E, Bernal MJ, et al. (2012) Human intestinal dendritic cells decrease cytokine release against *Salmonella* infection in the presence of *Lactobacillus paracasei* upon TLR activation. PLoS ONE 7: e43197.
49. Bermudez-Brito M, Muñoz-Quezada S, Gomez-Llorente C, Matencio E, Bernal MJ, et al. (2013) Cell-Free culture supernatant of *Bifidobacterium breve* CNCM I-4035 decreases pro-Inflammatory cytokines in human dendritic cells challenged with *Salmonella typhi* through TLR activation. PLoS ONE 8: e59370.
50. Ma X, Hua J, Li Z (2008) Probiotics improve high fat diet-induced hepatic steatosis and insulin resistance by increasing hepatic NKT cells. J Hepatol 49: 821–830.
51. Nanji AA, Khettry U, Sadrzadeh SM (1994) *Lactobacillus* feeding reduces endotoxemia and severity of experimental alcoholic liver (disease). Proc Soc Exp Biol Med 205: 243–247.
52. Li Z, Yang S, Lin H, Huang J, Watkins PA, et al. (2003) Probiotics and antibodies to TNF inhibit inflammatory activity and improve nonalcoholic fatty liver disease. Hepatology 37: 343–350.
53. Esposito E, Iacono A, Bianco G, Autore G, Cuzzocrea S, et al. (2009) Probiotics reduce the inflammatory response induced by a high-fat diet in the liver of young rats. J Nutr 139: 905–911.

2

Multiple Low-Dose Radiation Prevents Type 2 Diabetes-Induced Renal Damage through Attenuation of Dyslipidemia and Insulin Resistance and Subsequent Renal Inflammation and Oxidative Stress

Minglong Shao[1,2,3], Xuemian Lu[3], Weitao Cong[2,4], Xiao Xing[1,5], Yi Tan[2,6], Yunqian Li[7], Xiaokun Li[2,4], Litai Jin[2,4], Xiaojie Wang[4], Juancong Dong[1], Shunzi Jin[1]*, Chi Zhang[2,3]*, Lu Cai[2,6]

1 School of Public Health of Jilin University, Changchun, China, **2** Chinese-American Research Institute for Diabetic Complications, Wenzhou Medical University, Wenzhou, China, **3** Ruian Center of Chinese-American Research Institute for Diabetic Complications, the Third Affiliated Hospital of the Wenzhou Medical University, Wenzhou, China, **4** School of Pharmacy, Wenzhou Medical College, Wenzhou, China, **5** Changchun Institute for Food and Drug Control, Changchun, China, **6** Kosair Children's Hospital Research Institute at the Department of Pediatrics, University of Louisville, Louisville, Kentucky, United States of America, **7** Department of Neurosurgery, the First Hospital of Jilin University, Changchun, China

Abstract

Background: Dyslipidemia and lipotoxicity-induced insulin resistance, inflammation and oxidative stress are the key pathogeneses of renal damage in type 2 diabetes. Increasing evidence shows that whole-body low dose radiation (LDR) plays a critical role in attenuating insulin resistance, inflammation and oxidative stress.

Objective: The aims of the present study were to investigate whether LDR can prevent type 2 diabetes-induced renal damage and the underlying mechanisms.

Methods: Mice were fed with a high-fat diet (HFD, 40% of calories from fat) for 12 weeks to induce obesity followed by a single intraperitoneal injection of streptozotocin (STZ, 50 mg/kg) to develop a type 2 diabetic mouse model. The mice were exposed to LDR at different doses (25, 50 and 75 mGy) for 4 or 8 weeks along with HFD treatment. At each time-point, the kidney weight, renal function, blood glucose level and insulin resistance were examined. The pathological changes, renal lipid profiles, inflammation, oxidative stress and fibrosis were also measured.

Results: HFD/STZ-induced type 2 diabetic mice exhibited severe pathological changes in the kidney and renal dysfunction. Exposure of the mice to LDR for 4 weeks, especially at 50 and 75 mGy, significantly improved lipid profiles, insulin sensitivity and protein kinase B activation, meanwhile, attenuated inflammation and oxidative stress in the diabetic kidney. The LDR-induced anti-oxidative effect was associated with up-regulation of renal nuclear factor E2-related factor-2 (Nrf-2) expression and function. However, the above beneficial effects were weakened once LDR treatment was extended to 8 weeks.

Conclusion: These results suggest that LDR exposure significantly prevented type 2 diabetes-induced kidney injury characterized by renal dysfunction and pathological changes. The protective mechanisms of LDR are complicated but may be mainly attributed to the attenuation of dyslipidemia and the subsequent lipotoxicity-induced insulin resistance, inflammation and oxidative stress.

Editor: Zane Andrews, Monash University, Australia

Funding: This study was supported in part by a Young Scientist Award from the National Science Foundation of China (81000294, to CZ); the National Science Foundation of China (81370917, to CZ); the Research Development Fund of Wenzhou Medical University (QTJ13005, to CZ); the National Institutes of Health (1 R01 DK091338-01A1, to LC); a Start-up Fund for the Chinese-American Research Institute for Diabetic Complications from Wenzhou Medical University (to XL and LC); and the Zhejiang Provincial Natural Science Foundation (LQ12H07002, to WTC; LQ13H020005, to YW). The funders had no role in study design, data collection and analysis, decision to publish, or preparation of the manuscript.

Competing Interests: The authors have declared that no competing interests exist.

* E-mail: jinsz@jlu.edu.cn (SJ); zhangchi515@126.com (CZ)

Introduction

Diabetic nephropathy (DN) is one of the most severe complications of type 2 diabetes, which accounts for approximately 40% of all new cases who require renal replacement therapy [1,2]. DN initiates with early-stage diabetic kidney disease (DKD) characterized by renal dysfunction, and finally leading to fibrosis and glomerulosclerosis [3–6].

Although the pathogeneses of kidney disease in type 2 diabetes are complicated, dyslipidemia and the subsequent lipotoxicity are regarded as critical inducers of renal damage under diabetic conditions [7–9]. Dyslipidemia is characterized by abnormal lipid profiles [10,11], which contribute to progression of DKD [12]. Furthermore, dyslipidemia always leads to an imbalance between circulating and cytosolic fatty acid (FA) levels, which induce lipotoxicity [13].

Lipotoxicity underlies the insulin-deficient state, especially insulin resistance. Strong evidence showed that excessive FAs and their derivatives serve as signaling molecules that activate protein kinases [13]. These kinases can then impair insulin signaling, finally lead to insulin resistance [14,15]. It has been reported that lipotoxicity-induced insulin resistance plays a critical role in type 2 diabetes induced renal damage [16]. Moreover, insulin resistance directly induces relaxation of the afferent arteriole, resulting in glomerular hyperfiltration, angiogenesis and mesangial cell proliferation, then contributing to the development of DN [17,18]. Lipotoxicity also induces oxidative stress by production of reactive oxygen species (ROS) which causes damage to the glomeruli and glomerular glycocalyx and increases the permeability of the glomerular filtration barrier, which may contribute to the progression of DKD [19,20].

Inflammation is another key consequence of lipotoxicity in type 2 diabetes, which also strongly exacerbates kidney injury in type 2 diabetes characterized by increasing the release of multiple inflammatory factors [21,22]. Therefore, attenuation of dyslipidemia and the subsequent lipotoxicity might be a novel therapeutic strategy for DKD in type 2 diabetes.

Various therapeutic approaches have been investigated, but most if not all drugs need to be excreted via the kidney, which will further increase the renal working load in diabetic patients [23]. Based on this concern, low-dose ionizing radiation (LDR) as a non-invasive approach has been investigated to prevent chronic renal diseases [24,25]. Our previous study also determined that LDR significantly prevented renal damage in type 1 diabetic mice [23]. We also found that LDR prevented type 1 diabetes-induced renal oxidative stress via up-regulation of multiple anti-oxidants levels [26]. However, whether LDR can induce similarly beneficial effects on renal damage in type 2 diabetes is still unknown. To this end, we used the strategy of high-fat diet (HFD) feeding plus streptozotocin (STZ) injection to develop the type 2 diabetic mice models [27,28]. Then we investigated whether exposure to LDR could attenuate dyslipidemia, inflammation and oxidative stress and enhanced insulin sensitivity in type 2 diabetes.

Materials and Methods

Ethics Statement

The protocol was approved by the Committee on the Ethics of Animal Experiments of Jilin University, Jilin, China (Permit Number: 2007-0011). All surgery was performed under sodium pentobarbital anesthesia and all efforts were made to minimize suffering.

Animals and Induction of Type 2 Diabetes

Male C57BL/6J mice, 8 weeks old (18–22 g of body weight), were purchased from the experimental Animal Center of Beijing University of Medical Science (Beijing, China) and allowed to acclimate for 2 weeks. All mice were housed in the animal facility of the Jilin University Animal Center at 22°C with a 12:12-h light-dark cycle and free access to rodent chow and tap water.

In order to establish type 2 diabetic model, the combined strategy of a HFD (Shanghai SLAC laboratory Animal Co., Ltd., 40% of calories from fat) and STZ (Sigma Chemical, St. Louis, MO) treatment was applied in our study. The mice were fed with HFD for 12 weeks to induce obesity, characterized by abnormal glucose tolerance and insulin resistance. The age-matched nondiabetic mice were fed with a standard diet (SD, Shanghai SLAC laboratory Animal Co., Ltd., 10% of calories from fat). Then, the mice fed with HFD were intraperitoneally given a single injection of STZ at 50 mg/kg body weight. In addition, the mice fed with SD were given an injection of equivalent volume of citrate buffer. Blood glucose level was examined using a FreeStyle glucose meter (Abbott Diabetes Care, Alameda, CA) 3 days after the injection of STZ. Mice were considered diabetic when blood glucose exceeded 12 mmol/L. Next, mice were continued to feed with the corresponding diet for another 4 or 8 weeks.

Whole-body Low dose Rate X-ray Radiation

A 180-kVp X-ray generator (Model XSZ-Z20/20, China) was utilized to deliver radiation at dose rate of 12.5 mGy/min (120 kv, 13 mA). LDR was given to mice over whole body every other day at a dose of 25, 50 or 75 mGy for 4 or 8 weeks, respectively. Mice from both the diabetic and age-matched nondiabetic groups were randomly divided into the following groups: control group (Con), control plus 50 mGy group (Con/50 mGy), diabetes mellitus group (DM) and DM plus LDR at 25, 50 or 75 mGy (DM/25 mGy, DM/50 mGy, DM/75 mGy). The body weight, kidney weight and tibia length of the mice in all groups were examined at each time point.

Glucose Tolerance Test and Insulin Tolerance Test

To assess glucose tolerance, mice were intraperitoneally injected with D-glucose (1.5 g/kg) after an overnight fasting (12 h) with free access to water, and venous blood was collected 30 min before (time 0) and after injection at 0, 15, 30, 60 and 120 min from the tail of each mouse, and glucose was measured using a FreeStyle glucose meter. To assess insulin tolerance, a single dose of Novolin R regular insulin (Novo Nordisk A/S, Denmark) (0.5 units/kg or 1 unit/kg) was intraperitoneally administered to the mice after fasting for 4 h with free access to water, and the blood glucose level was measured as described above.

Measurements of Urine and Blood Metabolites

Twenty-four-hour urine collections were obtained by placing the mice in metabolic cages during the final 3 days before the mice were sacrificed. Urinary protein, urinary albumin and urinary creatinine were measured using enzyme-linked immunosorbent assay (ELISA) kits purchased from R&D (Itasea, MN) according to the manufacturer's instructions. Briefly, the kits assayed mouse urine protein or albumin and creatinine level in the sample, using purified mouse urinary protein, urinary albumin and urinary creatinine antibody to coat a 96-well plate. Different concentrations of standards, matrix blank and testing samples were added to wells after adding the specified volume of diluents. Followed by 30 min incubation at 37°C and washing, a horseradish peroxidase (HRP) conjugate reagent was added to the wells, except blank wells. After incubation and then washing, a peroxidase substrate-tetramethylbenzidine (TMB) was added to the wells and incubated for 10 min. Then stop solution was added and absorbance was measured at 450 nm within 10 min with a reference wavelength of 650 nm by an ELISA Reader (Molecular Devices MAX 190, USA). The concentration of target factors in the sample was calculated using a corresponding standard plot of the optical density vs. the concentration of the standards.

Blood samples were taken from the retro-orbital venous plexus and allowed to clot (kept still) at room temperature for 30 min. Serums were collected by centrifugation at 2,000×*g* for 20 min at 4°C. Serum triglycerides (TG), total cholesterol (CHO), high-density lipoprotein (HDL)-cholesterol and low-density lipoprotein (LDL)-cholesterol levels were determined using an Olympus

Au800 automatic biochemical analyzer (Olympus, Japan) at the Maternal and Child Health Hospital in Changchun, China.

Quantification of Renal Lipid and Lipid Peroxidation

For the measurement of TG and free fatty acid (FFA) content, 50–80 mg of renal tissue from each mouse was homogenized in 250 μL of buffer containing 150 mM NaCl and 10 mM Tris (pH 7.5), and extracted with 200 μL of methanol and 400 μL of chloroform. The chloroform layer containing TG was evaporated overnight and resuspended in 70% ethanol; TG and FFA content was measured using a commercial ELISA kit (R&D) at 450 nm and expressed relative to the protein content. To determine malondialdehyde (MDA) content, kidney tissues were homogenized in ice-cold 0.05 mM phosphate-buffered saline (PBS; pH 7.4, 1: 10 wt/vol) and centrifuged at 15,000×*g* for 15 min before the supernatants were collected. All these steps were performed at 4°C. The supernatants were then used for measurement of MDA according to the manufacturer's instructions (R&D). The protein levels of the samples were measured using the Coomassie Brilliant Blue G-250 method, with bovine serum albumin as the standard. The data were expressed as milligrams per gram of tissue or nanomoles per milligram of protein.

Total Protein Extraction and Western Blotting

Western blotting assays were performed as described previously [29]. Briefly, renal tissues were homogenized in lysis buffer. Proteins were collected by centrifugation at 12,000×*g* and 4°C. The total protein sample was run on 10.6% SDS-polyacrylamide gel electrophoresis, transferred onto nitrocellulose membranes and incubated in blocking buffer (5% milk and 0.5% bovine serum albumin) for 1 h at room temperature and then incubated overnight at 4°C with following primary antibodies: nuclear factor E2-related factor-2 (Nrf-2, 1: 1000), superoxide dismutase-1 (SOD-1, 1: 2000), NAD(P)H:quinone oxidoreductase-1 (NQO-1, 1: 1000), heme oxygenase-1 (HO-1, 1: 2000), 3-nitrotyrosine (3-NT, 1: 1000), intercellular adhesion molecule-1 (ICAM-1, 1: 2000), plasminogen activator inhibitor-1 (PAI-1, 1: 2000), tumor necrosis factor α (TNF-α, 1: 1000), which were purchased from Abcam (Cambridge, MA); total protein kinase B (*t*-Akt, 1: 2000), phosphorylated-Akt (*p*-Akt, 1: 1000) and β-actin (1: 2000), which were purchased from CST (Danvers, MA). After three washes with tris-buffered saline containing 0.05% Tween 20 (TBST), membranes were incubated with secondary horseradish peroxidase-conjugated antibody for 1 h at room temperature. Antigen-antibody complexes were then developed with an ECL kit (Amersham, Piscataway, NJ). The intensity of protein bands on blots were quantified by using Quantity one (Version 4.6.2, Bio-Rad, USA).

RNA Isolation and Real-time Quantitative Polymerase Chain Reaction (RT-PCR)

Total RNA was isolated from kidney tissues using TRIzol reagent according to the manufacturer's protocol (Invitrogen, Carlsbad, CA) and was quantified with a photometer Nanodrop 2000 (Thermo Scientific, San Jose, CA). The RNA samples were reverse transcribed into cDNA using a High-Capacity cDNA Reverse Transcription Kit (PE Applied Biosystems, Foster City, CA). The following primers were used for RT-PCR. ICAM-1: forward, 5′-GTGATGGCAGCCTCTTATGT-3′; and reverse, 5′-GGGCTTGTCCCTTGAGT TT-3′; PAI-1: forward, 5′-CTCCACAGCCTTTGTCATCT-3′; and reverse, 5′-ATTGTCTC TGTCGGGTTGTG-3′; TNF-α: forward, 5′-CTACCTTGTTGCCTCCTCTTT-3′; and reverse, 5′-GAGCAGAGGTTCAGTGATGTAG-3′; Nrf-2: forward, 5′-CTCCGTGGAGTCTTCCA TTTAC-3′; and reverse, 5′-GCACTATCTAGCTCCTCCATTTC-3′; SOD-1: forward, 5′-GGCAAAGGTGGAAATGAAGAAA-3′; and reverse, 5′-CTCAGACCACACAGGGAA TG-3′; NQO-1: forward, 5′-GAGAAGAGCCCTGATTGTACTG-3′; and reverse, 5′-ACC TCCCATCCTCTCTTCTT-3′; HO-1: forward, 5′-CTCCCTGTGTTTCCTTTCTCTC-3′; and reverse, 5′-CTGCTGGTTTCAAAGTTCAG-3′; β-actin: forward, 5′-AGGTATCCTGA CCCTGAAGTA-3′; and reverse, 5′-CACACGCAGCTCATTGTAGA-3′. RT-PCR was carried out in triplicate using the SYBR GREEN PCR master mix (Invitrogen, Carlsbad, CA) on a Stratagene MX3000p thermocycler (Agligent StrataGene, Santa Clara, CA). The amount of mRNA was calculated by the comparative CT method, which depends on the ratio of the amount of target genes to reference gene β-actin.

Histological Examination and Immunohistochemical Staining

The fixed kidney tissues were cut into 3-mm-thick blocks and embedded in paraffin and cut into 4-μm slices. After deparaffinization and rehydration, the sections were stained with hematoxylin and eosin (H&E) for general morphological examination, periodic acid Schiff (PAS) for evaluation of glomerulosclerosis, and Masson's trichrome-staining for indication of interstitial expansion. Glomerulosclerosis examination was done by a pathologist in a blinded manner as described previous [30,31]. Briefly, each slice randomly was selected five different fields containing at least fifty glomeruli, and the degree of glomerulosclerosis was divided into 4 grades from 0 to 4 according to the ratio of sclerosis lesions to each glomerulus (Grade 0, no changes; Grade 1, sclerotic area <1–25%; Grade 2, sclerotic area <26–50%; Grade 3, sclerotic area <51–75%; and Grade 4, sclerotic area <76–100%). The glomerulosclerosis index (GSI) was calculated with following formula: $GSI = [(N_1 \times 1)+(N_2 \times 2)+(N_3 \times 3)+(N_4 \times 4)]/n_{tot}$, where n_{tot} is the total number of glomeruli. Similarly, the extent of interstitial expansion was evaluated quantitatively by calculating tubular interstitial collagen-positive area (blue) for Masson's trichrome-staining using the Image-Pro plus 6.0 software (Media Cybernetics, Silver Spring, Maryland, USA). Twenty consecutive glomeruli were examined for each section, and the averaged percentages of the collagen-positive lesions were obtained for each mouse.

For immunohistochemical staining, the sections were blocked with Superblock buffer (Pierce, Rockford, IL) for 30 min and incubated with the primary antibodies at a 1: 200 dilution overnight at 4°C. Followed by three washes with PBS, sections were incubated with biotin-labeled secondary antibody (Sigma) for 1 h at room temperature. And signal was detected with diaminobenzidine (DAB) and developed according to manufacturer's instructions. Sections incubated with PBS in place of primary and second antibodies were used as blank controls.

Statistical Analysis

Data were collected from eight or nine mice in each group, and the results are presented as means ± standard error of the mean (SEM). Statistical analyses were performed using one-way or two-way ANOVA: post-hoc multiple comparisons, followed by Bonferroni with the GraphPad Prism 5.0 (GraphPad Software, San Diego, CA). Statistical significance was detected at the 0.05 level.

Results

Diabetic Animal Model and LDR Effects on Hyperglycemia and Insulin Resistance in Type 2 Diabetic Mice

Since clinical type 2 diabetes is always attributed to obesity in humans, in the present study the mice were fed with a HFD followed by a single injection of STZ to mimic human type 2 diabetes. Compared with SD-fed mice, HFD-fed mice exhibited a significant increase in body weight after treatment for 4 weeks, and the difference gradually increased in a time-dependent manner (Fig. 1A). Meanwhile, the glucose tolerance test and insulin tolerance test revealed that mice fed with HFD for 12 weeks exhibited obvious abnormal glucose tolerance (Fig. 1B) and insulin resistance (Fig. 1C). And hyperglycemia was subsequently induced by a single injection of STZ (Fig. 1D). After successful induction of the type 2 diabetic model, the diabetic mice and age-matched nondiabetic mice were randomly divided into groups with or without LDR treatment. As shown in Fig. 1E, F, exposure to LDR at any dose for 4 or 8 weeks had no impact on hyperglycemia in the type 2 diabetic mice, but 50 and 75 mGy treatment for 4 weeks significantly relieved insulin resistance (Fig. 1G). A similar beneficial effect was not observed at the 8-week time-point (Fig. 1H). This finding was also confirmed by calculating the area under the curve of the insulin tolerance test.

Since Akt plays critical role in regulating insulin sensitivity by mediating insulin-stimulated glucose metabolic signaling, we also examined the expression and phosphorylation of renal Akt among groups to identify whether LDR-induced insulin sensitivity increase was related to Akt activation (Fig. 1I). Results showed that neither diabetes nor LDR affected the expression of renal Akt expression; however, diabetes significantly decreased the phosphorylation of renal Akt, which was significantly reversed by LDR treatment for 4 weeks at 50 or 75 mGy, but not at 25 mGy. Exposure to LDR for 8 weeks also did not significantly affect the diabetic effect on Akt phosphorylation levels (Fig. 1I). This result is consistent with the patterns of IP ITT results (Fig. 1G, H).

The Effects of LDR on Type 2 Diabetes-induced Renal Hypertrophy and Dysfunction

As we know, the kidney is the target organ highly vulnerable to damage in type 2 diabetes. Therefore, we would investigate whether LDR can prevent diabetic-induced renal hypertrophy and dysfunction. We found diabetes significantly increased the kidney weight and decreased the body weight of the mice. However the tibia length of the mice in each group was unaffected. The ratio of kidney weight to tibia length strongly increased under diabetic condition. After exposure of the mice to LDR for 4 weeks, the magnitude of the ratio increase was slightly suppressed and the suppression became significantly once the LDR extended to 8 weeks (Table 1).

It is known that renal dysfunction manifests as an increase of the urinary volume, urinary protein and microalbumin (mAlb) and a decrease of urinary creatinine. We observed the above phenomenon in type 2 diabetic mice at both the 4- and 8-week time-points. Exposure of the mice to LDR for 4 weeks significantly prevented an increase of urinary protein and mAlb excretion. In contrast, urinary creatinine excretion was significantly increased after LDR treatment. However, the urinary volume was unaffected. In addition, the beneficial effects of LDR on diabetes induced renal dysfunction was largely diminished (Table 1).

LDR Prevented Type 2 Diabetes-induced Pathological Changes and Glomerulosclerosis in the Kidney

Generally, renal dysfunction reflects pathological changes in the diabetic kidney. Compared with the control group, mice in the Con/50 mGy group displayed a normal structure of glomerulus and renal tubules by H&E examination (Fig. 2A). However, the diabetic kidneys showed obvious Bowman's capsule adhesion, mesangial cell proliferation, mesangial matrix expansion and capillary collapse at the 4-week time-point. Simultaneously, renal tubular dilation and epithelial cell degeneration were also observed in the diabetic kidneys. Furthermore, there were some bubbles in the renal tubules, which were attributed to excessive lipid accumulation in the diabetic kidneys (Fig. 2A). Treatment with 50 mGy or 75 mGy for 4 weeks markedly attenuated the above pathological changes (Fig. 2A).

Meanwhile, kidney tissues were stained with PAS to detect glomerulosclerosis. As shown in (Fig. 2B and 2D). The glomerulosclerosis index was significantly increased in diabetic mice with a time-dependent manner. Exposure to LDR treatment for 4 weeks at 50 and 75 mGy, but not 25 mGy, greatly prevented glomerulosclerosis. However, the protective effect was attenuated once exposure of LDR extended to 8 weeks and only 25 mGy showed notable suppression on diabetes induced glomerulosclerosis.

Masson's trichrome staining showed significant accumulation of collagen in the kidneys of diabetic mice at the 4-week time-point, indicating the development of interstitial fibrosis (Fig. 2C, E). The collagen accumulation and fibrosis were more evident in the kidneys of diabetic mice at the 8-week time-point. Exposure to LDR at doses of 50 and 75 mGy significantly prevented the above phenomenon in type 2 diabetic mice at the 4-week time-point (Fig. 2C, E). The anti-fibrotic effect of LDR became weaker as time progressed to the 8-week time-point and only 25 mGy induced remarkably positive effects on the pathological changes under diabetic conditions (Fig. 2C, E).

LDR Prevented Systemic and Renal Dyslipidemia in Type 2 Diabetic Mice

Dyslipidemia is regarded as a main generator of type 2 diabetes-induced renal damage. Thus, a mechanistic study was carried out to investigate whether LDR can induce beneficial effects on the abnormal lipid profiles in type 2 diabetic mice. We found that under physiological conditions, there was no change in the lipid profiles in Con/50 mGy group (Table 2). In contrast, type 2 diabetes significantly increased plasma TG levels at the 4-week time-point, which was further enhanced at the 8-week time-point (Table 2). Although a dose of 25 mGy did not, LDR at 50 and 75 mGy for 4 weeks remarkably prevented increased plasma TG levels in diabetic mice (Table 2). However, the attenuation effect of LDR at these two doses vanished at the 8-week time-point (Table 2). In contrast, 25 mGy significantly lowered plasma TG under diabetic conditions at the 8-week time-point (Table 2). In addition, we also found that type 2 diabetes strongly increased the total CHO and LDL levels in the plasma at both the 4- and 8-week time-points. Exposure to LDR at any dose remarkably induced a decrease in the plasma LDL levels at the 4-week time-point (Table 2). However, at the 8-week time-point, only LDR at 25 mGy showed a preventive effect on plasma LDL levels in type 2 diabetes. The similar lowering effect due to LDR was not found on total plasma CHO levels at either time-point (Table 2). Furthermore, the results also showed that type 2 diabetes at the 4-week time-point did not, but at the 8-week time-point significantly decreased plasma HDL levels. In contrast, LDR at 50 and 75 mGy

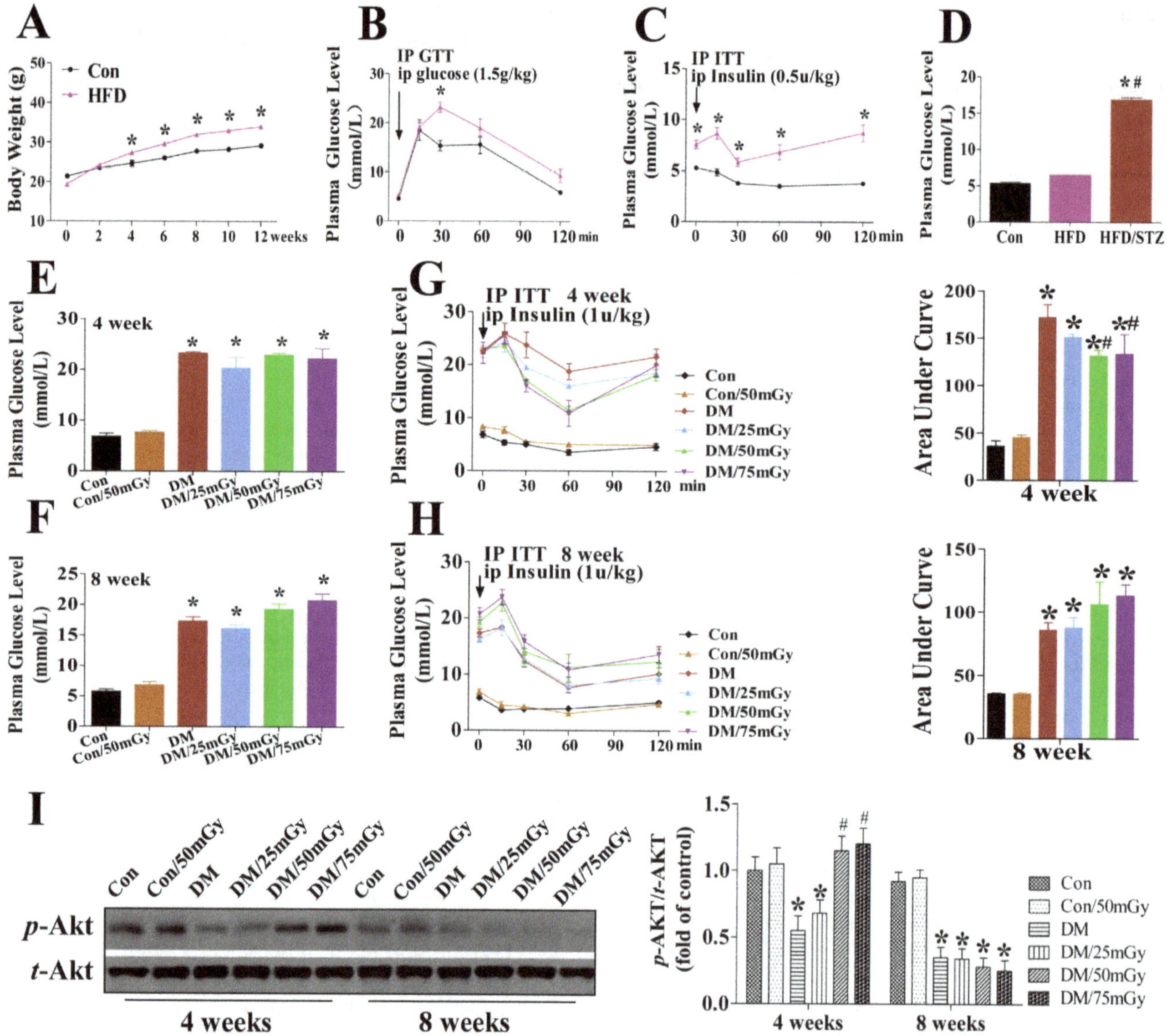

Figure 1. Induction of the type 2 diabetic mouse model and the effect of LDR on diabetes-induced hyperglycemia, insulin resistance and inactivation of Akt. The type 2 diabetic mouse model was established by a combination of a HFD and STZ treatment. C57BL/6J mice were fed with a HFD (40% of calories from fat) for 12 weeks to induce obesity (A), which exhibited abnormal blood glucose tolerance (B) and insulin resistance (C). After intraperitoneal injection of STZ (50 mg/kg), the type 2 diabetic mouse model was successfully induced with the characteristic of hyperglycemia (>12 mmol/L, D). The diabetic or control mice were irradiated with LDR at 25, 50, or 75 mGy over whole-body once every other day for the indicated times. The blood glucose levels and insulin tolerance at the 4-week time-point (E, G) and 8-week time-point (F, H) were examined. The *t*-Akt and *p*-Akt in kidneys were detected by western blotting assay (I). Data are presented as means ± SEM. n = 9 in diabetic group and n = 8 in each other group. **p*<0.05 vs. the corresponding control group; #*p*<0.05 vs. the corresponding DM group. Con, control mice; Con/50 mGy, control mice treated with 50 mGy; DM, diabetic mice without LDR treatment; DM/25 mGy, diabetic mice with LDR at 25 mGy; DM/50 mGy, diabetic mice with LDR at 50 mGy; DM/75 mGy, diabetic mice with LDR at 75 mGy.

remarkably increased plasma HDL levels at both the 4- and 8-week time-point; while 25 mGy showed the similar increasing effect on plasma HDL levels only observed at the 8-week time-point (Table 2).

Consistent with the plasma lipid profile examination in the kidney, increased renal TG and FFA levels were also observed in diabetic mice at both the 4- and 8-week time-points. LDR at 50 and 75 mGy, but not at 25 mGy, remarkably inhibited renal TG and FFA level increases in type 2 diabetic mice at the 4-week time-point (Table 2). The attenuation effect of LDR at these two doses vanished and only 25 mGy slightly prevented but significantly diabetes-induced renal TG increase at the 8-week time-point (Table 2).

LDR Attenuated Renal Inflammation in Type 2 Diabetic Mice

Dyslipidemia in type 2 diabetes always leads to lipotoxicity in the kidney, which can induce renal damage associated with the severe inflammation characterized by the release of multiple inflammatory factors. To define the effects of LDR on diabetes-induced renal inflammation, renal expression of ICAM-1 mRNA and protein was measured by RT-PCR (Fig. 3A) and western

Table 1. Assessment of renal function in mice fed a standard diet or a high-fat diet with sham-radiation or radiation.

		Nondiabetic mice		Type 2 diabetic mice			
		Low dose radiation					
Parameters	weeks	0 mGy	50 mGy	0 mGy	25 mGy	50 mGy	75 mGy
Body weight (g)	4	31.10±	29.66±	27.58±	29.80±	29.53±	28.90±
		0.9	1.05	0.84*	0.9	0.78	0.85*
	8	31.38±	30.46±	28.38±	30.20±	29.33±	29.23±
		1.08	1.2	0.45*	0.82	0.7	1.00*
Kidney weight (g)	4	0.43±	0.39±	0.67±	0.59±	0.53±	0.51±
		0.01	0.03	0.05*	0.03*	0.01	0.02#
	8	0.44±	0.39±	0.66±	0.58±	0.52±	0.51±
		0.02	0.03	0.06*	0.02*	0.06#	0.04#
Urinary volume (mL/24 h)	4	1.10±	1.10±	10.52±	10.30±	10. 20±	9.75±
		0.12	0.14	0.7	0.78	0.45	0.68
	8	1.15±	1.00±	10.80±	10.35±	10.50±	10.30±
		0.13	0.13	0.81	0.58	0.6	0.82
Urinary protein (μg/day)	4	98.3±	92.9±	1048.9±	885.5±	879.8±	848.5±
		1.9	2.3	15.8*	11.5*#	12.6*#	15.3*#
	8	105.9±	107.1±	1134.0±	923.2±	995.8±	967.5±
		1.2	1.5	22.5*	12.8*#	15.4*#	20.7*#
Urinary mAlb (μg/day)	4	6.1±	6.8±	318.2±	297.2±	194.5±	203.9±
		0.4	0.4	13.2*	10.2*	11.7*#	16.4 *#
	8	6.7±	7.2±	382.1±	295.5±	336.4±	378.8±
		0.3	0.4	18.0*	15.5*#	13.6*#	14.4*
Urinary creatinine (μmol/day)	4	40.6±	41.5±	360.9±	387.6±	397.4±	385.7±
		1.6	1	13.6*	16.8*#	13.4*#	15.3*#
	8	41.7±	38.5±	376.9±	386.5±	381.6±	370.8±
		1.5	1.1	16.2*	15.7*	11.5*	14.9*

Notes: Data were presented as means ± SEM. n = 9 in diabetic group and n = 8 in each other group. mAlb, microalbumin;
*$p<0.05$ vs. the corresponding control group;
#$p<0.05$ vs. the corresponding DM group;
&$p<0.05$ vs. the corresponding DM/25 mGy group.

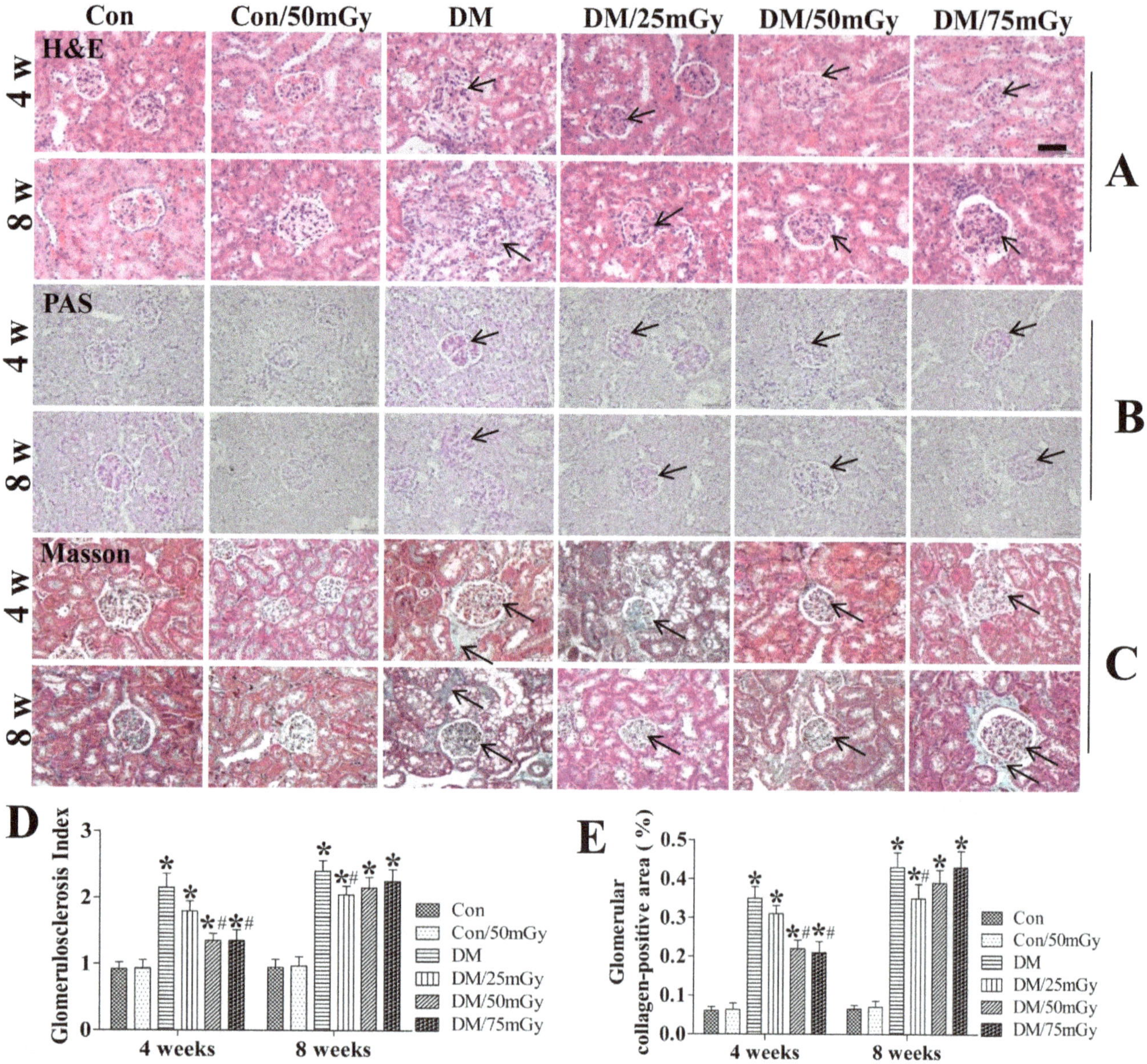

Figure 2. Exposure to LDR attenuated diabetes-induced histopathological changes in the kidneys of mice. Representative images of hematoxylin and eosin (H&E; panel A) staining, periodic acid-Schiff (PAS; panel B) staining, and Masson's trichrome staining (Masson; panel C) for detection of renal pathological changes, glomerulosclerosis and collagen deposition, respectively. 400× magnification. The glomerulosclerosis and collagen accumulation were examined in PAS or Masson stained slices respectively (D, E) and quantified using Image-Pro plus 6.0 software. Data are presented as means ± SEM. n = 9 in diabetic group and n = 8 in each other group. *$p<0.05$ vs. the corresponding control group; #$p<0.05$ vs. the corresponding DM group.

blotting assays (Fig. 3B), respectively. Diabetes induced strong increases in renal ICAM-1 at both the mRNA and protein levels at the 4-week time-point, which were further enhanced at the 8-week time-point. By immunohistochemical staining, diabetes-increased ICAM-1 was found to be expressed predominantly in the glomeruli (Fig. 3C), which was not observed in blank control group (no primary and secondary antibody, Fig. 3C). Multiple exposures of control mice to 50 mGy had no impact on renal ICAM-1 levels but significantly attenuated diabetes-induced ICAM-1 levels after treatment for 4 weeks (Fig. 3A, B). Simultaneously, compared with 25 mGy, LDR at 50 and 75 mGy further attenuated renal ICAM-1 levels in diabetic kidney (Fig. 3A, B). The anti-inflammatory effect of LDR became weaker at the 8-week time-point, although the preventive effect still existed (Fig. 3A, B).

Renal TNF-α expression was also found to be significantly increased in diabetic groups at the mRNA (Fig. 4A) and protein (Fig. 4B) levels in a time-dependent manner. The localization of increased TNF-α expression was found predominantly in tubules and less in the glomerulus (Fig. 4C). The positive staining of TNF-α was increased in diabetic group, which was much less in control group and was unobservable in blank control group (Fig. 4C). Under physiological conditions, control mice exposure to 50 mGy did not change the renal TNF-α level, which were significantly attenuated by LDR treatment at 50 and 75 mGy for 4 weeks in the diabetic kidneys (Fig. 4A, B). However, the anti-inflammatory

Table 2. Plasma and renal lipid metabolic parameters in mice fed a standard diet or a high-fat diet with sham-radiation or radiation.

		Nondiabetic mice		Type 2 diabetic mice			
		Low dose radiation					
Parameters	**weeks**	**0 mGy**	**50 mGy**	**0 mGy**	**25 mGy**	**50 mGy**	**75 mGy**
Plasma TG (mmol/L)	4	1.39±	1.25±	4.62±	4.11±	3.26±	3.37±
		0.12	0.14	0.19*	0.22*	0.24*#	0.18*#
	8	1.40±	1.20±	6.16±	4.72±	5.56±	5.70±
		0.13	0.12	0.28*	0.35*#	0.62*&	0.44*&
Plasma CHO (mmol/L)	4	3.12±	3.09±	4.60±	4.12±	4.32±	4.62±
		0.17	0.29	0.45*	0.30*	0.52*	0.43*
	8	3.24±	3.25±	4.86±	4.82±	4.78±	4.90±
		0.21	0.19	0.52*	0.48*	0.64*	0.45*
Plasma HDL (mmol/L)	4	1.79±	1.75±	1.78±	1.93±	2. 46±	2.49±
		0.14	0.20	0.19	0.24	0.36*#	0.20*#
	8	1.81±	1.88±	1.60±	2.45±	2.48±	2.23±
		0.18	0.22	0.17*	0.15*#	0.21*#	0.29*#
Plasma LDL (mmol/L)	4	0.29±	0.28±	0.46±	0.33±	0.35±	0.38±
		0.03	0.02	0.05*	0.05#	0.03#	0.03#
	8	0.31±	0.32±	0.53±	0.40±	0.52±	0.53±
		0.02	0.04	0.04*	0.03*	0.05*&	0.05*&
Renal TG (mg/g of tissue)	4	1.84±	1.78±	8.56±	7.65±	5.60±	5.45±
		0.10	0.10	0.95*	0.66*	0.45*#	0.58*#
	8	1.85±	1.90±	10.50±	8.86±	9.77±	10.64±
		0.20	0.14	0.70*	0.63*#	0.92*&	0.66*&
Renal FFA (mg/g of tissue)	4	7.85±	7.68±	14.65±	14.06±	10.26±	10.35±
		0.27	0.30	1.00*	0.88*	0.64*#	0.75*#
	8	7.95±	8.12±	17.62±	15.24±	16.78±	17.85±
		0.20	0.40	0.82*	1.05*	0.86*	0.95*

Notes: Data were presented as means ± SEM. n = 9 in diabetic group and n = 8 in each other group. TG, Triglyceride; FFA, free fatty acid; CHO, cholesterol; HDL, high-density lipoprotein; LDL, low-density lipoprotein.
*$p<0.05$ vs. the corresponding control group;
#$p<0.05$ vs. the corresponding DM group;
&$p<0.05$ vs. the corresponding DM/25 mGy group.

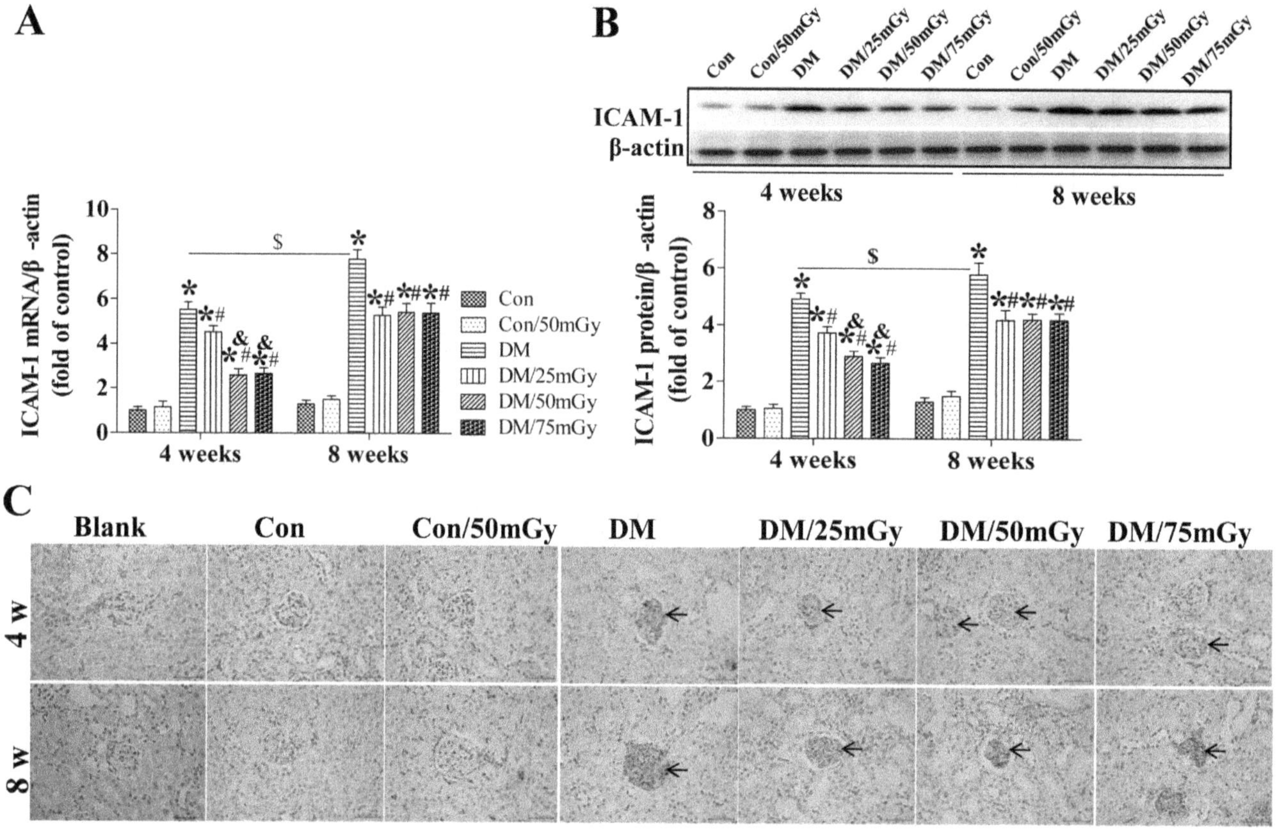

Figure 3. Effect of LDR on renal ICAM-1 levels in type 2 diabetic mice. Renal tissues from different groups were collected at the indicated times for measuring ICAM-1 expression at the mRNA (A) and protein (B) levels with RT-PCR and western blotting, respectively. (C) The location of ICAM-1 in the kidney was detected by immunohistochemical staining, at 400× magnification. Data are presented as means ± SEM. n = 9 in diabetic group and n = 8 in each other group. *$p<0.05$ vs. the corresponding control group; #$p<0.05$ vs. the corresponding DM group; &, $p<0.05$ vs. the corresponding DM/25 mGy; $, $p<0.05$ vs. DM group at the 4-week time-point.

effect of LDR at these two doses vanished at the 8-week time-point. Meanwhile, only 25 mGy induced an attenuation effect on renal TNF-α expression at both the mRNA and protein levels (Fig. 4A, B).

The proinflammatory cytokine PAI-1 is also profibrotic given its inhibition of the conversion of plasminogen to plasmin [32,33]. Moreover, in the present study, we found that exposure to LDR significantly prevented type 2 diabetes-induced inflammation and fibrosis. Therefore, we next determined whether the beneficial effect of LDR was associated with attenuation of renal PAI-1 expression at both the mRNA and protein levels. Real-time PCR and western blotting assays revealed that type 2 diabetes significantly up-regulated renal PAI-1 levels at the 4-week time-point, which were further strengthened at the 8-week time-point (Fig. 5A, B). Immunohistochemical staining confirmed our finding that diabetes-induced PAI-1 expression mainly located in the tubules which was less in the kidneys of nondiabetic mice and unobservable in blank control (Fig. 5C). Exposure to LDR at all doses remarkably attenuated renal PAI-1 levels at the 4-week time-point in diabetic mice. Furthermore, LDR at 50 and 75 mGy showed a greater attenuation effect than at 25 mGy; although the difference did not reach a level of significance (Fig. 5A, B). However, the beneficial effect of LDR at 50 and 75 mGy vanished at the 8-week time-point and only 25 mGy induced remarkable inhibition of the diabetes-caused renal PAI-1 expression increase (Fig. 5A, B).

LDR Prevented Renal Oxidative Stress in Type 2 Diabetic Mice

Oxidative stress is a common consequence of type 2 diabetes closely associated with lipotoxicity. It is also considered as the main pathogenesis of diabetic renal damage. Hence, we further identified the effect of LDR on lipotoxicity-induced oxidative damage measured by 3-NT as an index of nitrosative damage (Fig. 6A) and MDA as a classic oxidative damage marker (Fig. 6B). The results showed that both renal 3-NT and MDA had similar changing patterns among groups. Type 2 diabetes significantly increased their levels in the kidney at the 4-week time-point, and they were further enhanced at the 8-week time-point. LDR at 25 mGy did not, but at 50 and 75 mGy significantly attenuated renal 3-NT and MDA levels at the 4-week time-point under diabetic conditions (Fig. 6). A similar preventive effect of LDR was not found on the 3-NT level at the 8-week time-point; however, LDR at 25 mGy, rather than at 50 and 75, remarkably attenuated the renal MDA level at the same time-point (Fig. 6).

LDR Prevented Diabetic Downregulation of Renal Nuclear Factor E2-related Factor-2 (Nrf-2) Expression and Function

Nrf-2 is a key transcription factor that regulates intracellular redox balance and is a sensor of oxidative stress [34]. Next, we determined whether LDR-induced renal protection against oxidative damage was associated with up-regulation of renal

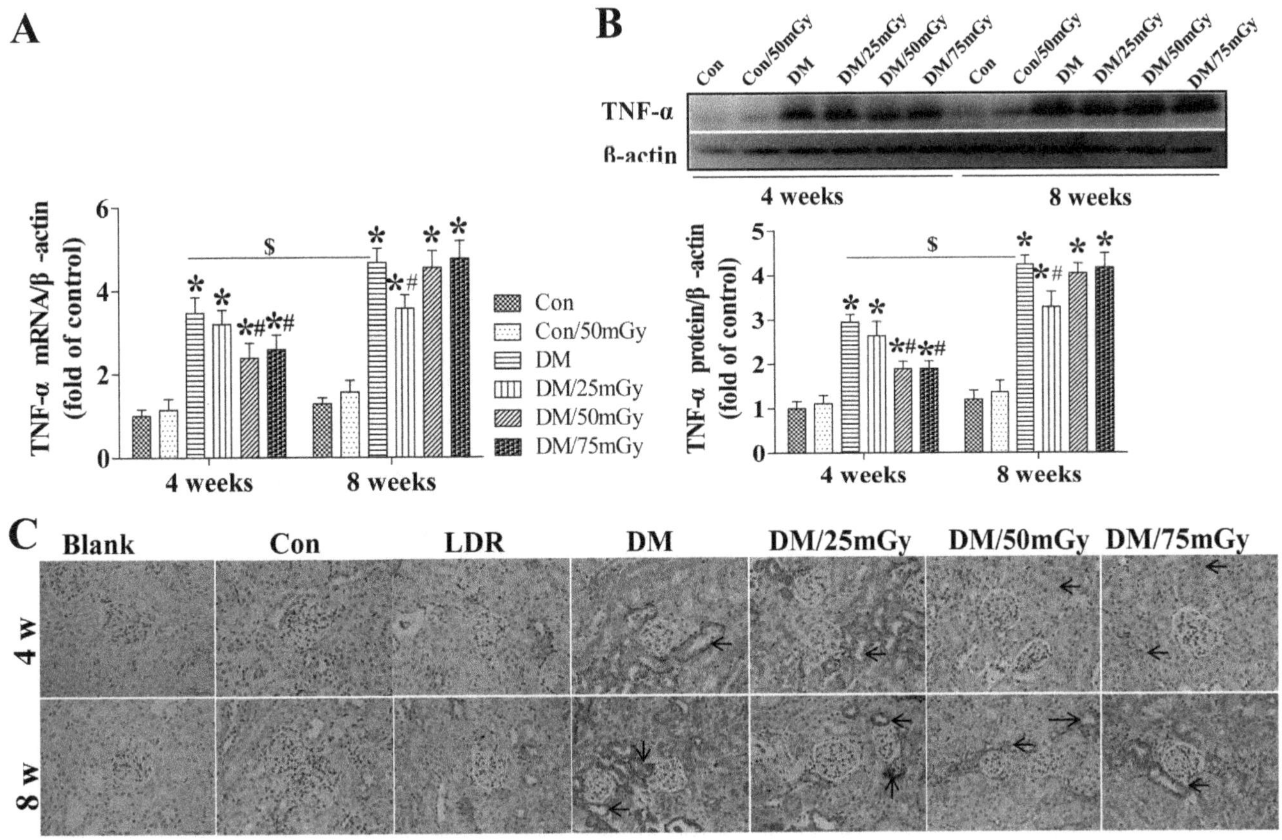

Figure 4. Effect of LDR on renal TNF-α levels in type 2 diabetic mice. Renal tissues from different groups were collected at the indicated times for measuring TNF-α expression at the mRNA (A) and protein (B) levels with RT-PCR and western blotting, respectively. (C) The location of TNF-α in the kidney was detected by immunohistochemical staining, at 400× magnification. Data are presented as means ± SEM. n = 9 in diabetic group and n = 8 in each other group. *$p<0.05$ vs. the corresponding control group; #$p<0.05$ vs. the corresponding DM group; \$, $p<0.05$ vs. DM group at the 4-week time-point.

Nrf-2 levels. The results showed that the expression of Nrf-2 at both the mRNA and protein levels significantly decreased in the kidneys of diabetic mice at the 4-week time-point, and the expression levels were further decreased at the 8-week time-point (Fig. 7A, B). Multiple exposures of diabetic mice to LDR at 25 mGy for 4 weeks did not, but 50 or 75 mGy almost completely prevented diabetic inhibition of renal Nrf-2 levels. Although exposure to LDR still up-regulated renal Nrf-2 levels after treatment for 8 weeks, the effect was weaker (Fig. 7A, B).

Immunohistochemical staining revealed that Nrf-2 expression was predominantly localized in the tubules and less in the glomerulus (Fig. 7C). However, no positive staining was observed in blank control group. The intensity of Nrf-2 staining was significantly reduced in the kidneys of diabetic mice, which was greatly reversed after LDR treatment for 4 weeks (Fig. 7C).

Since Nrf-2 is a transcription factor that positively regulates the expression of several downstream genes playing an important role in the prevention of oxidative stress and damage, we examined several of its downstream genes to functionally evaluate Nrf-2 in the diabetic kidneys with and without LDR treatment. Real-time PCR and western blotting assays disclosed that renal SOD-1 expression was significantly decreased in the diabetic group compared with the control group at the 4-week time-point and further decreased at the 8-week time-point (Fig. 8A, B). However, the decrease was completely reversed by exposure to LDR at all doses at both 4 and 8 weeks (Fig. 8A, B). Immunohistochemical staining confirmed our finding that exposure to LDR at all doses significantly preserved renal SOD-1 expression, located mainly in the tubules, in type 2 diabetic mice (Fig. 8C). And no positive staining was observed in blank control group.

In addition, we also examined other downstream targets of Nrf-2, HO-1 and NQO-1, which showed similar changing patterns as SOD-1 among groups. Renal HO-1 and NQO-1 levels were significantly decreased under diabetic conditions at both the 4- and 8-week time-points (Fig. 9). Exposure to LDR for both 4 and 8 weeks completely preserved the renal expression of both anti-oxidants. Although the beneficial effects were even among all doses of LDR at the 8-week time-point, 50 and 75 mGy further enhanced the protection compared with 25 mGy at the 4-week time-point.

Discussion

The study is the first one to demonstrate that multiple exposures to LDR, especially at 50 and 75 mGy for 4 weeks, significantly attenuated type 2 diabetes-induced DKD attributed to not only alleviation of systemic and renal dyslipidemia, but also suppression of the subsequent lipotoxicity via relieving insulin resistance, renal inflammation and oxidative damage.

The kidney is the main target organ that is attacked under conditions of type 2 diabetes, which leads to severe renal damage characterized by induction of renal dysfunction, fibrosis and glomerulosclerosis, finally causing DN [3–5]. Although the

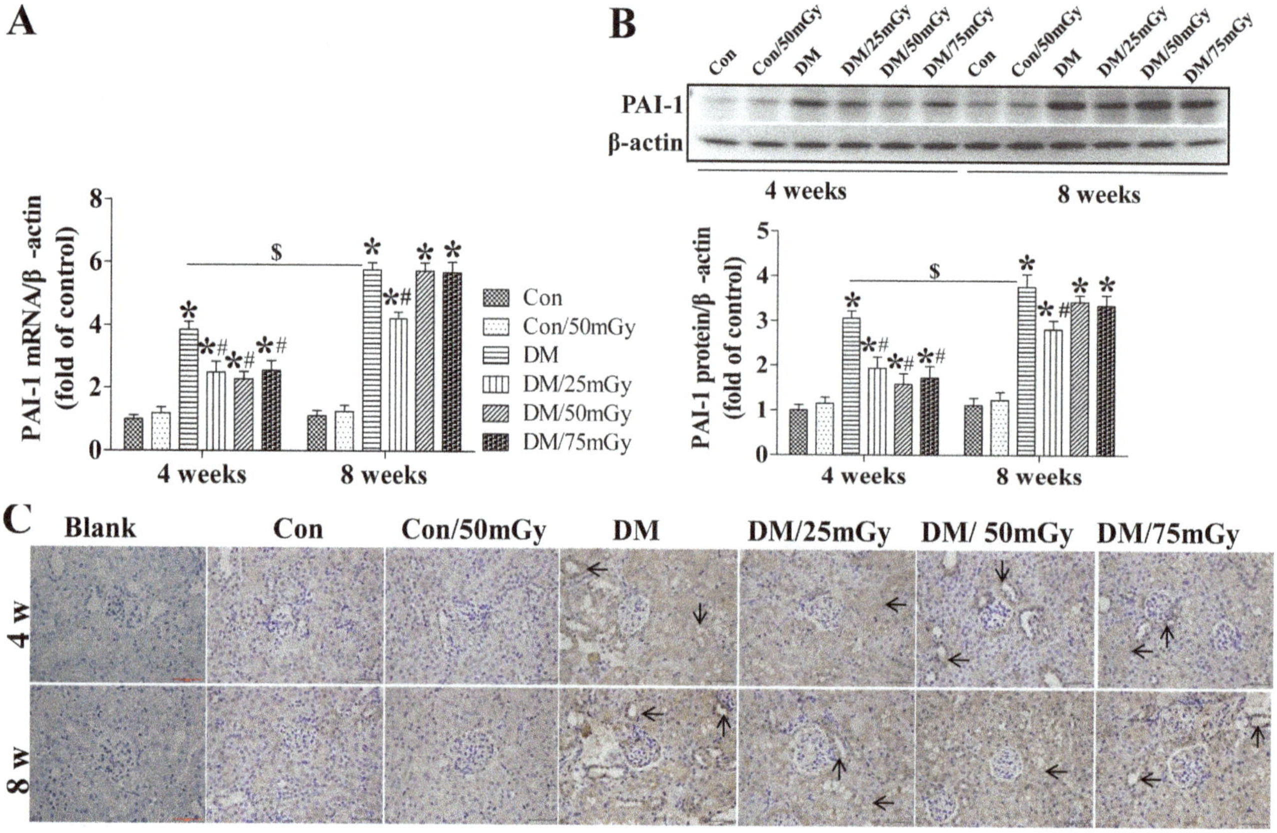

Figure 5. Effect of LDR on renal PAI-1 levels in type 2 diabetic mice. Renal tissues from different groups were collected at the indicated times for measuring PAI-1 expression at the mRNA (A) and protein (B) levels with RT-PCR and western blotting, respectively. (C) The location of PAI-1 in the kidney was detected by immunohistochemical staining, at 400× magnification. Data are presented as means ± SEM. n = 9 in diabetic group and n = 8 in each other group. *$p<0.05$ vs. the corresponding control group; #$p<0.05$ vs. the corresponding DM group; $, $p<0.05$ vs. DM group at the 4-week time-point.

pathogeneses of type 2 diabetes-induced renal damage are multiple and complicated, dyslipidemia and subsequent lipotoxicity play important roles in this pathological process and accelerate kidney injury [20,35,36]. Dyslipidemia is defined as abnormal lipid profiles characterized by an increase of plasma and tissue TG, LDL and total CHO levels, but a decrease of HDL levels [10,11]. Disturbances in lipoprotein metabolism contribute to atherogenic diathesis and possibly to progression of renal disease and impaired energy metabolism in DKD [12]. Diabetes-related dyslipidemia always leads to excessive lipid accumulation in the kidney, which causes severe renal damage through enhancement of insulin resistance, inflammation and oxidative stress [9,37,38]. In addition, insulin resistance induces the release of adipocytokines and relaxation of the afferent arteriole, resulting in glomerular hyperfiltration, angiogenesis, mesangial cell proliferation and renal damage [17,18]. The inflammatory response has been considered as one of the major mechanisms by which diabetic lipotoxicity causes renal oxidative injury, structural changes and dysfunction through the release of multiple inflammatory factors [39–41]. Moreover, lipotoxicity also induces excess lipid peroxidation products that stimulate transforming growth factor-β, thereby inducing oxidative stress by production of ROS and then causing renal function damage, which may contribute to the progression of DKD [19,20]. Therefore, finding a proper way to simultaneously prevent dyslipidemia and the subsequent lipotoxicity-induced insulin resistance, inflammation and oxidative stress might be an efficient candidate for DKD therapy.

Ionizing radiation is commonly considered to be harmful, which usually leads to DNA damage, cytotoxicity and tumorigenesis [42–45]. However, increasing evidence has demonstrated that exposure to radiation at a relatively low level resists radiation- or chemical-caused damage due to the protective mechanisms of stimulating cellular metabolic activities, enhancing immunity and increasing anti-oxidative action [46–49]. Additionally, it has been reported that LDR has the potential to modify the progression of chronic renal failure in rats [24,50]. Furthermore, our previous studies found that LDR significantly prevents type 1 diabetes-induced renal damage through attenuation of inflammation and oxidative stress [23,26]. Meanwhile, another advantage of LDR is its noninvasive characteristics, which cannot increase the working load of the kidney. Therefore, in the present study, we investigated whether LDR had the potential to prevent type 2 diabetes-induced renal damage and whether the protection was associated with attenuation of diabetes-induced dyslipidemia and lipotoxicity.

In order to test our hypothesis, the first mission for us was to establish a human-like type 2 diabetic mouse model. Although several genetically modified animal models are available to study type 2 diabetes, the patterns of disease initiation and development do not appear to be closely analogous to the clinical situation in humans [28,51]. Moreover, the observations derived from these highly inbred genetic strains may not always be satisfactorily extended to the human population as a whole because of the large heterogeneity in the latter. In addition, these animals are expensive and are not easily available for investigative purposes

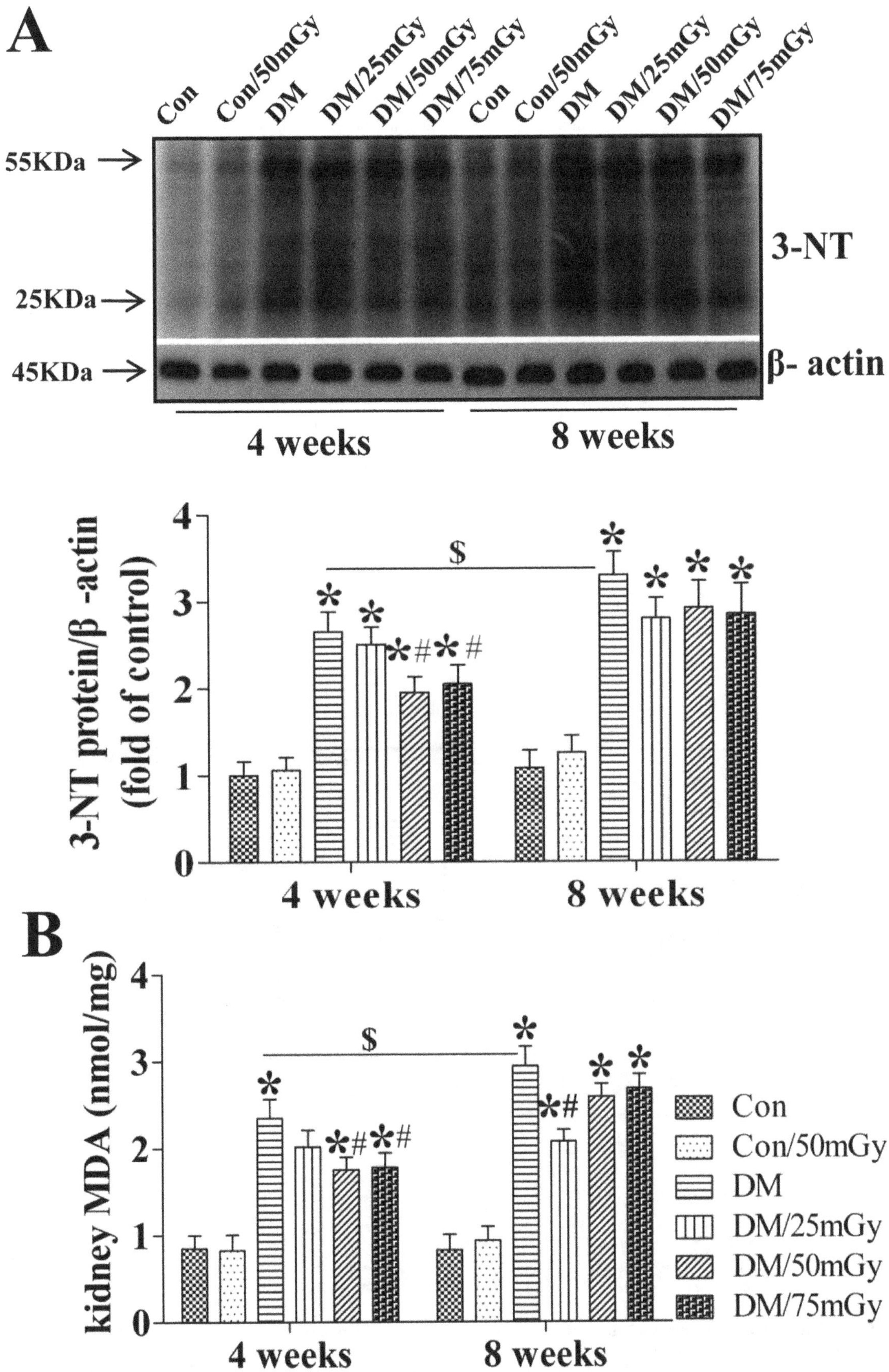

Figure 6. Effects of LDR on renal oxidative damage in type 2 diabetic mice. After control and diabetic mice with and without multiple exposures to LDR for 4 and 8 weeks, renal oxidative damage was examined by western blotting assays for the expression of 3-NT as an index of

protein nitration (A, B) and MDA by ELISA (C). Data are presented as means ± SEM. n = 9 in diabetic group and n = 8 in each other group. *$p<0.05$ vs. the corresponding control group; #$p<0.05$ vs. the corresponding DM group; $, $p<0.05$ vs. DM group at the 4-week time-point.

as well as regular screening experiments [28,52]. In humans, despite hereditary reasons, most type 2 diabetes cases are initiated by obesity. Therefore, we mimicked human-like type 2 diabetes by HFD/STZ strategy in C57BL/6J mice for which the type 2 diabetic mouse model was induced via HFD treatment for 12 weeks, followed by a single low-dose STZ injection of 50 mg/kg.

Once the type 2 diabetic model was successfully established, the diabetic or nondiabetic mice were exposed to LDR at 25, 50 or 75 mGy for 4 or 8 weeks. Then, the next question we have to answer is whether LDR can prevent type 2 diabetes-induced renal damage. Normally, the renal hypertrophy was determined by the ratio of kidney weight to body weight under the premise of constant body weight. But in our study the body weight varied among groups which will cause inaccurate conclusion. Therefore we used tibia length to replace the body weight, which was proximately even in each group. The results showed the ratio of kidney weight to tibia length was increased in diabetic group, which is a sign of renal hypertrophy. In addition, there was an increase of the urinary protein, mAlb excretion and a decrease of urinary creatinine excretion. Morphological studies also revealed that type 2 diabetes significantly induced renal pathological changes, including obvious Bowman's capsule adhesion, mesangial cell proliferation, mesangial matrix expansion, capillary wall thickness, capillary collapse, glomerulosclerosis and fibrosis. Meanwhile, abnormal lipid accumulation was also obvious in the kidney tissue of type 2 diabetic mice. However, most of the pathological changes induced by type 2 diabetes were prevented by exposure to LDR for 4 weeks. Although the beneficial effects of LDR were still observed at the 8-week time-point, the efficiency became weaker. Our findings implied that besides the single dose, the accumulated dose also plays a critical role in LDR-induced hormesis and beneficial effects on type 2 diabetes-induced renal damage. Despite the fact that each dose of radiation was equal in the groups treated for 4 or 8 weeks, the accumulated dose for 8 weeks was too high to further enhance the beneficial effects on diabetic renal damage compared with the 4-week time-point. After comprehensive evaluation of the renal protection among the three doses of LDR, we found that 50 and 75 mGy were more efficient than 25 mGy at the 4-week time-point. However, the above beneficial phenomenon was attenuated at the 8-week time-point; only LDR at 25 mGy showed great renal protection against type 2 diabetes at the 8-week time-point. The proper explanation might be that the accumulated dose of 50 mGy for 4 weeks and 25 mGy for 8 weeks were the same. Thus, both doses of LDR exhibited similar protection on diabetic renal damage.

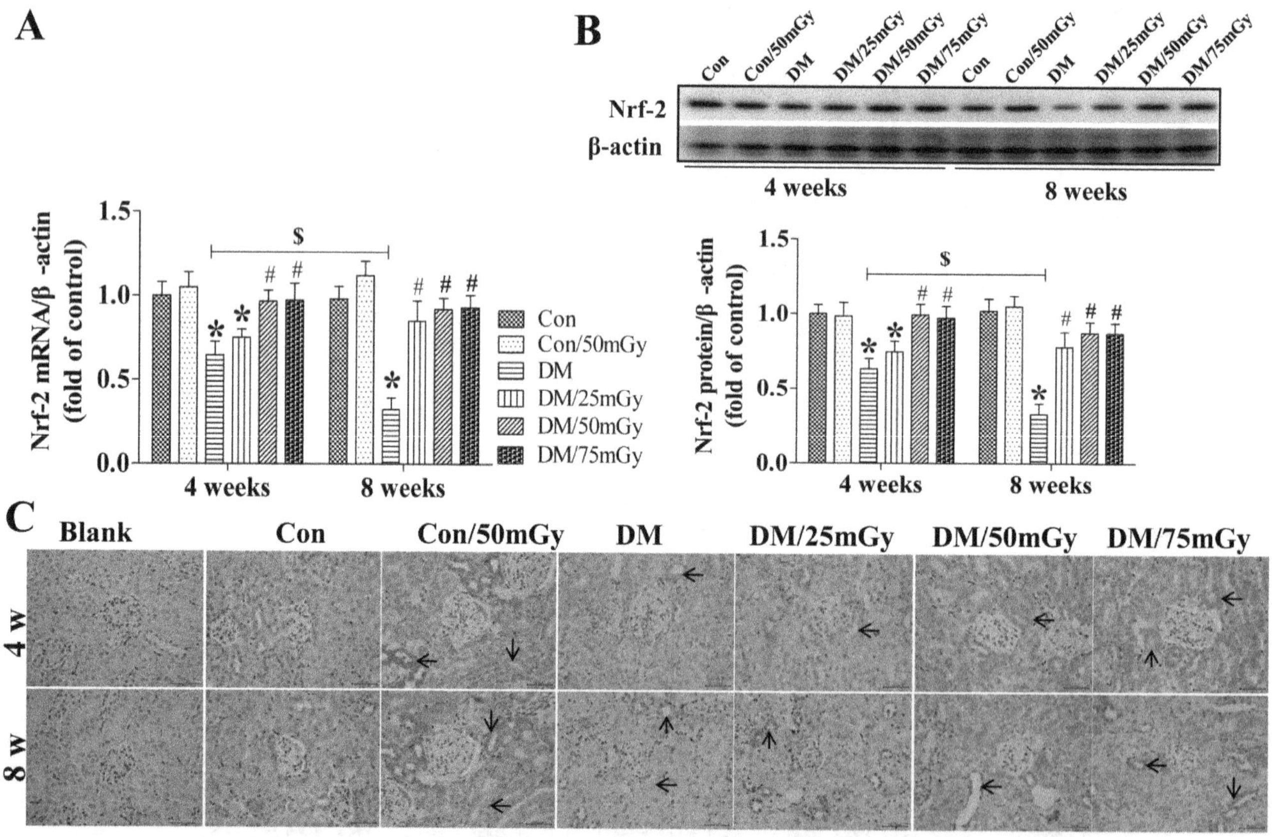

Figure 7. Effect of LDR on renal Nrf-2 levels in type 2 diabetic mice. Renal tissues from different groups were collected at the indicated times for measuring Nrf-2 expression at the mRNA (A) and protein (B) levels with RT-PCR and western blotting, respectively. (C) The location of Nrf-2 in the kidney was detected by immunohistochemical staining, at 400× magnification. Data are presented as means ± SEM. n = 9 in diabetic group and n = 8 in each other group. *$p<0.05$ vs. the corresponding control group; #$p<0.05$ vs. the corresponding DM group; $, $p<0.05$ vs. DM mice at the 4-week time-point.

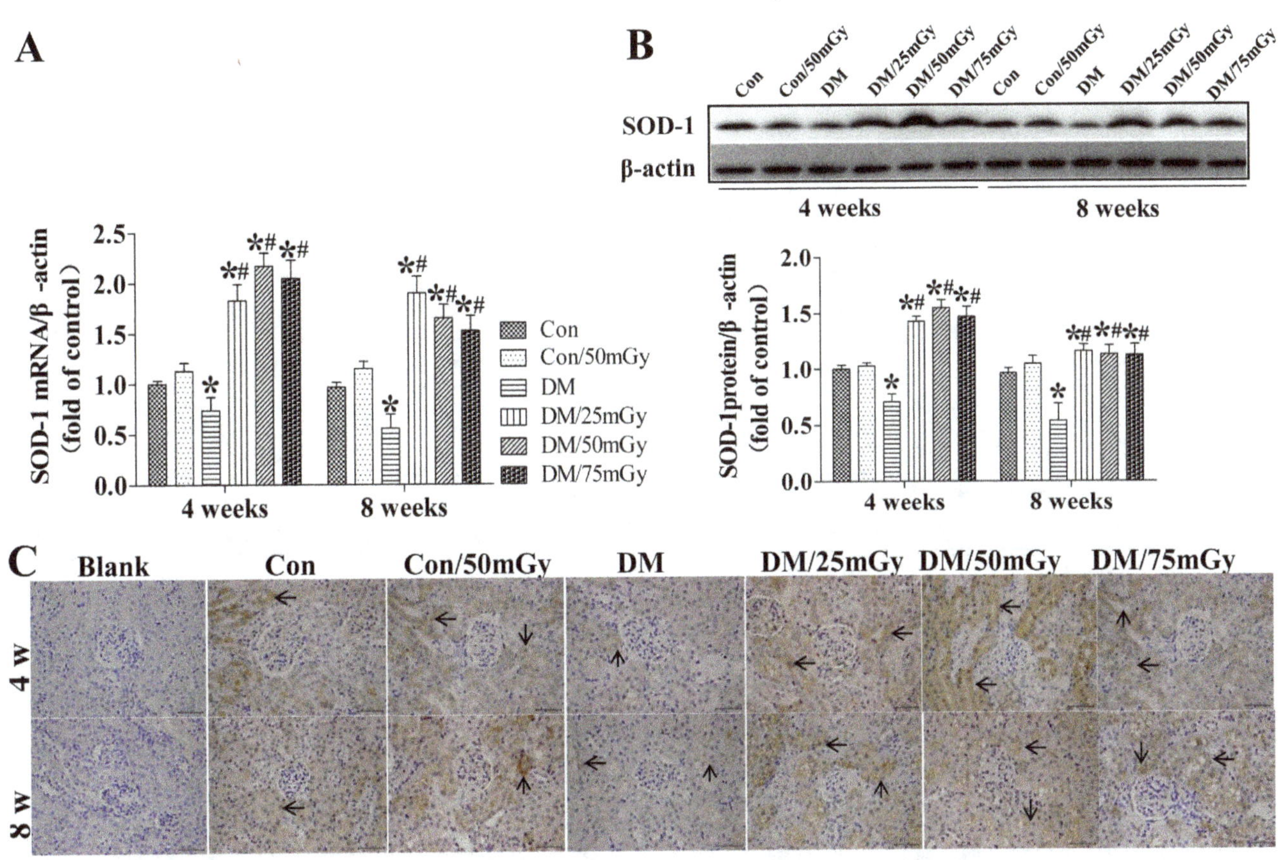

Figure 8. Effect of LDR on renal SOD-1 levels in type 2 diabetic mice. Renal tissues from different groups were collected at the indicated times for measuring SOD-1 expression at the mRNA (A) and protein (B) levels with RT-PCR and western blotting, respectively. (C) The location of SOD-1 in the kidney was detected by immunohistochemical staining, at 400× magnification. Data are presented as means ± SEM. n = 9 in diabetic group and n = 8 in each other group. *$p<0.05$ vs. the corresponding control group; #$p<0.05$ vs. the corresponding DM group; \$, $p<0.05$ vs. DM group at the 4-week time-point.

To date, we identified that LDR prevented type 2 diabetes-induced renal damage characterized by suppression of kidney hypertrophic response, attenuation of renal dysfunction and pathological changes; so, the protective mechanism of LDR remains to be elucidated. In our study, we found that LDR-induced renal protection against type 2 diabetes was independent of hypoglycemic effects but associated with improving insulin sensitivity, which might be attributed to activation of the Akt signaling pathway. Since insulin-induced glucose regulation was mainly mediated by the Akt signaling pathway, impairment of the Akt signaling pathway always leads to insulin resistance. In the literature, several studies have used *in vitro* models to show that LDR is able to stimulate cell survival signaling such as Akt phosphorylation [48,53]. Our previous study also determined that exposure to LDR significantly up-regulated the activation of the renal Akt signaling pathway in type 1 diabetic mice. Moreover, the Akt signaling pathway also plays an important role in preventing diabetes-induced renal cell death [54]. Similar anti-apoptotic effects of Akt in response to various pathogenic stimuli have also been extensively reported [55,56]. Therefore, we assumed that stimulation of the Akt signaling pathway by LDR in diabetic kidneys may be one of the possible mechanisms by which LDR prevents the development of DN.

Furthermore, strong evidence has demonstrated that besides hyperglycemia, lipotoxicity is another main pathogenesis of type 2 diabetes-induced insulin resistance by increasing the inhibition of serine phosphorylation of the key mediators of insulin receptor signaling [13–15]. Accordingly, we hypothesized that the renal protection of LDR might be related to the attenuation of lipotoxicity. Since lipotoxicity is the consequence of dyslipidemia, we next determined the systemic and renal lipid profiles. The results disclosed that type 2 diabetes-induced dyslipidemia in both the plasma and kidney was characterized by an increase of CHO, TG and LDL levels and a decrease of HDL levels. However, some of the abnormal lipid profiles were remarkably reversed by exposure to LDR, especially at 50 and 75 mGy. Although the lipid metabolic regulating effect was still observed at the 8-week time-point, the efficiency was getting weaker due to the high accumulated dose.

Dyslipidemia-induced lipotoxicity always leads to severe inflammation and oxidative stress, which also accelerates renal damage under diabetic conditions. Real-time PCR and western blotting assays revealed that type 2 diabetes significantly up-regulated the expression levels of inflammatory factors (ICAM-1, TNF-α and PAI-1) and nitrosative damage markers (3-NT and MDA) in the kidney. Exposure to LDR, especially at 50 and 75 mGy, for 4 weeks greatly prevented diabetes-induced inflammation and oxidative stress. Although LDR at 25 mGy induced less of an effect on anti-inflammatory and anti-oxidative stress at the 4-week time-point, the beneficial effect became significant at the 8-week time-point. This finding further confirmed that the accumulated dose is critical for LDR-induced renal protection

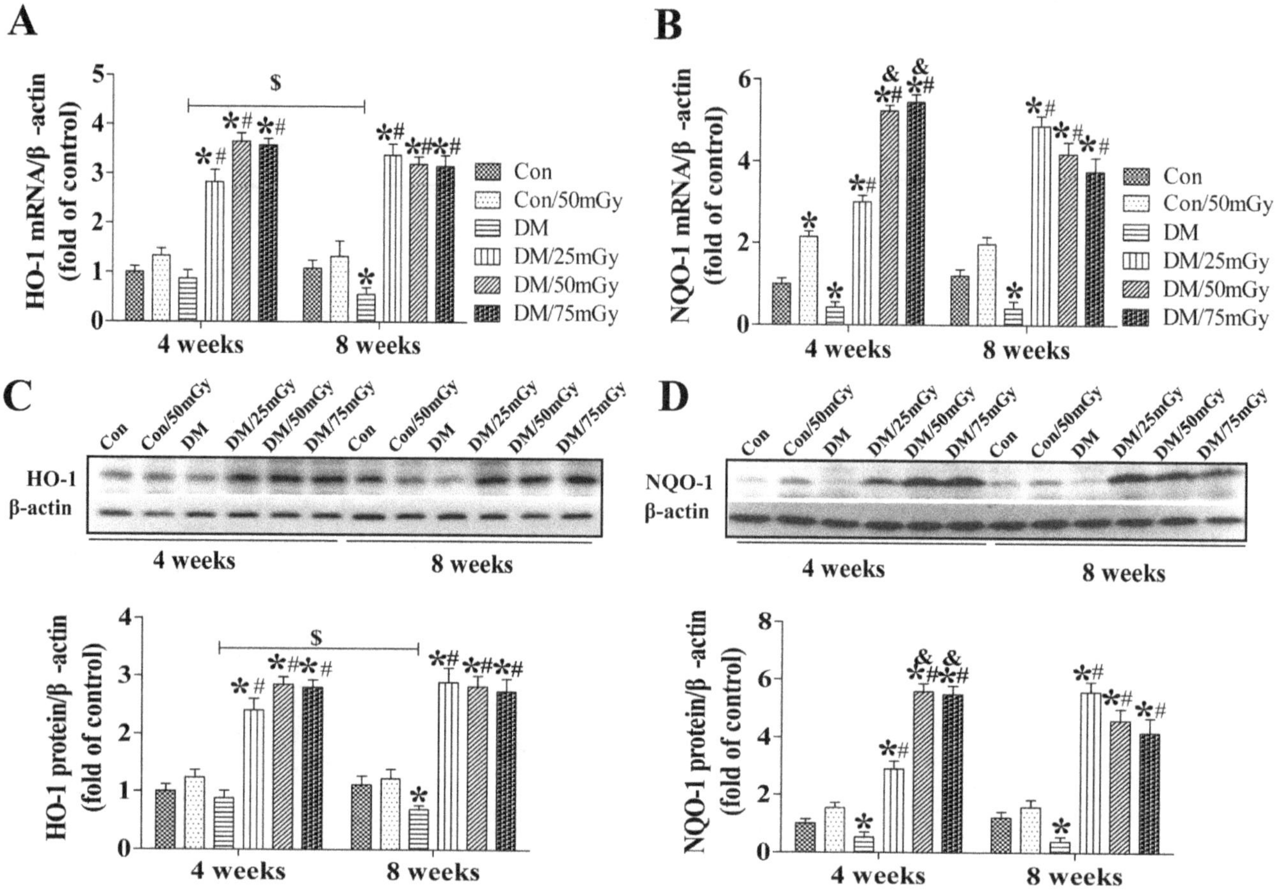

Figure 9. Effect of LDR on renal HO-1 and NQO-1 levels in type 2 diabetic mice. Renal tissues from different groups were collected at the indicated times for measuring HO-1 expression (A, C) and NQO-1 expression (B, D) levels at the mRNA and protein with RT-PCR and western blotting, respectively. Data are presented as means ± SEM. n = 9 in diabetic group and n = 8 in each other group. **p*<0.05 vs. the corresponding control group; #*p*<0.05 vs. the corresponding DM group; $, *p*<0.05 vs. DM group at the 4-week time-point.

against inflammation and oxidative stress induced by type 2 diabetes. In the present study, LDR prevented most of the renal pathological changes only with the total dose ranging from 700 mGy (50 mGy for 4 weeks) to 1035 mGy (75 mGy for 4 weeks). A dose that is either too low or too high will reduce the protective effect of LDR.

Finally, we explored the mechanism of LDR-induced anti-oxidative stress. Our previous study has indicated that LDR protection of rat testes from diabetes-induced oxidative damage occurred along with an up-regulation of testicular superoxide dismutase levels [57]. Recently, we also reported that LDR-induced up-regulation of multiple renal antioxidant levels was mediated by Nrf-2 expression in the kidney [26]. Nrf-2 is a key transcription factor that regulates the intracellular redox balance and is a sensor of oxidative stress. SOD-1, NQO-1 and HO-1 are all well-studied Nrf-2 target genes that are up-regulated through the antioxidant response regulatory element in response to oxidative stress [26,29,58]. In the present study, we found that type 2 diabetes significantly down-regulated the expression of renal Nrf-2 and the downstream targets SOD-1, HO-1 and NQO-1, which were remarkably reversed by exposure to LDR, especially at 50 or 75 mGy for both 4 and 8 weeks. This study answered our question that LDR protects the kidney from type 2 diabetes-induced oxidative damage associated with up-regulation of Nrf-2 and the downstream target oxidants. It is interesting that the antioxidant expression in each DM/LDR group was much higher than in Con, Con/50 mGy or DM group. Why does this phenomenon appear? We suspected that under normal condition, oxidative stress is just kept at low level and unharmful to the kidney. However, under diabetic condition, renal oxidative stress significantly increased attributed to up-regulation of ROS production and down-regulation of the anti-oxidants expressions [26,59–64]. LDR induced increase of antioxidants is not only to compensate the decrease of renal anti-oxidants expression induced by diabetes [26,65], but also to neutralize the ROS production in diabetic kidney [66–69]. Therefore, the expressions of multiple anti-oxidants in the kidney were significantly higher than in Con or DM groups.

Conclusion

In summary, we showed for the first time that exposure of mice to LDR significantly prevented type 2 diabetes-induced renal damage through attenuation of renal hypertrophy, dysfunction and pathological changes. The mechanistic study demonstrated that the protection was independent of blood glucose level reduction but was attributed to the suppression of dyslipidemia and the subsequent lipotoxicity-induced insulin resistance, inflammation and oxidative stress. The beneficial effects of LDR on renal damage were associated with activation of the Akt signaling pathway and up-regulation of Nrf-2 expression and function. In the present study, we also found that both the single and accumulated doses play a critical role in LDR-induced renal protection; either too low or too high of a dose will reduce the efficiency. Although potential long-term mild toxic effects should be considered for diabetic patients who may develop severe DN earlier than the occurrence of the late adverse effects of LDR. Furthermore, given that whole body exposure to LDR is so easy and convenient to perform, this method may provide a novel therapeutic approach for diabetic patients in the near future.

Author Contributions

Conceived and designed the experiments: CZ SJ LC. Performed the experiments: MS WC XX YT YL XW JD. Analyzed the data: CZ LJ XKL LC SJ. Contributed reagents/materials/analysis tools: MS XML XKL LC. Wrote the paper: CZ SJ LC.

References

1. Burrows NR, Li Y, Williams DE (2008) Racial and ethnic differences in trends of end-stage renal disease: United States, 1995 to 2005. Adv Chronic Kidney Dis 15: 147–152.
2. Iseki K (2008) Chronic kidney disease in Japan. Intern Med 47: 681–689.
3. Meguro S, Tomita M, Kabeya Y, Katsuki T, Oikawa Y, et al. (2012) Factors Associated with the Decline of Kidney Function Differ among eGFR Strata in Subjects with Type 2 Diabetes Mellitus. Int J Endocrinol 2012: 687867.
4. Heerspink HJ, de Zeeuw D (2011) The kidney in type 2 diabetes therapy. Rev Diabet Stud 8: 392–402.
5. Franceschini N, Shara NM, Wang H, Voruganti VS, Laston S, et al. (2012) The association of genetic variants of type 2 diabetes with kidney function. Kidney Int 82: 220–225.
6. Toblli JE, Ferrini MG, Cao G, Vernet D, Angerosa M, et al. (2009) Antifibrotic effects of pioglitazone on the kidney in a rat model of type 2 diabetes mellitus. Nephrol Dial Transplant 24: 2384–2391.
7. McKay GJ, Savage DA, Patterson CC, Lewis G, McKnight AJ, et al. (2013) Association analysis of dyslipidemia-related genes in diabetic nephropathy. PLoS One 8: e58472.
8. Jisieike-Onuigbo NN, Unuigbe EI, Kalu OA, Oguejiofor CO, Onuigbo PC (2011) Prevalence of dyslipidemia among adult diabetic patients with overt diabetic nephropathy in Anambra state south-east Nigeria. Niger J Clin Pract 14: 171–175.
9. Murea M, Freedman BI, Parks JS, Antinozzi PA, Elbein SC, et al. (2010) Lipotoxicity in diabetic nephropathy: the potential role of fatty acid oxidation. Clin J Am Soc Nephrol 5: 2373–2379.
10. Bonnet F, Cooper ME (2000) Potential influence of lipids in diabetic nephropathy: insights from experimental data and clinical studies. Diabetes Metab 26: 254–264.
11. Hirano T (1999) Lipoprotein abnormalities in diabetic nephropathy. Kidney Int Suppl 71: S22–24.
12. Bobulescu IA (2010) Renal lipid metabolism and lipotoxicity. Curr Opin Nephrol Hypertens 19: 393–402.
13. Harjai KJ (1999) Potential new cardiovascular risk factors: left ventricular hypertrophy, homocysteine, lipoprotein(a), triglycerides, oxidative stress, and fibrinogen. Ann Intern Med 131: 376–386.
14. Petersen KF, Shulman GI (2006) Etiology of insulin resistance. Am J Med 119: S10–16.
15. Qatanani M, Lazar MA (2007) Mechanisms of obesity-associated insulin resistance: many choices on the menu. Genes Dev 21: 1443–1455.
16. Gum RJ, Gaede LL, Koterski SL, Heindel M, Clampit JE, et al. (2003) Reduction of protein tyrosine phosphatase 1B increases insulin-dependent signaling in ob/ob mice. Diabetes 52: 21–28.
17. Miller AW, Dimitropoulou C, Han G, White RE, Busija DW, et al. (2001) Epoxyeicosatrienoic acid-induced relaxation is impaired in insulin resistance. Am J Physiol Heart Circ Physiol 281: H1524–1531.
18. Piqueras L, Reynolds AR, Hodivala-Dilke KM, Alfranca A, Redondo JM, et al. (2007) Activation of PPARbeta/delta induces endothelial cell proliferation and angiogenesis. Arterioscler Thromb Vasc Biol 27: 63–69.
19. Yang RL, Shi YH, Hao G, Li W, Le GW (2008) Increasing Oxidative Stress with Progressive Hyperlipidemia in Human: Relation between Malondialdehyde and Atherogenic Index. J Clin Biochem Nutr 43: 154–158.
20. Rutledge JC, Ng KF, Aung HH, Wilson DW (2010) Role of triglyceride-rich lipoproteins in diabetic nephropathy. Nat Rev Nephrol 6: 361–370.
21. Pradhan AD, Manson JE, Rifai N, Buring JE, Ridker PM (2001) C-reactive protein, interleukin 6, and risk of developing type 2 diabetes mellitus. JAMA 286: 327–334.
22. Skrha J (2003) Pathogenesis of angiopathy in diabetes. Acta Diabetol 40 Suppl 2: S324–329.
23. Zhang C, Tan Y, Guo W, Li C, Ji S, et al. (2009) Attenuation of diabetes-induced renal dysfunction by multiple exposures to low-dose radiation is associated with the suppression of systemic and renal inflammation. Am J Physiol Endocrinol Metab 297: E1366–1377.
24. Aunapuu M, Pechter U, Gerskevits E, Marjamagi MM, Suuroja S, et al. (2004) Low-dose radiation modifies the progression of chronic renal failure. Ann Anat 186: 277–282.
25. van Kleef EM, Zurcher C, Oussoren YG, Te Poele JA, van der Valk MA, et al. (2000) Long-term effects of total-body irradiation on the kidney of Rhesus monkeys. Int J Radiat Biol 76: 641–648.
26. Xing X, Zhang C, Shao M, Tong Q, Zhang G, et al. (2012) Low-dose radiation activates Akt and Nrf2 in the kidney of diabetic mice: a potential mechanism to prevent diabetic nephropathy. Oxid Med Cell Longev 2012: 291087.
27. Gilbert ER, Fu Z, Liu D (2011) Development of a nongenetic mouse model of type 2 diabetes. Exp Diabetes Res 2011: 416254.
28. Srinivasan K, Viswanad B, Asrat L, Kaul CL, Ramarao P (2005) Combination of high-fat diet-fed and low-dose streptozotocin-treated rat: a model for type 2 diabetes and pharmacological screening. Pharmacol Res 52: 313–320.
29. Zhao Y, Tan Y, Dai J, Li B, Guo L, et al. (2011) Exacerbation of diabetes-induced testicular apoptosis by zinc deficiency is most likely associated with oxidative stress, p38 MAPK activation, and p53 activation in mice. Toxicol Lett 200: 100–106.
30. Ji H, Pesce C, Zheng W, Kim J, Zhang Y, et al. (2005) Sex differences in renal injury and nitric oxide production in renal wrap hypertension. Am J Physiol Heart Circ Physiol 288: H43–47.
31. Song Y, Li C, Cai L (2004) Fluvastatin prevents nephropathy likely through suppression of connective tissue growth factor-mediated extracellular matrix accumulation. Exp Mol Pathol 76: 66–75.
32. Zhao W, Ahokas RA, Weber KT, Sun Y (2006) ANG II-induced cardiac molecular and cellular events: role of aldosterone. Am J Physiol Heart Circ Physiol 291: H336–343.
33. Marney AM, Brown NJ (2007) Aldosterone and end-organ damage. Clin Sci (Lond) 113: 267–278.
34. Adair LS (2008) Child and adolescent obesity: epidemiology and developmental perspectives. Physiol Behav 94: 8–16.
35. Athyros VG, Mitsiou EK, Tziomalos K, Karagiannis A, Mikhailidis DP (2010) Impact of managing atherogenic dyslipidemia on cardiovascular outcome across different stages of diabetic nephropathy. Expert Opin Pharmacother 11: 723–730.
36. Kim MY, Lim JH, Youn HH, Hong YA, Yang KS, et al. (2013) Resveratrol prevents renal lipotoxicity and inhibits mesangial cell glucotoxicity in a manner dependent on the AMPK-SIRT1-PGC1alpha axis in db/db mice. Diabetologia 56: 204–217.
37. Wahba IM, Mak RH (2007) Obesity and obesity-initiated metabolic syndrome: mechanistic links to chronic kidney disease. Clin J Am Soc Nephrol 2: 550–562.
38. Chung HW, Lim JH, Kim MY, Shin SJ, Chung S, et al. (2012) High-fat diet-induced renal cell apoptosis and oxidative stress in spontaneously hypertensive rat are ameliorated by fenofibrate through the PPARalpha-FoxO3a-PGC-1alpha pathway. Nephrol Dial Transplant 27: 2213–2225.
39. Lin J, Glynn RJ, Rifai N, Manson JE, Ridker PM, et al. (2008) Inflammation and progressive nephropathy in type 1 diabetes in the diabetes control and complications trial. Diabetes Care 31: 2338–2343.
40. Navarro-Gonzalez JF, Mora-Fernandez C (2008) The role of inflammatory cytokines in diabetic nephropathy. J Am Soc Nephrol 19: 433–442.
41. Rivero A, Mora C, Muros M, Garcia J, Herrera H, et al. (2009) Pathogenic perspectives for the role of inflammation in diabetic nephropathy. Clin Sci (Lond) 116: 479–492.
42. Pinar B, Lara PC, Lloret M, Bordon E, Nunez MI, et al. (2007) Radiation-induced DNA damage as a predictor of long-term toxicity in locally advanced breast cancer patients treated with high-dose hyperfractionated radical radiotherapy. Radiat Res 168: 415–422.
43. Hellman B, Brodin D, Andersson M, Dahlman-Wright K, Isacsson U, et al. (2005) Radiation-induced DNA-damage and gene expression profiles in human lung cancer cells with different radiosensitivity. Exp Oncol 27: 102–107.
44. Popanda O, Ebbeler R, Twardella D, Helmbold I, Gotzes F, et al. (2003) Radiation-induced DNA damage and repair in lymphocytes from breast cancer patients and their correlation with acute skin reactions to radiotherapy. Int J Radiat Oncol Biol Phys 55: 1216–1225.
45. Palyvoda O, Mukalov I, Polanska J, Wygoda A, Drobot L, et al. (2002) Radiation-induced DNA damage and its repair in lymphocytes of patients with head and neck cancer and healthy donors. Anticancer Res 22: 1721–1725.
46. Cai L (1999) Research of the adaptive response induced by low-dose radiation: where have we been and where should we go? Hum Exp Toxicol 18: 419–425.
47. de Toledo SM, Asaad N, Venkatachalam P, Li L, Howell RW, et al. (2006) Adaptive responses to low-dose/low-dose-rate gamma rays in normal human fibroblasts: the role of growth architecture and oxidative metabolism. Radiat Res 166: 849–857.
48. Kim CS, Kim JK, Nam SY, Yang KH, Jeong M, et al. (2007) Low-dose radiation stimulates the proliferation of normal human lung fibroblasts via a transient activation of Raf and Akt. Mol Cells 24: 424–430.

49. Liu G, Gong P, Bernstein LR, Bi Y, Gong S, et al. (2007) Apoptotic cell death induced by low-dose radiation in male germ cells: hormesis and adaptation. Crit Rev Toxicol 37: 587–605.
50. Pathak CM, Avti PK, Kumar S, Khanduja KL, Sharma SC (2007) Whole body exposure to low-dose gamma radiation promotes kidney antioxidant status in Balb/c mice. J Radiat Res 48: 113–120.
51. Srinivasan K, Ramarao P (2007) Animal models in type 2 diabetes research: an overview. Indian J Med Res 125: 451–472.
52. Luo J, Quan J, Tsai J, Hobensack CK, Sullivan C, et al. (1998) Nongenetic mouse models of non-insulin-dependent diabetes mellitus. Metabolism 47: 663–668.
53. Gaipl US, Meister S, Lodermann B, Rodel F, Fietkau R, et al. (2009) Activation-induced cell death and total Akt content of granulocytes show a biphasic course after low-dose radiation. Autoimmunity 42: 340–342.
54. Rane MJ, Song Y, Jin S, Barati MT, Wu R, et al. (2010) Interplay between Akt and p38 MAPK pathways in the regulation of renal tubular cell apoptosis associated with diabetic nephropathy. Am J Physiol Renal Physiol 298: F49–61.
55. Lee S, Chanoit G, McIntosh R, Zvara DA, Xu Z (2009) Molecular mechanism underlying Akt activation in zinc-induced cardioprotection. Am J Physiol Heart Circ Physiol 297: H569–575.
56. Matheny RW Jr, Adamo ML (2010) PI3K p110 alpha and p110 beta have differential effects on Akt activation and protection against oxidative stress-induced apoptosis in myoblasts. Cell Death Differ 17: 677–688.
57. Zhao H, Xu S, Wang Z, Li Y, Guo W, et al. (2010) Repetitive exposures to low-dose X-rays attenuate testicular apoptotic cell death in streptozotocin-induced diabetes rats. Toxicol Lett 192: 356–364.
58. Tan Y, Ichikawa T, Li J, Si Q, Yang H, et al. (2011) Diabetic downregulation of Nrf2 activity via ERK contributes to oxidative stress-induced insulin resistance in cardiac cells in vitro and in vivo. Diabetes 60: 625–633.
59. Forbes JM, Coughlan MT, Cooper ME (2008) Oxidative stress as a major culprit in kidney disease in diabetes. Diabetes 57: 1446–1454.
60. Bagby SP (2007) Diabetic nephropathy and proximal tubule ROS: challenging our glomerulocentricity. Kidney Int 71: 1199–1202.
61. Tan AL, Forbes JM, Cooper ME (2007) AGE, RAGE, and ROS in diabetic nephropathy. Semin Nephrol 27: 130–143.
62. Soetikno V, Watanabe K, Sari FR, Harima M, Thandavarayan RA, et al. (2011) Curcumin attenuates diabetic nephropathy by inhibiting PKC-alpha and PKC-beta1 activity in streptozotocin-induced type I diabetic rats. Mol Nutr Food Res 55: 1655–1665.
63. Li B, Liu S, Miao L, Cai L (2012) Prevention of diabetic complications by activation of Nrf2: diabetic cardiomyopathy and nephropathy. Exp Diabetes Res 2012: 216512.
64. Cui W, Li B, Bai Y, Miao X, Chen Q, et al. (2013) Potential role for Nrf2 activation in the therapeutic effect of MG132 on diabetic nephropathy in OVE26 diabetic mice. Am J Physiol Endocrinol Metab 304: E87–99.
65. Calabrese EJ (2013) Low doses of radiation can enhance insect lifespans. Biogerontology 14: 365–381.
66. Blokhina O, Virolainen E, Fagerstedt KV (2003) Antioxidants, oxidative damage and oxygen deprivation stress: a review. Ann Bot 91 Spec No: 179–194.
67. San Miguel SM, Opperman LA, Allen EP, Svoboda KK (2011) Reactive oxygen species and antioxidant defense mechanisms in the oral cavity: a literature review. Compend Contin Educ Dent 32: E10–15.
68. Karihtala P, Soini Y (2007) Reactive oxygen species and antioxidant mechanisms in human tissues and their relation to malignancies. APMIS 115: 81–103.
69. Mantovani G, Maccio A, Madeddu C, Mura L, Massa E, et al. (2003) Reactive oxygen species, antioxidant mechanisms, and serum cytokine levels in cancer patients: impact of an antioxidant treatment. J Environ Pathol Toxicol Oncol 22: 17–28.

3

Adipose Overexpression of Heme Oxygenase-1 does not Protect against High Fat Diet-Induced Insulin Resistance in Mice

Jun-Yuan Huang[1,2], Ming-Tsai Chiang[2], Lee-Young Chau[1,2*]

1 Institute of Biomedical Sciences, Academia Sinica, Taipei, Taiwan, Republic of China, 2 Graduate Institute of Life Sciences, National Defense Medical Center, Taipei, Taiwan, Republic of China

Abstract

Heme oxygenase-1 (HO-1) is a stress-responsive enzyme with potent anti-oxidant and anti-inflammatory activities. Previous studies have shown that systemic induction of HO-1 by chemical inducers reduces adiposity and improves insulin sensitivity. To dissect the specific function of HO-1 in adipose tissue, we generated transgenic mice with adipose HO-1 overexpression using the adipocyte-specific aP2 promoter. The transgenic (Tg) mice exhibit similar metabolic phenotype as wild type (WT) control under chow-fed condition. High fat diet (HFD) challenge significantly increased the body weights of WT and Tg mice to a similar extent. Likewise, HFD-induced glucose intolerance and insulin resistance were not much different between WT and Tg mice. Analysis of the adipose tissue gene expression revealed that the mRNA levels of adiponectin and interleukin-10 were significantly higher in chow diet-fed Tg mice as compared to WT counterparts, whereas HFD induced downregulation of adiponectin gene expression in both Tg and WT mice to a similar level. HFD-induced proinflammatory cytokine expression in adipose tissues were comparable between WT and transgenic mice. Nevertheless, immunohistochemistry and gene expression analysis showed that the number of infiltrating macrophages with preferential expression of M2 markers was significantly higher in the adipose tissue of obese Tg mice than WT mice. Further experiment demonstrated that myeloid cells from Tg mice expressed higher level of HO-1 and exhibited greater migration response toward chemoattractant in vitro. Collectively, these data indicate that HO-1 overexpression in adipocytes does not protect against HFD-induced obesity and the development of insulin resistance in mice.

Editor: Jörg Hermann Fritz, McGill University, Canada

Funding: This work was supported by a grant (NSC-97-2320-B-001-010-MY3) from the National Science Council of Taiwan (http://web1.nsc.gov.tw/). The funder had no role in study design, data collection and analysis, decision to publish, or preparation of the manuscript.

Competing Interests: The authors have declared that no competing interests exist.

* E-mail: lyc@ibms.sinica.edu.tw

Introduction

Adipose tissue is a primary site in the body to store energy in the form of triglyceride [1] When dietary energy intake persistently exceeds energy expenditure, the adipose tissue can expand through hypertrophy of the existing adipocytes and generation of new adipocytes, leading to the development of obesity [2]. Obesity caused by the sedentary life style and Western diet has become a prevalent health problem associated with increased incidence of insulin resistance, which is a major risk factor for type II diabetes and cardiovascular diseases [3]. Substantial works have revealed that obesity is associated with systemic oxidative stress and low-grade inflammation [4–5]. Adipocytes express a number of proinflammatory cytokines, including tumor necrosis factor-α (TNF-α), interleukin-6 (IL-6), and monocyte chemotactic protein-1 (MCP-1), which are upregulated in the adipose tissues of obese subjects [6]. In contrast, the expression of adiponectin, the adipocyte-derived adipokine with potent function in regulating insulin sensitivity, is downregulated during obesity [6]. In parallel, macrophage infiltration is increased in the adipose tissues and contributes to the adipose inflammation and the development of insulin resistance in obesity. Moreover, the adipose tissue macrophages have been shown to exhibit in two different phenotypes, the classically activated M1 or alternatively activated M2 macrophages [7–9]. The resident macrophages in lean adipose tissues are primarily in M2 state, which expresses immunosuppressive interleukin-10 (IL-10) but downregulates inducible nitric oxide synthase (iNOS) [7–9]. Obesity promotes adipose macrophage accumulation with a phenotypic switch to M1 phenotype expressing CD11c and proinflammatory cytokines [7–9].

Heme oxygenase-1 (HO-1) is a stress-inducible enzyme catalyzing the oxidative degradation of heme to release free iron, carbon monoxide (CO), and biliverdin [10]. In addition to its primary role in heme catabolism, numerous studies have supported the vital function of HO-1 in various pathophysiological states associated with cellular stress. It has been shown that HO-1 protects cardiovascular system against various insults by virtue of the anti-oxidant properties of the biliverdin and its metabolite, bilirubin, and the anti-inflammatory effect of CO, suggesting that HO-1 is a potential therapeutics for cardiovascular diseases [10]. HO-1 has been shown to highly express in the white adipose tissue (WAT) of genetic and high fat-diet (HFD)-induced obese mice [11–12]. However, the pathophysiological role of adipose HO-1 during obesity and the development of insulin resistance has not yet been fully characterized. Over the past few years, there were studies showing that systemic induction of HO-1 by treatment with HO-1 inducer, hemin or cobalt protoporphyrin, in ob/ob mice or Zucker diabetic rats reduced adiposity and improved insulin sensitivity [13–15]. The protective effect of systemic HO-1 induction was attributed to an increase in adiponectin expression, enhanced AMP kinase activation in both adipocytes and skeletal muscles, and suppression of adipogenesis and inflammatory cytokine expression. Nevertheless, a study has shown that the endogenous HO-derived CO was increased and promoted hypertension and endothelial dysfunction in obese Zucker rats [16]. More recently, a study from our group also demonstrated that hematopoietic HO-1 expression promoted macrophage infiltration in adipose tissue and the development of insulin resistance [12], indicating that HO-1 may impact this complicated disease through its differential effects on various cell compartments. To dissect the potential discrete roles of HO-1 in different cell types implicated in the metabolic disease, here we generated transgenic mice overexpressing HO-1 in adipocytes to study the effect of adipocyte HO-1 on diet-induced adiposity and insulin resistance.

Materials and Methods

Ethics Statement

All experimental procedures with animals were approved by the Institutional Animal Care and Utilization Committee of the Academia Sinica, Taiwan (Protocol #: RMiIBMCL2008070).

Animals

DNA fragment encoding human full length HO-1 was amplified by the polymerase chain reaction (PCR) from pAdCMV-HO-1 [17] and subcloned into mouse pBS aP2 promoter polyA plasmid (Addgene). The transgene consisting of 5.4 kb of the aP2 gene promoter, the human HO-1 cDNA and a polyadenylation sequence was cut from the vector with ClaI and SacII restriction enzymes and subjected to pronuclear microinjection. The HO-1 transgenic (Tg) mice in C57BL/6J genetic background were generated by Level Biotechnology (New Taipei City, Taiwan R.O.C). HO-1 Tg founders were then bred to generate F1 Tg mice and subjected to Southern blot and PCR analysis to check the transgene expression. The Tg F2 offspring was generated by crossing the F1 Tg mice with wild type (WT) C57BL/6J mice and their descendants were used in the experiments. In diet-induced obesity, 8 weeks old WT and HO-1 Tg male mice were divided into two groups and fed either a regular chow (10 kcal% fat, 5058, LabDiet) or a high fat diet (60 kcal% fat, D12492, Research Diets) for 12 weeks. All mice were kept on a 12 h light-dark cycle and allowed free access to food and water.

Isolation of Genomic DNA and Genotyping

Mouse tail snip (~0.5 cm) was incubated in 700 µl of lysis buffer containing 50 mM Tris-HCl pH 8.0, 100 mM EDTA, 0.5% SDS and 360 µg proteinase K at 55°C for 18 h. Samples were then mixed with 700 µl of phenol/chloroform/isoamyl alcohol (25:24:1), vortexed for 3 min at room temperature, and centrifuged at 15,500×g for10 min at 4°C. The upper layer was transferred to a new tube, mixed with equal volume of chloroform/isoamyl alcohol (24:1) and vortexed for 3 min at room temperature. Then the sample was centrifuged at 15,500×g for 10 min at 4°C, and the upper layer was removed and mixed with equal volume of isopropanol. After gently mixing, the genomic DNA was pelleted by centrifugation at 15,500×g for 10 min, rinsed once with 75% alcohol, air dried, and resuspended in 100 µl ddH$_2$O. Genotyping PCR was performed by using 50 ng genomic DNA, 62.5 pmole primer, 10 nmole dNTPs and 2.5 U FastStart Taq DNA polymerase (Roche). The primer used were:5′ -primer, 5′-ATTGCCCAGAAAGCCCTGGACC-3′ and 3′-primer, 5′-GATCCGAATTCGCCCTATAG-3′. The PCR condition was 94°C 5 min; 35 cycles of 94°C 30 sec, 50°C 30 sec, and 72°C 30 sec; then 72°C 7 min.

Southern Blot Analysis

Mouse genomic DNA (10 µg) was digested with SacI at 37°C for 2 h. Copy number standards were prepared by mixing WT mice genomic DNA with known amount of transgene plasmid DNA followed by SacI digestion. Following 1% agarose gel electrophoresis, gel was soaked in denaturation buffer containing 0.5 N NaOH and 1.5 M NaCl for 40 min and then in neutralization buffer containing.5 M Tris-HCl, pH7.5 and 3 M NaCl for another 40 min. DNA was then transferred to Hybond-N+ membrane (GE Healthcare Life Sciences) by vacuum blotting system (VacuGene XL, Pharmacia LKB) for 5 hr. The DNA was fixed to membrane by UV crosslinking. Southern blot analysis was performed using Digoxigenin (DIG) High Prime DNA Labeling and Detection Starter Kit II (Roche) according to the manufacturer's instruction. To prepare the DIG-labeled DNA probe, 1 µg of a human HO-1 cDNA fragment (~0.7 kb) was first denatured by boiling in water for 10 min and then cooled down on ice. The denatured DNA was incubated with 4 µl DIG-High Prime at 37°C for 20 h. The reaction was stopped by adding 2 µl of 0.2 M EDTA (pH 8.0) and heating to 65°C for 10 min. The labeling efficiency was determined by comparing with the serial diluted DIG-labeled control DNA. To perform the Southern blot analysis, the membrane was preincubated with 10 ml of pre-heat DIG Easy Hyb (Roche) at 42°C for 30 min in the hybridization bag. The DIG-labeled DNA probe specific for human HO-1 cDNA (25 ng/ml) was then added to the hybridization bag. After overnight incubation at 42°C, the membrane was washed twice with buffer containing 2× saline-sodium citrate buffer (SSC) and 0.1% SDS for 5 min at room temperature, followed by wash twice with buffer containing 0.5× SSC and 0.1% SDS for 15 min at 60°C. Subsequently, the membrane was rinsed once with buffer A (0.1 M maleic acid, pH 7.5, 0.15 M NaCl, and 0.3% Tween-20), and incubated with blocking solution (Roche) and then antibody solution (anti-DIG-AP conjugate, 1/10,000 in blocking solution) for 30 min at room temperature, respectively. After two washes with buffer A for 15 min/wash, membrane was equilibrated in detection buffer (0.1 M Tris-HCl pH 9.5 and 0.1 M NaCl) for 5 min. The chloro-5-substituted adamantyl-1,2-dioxetane phosphate was applied to the membrane and the luminescence signal was detected by X-ray film exposure.

Metabolic Parameter Analysis

Blood glucose level was measured using automatic blood glucose meter (ACCU-CHEK Advantage, Roche, IN, USA). Serum insulin level was measured with mouse insulin ELISA kit (Millipore). Cholesterol and triglyceride concentrations were measured by FUJI DRI-CHEM clinical chemistry analyzer (FUJIFILM, Tokyo, Japan). Glucose tolerance test was performed by intraperitoneal (i.p.) injection of glucose (1g/kg of body weight) in mice fasted for 16 h. For insulin tolerance test, mice fasted for 6 h received i.p.injection of insulin (1.3 U/kg of body weight). Blood samples were drawn from the tail vein at the indicated time point and glucose concentration was measured with an automatic blood glucose meter.

Peritoneal Macrophage Isolation

Mice received i.p. injection of 3 ml 3% thioglycollate. After 4 days, peritoneal macrophages were isolated by washing the peritoneal cavity with RPMI 1640 medium containing 0.5% bovine serum albumin (BSA). Cells were then plated on cell culture plate. After 4 h incubation, the nonadherent cells were removed by washing with culture medium and the adherent cells used as peritoneal macrophages.

Real-time Quantitative PCR

Total RNA were isolated with TRIzol reagent. Reverse transcription was performed by using 2 μg of DNase I-treated total RNA, 100 ng random hexamers, 10 nmole dNTPs and 200 U Superscript III reverse transcriptase. Real-time quantitative PCR was performed with LightCycler FastStart DNA Master^{PLUS} SYBR Green I kit (Roche) on a LightCycler Carousel-Based System (Roche Applied Science, IN, USA). 36B4 was used as an internal control. The primer pairs were TNFα (5′-AGACCCT-CACACTCAGA-3′ and 5′-CCTTGTCCCTTGAAGAGAAC-3′), IL-6 (5′-GAGGATACCACTCCCAACAGACC-3′ and 5′-AAGTGCATCATCGTTGTTCATACA-3′), vascular endothelial growth factor (VEGF) (5′-CAGGCTGCACCCACGACA-GAAG-3′ and 5′-CTATGTGCTGGCTTTGGTGAGGTTT-3′), sromal cell-derived factor-1 (SDF-1) (5′-ATGGACGC-CAAGGTCGTCGCC-3′ and 5′-TTACTTGTT-TAAAGCTTTCTC-3′), MCP-1 (5′-CTTCTGGGCCTGCTGTTCA -3′ and 5′-CCAGCCTACT-CATTGGGATCA-3′), adiponectin (5′-GCAGAGATG GCACTCCTGGA-3′ and 5′-CCCTTCAGCTCCTGT-CATTCC-3′), F4/80 (5′-TTTCCTCGCCTGCTTCTTC-3′ and 5′-CCCCGTCTCTGTATTCAACC-3′), interleukin-10 (IL-10) (5′-GGTTGCCAAGCCTTATCGGA-3′ and 5′-AC-CTGCTCCACTGCCTTG CT-3′), CD11c (5′-GAGAGCCCA-GACGAAGACAG-3′ and 5′-CCATTTGCTTCCTCCAACAT-3′), Mannose receptor (MR) (5′-GCAAATGGAGCC GTCTGTGC-3′ and 5′-CTCGTGGATCTCCGTGACAC-3′), iNOS (5′- TGCATGGACCAGTATAAGGCAAGC-3′ and 5′-GCTTCTGGTCGATGTCATGAGCAA-3′), macrophage galactose-type C-type lectin 1 (Mgl1) (5′- TGAGAAAGGCTTTAA-GAACTGGG-3′ and 5′- GACCACCTGTAGTGATGTGGG-3′) and 36B4 (5′-CCCACTTACTGAAAAGG-3′ and 5′-GGCGGGATTAGTCGAA-3′).

Western Blot Analysis

Tissues or cells were lysed in buffer containing 50 mM Tris, pH 7.4, 150 mM NaCl, 1% Nonidet P-40, 0.25% sodium deoxycholate, 1 mM EDTA, 1 mM PMSF and 1% protease inhibitor, followed by centrifugation at 15,500×g for 10 min at 4°C. The tissue or cell lysates (supernatants) were collected and the protein concentrations determined. The protein samples were separated by electrophoresis in 10% SDS-polyacrylamide gel and transferred to Immobilon-P Membrane (Millipore). After blocking with 5% skim milk in Tris-buffered saline containing 0.1% Tween-20 (TBST), the membrane was incubated with rabbit anti-HO-1 antibody [18](1:2000 dilution) or goat anti-Mgl1 antibody (R&D systems; 1:1000 dilution) in TBST containing 1% skim milk for 2 h at room temperature. The membrane was then washed with TBST for three times and incubated with horseradish peroxidase (HRP)-conjugated anti-rabbit ((Santa Cruz; 1:3000 dilution) or anti-goat (Santa Cruz; 1:2000 dilution) secondary antibody in TBST containing 5% skim milk for another 1 h. After three washes with TBST, antigen-antibody complex was detected using Western Lightning Plus-ECL (PerkinElmer). To repobe the membrane with anti-GAPDH antibody (Santa Cruz; 1:3000 dilution), the membrane was incubated in stripping buffer containing 62.5 mM Tris-HCl, pH 6.8, 2% SDS, and 100 mM 2-mercaptoethanol at 55°C for 30 min with shaking. After washing with TBST for three times, the membrane was blocked and incubated with antibody as described above. For immunoblot quantification, the X-film was scanned by ScanMaker 8700 (MICROTEK, Hsinchu, Taiwan) and images were analyzed using MetaMorph image analysis software. The band intensity of target protein was normalized by dividing its intensity value with the value of the internal control protein (GAPDH) band in the same lane of the blot. Data were presented as the normalized intensities of at least 3 mice in each group.

HO Activity Measurement

Epididymal adipose tissue was homogenized in ice cold buffer containing 0.1 M K_3PO_4 pH 7.4, 1 mM EDTA and 0.5 mM PMSF, and centrifuged at 15,500×g for 10 min at 4°C. The supernatant was removed and 1 mg of proteins were incubated in 200 μl of buffer containing 0.1 M K_3PO_4, pH 7.4, 1.5 mg of rat liver cytosol, 50 μM hemin, 1 mM NADPH, 2 mM glucose-6-phosphate and 0.3 units of glucose-6-phosphate dehydrogenase. The mixture was incubated in the dark for 1 h at 37°C. Bilirubin was then extracted with 1 ml chloroform and determined by the absorbance difference between 464 and 530 nm with an extinction coefficient of 40/mM*cm.

ELISA

The adipokine levels in mouse serum samples and adipose tissue lysates were determined using the indicated ELISA kits (R&D Systems) according to the manufacturer's instructions. For tissue adipokine levels, data were represented as the amount of cytokine per 100 μg of tissue lysates.

Immunohistochemistry

Adipose tissue was fixed in Bouin's solution for 16 h with shaking (30 rpm) at room temperature and embedded in paraffin. The 5 μm sections were deparaffinized in xylene and rehydrated. The endogenous peroxidase activity was depleted with 3% H_2O_2 for 10 min at room temperature. For immunostaining of F4/80, sections were first blocked with phosphate-buffered saline (PBS) containing 5% normal goat serum for 30 min at 37°C, followed by incubation with mouse anti-F4/80 antibody (eBioscience; 1:300 dilution) in PBS for 1 h at 37°C. The sections were washed three times with PBS, and then incubated with HRP-conjugated goat anti-mouse (Santa Cruz; 1:300 dilution) secondary antibody in PBS for 1 h at room temperature. After three washes with PBS, the sections were incubated with 0.1% 3,3′-diaminobenzidine (DAB) solution. The nuclei were counterstained with hematoxylin for 5 min at room temperature. The pictures were taken in four different fields per section (x 100) under a light microscope. The extent of macrophage infiltration was calculated as the percentage of adipocytes surrounded by a F4/80-positive crown-like structure in the total adipocytes in each field. For detection of Mgl1 expression, sections were blocked with PBS containing 5% donkey serum (Jackson ImmunoResearch), followed by incubation with goat anti-Mgl1 (R&D systems; 1:100 dilution) in PBS for 1 h at 37°C. After 3 washes, the sections were incubated with HRP-conjugated donkey anti-goat (Santa Cruz; 1:200) secondary antibody in PBS for 1 h at room temperature, washed, and incubated with 0.1% DAB for antigen detection. For immunostaining of the vasculature, sections were incubated with 20 μg/ml of proteinase K (Sigma-Aldrich) at room temperature for 5 min. After a PBS wash, the sections were blocked with 5% normal goat serum, followed by incubation overnight at 4°C with antibody against CD31 (BD Pharmingen;1:100 dilution). After three PBS washes, the sections were incubated with FITC-conjugated secondary antibody (Invitrogen;1:200 dilution) at room temperature for 1 h in the dark, followed by washing, and examined by fluorescence microscopy. Vascular density was calculated as described previously [12]. Briefly, the CD31 immunofluorescence images were taken from 4 different fields per section under a fluorescence microscope (x 200 magnification). MetaMorph image analysis software (Molecular Devices) was used for image analysis. The $CD31^+$ area in each field was calculated as [($CD31^+$ signal − background (FITC-goat anti-rat IgG))/total pixels] × 0.6183 mm^2 (the total real area under 200× magnification). The vascular density was defined as $CD31^+$ area per field ($\times 10^{-6}/um^2$). The normalized vascular density was calculated by dividing the $CD31^+$ area with the total number of adipocytes per area. The adipocyte density was calculated by counting the number of adipocytes per area ($\times 10^{-6}/um^2$).

Isolation of $CD11b^+$ Myeloid Cells

Mouse spleen was minced into pieces in 2 ml serum free RPMI medium containing 0.5% BSA. The clumps were further dispersed by gently pipetting up and down several times. The cell suspension was then passing through a 70 μm cell strainer into a 50 ml tube, followed by centrifugation at 400×g for 5 min. The cell pellet was subjected to red blood cell lysis in ammonium chloride solution (BD Pharm Lyse™) for 5 min at room temperature. After washing once with PBS containing 2% fetal bovine serum (FBS) (PBS/2% FBS), cells were spin down at 300×g for 5 min at 4°C, and resuspended at a density of 1×10^8 cells/ml in PBS/2% FBS. $CD11b^+$ cells were enriched using the EasySep mouse CD11b positive selection kit (18770, Stemcell Tech) following the manufacturer's instruction, and confirmed by flow cytometry.

In vitro Migration Assay

Cell migration was performed using 24 well Transwell with a pore size of 5 μm (Corning). Briefly, $CD11b^+$ cells (1×10^5) isolated from WT and HO-1 Tg mice were suspended in serum free RPMI 1640 medium containing 0.5% BSA and added into the upper chambers. The lower chambers were filled with medium supplemented with 10 ng/ml of MCP-1. To test the effect of HO-1 inhibition, tin protoporphyrin IX (SnPP) was added into both upper and lower chambers to a final concentration of 10 μM prior to the addition of MCP-1 to the lower chambers. After 4 h incubation, unmigrated cells were wiped off the upper side of the filter with a cotton swab. The migrated cells on the lower side were fixed with 4% paraformaldehyde for 10 min, stained with Giemsa for 2 h, and counted under light microscope.

Statistical Analysis

Results were expressed as the means ±S.E. Differences between groups were examined for statistical significance using Student's t test or ANOVA. A *P*-value < 0.05 was considered statistically significant.

Results

Generation of Transgenic Mice with Adipose Overexpression of Human HO-1

In an attempt to elucidate the effect of HO-1 on adipose remodeling and the development of insulin resistance during obesity, we used the adipocyte-specific aP2 promoter to generate Tg mice carrying human HO-1 gene. Three Tg mouse lines carrying various copy numbers of HO-1 gene were obtained (Fig. 1A). As assessed by Western blot analysis (Fig. 1B), the levels of HO-1 protein expression in epididymal WAT was significantly higher in the Tg mouse lines carrying 6~8 (Tg-2) and >20 copies (Tg-3) of HO-1 gene as compared to that of WT control. To confirm that the HO-1 transgene is functionally active, we performed the HO enzymatic activity assay. As shown in Figure 1C, the HO activity of WAT was substantially higher in these two Tg mouse lines carrying the high copies of transgene. When HO-1 expressions in other tissues were examined, the results showed that HO-1 transgene overexpression was also noted in the interscapular brown fat tissue (BAT) of Tg mice (Fig. 1D). Whereas, HO-1 expressions in non-fat tissues, including heart, skeletal muscle, brain, liver, kidney, lung, did not show significant differences between WT and Tg mice (Fig. 1D). Since aP2 gene has been shown to be induced in activated macrophages [18–19], experiment was also performed to examine whether there is a leaked transgene expression in macrophages of Tg mice. As illustrated in Figure 1E and 1F, HO-1 protein expression was much higher in the peritoneal macrophages isolated from Tg mice as compared to WT counterparts.

Tg Mice Exhibit a Metabolic Phenotype Similar to WT Mice

Figure 2A and 2B showed that the body weight gains of the Tg mice, Tg-2 and Tg-3 lines, respectively, were similar to their WT littermates when placed on regular chow (RC) diet for over 12 weeks. Likewise, food intake and serum concentrations of glucose, lipid, and insulin of Tg mice (Tg-3) and WT littermates were comparable (Table 1). Glucose tolerance test (GTT) and insulin tolerance test (GTT) again demonstrated no significant difference in insulin sensitivity between the lean Tg mice of either line and their WT counterparts (Fig. 2C and 2D). To investigate whether adipose HO-1 overexpression has an impact on diet-induced obesity and insulin resistance, Tg mice and their WT littermates were fed with HFD. As shown in Figure 2A and 2B, the body weight gains of both Tg mouse lines were similar to those of their respective WT controls. The serum glucose and insulin levels were significantly increased by HFD feeding to similar extents between the Tg and WT mice (Table 1). When these HFD-fed mice were subjected to GTT and ITT, the results again showed that both Tg lines of mice exhibited similar glucose intolerance and insulin resistance as compared to their WT counterparts (Fig. 2E and 2F). When the serum levels of adipokines, including adiponectin, leptin, IL-6, TNF-α, and MCP-1 in HFD-fed WT and Tg mice were determined, no significant difference was found between these two groups of mice (Fig. 3).

Effect of HO-1 on Adipose Gene Expression in Tg Mice

HO-1 has been shown to modulate cytokine expression. To examine whether HO-1 overexpression in adipocytes affects adipokine gene expression, we performed quantitative real-time PCR with total RNAs isolated from the WAT of 20 weeks old male Tg mice (Tg-3) and the WT control placed on chow diet. As shown in Figure 4A, the adiponectin and IL-10 gene expression levels were significantly greater in WAT of lean Tg mice as compared to WT control. Nevertheless, the expression levels of TNF-α, IL-6, MCP-1, VEGF and SDF-1 were not significantly different between WT and Tg mice. Moreover, the gene expression levels of macrophage markers, including F4/80, CD11c, and iNOS, in lean WT and Tg mice were comparable as shown in the same figure. Nevertheless, the expression of Mgl1, a marker for M2 macrophages, was significantly higher in the adipose tissue of Tg mice as compared to WT controls, suggesting that adipose HO-1 overexpression may increase the polarization of adipose resident macrophages toward M2 phenotype even in

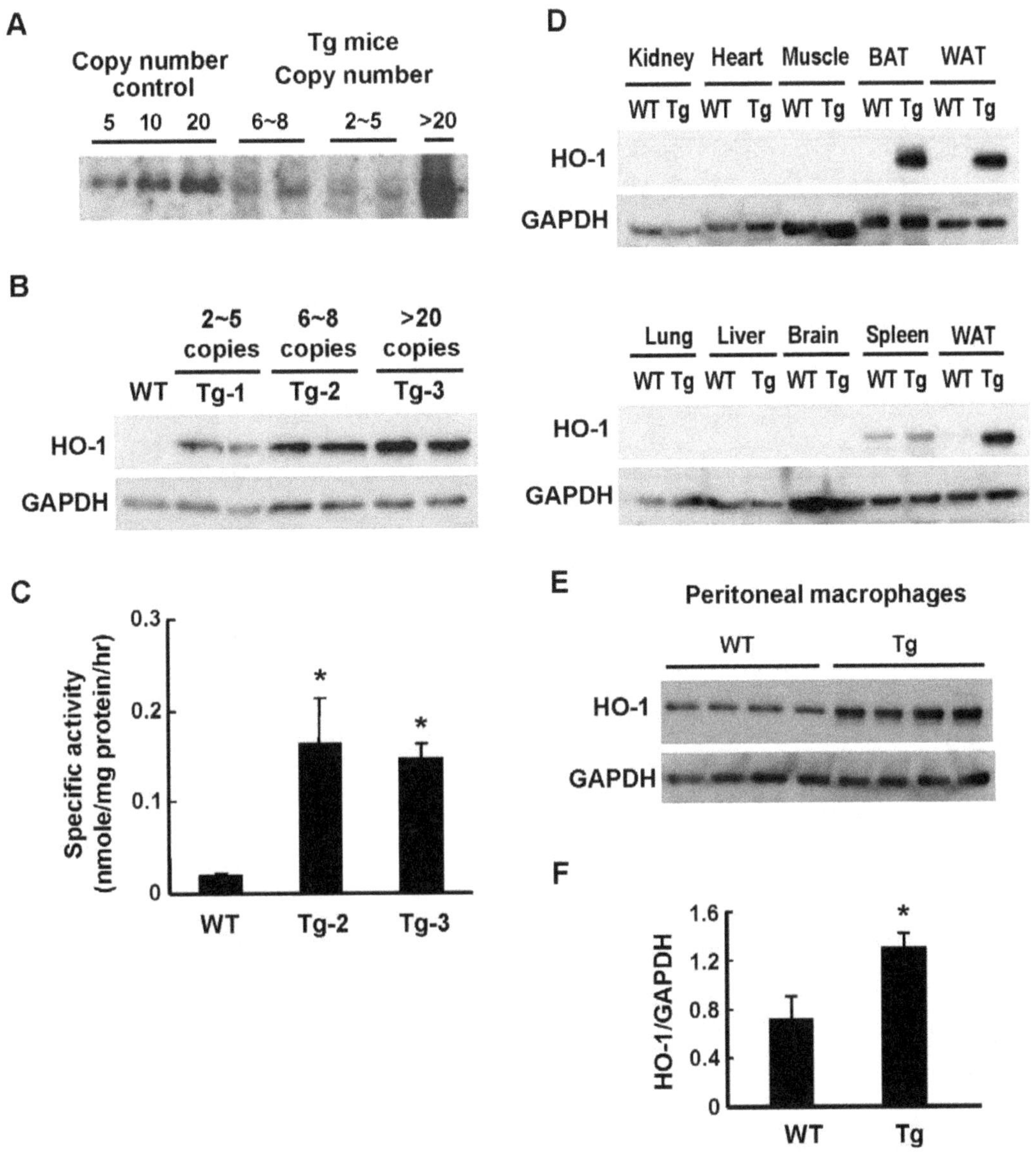

Figure 1. Generation of aP2-HO-1 Tg mice. A, Southern blot analysis of SacI-digested mouse genomic DNA from three lines of aP2-HO-1 Tg mice. The copy numbers of each line were estimated to be 2~5, 6~8 and >20 copies, respectively. B, HO-1 expressions in adipose tissues from three lines of aP2-HO-1 Tg mice were examined by Western blot analysis. C, Adipose HO-1 activities in WT and HO-1 Tg mice were determined. Data shown are means ± SE. *$P<0.05$ vs. WT. The number of mice in each group was four. D, HO-1 expressions in various tissues of WT and Tg mice examined by Western blot analysis. WAT, epididymal white adipose tissue; BAT, interscapular brown adipose tissue. E, HO-1 expressions in thioglycollate-induced peritoneal macrophages isolated from WT and Tg mice (n = 4/group) were examined. F, HO-1 protein levels of peritoneal macrophages were quantified by densitometry. *$P<0.05$ vs the WT group.

the lean state. As demonstrated in the same figure, HFD caused a significant down regulation of adiponectin gene expression to a similar level in both WT and Tg mice. VEGF expression was also down-regulated in obese WAT, but its level was greater in obese Tg mice as compared to that of WT counterparts. The expressions of TNF-α, IL-6, IL-10, MCP-1, and SDF-1 in WAT were markedly induced by HFD. Interestingly, the levels of IL-10 and SDF-1 mRNAs induced were significantly higher in obese Tg mice as compared to WT controls. When the expression level of F4/80, an index of macrophage infiltration in WAT, was examined, the result showed that HFD-induced increase of F4/80 expression was much greater in Tg mice than WT controls. Although the expressions of CD11c and iNOs, the markers of M1 macrophages, were also significantly increased in both groups of mice after HFD feeding, the levels were not significantly different between these two groups. However, when the expression levels of MR and Mgl-1, the markers of M2 macrophages, were assessed, the data showed that their mRNAs were much higher in obese Tg mice than WT counterparts. Consistent with the mRNA expression levels, the levels of TNF-α, and MCP-1 proteins determined by ELISA did not show significant difference in the WAT of HFD-fed WT and Tg mice (Fig. 4B). However, the protein level of IL-10 was substantially greater in the WAT of HFD-fed Tg mice as compared to WT counterparts (Fig. 4B).

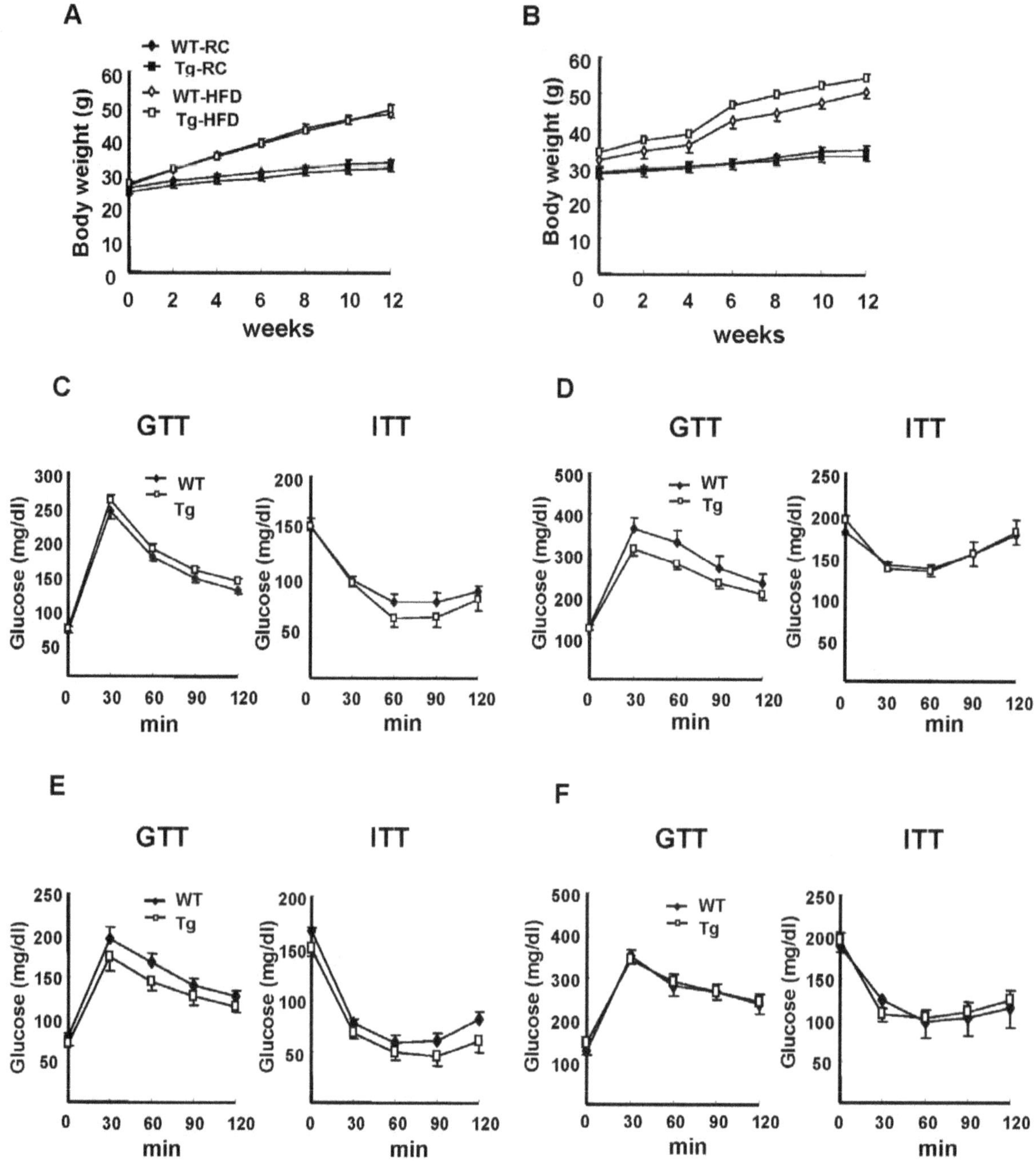

Figure 2. Tg mice exhibit similar metabolic phenotype as WT mice. A &B, HO-1 Tg (Tg-2 line, A; Tg-3 line, B) mice and their corresponding WT littermates were fed with a regular chow (RC) or HFD as indicated for 12 weeks. The body weights were measured every other week. The number of mice in each group was six to eight. C-F, WT and Tg mice (C&D,Tg-2 line; E&F, Tg-3 line) were fed with RC (C&E) or HFD (D&F) for 12 weeks, then the GTT and ITT assays were performed. The number of mice in each group was six to eight.

HFD Promotes Angiogenesis and Macrophage Infiltration in WAT of Tg Mice

Histological examination of the visceral WAT of these mice after 12 weeks of HFD feeding revealed the enlargement of adipocytes and the decrease in the adipocyte density, which were not significantly different between WT and Tg groups (Fig. 5A and 5B). Immunostaining experiment performed using specific antibody against endothelial marker, CD31, demonstrated that the adipose vascular density was substantially higher in HFD-fed Tg mice as compared to that of WT counterparts. (Fig. 5C and 5D). When the immunostaining experiment was performed with F4/80 antibody, the results showed that the extent of macrophage infiltration, characterized by a crown-like structure surrounding dead adipocytes, in the WAT was significantly higher in HFD-fed Tg mice than in WT controls (Fig. 6A and 6B), which was consistent with the levels of F4/80 gene expression shown in Figure 4A. To examine whether the macrophages of HFD-fed Tg mice preferentially expressed M2 marker, Mgl1, we also performed immunostaining using antibody against Mgl1. As

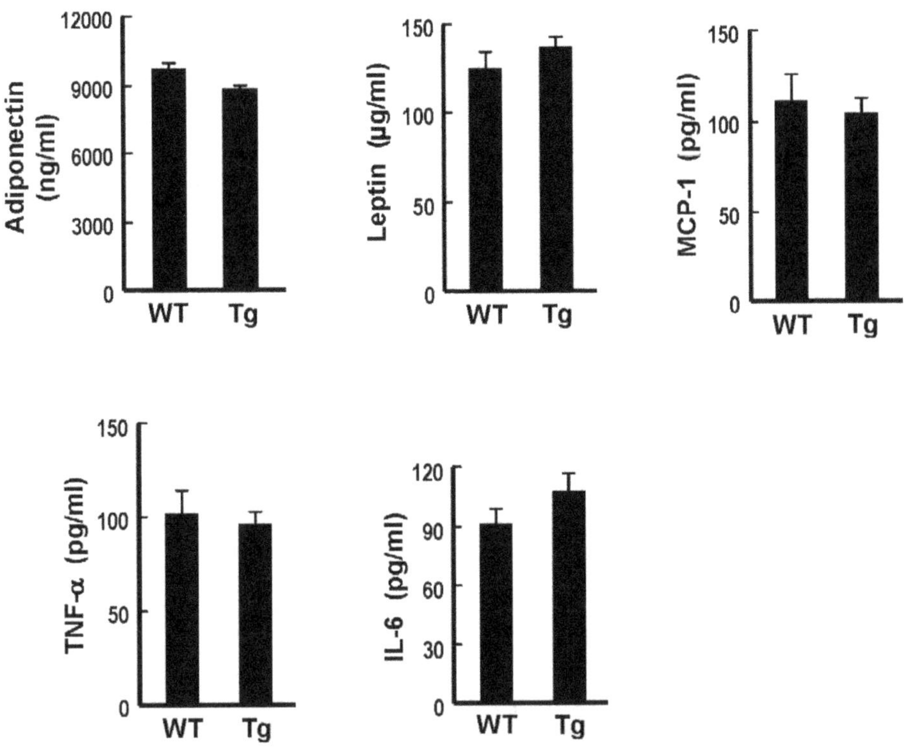

Figure 3. Serum adipokine levels in HFD-fed WT and Tg mice. Serum samples were collected from WT and Tg mice fed with HFD for 12 weeks, and the indicated adipokine levels were then determined by ELISA kits. The numbers of mice in WT and Tg groups were six and eight, respectively.

shown in Figure 6C, the positive immunostain for Mgl1 was more prominent in WAT of Tg mice than that of WT mice. Western blot analysis again demonstrated higher Mgl1 protein levels in the WAT lysates of Tg mice than WT counterparts (Fig. 6D and 6E).

Table 1. Metabolic parameters of the WT and HO-1 Tg mice.

Diet	RC		HFD	
genotype	**WT (n = 8)**	**Tg (n = 8)**	**WT (n = 6)**	**Tg (n = 8)**
Body weight (g)	34.31±1.29	32.83±1.52	52.42±0.92[a]	55.95±1.24[a]
Food intake (g/d/mouse)	3.7±0.22	3.51±0.3	2.87±0.35[a]	2.87±0.14[a]
Liver (g)	1.36±0.08	1.31±0.07	2.43±0.34[a]	2.56±0.16[a]
eWAT (g)	1.75±0.2	1.36±0.21	4.51±0.43[a]	4.43±0.16[a]
Serum cholesterol (mg/dl)	108.25±4.29	99.25±1.63	230±13.73[a]	240.5±10.18[a]
Serum triglyceride (mg/dl)	66.5±5.18	88.5±8.54	66±6.02	57.88±2.52[a]
Serum glucose (mg/dl)	78.25±4.36	70.25±3.45	125.17±7.35[a]	144±8.49[a]
Serum insulin (ng/ml)	0.95±0.25	0.72±0.25	4.81±1.1[a]	6±2.13[a]

The number of animals in each group is indicated in parenthesis. Eight weeks old WT or Tg mice were fed with regular chow (RC) or high fat diet (HFD). At 12 weeks on the diets, serum samples were collected, and body weight, liver and epididymal white adipose tissue (eWAT) weights were determined. Data are expressed as the mean ± SEM.

[a]Significant difference between different diets within the same genotype.

Myeloid Cells of Tg Mice Exhibit Greater Migration Response Toward Chemoattractant

We recently reported that HO-1 expression in monocytes/macrophages promotes chemoattractant-induced cell migration response [12]. To examine whether the increased adipose macrophage infiltration in HFD-fed Tg mice is due to the enhanced migration of myeloid cells to obese adipose tissue, we performed in vitro transwell migration assay using splenic CD11b$^+$ myeloid cells isolated from Tg and WT mice. Similar to the peritoneal macrophages, CD11b$^+$ cells of Tg mice expressed higher HO-1 than the WT counterparts (Fig. 7A and 7B). Although the basal migration response was comparable between WT and Tg myeloid cells, the migration response induced by MCP-1 was significantly greater in Tg group as compared to that of WT group (Fig. 7C). When cells were treated with 10 μM of SnPP, a HO inhibitor, MCP-1-induced migration response was markedly attenuated (Fig. 7C). Moreover, the difference in the migration response between cells of WT and Tg mice was abolished, supporting the role of HO-1 in the greater migration of myeloid cells of Tg mice.

Discussion

Earlier studies have shown that chemical-induced systemic HO-1 overexpression inhibits obesity and improves insulin sensitivity in diabetic animals [13–15]. However, in the present study we found that the body weight or epidermal fat mass of lean Tg mice was not significantly different from that of WT mice. Although Tg mice (Tg-3 line) gained some more weight (~6%) as compared to WT mice after HFD feeding, again the increases in the fat mass of both groups of mice were comparable. We reasoned that aP2 gene promoter is activated in the terminal differentiated adipocytes,

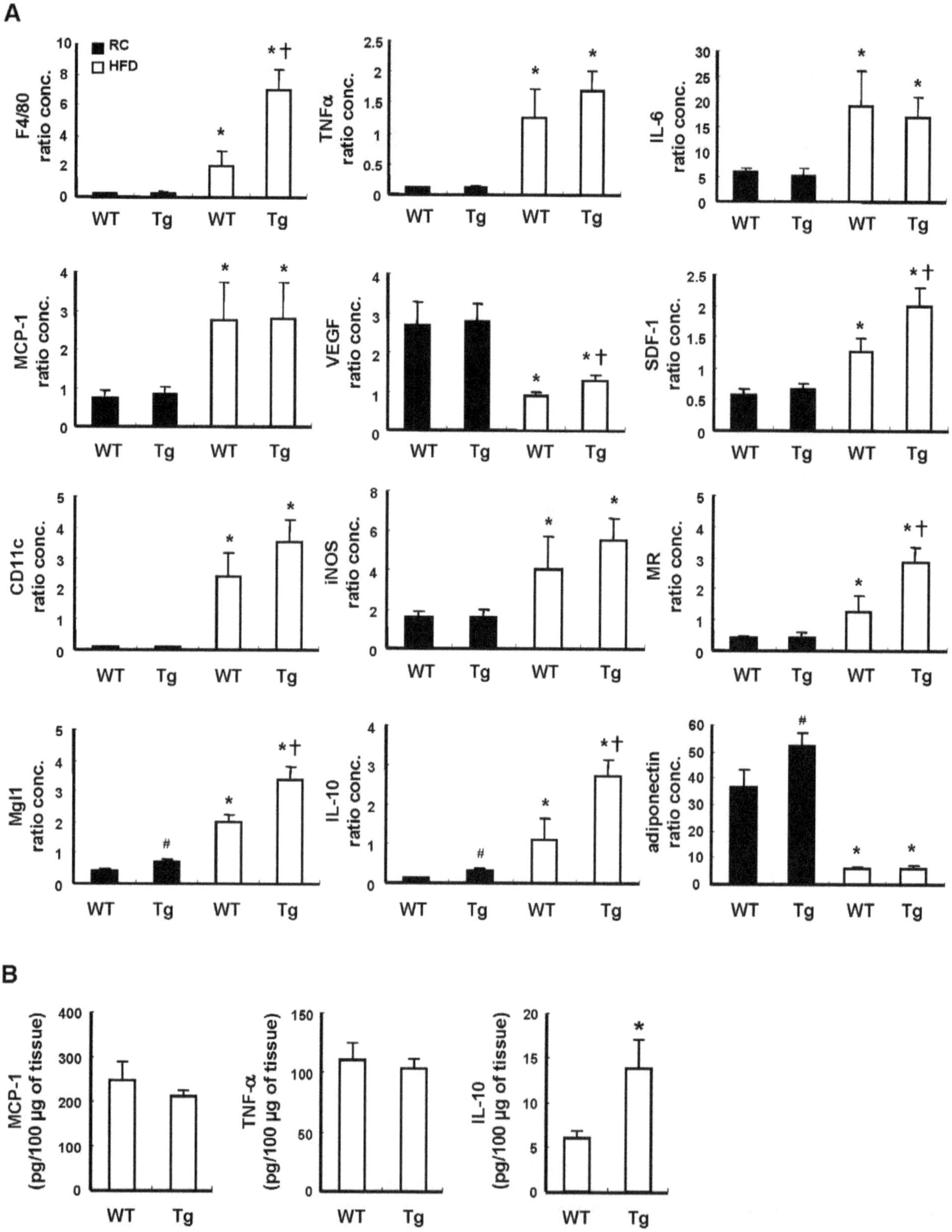

Figure 4. Adipokine gene expression in WT and Tg mice. WT and Tg mice were fed with a RC diet or HFD for 12 weeks, then the animals were killed and their visceral adipose tissues were collected. A, The expressions of the indicated genes in the adipose tissues were then analyzed by quantitative PCR. The expression level of 36B4 was used as an internal control for normalization. The number of mice in each group was six to eight. $^{\#}P<0.05$ vs RC-fed WT group; $^{*}P<0.05$ vs the RC-fed group of the same genotype; $^{\dagger}P<0.05$ vs HFD-fed WT group. B, The levels of indicated adipokines in the WAT lysates of HFD-fed WT and Tg mice were determined by ELISA. The numbers of mice in WT and Tg groups were six and eight, respectively. $^{*}P<0.05$ vs WT group.

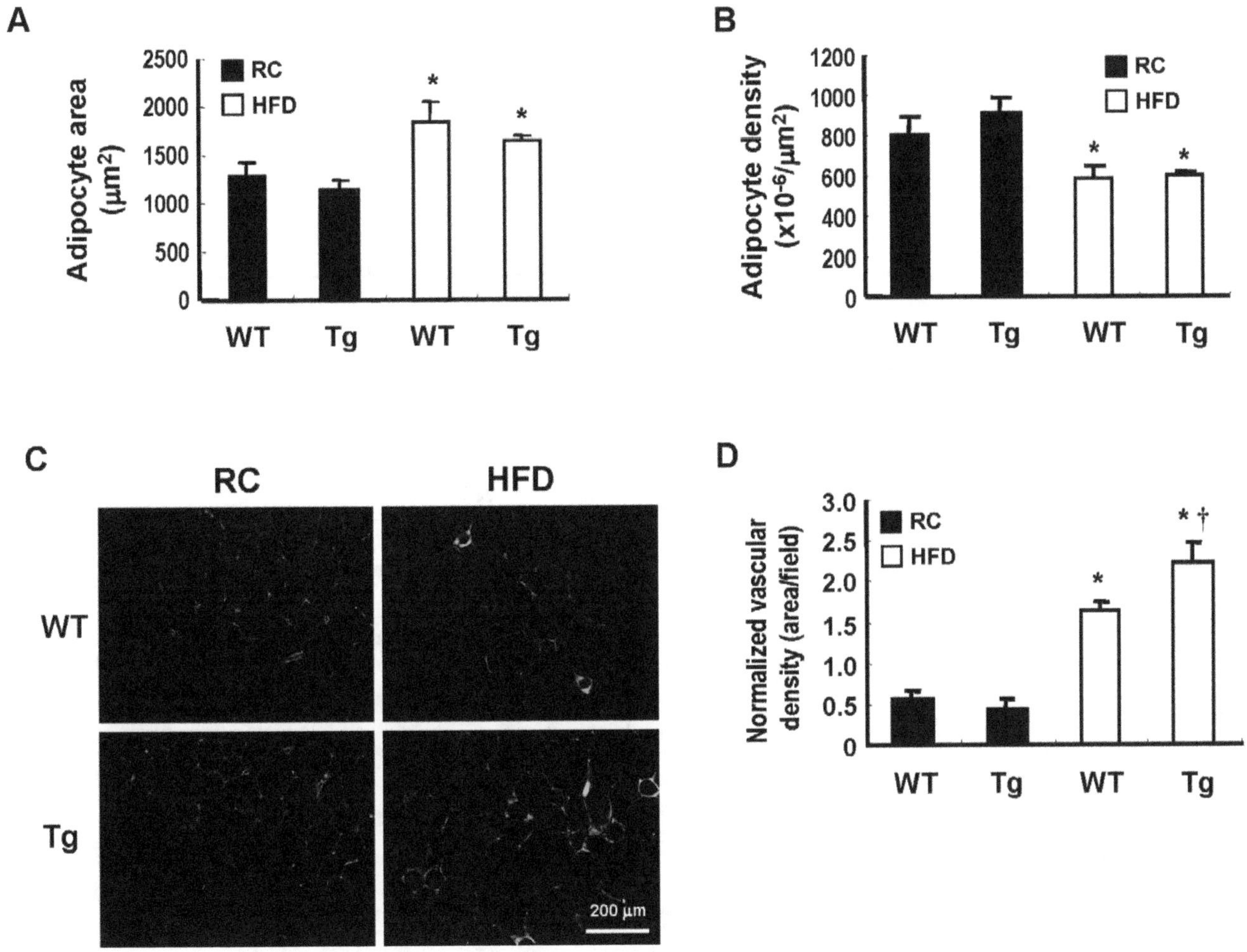

Figure 5. Effect of HFD on adipocyte hypertrophy and vascularization in visceral adipose tissues of WT and Tg mice. WT and Tg mice were fed with a RC or HFD for 12 weeks, and then sacrificed. A, The adipocyte size in the visceral adipose tissue sections of each group was analyzed. *$P<0.05$ vs the RC-fed WT group of the same genotype. B, The adipocyte density was calculated by counting the number of adipocyte per area. *$P<0.05$ vs the RC-fed group of the same genotype. C, The WAT sections were immunostained with antibody against CD31 as described in Materials and Methods. D, The normalized vascular density was quantified as the CD31-positve area divided by adipocyte density per filed. The number of animals in each group was five to six. *$P<0.05$ vs the RC-fed group of the same genotype; $^{\dagger}P<0.05$ vs HFD-fed WT group.

therefore HO-1 transgene expression driven by aP2 gene promoter is not induced in the adipocyte progenitor cells in the Tg mice. In this case, HO-1 has no effect on the increased adipogenesis during HFD feeding in Tg mice. In subsequent experiment, we demonstrated that adipose overexpression of HO-1 did not provide salutary effect to protect mice from HFD-induced insulin resistance. We speculate that the discrepancy between our study and previous reports is caused by the differential involvement of tissues with HO-1 overexpression. In previous studies by others, chemical-induced HO-1 was not only expressed in adipocytes but also in non-adipose tissues. The effects of HO-1 on other tissues, such as liver and skeletal muscle, and their interplays with adipose tissue might contribute to the protective effect of HO-1 inducer observed in their experimental settings. However, more recently the same group reported that HFD caused down regulation of HO-1 in adipose tissue and the induction of HO-1 expression in adipocytes mediated by the intracardial injection of lentivirus bearing aP2-promoter driven human HO-1 gene was able to attenuate adiposity and vascular dysfunction in HFD-fed mice [20]. Again, their results are contradictory to the present findings with HO-1 Tg mice. The reasons for such discrepancy are unclear at the present time.

Histological examination of the adipose tissues revealed that the adipocyte hypertrophy observed in HFD-fed WT and Tg mice did not show significant difference. Whereas, immunohistochemical staining of endothelial cell marker, CD31, demonstrated that HFD-induced increase of adipose vascular density was much greater in Tg mice in the WAT of this group of mice. This observation was consistent with early works showing that HO-1 overexpression promotes angiogenesis [21–22]. When immunostaining experiment was performed with antibody against macrophage marker, F4/80, the results demonstrated that adipose macrophage infiltration was more prominent in HFD-fed Tg mice than WT mice. Likewise, quantitative PCR also confirmed the higher gene expression of F4/80 in HFD-fed mice as compared to WT counterparts. Nevertheless, when the expression profiles of adipokine genes linked to inflammation were analyzed, the results showed that the expressions of proinflmmatory cytokines, such as TNF-α and IL-6, in obese adipose tissues did not show significant difference between HFD-fed Tg and WT mice. To investigate the polarity of infiltrated macrophages, the relative expression levels of

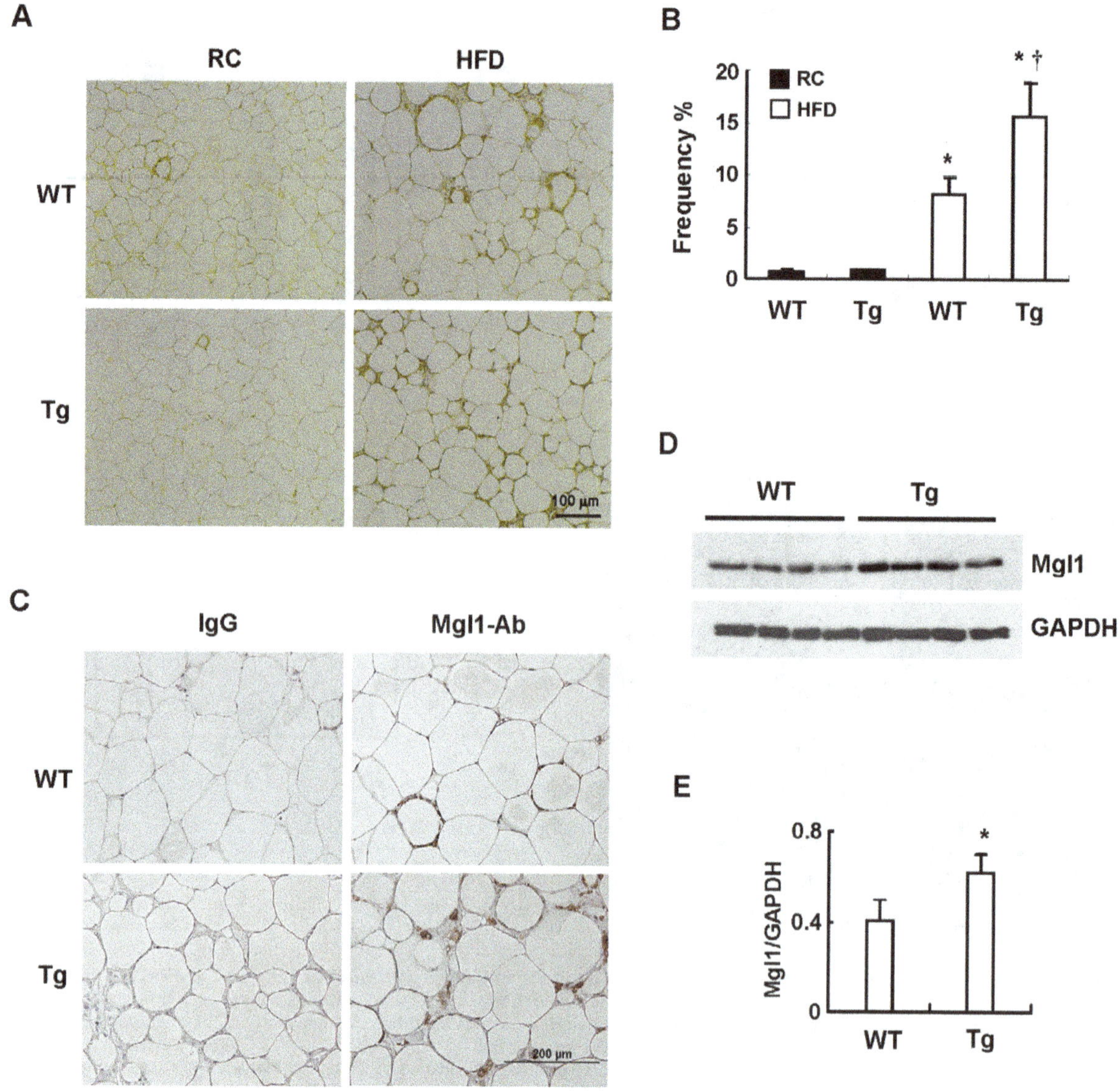

Figure 6. Effect of HFD on macrophage infiltration in visceral adipose tissues of WT and Tg mice. WT and Tg mice were fed with a RC or HFD for 12 weeks, and then sacrificed. A, The WAT sections were subjected to immunostaining using antibody against F4/80 as described in Materials and Methods. B, F4/80-positive macrophages were quantified as the percentage of adipocytes surrounded by a crown-like structure in the total adipocytes. The number of animals in each group was five to six. **P*<0.05 vs the RC-fed group of the same genotype; †*P*<0.05 vs HFD-fed WT group. C, The WAT sections of HFD-fed WT and Tg mice were immunostained with antibody against Mgl1 as described in Materials and Methods. D, The Mgl1 expression levels in WAT tissues of HFD-fed WT and Tg mice were examined by Western blot analysis. E, The Mgl1 protein levels were quantified by densitometry. The number of animals in each group was four. **P*<0.05 vs the WT group.

M1 and M2 macrophage markers were also assessed. The results showed that the expressions of CD11c and iNOS, the markers of M1 macrophages, were significantly induced by HFD in the adipose tissues of WT and Tg mice. However, the differences were not statistically different between two groups of mice. On the other hand, the increased expressions of MR and Mgl1, markers of M2 macrophages, were significantly greater in HFD-fed Tg mice as compared to WT mice. Immunostaining experiment and Western blot analysis again confirmed the higher expression of Mgl1 in WAT of HFD-fed Tg mice. These findings indicate that the macrophages recruited to obese adipose tissue of Tg mice are preferentially polarized toward M2 phenotype, which may explain why the higher degree of macrophage infiltration did not further augment adipose tissue inflammation in obese Tg mice. Notably, Mgl 1 expression was also much higher in the adipose tissue of lean Tg mice as compared to their WT counterparts, although the levels of F4/80 expression in both groups of mice were comparable. These observations suggest the possibility that HO-1 overexpression has an effect on the expression of adipocyte-derived Th2 cytokines, which are known to modulate macrophage alternative activation, in both lean and obese states [8] [23]. We paid particular interest in the expression of IL-10, which has been shown to be up-regulated by HO-1 [24] and has an effect to promote M2 polarization of adipose macrophages in obese animals [8]. As revealed by the gene expression analysis, IL-10 expression was significantly greater in the adipose tissue of Tg mice as compared to WT mice even in the lean state. HFD feeding led to markedly increase in adipose IL-10 gene expression in both

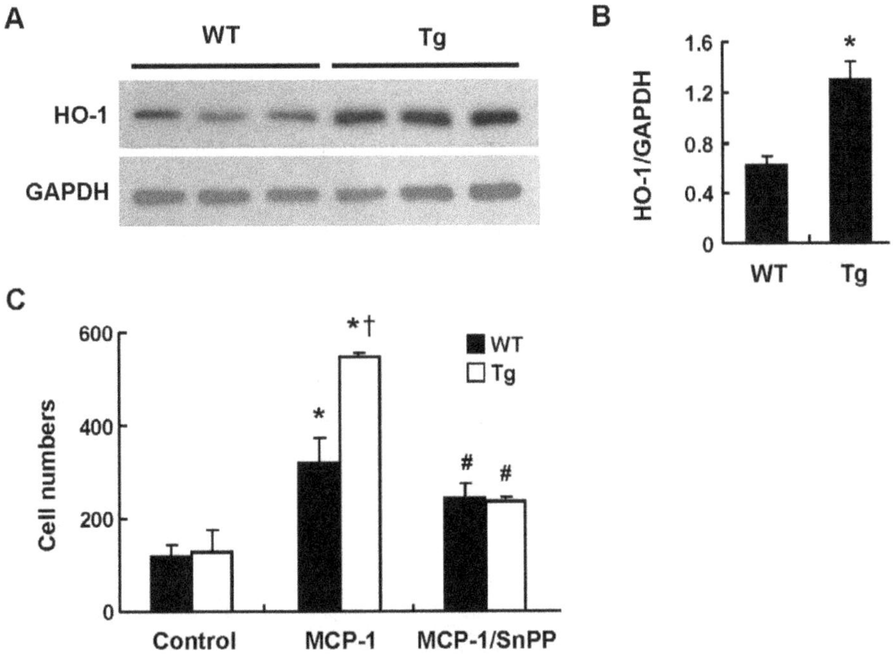

Figure 7. Myeloid cells of Tg mice exhibit greater migration response toward MCP-1. Splenic CD11b$^+$ cells were isolated from WT or Tg mice. A, HO-1 expression level in each individual mouse was examined by Western blot analysis. B, HO-1 levels were quantified by densitometry (n = 3/group). *$P<0.05$ vs the WT group. C, CD11b$^+$ cells isolated from each individual mouse were tested for their migration response toward 10 ng/ml of MCP-1 in the absence or presence of 10 μM SnPP. The number of mice in each group was three. *$P<0.02$ vs control group of the same genotype; $^{\dagger}P<0.02$ vs WT CD11b$^+$ cells receiving MCP-1 treatment; $^{\#}P<0.02$ vs MCP-1-treated alone group of the same genotype.

WT and Tg mice. Again, both mRNA and protein levels of IL-10 expression induced by HFD was significantly greater in Tg mice than that in WT mice, suggesting that the higher content of M2 macrophages in the adipose tissue of obese Tg mice is likely mediated by the higher expression of IL-10.

Adiponectin is an insulin sensitizing adipokine specifically produced by adipocytes [6]. Its expression was inversely correlated with obesity and insulin resistance in experimental animals and human patients. It was found that adiponectin gene expression in lean Tg mice was significantly higher than the WT counterparts. This observation was consistent with previous reports showing that HO-1 increases adponection expression [13–15]. However, HFD feeding downregulated adiponectin expression in both WT and Tg mice to a similar level. Studies have shown that the inflammatory cytokines, such as TNF-α and IL-6, suppress adiponectin expression [6]. It is envisaged that the suppressive effect of inflammatory cytokines produced during obesity might surpass the promoting effect of HO-1 on adiponection gene expression in HFD-fed Tg mice. The failure to sustain high expression of adiponectin by HO-1 in obese state may contribute to the ineffective protection of Tg mice from the development of insulin resistance.

Although HO-1 transgene expression was primarily detected in the adipose tissues of Tg mice, we found a leaky expression of HO-1 transgene in myeloid cells in these mice. The expression of transgene in adipocytes and myeloid cells were also reported in other transgenic mice using the ap2 promoter [18–19]. Consistent with our early report showing that HO-1 promotes chemoattractant-induced myeloid cell migration [12], we demonstrated that myeloid cells isolated from Tg mice exhibited greater migration response toward MCP-1 than their WT counterparts. It is conceivable that the effect of HO-1 on myeloid cell migration may underlie the enhanced adipose macrophage infiltration in HFD-fed Tg mice. On the other hand, the expression levels of VEGF and SDF-1, but not MCP-1, in the adipose tissue of HFD-fed Tg mice were found to be much higher than their WT counterparts. As VEGF and SDF-1 are potent chemoattractants for myeloid cells [25–26], their high expression may also promote the recruitment of more monocytes/macrophages toward adipose tissue in obese Tg mice.

In conclusion, the present study demonstrated that HO-1 overexpression in adipocytes did not protect mice from obesity and the development of insulin resistance. HO-1 increased adiponectin expression in the adipose tissue of Tg mice in the lean state. However, it did not prevent the down regulation of adiponectin during obesity. Moreover, HO-1 transgene was also expressed in myeloid cells and likely promoted adipose macrophage infiltration in HFD-fed Tg mice. Although the adipose macrophages exhibit preferentially M2 phenotype in the obese Tg mice, they did not seem to improve the adipose inflammation state and the development of insulin resistance during obesity in Tg mice.

Acknowledgments

We thank the Taiwan Mouse Clinic Core (NSC97-3112-B001-025) funded by the National Research Program for Genomic Medicine at the National Science Council of Taiwan for technical support.

Author Contributions

Conceived and designed the experiments: LYC. Performed the experiments: JYH MTC. Analyzed the data: JYH MTC. Wrote the paper: LYC.

References

1. Kersten S (2001) Mechanisms of nutritional and hormonal regulation of lipogenesis. EMBO Rep 2: 282–286.
2. Spiegelman BM, Flier JS (2001) Obesity and the regulation of energy balance. Cell 104: 531–543.
3. Mozaffarian D, Hao T, Rimm EB, Willett WC, Hu FB (2011) Changes in diet and lifestyle and long-term weight gain in women and men. N Engl J Med 364: 2392–2404.
4. Hotamisligil GS (2006) Inflammation and metabolic disorders. Nature 444: 860–867.
5. Schenk S, Saberi M, Olefsky JM (2008) Insulin sensitivity: modulation by nutrients and inflammation. J Clin Invest 118: 2992–3002.
6. Ouchi N, Parker JL, Lugus JJ, Walsh K (2011) Adipokines in inflammation and metabolic disease. Nat Rev Immunol 11: 85–97.
7. Lumeng CN, Bodzin JL, Saltiel AR (2007) Obesity induces a phenotypic switch in adipose tissue macrophage polarization. J Clin Invest 117: 175–184.
8. Fujisaka S, Usui I, Bukhari A, Ikutani M, Oya T, et al. (2009) Regulatory mechanisms for adipose tissue M1 and M2 macrophages in diet-induced obese mice. Diabetes 58: 2574–2582.
9. Morris DL, Singer K, Lumeng CN (2011) Adipose tissue macrophages: phenotypic plasticity and diversity in lean and obese states. Curr Opin Clin Nutr Metab Care 14: 341–346.
10. Abraham NG, Kappas A (2008) Pharmacological and clinical aspects of heme oxygenase. Pharmacol Rev 60: 79–127.
11. Soukas A, Cohen P, Socci ND, Friedman JM (2000) Leptin-specific patterns of gene expression in white adipose tissue. Genes Dev 14: 963–980.
12. Huang JY, Chiang MT, Yet SF, Chau LY (2012) Myeloid heme oxygenase-1 haploinsufficiency reduces high fat diet-induced insulin resistance by affecting adipose macrophage infiltration in mice. PLoS One 7: e38626.
13. Li M, Kim DH, Tsenovoy PL, Peterson SJ, Rezzani R, et al. (2008) Treatment of obese diabetic mice with a heme oxygenase inducer reduces visceral and subcutaneous adiposity, increases adiponectin levels, and improves insulin sensitivity and glucose tolerance. Diabetes 57: 1526–1535.
14. Nicolai A, Li M, Kim DH, Peterson SJ, Vanella L, et al. (2009) Heme oxygenase-1 induction remodels adipose tissue and improves insulin sensitivity in obesity-induced diabetic rats. Hypertension 53: 508–515.
15. Ndisang JF, Lane N, Jadhav A (2009) The heme oxygenase system abates hyperglycemia in Zucker diabetic fatty rats by potentiating insulin-sensitizing pathways. Endocrinology 150: 2098–2108.
16. Johnson FK, Johnson RA, Durante W, Jackson KE, Stevenson BK, et al. (2006) Metabolic syndrome increases endogenous carbon monoxide production to promote hypertension and endothelial dysfunction in obese Zucker rats. Am J Physiol Regul Integr Comp Physiol 290: R601–608.
17. Juan SH, Lee TS, Tseng KW, Liou JY, Shyue SK, et al. (2001) Adenovirus-mediated heme oxygenase-1 gene transfer inhibits the development of atherosclerosis in apolipoprotein E-deficient mice. Circulation 104: 1519–1525.
18. Makowski L, Boord JB, Maeda K, Babaev VR, Uysal KT, et al. (2001) Lack of macrophage fatty-acid-binding protein aP2 protects mice deficient in apolipoprotein E against atherosclerosis. Nat Med 7: 699–705.
19. Koliwad SK, Streeper RS, Monetti M, Cornelissen I, Chan L, et al. (2010) DGAT1-dependent triacylglycerol storage by macrophages protects mice from diet-induced insulin resistance and inflammation. J Clin Invest 120: 756–767.
20. Cao J, Peterson SJ, Sodhi K, Vanella L, Barbagallo I, et al. (2012) Heme oxygenase gene targeting to adipocytes attenuates adiposity and vascular dysfunction in mice fed a high-fat diet. Hypertension 60: 467–475.
21. Dulak J, Deshane J, Jozkowicz A, Agarwal A (2008) Heme oxygenase-1 and carbon monoxide in vascular pathobiology: focus on angiogenesis. Circulation 117: 231–241.
22. Kim YM, Pae HO, Park JE, Lee YC, Woo JM, et al. (2011) Heme oxygenase in the regulation of vascular biology: from molecular mechanisms to therapeutic opportunities. Antioxid Redox Signal 14: 137–167.
23. Kang K, Reilly SM, Karabacak V, Gangl MR, Fitzgerald K, et al. (2008) Adipocyte-derived Th2 cytokines and myeloid PPARdelta regulate macrophage polarization and insulin sensitivity. Cell Metab 7: 485–495.
24. Bach FH (2005) Heme oxygenase-1: a therapeutic amplification funnel. FASEB J 19: 1216–1219.
25. Hiratsuka S, Minowa O, Kuno J, Noda T, Shibuya M (1998) Flt-1 lacking the tyrosine kinase domain is sufficient for normal development and angiogenesis in mice. Proc Natl Acad Sci U S A 95: 9349–9354.
26. Schioppa T, Uranchimeg B, Saccani A, Biswas SK, Doni A, et al. (2003) Regulation of the chemokine receptor CXCR4 by hypoxia. J Exp Med 198: 1391–1402.

Celecoxib Ameliorates Non-Alcoholic Steatohepatitis in Type 2 Diabetic Rats via Suppression of the Non-Canonical Wnt Signaling Pathway Expression

Feng Tian[1]*, Ya Jie Zhang[1], Yu Li[2], Ying Xie[1]

1 Department of Gastroenterology, Shengjing Hospital of China Medical University, Shenyang, Liaoning Province, China, **2** Department of Gastroenterology, Third People's Hospital of Dalian city, Dalian, Liaoning Province, China

Abstract

Our aim was to test whether pharmacological inhibition of cycloxygenase-2 (COX-2) reverses non-alcoholic steatohepatitis (NASH) in type 2 diabetes mellitus (T2DM) rats via suppression of the non-canonical Wnt signaling pathway expression. Twenty-four male Sprague-Dawley rats were randomly distributed to two groups and were fed with a high fat and sucrose (HF-HS) diet or a normal chow diet, respectively. After four weeks, rats fed with a HF-HS diet were made diabetic with low-dose streptozotocin. At the 9th week the diabetic rats fed with a HF-HS diet or the non-diabetic rats fed with a normal chow diet were further divided into two subgroups treated with vehicle or celecoxib (a selective COX-2 inhibitor, 10 mg/Kg/day, gavage) for the last 4 weeks, respectively. At the end of the 12th week, rats were anesthetized. NASH was assessed by histology. Related cytokine expression was measured at both the protein and gene levels through immunohistochemistry (IHC), Western blot and real-time PCR. T2DM rats fed with a HF-HS diet developed steatohepatitis and insulin resistance associated with elevated serum alanine aminotransferase (ALT), aspartate aminotransferase (AST), insulin levels and the non-alcoholic fatty liver disease (NAFLD) activity score (NAS). The expression of Wnt5a, JNK1, NF-κB p65, and COX-2 were all significantly increased in the T2DM-NASH group compared with the control and control-cele group. Hepatic injury was improved by celecoxib in T2DM-NASH-Cele group indicated by reduced serum ALT and AST levels and hepatic inflammation was reduced by celecoxib showed by histology and the NAFLD activity score (NAS). Serum related metabolic parameters, HOMA-IR and insulin sensitivity index were all improved by celecoxib. The expression of Wnt5a, JNK1, NF-κB p65, and COX-2 expression were all suppressed by celecoxib in T2DM-NASH-Cele group. The results of the present study indicated that celecoxib ameliorated NASH in T2DM rats via suppression of the non-canonical Wnt5a/JNK1 signaling pathway expression.

Editor: Yu Wang, The University of Hong Kong, Hong Kong

Funding: The article was supported by Science and Technology Program of Liaoning Province(2010225034). The funders had no role in study design, data collection and analysis, decision to publish, or preparation of the manuscript.

Competing Interests: The authors have declared that no competing interests exist.

* E-mail: tianfeng@sj-hospital.org

Introduction

Non-alcoholic steatohepatitis (NASH) is one of the most frequent causes of abnormal liver function and correlates with central adiposity, insulin resistance, dyslipidemia, and T2DM [1]. In diabetes patients, NASH is more frequent than in the general people by about 3-fold [2]. T2DM might be an independent risk factor for the progression of non-alcoholic fatty liver disease (NAFLD) from simple steatosis to NASH and fibrosis [3–4]. The mechanisms by which diabetes aggravates the progression of NASH mainly include insulin resistance, insulin deficiency, inflammatory response, and oxidative stress mediated by cytokines and chemokines [4–5]. However, the role of cytokines and chemokines on the development of NASH remains poorly understood and therapeutic options are limited.

Growing evidence support the notion that among the pro-inflammatory mediators that have been upregulated in NAFLD is cyclooxygenase2 (COX-2). Accordingly, NASH development can be protected against by treatment with COX-2 inhibitors [6–9]. Hepatic nuclear factor-κB (NF-κB) with downstream consequences including COX-2, TNF-α, and IL-6 were increased and aggravated inflammation in NASH [6–7]. COX-2 inhibitors reduced COX-2 expression by inhibiting NF-κB expression and activation [10]. Despite of these studies, there was hardly any research which indicated the role of COX-2 in the diabetic model of NASH and whether inhibiting COX-2 reversed diabetes-related NASH.

Recent evidence has implicated a direct role of disturbed Wnt signaling on metabolic syndrome including obesity, insulin resistence and T2DM [11]. The Wnt signaling pathways are involved the process of metabolic disorders including inflammatory response and insulin resistance [11]. However, studies about the role of Wnt pathway in hepatic metabolism has been largely ignored, especially for the non-canonical Wnt pathway. Hepatocyte-specific loss of β-catenin led to increased susceptibility to developing steatohepatitis and fibrosis in the mice fed with the MCD diet [12], which suggested the protective effect of the canonical Wnt/β-catenin signaling. Although Ouchi et al [13] showed that increased non-canonical Wnt5a/JNK1 pathway expression in adipose tissue led to enhanced insulin resistance and fatty liver, the influence of hepatic Wnt5a signaling pathway on NASH is still not researched and remains unknown at present.

As shown by recent reports, Wnt5a can induce NF-κB activity and NF-κB can upregulate Wnt5a expression [14–15]. COX-2 can be upregulated by NF-κB [7] and COX-2 inhibitors can inactivate NF-κB pathway [10]. These studies prompt the interaction among these cytokines. All of findings above triggered us to clarify the pathogenetic role exerted by the non-canonical Wnt5a/JNK1 pathway, NF-κB, and COX-2 in NASH development. We investigated their protein and mRNA levels in liver tissues. And we preliminarily analysed whether there was interaction among these cytokines. Ultimately we aimed to determine if the protective effect of the selective COX-2 inhibitor, celecoxib, on T2DM-related NASH was associated with expression changes of these cytokines.

Methods

Ethics Statement

All animal experimental protocols were approved by the ethics committee of Shengjing Hospital of China Medical University and conducted in accordance with their guidelines.

Animals and experimental design

Twenty-four male Sprague Dawley rats were purchased from China Medical University at 5–6 weeks of age. After one week acclimatization, rats were randomly distributed into two groups: (1) control rats were fed with a normal chow diet (CHOW; 5%kcal fat, with total calorific value 25 kJ/kg) (n = 12), and (2) rats were fed with a high fat and sucrose diet (HF-HS; 33%kcal fat, 54%kcal carbohydrate, with total calorific value 41.4 kJ/kg) (n = 12). After four weeks of diets, the HF-HS group were rendered T2DM with low dose streptozotocin (STZ; Sigma) intraperitoneally (30 mg/kg of body weight). After one week, blood glucose was measured from tail vein using point of care blood glucose monitoring system(Accu-Chek Advantage, Roch Diagnostics, USA). The rats with blood glucose <16.7 mmol/L were injected with STZ again (30 mg/kg). The blood glucose and body weight were measured every week. Four weeks following the STZ injections, rats with blood glucose levels of ≥16.7 mmol/L were considered diabetic. In order to determine the capacity of celecoxib to prevent NASH, four subgroups were formed and treated respectively with vehicle (saline, gavage, daily) as the control group or the T2DM-NASH group and celecoxib (10 mg/kg/, gavage, daily; Pfizer, New York, NY) as the control-Cele group or the T2DM-NASH-Cele group for four weeks. At the end of the 12th week, rats were anesthetised with chloral hydrate (3 ml/kg of body weight) and terminated by exsanguination.

Blood sampling and analysis

Blood was obtained by abdominal aortic puncture and separated by centrifugation (1500 rpm, 20 min) for serum. Serum alanine aminotransferase (ALT), aspartate aminotransferase (AST), glucose, low-density lipoprotein (LDL), and high-density lipoprotein (HDL) concentrations were determined using an automatic biochemical analyzer (ci16200, Abbott, USA). Serum insulin was determined with an Insulin Radioimmunoassay Kit (HTA Co. Ltd, People's Republic of China).

Assessment of insulin resistance

To assess insulin sensitivity, insulin tolerance test (ITT) was conducted at 11 weeks. Rats fasted for 6 h were injected i.p. with rh insulin (0.5 U/kg of body weight). Blood glucose was measured from tail vein using point of care blood glucose monitoring system (Accu-Chek Advantage, Roch Diagnostics, USA) at 0, 30, 60, 90, and 120 min after insulin administration. The change in Area Under the Curve (AUC) was compared with the AUC obtained for the T2DM-NASH group (normalized to 100%). The homeostasis model assessment of insulin resistance (HOMA-IR) method was used to calculate insulin resistance as [fasting insulin (mIU/L)×fasting glucose (mmol/L)]/22.5. The insulin sensitivity index (ISI) was assessed by ln {1/[fasting insulin (mIU/L)×fasting glucose (mmol/L)]}.

Histological examination

Livers were fixed in 10% buffered formalin, processed, and embedded in paraffin for Hematoxylin–Eosin staining (H&E). Histological scoring was graded by pathologists (blinded to the goups) for hepatic steatosis, lobular inflammation, ballooning, and fibrosis in accordance with the 2011 programme for diagnosis and treatment of non-alcoholic steatohepatitis called the NAFLD activity score (NAS), issued by the USA CRN [16]. NASH was diagnosed if NAS (total scores) was greater than four.

Immunohistochemistry(IHC)

Immunostaining was performed on 3 μm sections after deparaffinization. Microwave or high pressure antigen retrieval was performed in citrate buffer pH 6.0 for 10 min prior to peroxidase quenching with 3% H_2O_2 in phosphate-buffered saline (PBS) for 10 min. The sections were then washed in water and preblocked with normal goat or rabbit serum for 10 min. Then, slides were incubated, respectively, with anti-Wnt5a (Abcam, USA), anti-JNK1 (Santa Cruz Biotechnology, USA), anti-NF-κB p65 (Santa Cruz Biotechnology, USA), and anti-COX-2 (Santa Cruz Biotechnology, USA) (final concentrations 1:100, 1:100, 1:200, 1:320, respectively) for over-night at 4°C. The sections were then incubated with biotinylated secondary antibodies (1:400) for 20 min. Following a washing step with PBS, the avidin–biotin complex was applied. Finally, the sections were rinsed in PBS, developed with diaminoben-zidine tetrahydrochloride substrate for 3 min and counterstained with hematoxylin. Five fields with a final magnification of ×400 were randomly selected for each rat liver, and the Integral Optical Density(IOD) were analyzed by Image Pro Plus 6.0 software.

Western blotting

Liver tissue was homogenized in RIPA Lysis Buffer containing PMSF (a protease inhibitor (Beyotime Institute of Biotechnology), and total protein concentrations were determined by bicinchoninic acid protein assay (Boster). About 50 micrograms of protein were loaded on 5–10% gradient gels. Proteins were transferred to a PVDF membrane(Thermo Scientific) for 70 min at 100 V. The membranes were incubated in blocking buffer for 2 hours before the addition of primary antibody including Wnt5a (Abcam, USA), JNK1 (Santa Cruz Biotechnology, USA), NF-κB p65 (Abcam, USA) and COX-2 (Proteintech Group, PTG, USA). All of the primary antibodies were used at a 1:400 dilution. All secondary antibodies were diluted 1:1000 except for anti-NF-κB p65, which was diluted 1:3000. Proteins were detected via enhanced chemiluminescence (Beyotime Institute of Biotechnology), and the intensity of protein bands were quantified using the Quantity One software (Bio-Rad, USA).

Quantitative real-time polymerase chain reaction

Total RNA was extracted from liver tissue (100 mg) with TRIzol reagent (Takara, Japan). RNA amount and quality was determined using a Nanodrop spectrophotometer. Total RNA (500 ng) was then reverse-transcribed to cDNA using the Reverse Transcription System from TaKaRa (Japan). cDNA (200 ng) was used in each PCR reaction. Real-time quantitative PCR was performed with an ABI Prism 7500 Sequence Detection System (Applied Biosystems, Foster City, CA) with SYBR Green reagents. The housekeeping gene β-actin was used as a reference gene for normalization. Primers sequences were as follows: Wnt5a: F: 5′-GCTTCAACTCCCCAACCA-3′, R: 5′-CTCG-CAGCCGTC-CATC-3′; NF-κB p65: F: 5′-CGACGTATTGCTGTGCCTTC-3′, R: 5′-TTGAGAT-CTGCCCAGGTGGTA-3′; COX-2: F: 5′-CGGAGAGGAGAAGTGGGGTTTAG-3′, R: 5′-TGA-AAGA-GGCGAAGGGACA-3′; β-actin: F: 5′-GGAGATTACTGCC-CTGGCTCCTA-3′, R: 5′-GACTCATCGTACTCCTGCT-TGCTG-3′. For each gene, relative change in steady state mRNA in samples was determined using the $2^{-\Delta\Delta CT}$ method, corrected for the housekeeper.

Statistical analysis

The results are presented as the mean±SD. Comparisons between two groups were analyzed via Student's *t*-test, and comparisons between more than two groups were analyzed via one-way ANOVA to identify differences among means. A probability of $P<0.05$ was taken to indicate a significant difference between means.

Results

Celecoxib reduced liver weight index and increased EAW/BW

Rats fed with a HF-HS diet showed significantly lower body weight (BW); but higher liver weight index than rats fed with a CHOW diet (Table 1). Although no significant difference between the T2DM-NASH group and T2DM-NASH-Cele group was found in BW and liver weights, the liver weight index did make a difference (Table 1). We observed increased central lipolysis in the T2DM-NASH group as shown by significantly lower EAW/BW, compared with the rats fed with a CHOW diet. In the T2DM-NASH-Cele group, celecoxib increased EAW/BW compared with the T2DM-NASH group (Table 1).

Effect of celecoxib on serum metabolic parameters

Rats in the T2DM-NASH group exhibited impaired metabolic function as shown by increased serum glucose, triglyceride, LDL-cholesterol, and decreased HDL-cholesterol concentrations. In the T2DM-NASH-Cele group, celecoxib improved and reduced these observed values and had lower concentrations compared with the T2DM-NASH group, except for serum HDL-cholesterol (Table 2). Our work noted serum ALT and AST concentrations were extremely elevated in rats fed with a HF-HS diet, which further confirmed the model of steatohepatitis. In the T2DM-NASH-Cele group, celecoxib treatment significantly lowered serum ALT and AST concentrations compared with the T2DM-NASH group (Table 2).

Celecoxib treatment ameliorated insulin sensitivity

Insulin resistance was induced in the T2DM-NASH group as shown by hyperinsulinemia, increased HOMA-IR, and decreased insulin sensitivity index (ISI) as compared with the control group and the control-cele group (Table 2; Fig. 1A and B). Compared to the T2DM-NASH group, celecoxib significantly reduced insulin levels and HOMA-IR and increased ISI in the T2DM-NASH-Cele group (Table 2; Fig. 1A and B). Furthermore, the T2DM-NASH group rats displayed reduced response to exogenous insulin in the insulin tolerance test (ITT) and increased glucose AUC value by about 82% than the control and control-cele groups (Table 2; Fig. 1C). Treatment with celecoxib significantly improved the insulin sensitivity and reduced the glucose AUC by about 31% in the T2DM-NASH-Cele group (Table 2; Fig. 1C).

T2DM rats fed with a HF-HS diet manifested NASH and celecoxib reversed NASH

The control group had normal liver morphology and no steatosis (Fig. 2A, E and I), the same as the control-cele group (Fig. 2B, F and J). The T2DM-NASH group exhibited significant non-alcoholic steatohepatitis by histological examination (Fig. 2C, G and K). However, the T2DM-NASH-Cele group appeared mild steatotic and steatohepatitis by histological examination that was comparable with the T2DM-NASH group (Fig. 2D, H and L). By the method of the NAFLD activity score (NAS) liver sections from the T2DM-NASH group showed severe steatosis, moderate lobular inflammation, and diffuse hepatocyte ballooning; NAS (total scores) was greater than four. In the celecoxib treatment group, steatosis, lobular inflammation, and NAS (total scores) were markedly reduced; however, celecoxib didn't make a significant change of ballooning degeneration compared with the T2DM-NASH group (Fig. 2M, N, O and P).

Increased Wnt5a/JNK1 expression in liver tissues from the T2DM-NASH group and suppressed by celecoxib

To test whether hepatic Wnt5a/JNK1 pathway involves in the mechanism of NASH, we examined their expression by different methods. IHC staining for Wnt5a and JNK1 in livers from the T2DM-NASH group were both strongly positive (Fig. 3C and G), whereas they were almost negative in the control group (Fig. 3A and E) and the control-cele group (Fig. 3B and F). The Integral Optical Density (IOD) of Wnt5a and JNK1 in the T2DM-NASH group were both significantly higher than those in the control goup and the control-cele group (Figure 3Q and R). Celecoxib treatment significantly reduced the IOD of Wnt5a and JNK1 in the T2DM-NASH-Cele group (Figure 3Q and R). Western blot

Table 1. Basic parameters in four groups.

	CHOW diet		HF-HS diet	
Group	**control**	**control-cele**	**T2DM-NASH**	**T2DM-NASH-Cele**
Body weight(BW)(g)	588.6±10.5	562.8±29.46	394.0±17.79*	425.8±18.75
Liver weight index(%)	2.39±0.41	2.8±0.14	7.13±0.47*	5.87±0.80▲
EAW/BW(%)	1.97±0.27	2.07±0.26	1.02±0.23*	1.6±0.36▲

*$P<0.01$ *vs.* the control group and the control-cele group;
▲$P<0.05$ *vs.* the T_2DM-NASH group.

Table 2. Serum metabolic parameters in four groups.

	CHOW diet		HF-HS diet	
Group	control	control-cele	T_2DM-NASH	T_2DM-NASH-Cele
Serum glucose(mmol/L)	6.25±1.28	6.15±0.70	31.21±0.86*	22.29±0.82△
Serum insulin(mIU/L)	15.31±1.47	14.51±1.3	28.66±3.97*	19.56±3.09△
ITT (glucose AUC) (%change from the T2DM-NASH group)	17.65±2.52	17.03±3.01	100.00±3.58*	68.71±3.76△
Serum triglycerides(mmol/L)	0.18±0.08	0.26±0.03	0.91±0.04*	0.49±0.08△
Serum LDL-cholesterol (mmol/L)	0.24±0.07	0.30±0.08	11.94±0.21*	2.31±0.85△
Serum HDL-cholesterol (mmol/L)	1.24±0.17	1.11±0.10	0.94±0.07	1.11±0.11
Serum ALT(U/L)	33.00±4.06	36.8±2.39	301.80±5.40*	88.80±13.07△
Serum AST(U/L)	76.6±7.64	80.2±6.42	345.4±9.63*	99.8±20.51△

*$P<0.01$ *vs.* the control group and the control-cele group;
△$P<0.01$ *vs.* the T_2DM-NASH group.

analysis showed that hepatic Wnt5a, JNK1 p54 and JNK1 p46 protein levels in the T2DM-NASH group were significantly increased compared with those of the control group and control-cele group (Fig. 4A and B), as was hepatic Wnt5a mRNA (Fig. 5A). Consistent with the protective effect, celecoxib administration supressed the expression of Wnt5a and JNK1. Hepatic Wnt5a, JNK1 p54 and JNK1 p46 protein levels of the T2DM-NASH-Cele group were all strongly reduced than those from the T2DM-NASH group (Fig. 4A and B), as was hepatic Wnt5a mRNA (Fig. 5A).

NF-κB and COX-2 were activated in liver tissues from the T2DM-NASH group and were reduced by celecoxib

We tested whether NF-κB was activated in the model of T2DM-NASH. Consistent with the current findings, hepatic NF-κB p65 protein level was significantly increased in the T2DM-NASH group (Fig. 3K and S; Fig. 4C) compared with the control group (Fig. 3I and M) and the control-cele group(Fig. 3J and N). Celecoxib determined a decrease of the NF-κB p65 protein in the T2DM-NASH-Cele group (Fig. 3L and S; Fig. 4C). In the T2DM-NASH group, more hepatocytes nucleus were stained (Fig. 3K). In the T2DM-NASH-Cele group, the nuclei were slightly stained (Fig. 3L), which indicated that celecoxib administration supressed nuclear translocation of NF-κB p65. However, we detected no significant difference of NF-κB p65 mRNA in the T2DM-NASH group (Fig. 5B) compared with the control group and the control-cele group. Celecoxib just slightly reduced NF-κB p65 mRNA in the T2DM-NASH-Cele group (Fig. 5B). The IHC and Western blotting showed that hepatic COX-2 protein level was significantly increased in the T2DM-NASH group (Fig. 3O and T; Fig. 4D), as was hepatic COX-2 mRNA (Fig. 5C). Hepatic COX-2 protein and mRNA levels were both obviously decreased by celecoxib in the T2DM-NASH-Cele group (Fig. 3P and T; Fig. 4D; Fig. 5C).

Discussion

In this study, a HF-HS diet added to T2DM induction was shown to cause the model of diabetes-related NASH where both the pathophysiology and liver pathology closely resembled human NASH established with T2DM. In the T2DM-NASH group, while hyperinsulinemia was observed to indicate the predomination of insulin resistance, hyperglycemia showed relative insulin deficiency. Insulin resistance and insulin deficiency of adipose tissue cause increased central lipolysis and elevated circulating free fatty acids, with resulting increased hepatic delivery and uptake [17]. In the T2DM-NASH group we observed a marked reduction of EAW/BW and a significant increase of liver weight index, implicating enhanced adipose lipolysis and hepatic intake. The increased circulating triglyceride and LDL-cholesterol were consistent with increased lipolysis. As expected, we observed decreased HDL-cholesterol in the T2DM-NASH group, which is the characteristic of NAFLD [18].

An early study has shown that high doses of salicylates, a kind of Nonsteroidal anti-inflammatory drugs (NSAIDs) reverse hyperglycemia, hyperinsulinemia, and dyslipidemia in obese rodents by sensitizing insulin signaling [19]. Hence, we detected the role of celecoxib, an NSAID that is a selective COX-2 inhibitor, on the development of T2DM-related NASH. In the T2DM-NASH-Cele

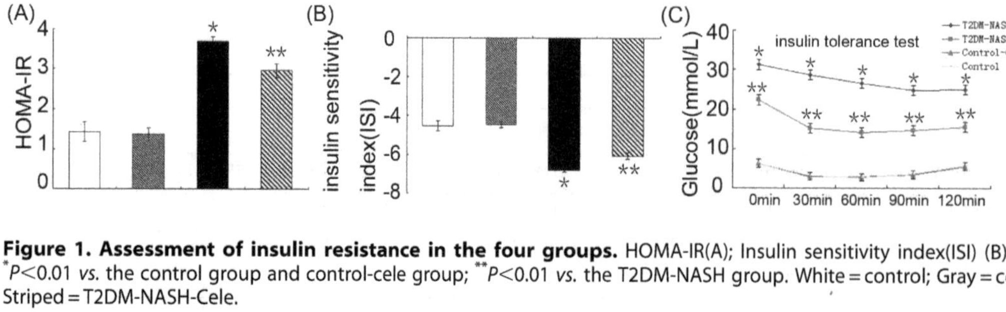

Figure 1. Assessment of insulin resistance in the four groups. HOMA-IR(A); Insulin sensitivity index(ISI) (B); insulin tolerance test (ITT) (C). *$P<0.01$ *vs.* the control group and control-cele group; **$P<0.01$ *vs.* the T2DM-NASH group. White = control; Gray = control-cele; Black = T2DM-NASH; Striped = T2DM-NASH-Cele.

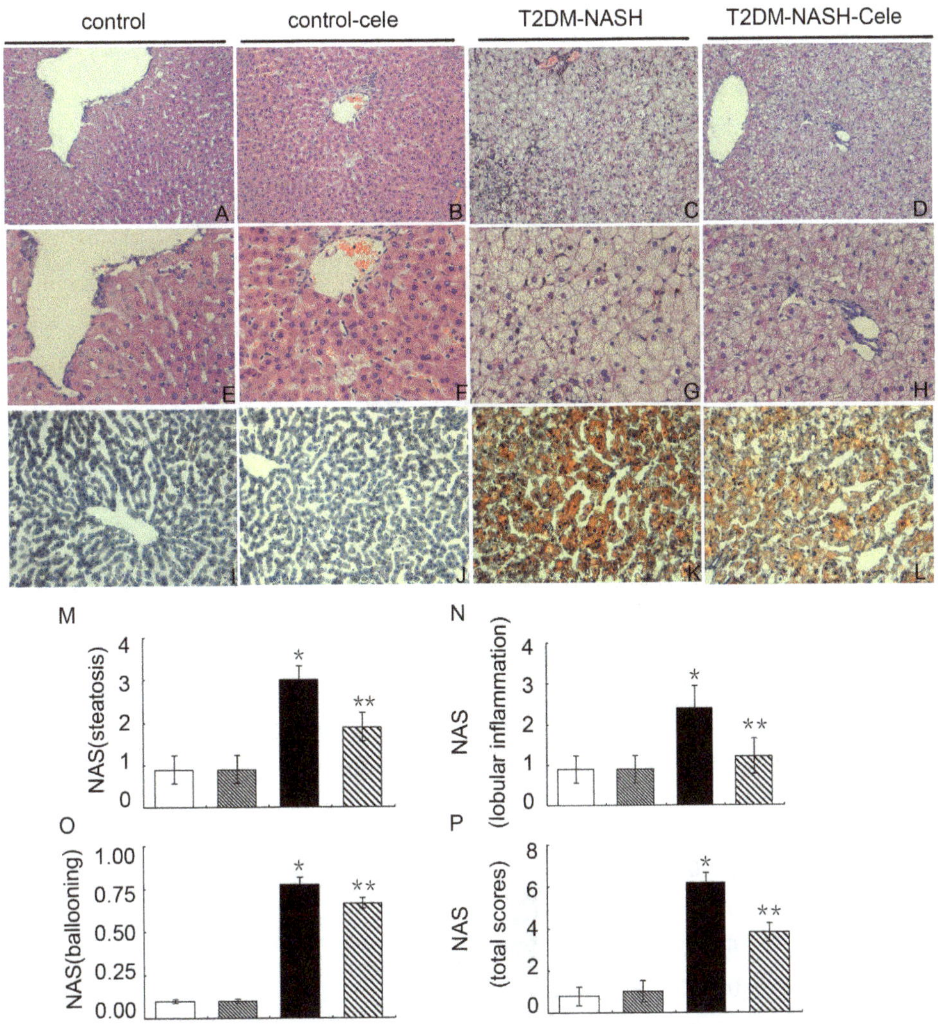

Figure 2. T_2DM rats fed with a HF-HS diet developed severe steatohepatitis. H&E-stained livers ((A–D; ×200) and (E–H; ×400)). Oil Red-O staining of livers lipid accumulation (I–L; ×200). The results of NAFLD activity score (NAS) (M–P). Quantification results of steatosis (M), lobular inflammation (N), ballooning (O), NAS total scores (P). *$P<0.01$ *vs.* the control group and the control-cele group; **$P<0.01$ *vs.* the T2DM-NASH group. White = control; Gray = control-cele; Black = T2DM-NASH; Striped = T2DM-NASH-Cele.

group, we observed that celecoxib weakened central lipolysis indicated by increased EAW/BW and decreased liver weight index, compared with the T2DM-NASH group.Besides, we observed that celecoxib ameliorated insulin resistence, including reduced serum insulin level, HOMA-IR, glucose AUC and increased insulin sensitivity in the T2DM-NASH-Cele group. Also, celecoxib ameliorated dyslipidemia, including reduction of serum triglyceride and LDL-cholesterol levels. However, there was no obvious effect on HDL-cholesterol. The mechanism about the improvement of dyslipidemia needs to be further explored.Another benefit of celecoxib in our data were considerable improvement of liver steatosis and inflammation indicated by reduction of NAFLD activity score (NAS). Celecoxib alle-viated liver injury showed by reduction of serum ALT and AST levels. All of these events might be causally related to changes of cytokines we tested.

We monitored COX-2 expression because it is a key enzyme in activating the inflammatory response. And inflammation caused by COX-2 activation in fat and liver tissue plays a pivotal role in the development of insulin resistance and NAFLD [6,8]. The present study further examined that the driving effect of COX-2 mediated inflammation in the development of NASH in diabetic rats. Alternatively, celecoxib reduced COX-2 expression and ameliorated NASH, consistently with the current literatures. Earlier studies identified NF-κB as a key regulator of hepatic inflammatory recruitment and liver injury in NASH [20,21]. COX-2 is regulated by NF-κB because COX-2 gene promoter has two binding sites for NF-κB which works as a positive regulator of COX-2 gene during inflammatory response [22]. Also, COX-2 inhibitors had been observed to suppress COX-2 expression through NF-κB inactivation pathway [23]. And in our research, we found that NF-κB protein level was significantly increased in the T2DM-NASH group, and nuclear translocation of p65 was reduced by celecoxib in the T2DM-NASH-Cele group. However, NF-κB mRNA level had no significant difference. Possibly, it didn't respond adequately to metabolic stress at the gene level.

Recently, the role of Wnt signaling pathway facing to the metabolic stress has been paid for attention. The canonical Wnt/β-catenin signaling resists adipogenesis and improves glucose tolerance and insulin sensitivity [24–27]. Schulte DM et al [28] showed that the non-canonical Wnt5a might act as an important pro-inflammatory molecule in low grade inflammation of adipose

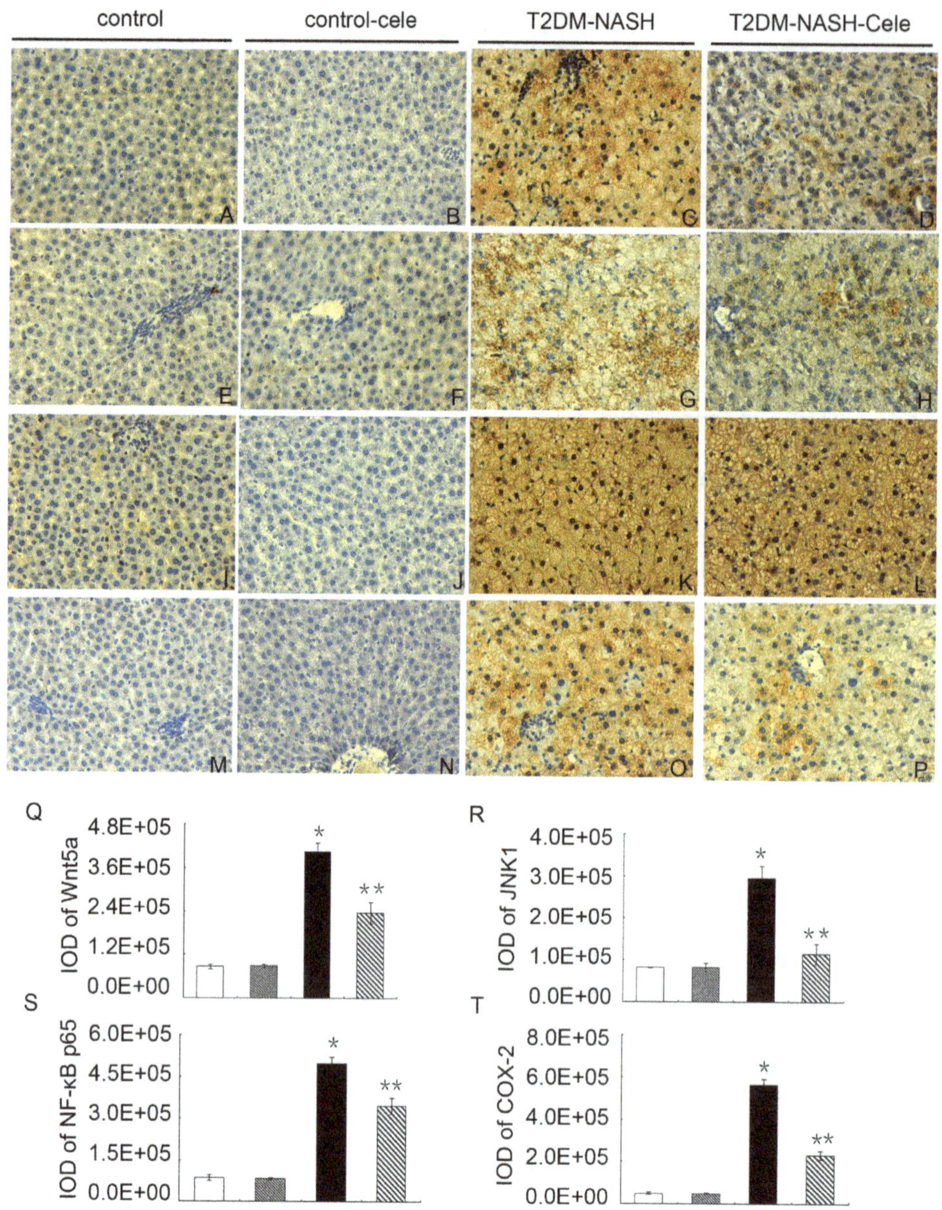

Figure 3. Immunohistochemistry(IHC) staining for Wnt5a, JNK1, NF-κB p65, and COX-2. IHC staining for Wnt5a (A–D; ×400); IHC staining for JNK1 (E–H; ×400); IHC staining for NF-κB p65 (I–L; ×400); IHC staining for COX-2 (M–P; ×400). The Integral Optical Density(IOD) of Wnt5a (Q), JNK1 (R), NF-κB p65 (S); COX-2 (T). *$P<0.01$ *vs.* the control group and the control-cele group; **$P<0.01$ *vs.* the T2DM-NASH group. White = control; Gray = control-cele; Black = T2DM-NASH; Striped = T2DM-NASH-Cele.

tissue in obese humans. However, the role of Wnt signaling pathway in NAFLD is less researched. The canonical Wnt/β-catenin signaling may confer a protective effect on the liver in the face of metabolic stress. Hepatocyte-specific loss of β-catenin led to increased susceptibility to developing steatohepatitis and fibrosis in the mice fed with the MCD diet [12]. The protection mechanism could be the role of β-catenin maintaining mitochondrial function and regulating ATP production, which is the principle energy source for lipid and glucose oxidative metabolism [29,30]. However, little is known about the role of non-canonical Wnt5a signaling pathway on the development of NASH. These observations prompt us to investigate changes of Wnt5a expression in the liver. To our knowledge, this is the first report that shows a significant correlation between hepatic increased Wnt5a protein and mRNA expression and development of NASH, especially associated with T2DM in the liver tissue. JNK was a downstream target of the non-canonical Wnt signaling pathway [31]. Activation of JNK1 is associated with hepatic triglyceride accumulation and insulin resistance in rats fed a high-fat diet [32]. Ouchi et al [13] showed that Wnt5a upregulated JNK1 expression in fat tissues and exacerbated hepatic steatosis in obesity mice. Inhibition of Wnt5a/JNK1 axis improved insulin sensitivity and metabolic function. Consistently, in our study, we discovered that the protein levels of JNK1 at p54 and p46 subunit were both significantly increased in the T2DM-NASH group. All the data indicated the non-canonical Wnt5a/JNK1 signaling was highly expressed in the model of T2DM-related NASH, probably involving in the process of development of T2DM-related NASH.

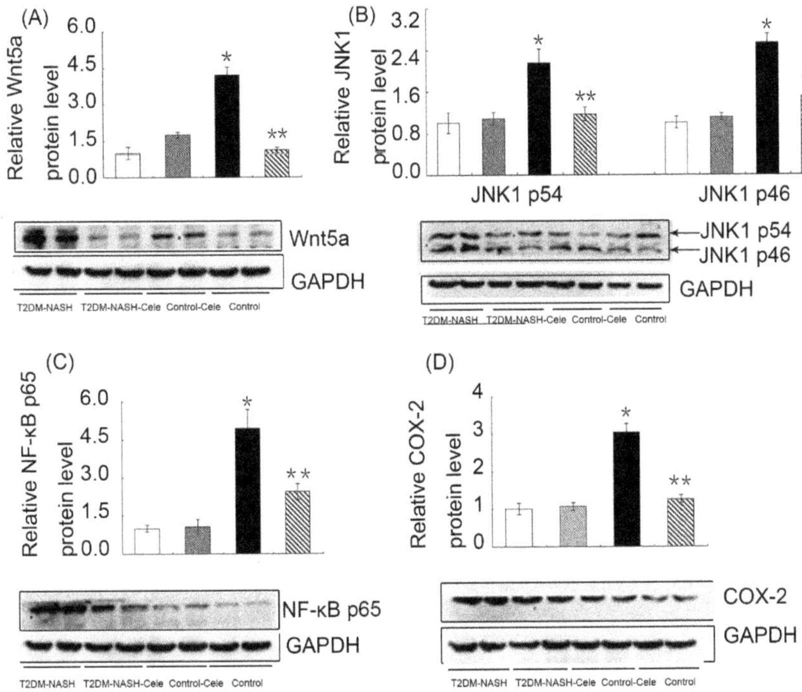

Figure 4. Western blot analysis of Wnt5a, JNK1, NF-κB p65, and COX-2 protein expression. Representative western blot images and quantitative analysis of Wnt5a (A), JNK1 p54 and p46 (B), NF-κB p65 (C), and COX-2 (D). GAPDH was used as a loading control. $^{*}P<0.01$ *vs.* the control group and the control-cele group; $^{**}P<0.01$ *vs.* the T2DM-NASH group. White = control; Gray = control-cele; Black = T2DM-NASH; Striped = T2DM-NASH-Cele.

Another striking finding was that celecoxib significantly reduced the expression of Wnt5a at both protein and mRNA level accompanied with protective effect of celecoxib on the development of T2DM-related NASH in the T2DM-NASH-Cele group. As for JNK1, celecoxib decreased the levels of JNK1 at p54 and p46 subunit in the T2DM-NASH-Cele group, consistently with the current study [33]. Our current data indicated that protective effect of celecoxib was probably related to its suppression of the Wnt5a and JNK1 expression and there was interaction between celecoxib and the Wnt5a/JNK1 signaling. Recent reports showed that there was direct synergetic interaction between COX-2 and Wnt/β-catenin signaling cascades. Likely, in the COX-2 promoter there was TBE Site II and β-catenin could bind to this promoter region to regulate COX-2 expression [34]. And one of the bioactive products of COX-2, prostaglandin E2 could activate components of the canonical Wnt signaling through inducing phosphorylation of GSK-3β, ultimately promoting the activity of β-catenin [35,36]. Celecoxib can inhibit Wnt/β-catenin activity through inducing decreased activity of GSK-3β [37]. However, there is no research about the crosstalk between non-canonical Wnt signaling and COX-2. In our research, we found that increased expression of Wnt5a and COX-2 were in parallel in the liver of T2DM-NASH rats, which can be both reduced by celecoxib. These observations demonstrate that COX-2 is directly involved in the regulation of Wnt5a by celecoxib. We supposed NF-κB might play the bridge role on connecting Wnt5a and COX-2. NF-κB can upregulate Wnt5a because there is NF-κB-binding site within Wnt5a promoter B [14]. And Wnt5a can induce NF-κB activity through Wnt5a/ROR1/Ca^{2+} pathway [15]. Herein, we inferred that increased Wnt5a upregulated COX-2 expression to mediate hepatic inflammation by activating NF-κB. And celecoxib might reduce Wnt5a through inactivating NF-κB. The molecular mechanisms underlying remain to be elucidated.

In summary, we first identified increased hepatic Wnt5a expression accompanying activation of JNK1, NF-κB, and COX-2 was associated with the development of T2DM-NASH. Treatment with the selective COX-2 inhibitor celecoxib ameliorated T2DM-related NASH as shown by anti-inflammatory activity and restraining insulin resistance, probably via suppression

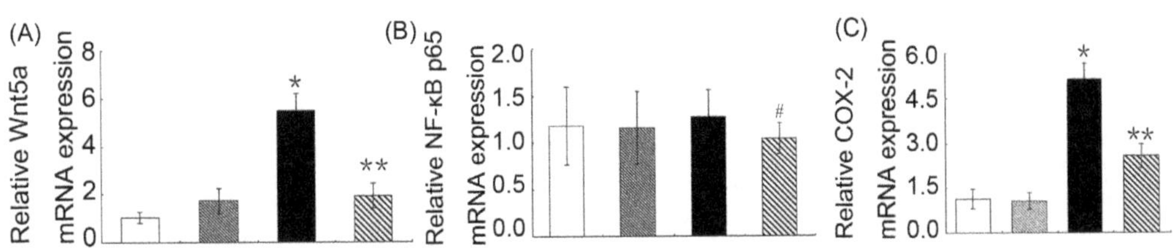

Figure 5. Real-time pcr analysis of Wnt5a, NF-κB p65, and COX-2 mRNA expression. Quantitative analysis of Wnt5a mRNA (A), NF-κB p65 mRNA (B), COX-2 mRNA (C). β-actin was used as a control. $^{*}P<0.01$ *vs.* the control group and the control-cele group; $^{**}P<0.01$ *vs.* the T2DM-NASH group. $^{\#}P<0.05$ *vs.* the T2DM-NASH group. White = control; Gray = control-cele; Black = T2DM-NASH; Striped = T2DM-NASH-Cele.

of the non-canonical Wnt5a/JNK1 signaling pathway and NF-κB. The mechanism by which celecoxib regulates Wnt5a expression via COX-2 needs further investigation and our results may suggest a new molecule mechanism in therapy strategy.

Author Contributions

Conceived and designed the experiments: FT. Performed the experiments: YJZ YL. Analyzed the data: YJZ YX FT. Contributed reagents/materials/analysis tools: YJZ YL YX. Wrote the paper: YJZ FT.

References

1. Musso G, Gambino R, Cassader M (2010) Non-alcoholic fatty liver disease from pathogenesis to management: an update. Obes Rev 11:430–45.
2. Clark JM (2006) The epidemiology of nonalcoholic fatty liver disease in adults. J Clin Gastroenterol 40 Suppl 1:S5–10.
3. Rivera CA (2008) Risk factors and mechanisms of non-alcoholic steatohepatitis. Pathophysiology 15:109–14.
4. Lo L, McLennan SV, Williams PF, Bonner J, Chowdhury S, et al. (2011) Diabetes is a progression factor for hepatic fibrosis in high fat fed mouse obesity model of non-alcoholicsteatohepatitis. J Hepatol 55:435–44.
5. Braunersreuther V, Viviani GL, Mach F, Montecucco F (2012) Role of cytokines and chemokines in non-alcoholic fatty liver disease. World J Gastroenterol 18:727–35.
6. Yu J, Ip E, Dela Peña A, Hou JY, Sesha J, et al. (2006) COX-2 induction in mice with experimental nutritional steatohepatitis: Role as pro-inflammatory mediator. Hepatology 43:826–36.
7. Leclercq IA, Farrell GC, Sempoux C, dela Peña A, Horsmans Y (2004) Curcumin inhibits NF-kappaB activation and reduces the severity of experimental steatohepatitis in mice. J Hepatol 41:926–934.
8. Hsieh PS, Jin JS, Chiang CF, Chan PC, Chen CH, et al. (2009) COX-2-mediated Inflammation in Fat Is Crucial for Obesity-linked Insulin Resistance and Fatty Liver. Obesity(Silver Spring) 17:1150–7.
9. Wu HT, Chen W, Cheng KC, Yeh CH, Shen KH, et al. (2010) Indomethacin activates peroxisome proliferator-activated receptor γ to improve insulin resistance in cotton pelletgranuloma model. Horm Metab Res 42:775–80.
10. Vaish V, Tanwar L, Sanyal SN (2010) The role of NF-κB and PPARγ in experimentally induced colorectal cancer and chemoprevention by cyclooxygenase-2 inhibitors. Tumour Biol 31:427–36.
11. Kikuchi A, Yamamoto H, Sato A, Matsumoto S (2012) Wnt5a: its signaling, functions and implication in diseases. Acta Physiol (Oxf) 204:17–33.
12. Behari J, Yeh TH, Krauland L, Otruba W, Cieply B, et al. (2010) Liver-specific beta-catenin knockout mice exhibit defective bile acid and cholesterol homeostasis and increased susceptibility to diet-induced steatohepatitis. Am J Pathol 176:744–53.
13. Ouchi N, Higuchi A, Ohashi K, Oshima Y, Gokce N, et al. (2010) Sfrp5 is an anti-inflammatory adipokine that modulates metabolic dysfunction in obesity.Science 329:454–7.
14. Katoh M,Katoh M (2009) Transcriptional mechanisms of WNT5A based on NF-κB, Hedgehog, TGFβ, and Notch signaling cascades. Int J Mol Med 23:763–9.
15. Fukuda T, Chen L, Endo T, Tang L, Lu D, et al.(2008) Antisera induced by infusions of autologous Ad-CD154-leukemia B cells identify ROR1 as an oncofetal antigen and receptor for Wnt5a. Proc Natl Acad Sci U S A 105:3047–52.
16. Brunt EM, Kleiner DE, Wilson LA, Belt P, Neuschwander-Tetri BA, et al.(2011) Nonalcoholic fatty liver disease (NAFLD) activity score and the histopathologic diagnosis in NAFLD: distinct clinicopathologic meanings. Hepatology 53:810–20.
17. Sheth SG, Gordon FD, Chopra S (1997) Nonalcoholic steatohepatitis. Ann Intern Med 126:137–145.
18. Chatrath H, Vuppalanchi R, Chalasani N (2012) Dyslipidemia in patients with Nonalcoholic fatty liver disease. Semin Liver Dis 32:22–9.
19. Yuan M, Konstantopoulos N, Lee J, Hansen L, Li ZW, et al. (2001) Reversal of obesity-and diet-induced insulin resistance with salicylates or targeted disruption of Ikkbeta. Science 293:1673–7.
20. Dela Peña A, Leclercq I, Field J, George J, Jones B, et al. (2005) NF-kappaB activation,rather than TNF, mediates hepatic inflammation in a murine dietary model of steatohepatitis. Gastroenterology 129:1663–74.
21. Boden G, She P, Mozzoli M, Cheung P, Gumireddy K, et al. (2005) Free fatty acids produce insulin resistance and activate the proinflammatory nuclear factor-kappaB pathway in rat liver. Diabetes 54: 3458–65.
22. Vandoros GP, Konstantinopoulos PA, Sotiropoulou-Bonikou G, Kominea A, Papachristou GI, et al. (2006) PPAR-gamma is expressed and NF-κ B pathway is activated and correlates positively with COX-2 expression in stromal myofibroblasts surrounding colon adenocarcinomas,J Cancer Res Clin Oncol 132:76–84.
23. BenitahSA ValerónPF, LacalJC (2003) ROCK and nuclear factor-κ B-dependent activation of cyclooxygenase-2 by Rho GTPases:effects on tumor growth and therapeutic consequences. Mol Biol Cell 14:3041–54.
24. Kawai M, Mushiake S, Bessho K, Murakami M, Namba N, et al. (2007) Wnt/Lrp/beta-catenin signaling suppresses adipogenesis by inhibiting mutual activation of PPARgamma and C/EBPalpha. Biochem Biophys Res Commun 363:276–282.
25. Ross SE, Hemati N, Longo KA, Bennett CN, Lucas PC, et al. (2000) Inhibition of adipogenesis by Wnt signaling. Science 289:950–3.
26. Gustafson B, Smith U (2006) Cytokines promote Wnt signaling and inflammation and impair the normal differentiation and lipid accumulation in 3T3-L1 preadipocytes. J Biol Chem 281:9507–16.
27. Abiola M, Favier M, Christodoulou-Vafeiadou E, Pichard AL, Martelly I, et al. (2009) Activation of Wnt/beta-catenin signaling increases insulin sensitivity through a reciprocal regulation of Wnt10b and SREBP-1c in skeletal muscle cells. PLoS One 4:e8509.
28. Schulte DM, Müller N, Neumann K, Oberhäuser F, Faust M, et al. (2012) Pro-inflammatory wnt5a and anti-inflammatory sFRP5 are differentially regulated by nutritionalfactors in obese human subjects. PLoS One 7: e32437.
29. Lehwald N, Tao GZ, Jang KY, Papandreou I, Liu B, et al. (2012) β-Catenin Regulates Hepatic Mitochondrial Function and Energy Balance in Livers of Mice. Gastroenterology 143:754–64.
30. Morris EM, Rector RS, Thyfault JP, Ibdah JA (2011) Mitochondria and redox signaling in steatohepatitis. Antioxid Redox Signal 15:485–504.
31. Veeman MT, Axelrod JD, Moon RT (2003) A second canon. Functions and mechanisms of beta-catenin-independent Wnt signaling. Dev Cell 5:367–77.
32. Samuel VT, Liu ZX, Qu X, Elder BD, Bilz S, et al. (2004) Mechanism of hepatic insulin resistance in non-alcoholic fatty liver disease. J Biol Chem 279:32345–32353.
33. Lu S, Archer MC (2007) Celecoxib decreases fatty acid synthase expression via down-regulation of c-Jun N-terminal kinase-1. Exp Biol Med (Maywood) 232:643–53.
34. Nuñez F, Bravo S, Cruzat F, Montecino M, De Ferrari GV (2011) Wnt/β-catenin signaling enhances cyclooxygenase-2(COX2) transcriptional activity in gastric cancer cells. PLoS One 6:e18562.
35. Buchanan FG, DuBois RN (2006) Connecting COX-2 and Wnt in cancer.Cancer Cell 9:6–8.
36. Castellone MD, Teramoto H, Williams BO, Druey KM, Gutkind JS (2005) Prostaglandin E2 promotes colon cancer cell growth through a Gs-axin-beta-catenin signaling axis. Science 310:1504–10.
37. Tuynman JB, Vermeulen L, Boon EM, Kemper K, Zwinderman AH, et al. (2008) Cyclooxygenase-2 inhibition inhibits c-Met kinase activity and Wnt activity in colon cancer. Cancer Res 68:1213–20.

Elevated Peripheral Frequencies of Th22 Cells: A Novel Potent Participant in Obesity and Type 2 Diabetes

Ruxing Zhao[1,2,3], Dongqi Tang[3], Shounan Yi[4], Wenjuan Li[1], Chuanlong Wu[1], Yiran Lu[1], Xinguo Hou[1], Jun Song[1], Peng Lin[1], Li Chen[1,2*¶], Lei Sun[1,2*¶]

1 Department of Endocrinology, Qilu Hospital, Shandong University, Jinan, China, **2** Institute of Endocrinology and Metabolism, Shandong University, Jinan, China, **3** Research Center for Cell Therapy, Key Laboratory of Cardiovascular Remodeling and Function Research, Qilu Hospital, Shandong University, Jinan, China, **4** Centre for Transplant and Renal Research, Westmead Millennium Institute, The University of Sydney at Westmead Hospital, Westmead, New South Wales, Australia

Abstract

Objective: Chronic low-grade inflammation has long been recognized as the central link between obesity and type 2 diabetes (T2D). The novel subset of T helper (Th) cells, Th22, plays an emerging role in chronic inflammation. We investigated the potential association between Th22 and the pathogenesis of obesity and T2D.

Methods: Ninety T2D inpatients (T2D group), 30 healthy participants with BMI ranged from 19 to 23.9 kg/m2 (CTL group) and 30 metabolically healthy obese controls with BMI $\geq$ 30 kg/m2 (MHO group) were employed in our study. Peripheral frequencies of Th22 and Th1 and Th17 cells were determined by flow cytometry based on their specific cytokine patterns. Cytokine levels in fresh plasma were quantified by ELISA.

Results: Compared to that in CTL group (1.18±0.06%, n = 28), peripheral frequency of Th22 cells was significantly increased in MHO group (1.88±0.10%, n = 30) and in T2D group (2.247±0.10%, n = 89). There was a consistent notable increase in plasma interleukin (IL)-22 of T2D patients [47.56 (30.55–76.89) pg/mL] as compared with that of MHO group [36.65 (29.52–55.70) pg/ml; $*P<0.0001$] and CTLs [36.33 (31.93–40.62) pg/mL; $*P<0.0001$]. Furthermore, other than Th1/Th17, previously frequently described participants in obesity and T2D, there was a strong correlation between Th22 frequency and the homeostasis model of assessment for insulin resistance index ($r = 0.6771$, $*P<0.0001$) and HOMA for β-cell function ($r = -0.7264$, $*P<0.0001$).

Conclusions: There were increased Th22 frequencies and IL-22 levels in obesity and T2D. Elevated Th22 and IL-22 also aided in the differentiation of MHO from T2D patients. The notable correlation implied that Th22 might play a more determinant role in both insulin resistance and β-cell impairment.

Editor: Jean-Marc A. Lobaccaro, Clermont Université, France

Funding: This study was financially supported by the National Natural Science Foundation of China (Grant No.81000326; 81100617), China Postdoctoral Science Foundation (Grant No. 2012M521354), Jinan Overseas Students Pioneer plan (Grant No.20100205;20110407), The Special Fund of Clinical Research of Chinese Medical Association(Grant No.12030420342), Shandong International Scientific Corporation Plan(Grant No.2012GGE27126), Shandong Natural Science Foundation (Grant No.ZR2012HM014), Shandong Provincial Health& Medical Development Project (Grant No.2011HD005), National Key Technology R&D Program Grant No.2009BAI80B04). The funders had no role in study design, data collection and analysis, decision to publish, or preparation of the manuscript.

Competing Interests: The authors have declared that no competing interests exist.

* E-mail: sduchenli@gmail.com (LC); sunlei1@medmail.com.cn (LS)

¶ These authors contributed equally to this work.

Introduction

Parallel to type 2 diabetes (T2D), obesity has become a worldwide epidemic concern [1]. Obesity-associated insulin resistance is the key pathological change that leads to T2D. T2D develops when exhausted islet β cells fail to compensate for the increased need for insulin to maintain glucose homeostasis [2]. Evidence from the past decade unequivocally indicates that chronic low-grade inflammation is the major underlying link between these two disorders [3–5]. In fact, apart from the long list of metabolic disorders, obesity is frequently reported with an apparent increased prevalence of autoimmune and inflammatory disorders, e.g., asthma [6], rheumatic diseases [7], inflammatory bowel disease [8], and so on. These clinical observations strengthen the case for immunologic imbalance possibly underlying or at least being closely linked to the aggravating metabolic disturbances resulting from nutrition overload. Adipose tissue macrophage accumulation was the first well-described inflammatory participant in obesity, whose recruitment and pro-inflammatory polarization directly contribute to inflammatory status [9,10]. More recently, Wu et al. [11] and Kintscher et al. [12] extended those observations to cells of adaptive immunity. They suggested that T lymphocyte accumulation occurs in adipose tissue prior to that of macrophages. Moreover, T-cell infiltration accompanied the initiation of insulin resistance and impaired glucose tolerance [11–13]. Taken together, these studies indicated that T-cell groups are important regulators of inflammation in both rodent models and obesity and T2D patients.

An appropriate balance between pro-inflammatory and anti-inflammatory T-cell subsets is essential to maintain immune homeostasis and avoid inflammatory diseases. Previous studies in a rodent model of T2D identified an elevation of T helper (Th)1 and Th17 subsets accompanied by a significant decrease of regulatory T cells (Tregs), which may directly trigger activation of innate immunity and thus inflammation, and contribute greatly to insulin resistance [14,15]. A subsequent study confirmed that there was a skewed pro-inflammatory T-cell compartment in the peripheral blood of T2D patients [16]. In addition, correlation analysis between pro-inflammatory T-cell frequencies and clinical indicators of disease severity has provided fundamental insights into the notion that the imbalance of T-cell subsets is responsible for the development of obesity and T2D [17].

To date, substantial progress in understanding the interactions and counterbalance between helper T-cells in inflammatory status suggests the possibility that new helper T subsets may also play a role in either feedback regulation of immune/inflammatory cell polarization or direct instruction to tissue cells. Recently identified as a distinct lineage of $CD4^+$ T cells characterized by their production of interleukin-22 (IL-22), Th22 cells are emergent constitutor in autoimmune and inflammatory diseases [18]. Th22 cells have a specific $CCR4^+$ $CCR6^+$ $CCR10^+$ phenotype and do not express IL-17, CCL20, IL-23R, CD161 (Th17 markers), IL-4 (Th2 marker), or IFN-γ (Th1 marker) [19]. Aryl hydrocarbon receptor is the key transcription factor determining the lineage commitment of Th22 cells from naïve $CD4^+$ T (Th0) cells, whose activation can be positively regulated by IL-6 and TNF-α [18,20]. It has been proven that IL-22, a cytokine predominantly secreted by Th22 cells, is upregulated in many chronic inflammatory diseases [21]. Accumulating evidence supports an important and complicated role for Th22 cells in chronic inflammation and autoimmune diseases such as psoriasis, rheumatoid arthritis, ankylosing spondylitis, immune thrombocytopenia, Graves' diseases [22–25], and the like. Although the skewed pro-inflammatory phenotype of $CD4^+$ T subsets that include Th1, Th17, and Treg cells is frequently reported, there is no study at present on the frequencies and function status of Th22 cells in obesity and T2D patients. In the present study, we determined the frequencies of peripheral Th22, Th1, and Th17 cells and plasma levels of the cytokines IL-22, IFN-γ, IL-17, IL-6, and TNF-α. The relevance between Th22 cells and clinical patient data was evaluated.

Research Design and Methods

Subjects and ethics statement

Enrollment took place between April 2012 and January 2013 in Qilu Hospital, Shandong University, China. Subjects were assigned to three groups. The T2D group comprised clinically definite T2D inpatients from the Qilu Hospital Department of Endocrinology. Healthy (CTL; BMI: 19–23.9 kg/m^2) and metabolically healthy obese (MHO; BMI ≥ 28 kg/m^2) control groups were formed with volunteers from the community and hospital staff. Subjects in the MHO group had increased weight but normal glucose tolerance and lipid profiles. A detailed clinical record was registered for each subject, including history of disease and physical and laboratory examinations. Exclusion criteria were any signs of autoimmune disorders, recent infections, tumors, fever of any cause, and significantly elevated erythrocyte sedimentation rate. Participants did not receive immunosuppressive or immunomodulatory drugs for at least three months during sampling. The Medical Ethical Committee of Qilu Hospital approved this study. A signed consent form was obtained from each participant. Baseline clinical parameters are summarized in Table 1.

Table 1. Demographic characteristics of participants.

	CTL	MHO	T2D
Number	30	30	90
BMI (kg/m^2)	22.19±0.24	30.37±0.45	24.89±0.47
Age (year)	44.43±1.75	42.47±2.18	54.36±1.18
Sex (female/male)	14/16	13/17	43/47
FBG (mM)	5.19±0.08	5.29±0.08	10.63±0.28
2 h BG (mM)	5.81±0.23	5.98±0.13	12.25±0.40
FINS (IU/mL)	7.44±0.45	11.54±0.77	11.34±0.79
2 h INS (IU/mL)	n.a.	43.96±1.83	37.14±2.27
ICA/GAD/IAA	n.a.	n.a.	Negative
Duration of illness (year)	n.a.	n.a.	6.14±1.63

FBG: Fasting blood glucose; 2 h BG: blood glucose level 2 h after a meal;
FINS: fasting insulin level; 2 h INS: insulin level 2 h after a meal;
ICA: islet cell antibodies;
GAD: autoantibody for glutamate decarboxylase;
IAA: insulin antibodies
n.a: not applicable

Sample preparation

Fasting peripheral blood samples were obtained from each donor between 7 and 9 a.m. All samples were processed within 2 h after collection. Blood (6 mL) for further incubation or isolation was drawn into BD Vacutainer® Heparin (sodium) Tubes (BD, Franklin Lakes NJ, USA). Heparinized peripheral whole blood (400 µL) diluted with an equal volume of RPMI 1640 medium containing 50 ng/mL phorbol myristate acetate (PMA), 2 µg/mL ionomycin, and 3.4 µg/mL monensin (Sigma-Aldrich, St. Louis, MO, USA) was incubated for 4.5 h at 37°C in 5% CO_2. PMA and ionomycin function synergistically as T-cell activators through non–antigen-specific activation of PKC and by increasing intracellular Ca^{2+}, mimicking signals induced by the T-cell receptor complex. Monensin, a protein transport inhibitor, leads to intracellular cytokine accumulation, thus facilitating subsequent detection by flow cytometric analysis.

Cell staining and flow cytometric analysis

Stimulated whole blood was stained for flow cytometric study to identify cytokine-producing cells. After incubation, 100 µL blood was stained with PerCP-Cy5.5–conjugated anti-human CD4 monoclonal antibodies (clone: OKT4, Cat.: 85-45-0048-42) at room temperature for 20 min. The sample was then treated with an equal volume of Fix-Perm reagent A for 15 min, and then washed with pre-cooled washing buffer. Subsequently, Fix-Perm reagent B was added for further permeabilization for intracellular staining and erythrocyte lysis. The sample was incubated for 20 min together with PE-conjugated anti–IFN-γ monoclonal antibodies (clone: 4S.B3, Cat.: 85-11-7319-82), FITC-conjugated anti–IL-17A monoclonal antibodies (clone: eBio64D, Cat.: 85-11-7179-42), and eFluro680-conjugated anti–IL-22 monoclonal antibodies (clone: 22URTI, Cat.: 85-50-7229-42). Isotope controls were used for each staining procedure as negative controls and for fluorescence compensation. All antibodies were from eBioscience, San Diego, CA, USA. Fix-Perm reagents were from Invitrogen (Carlsbad, CA, USA). All samples were washed and collected using BD Accuri C6 Flow Cytometer. Data were analyzed with FlowJo 7.6.

Quantification of plasma cytokines by using enzyme-linked immunoassay

The plasma levels of Th1/Th17/Th22-predominantly secreted cytokines IFN-γ, IL-22, IL-17A, and the cytokines previously reported as major drivers of Th22 commitment from Th0 cells, i.e., IL-6 and TNF-α, were determined with a quantitative sandwich ELISA according to the manufacturer's recommendations (Multisciences, CN). The minimum detectable concentration of IFN-γ, IL-22, IL-17A, IL-6 and TNF-α is 0.30, 2.56, 0.55, 0.37, 0.42 pg/ml respectively.

Statistical analysis

Results are expressed as mean ± SEM or median (range). Differences in Th22, Th17, and Th1 cell frequencies; plasma cytokine levels; and expression of specific transcription factors in PBMC among T2D, MHO patients, and CTLs were determined by using ANOVA, and differences between two groups were determined by using the Newman–Keuls multiple comparison test (q test). Data not normally distributed were analyzed with the Kruskal–Wallis test (H test) and Dunn test. Odds ratio was calculated in a 2×2 arranged table with Fisher's exact test. The Pearson or Spearman correlation test was used for correlation analysis depending on data distribution. Partial correlation analysis was conducted to role out confounding factors. SPSS 18.0 or GraphPad Prism 5.0 were used to perform all tests and generate values. A P-value of less than 0.05 was considered statistically significant.

Results

Circulating Th22 cells increased in tandem with Th1/Th17 cell frequencies in MHO and T2D patients

The peripheral frequencies of Th22, Th1, and Th17 cells were analyzed based on their specific cytokine patterns after 5-h stimulation in the presence of PMA, ionomycin, and monensin. The gating procedure and typical dot plots in defining the expression of circulating Th22 ($CD4^+$ $IFN\gamma^-IL\text{-}17^-IL\text{-}22^+$), Th1 ($CD4^+$ $IFN\gamma^+$), and Th17 ($CD4^+$ $IFN\gamma^-IL\text{-}17^+$) cells are depicted in Figure 1. Compared to CTLs (1.18±0.06%, n = 28), the frequency of peripheral Th22 cells was significantly increased (1.59 folds) in MHO (1.88±0.10%, n = 30; $*P<0.0001$) and (1.90 folds) T2D patients (2.247±0.10%, n = 89; $*P<0.0001$). Even higher percentages (1.31 folds) of Th22 cells were observed in T2D compared to MHO patients ($*P<0.05$) (Fig. 2A).

To further evaluate the increased risk associated with elevated Th22 for health people to develp obesity and for obese people to develop diabetes respectively, the odds ratio was calculated in a 2×2 table (with continuity correction of 0.5 to each cell when needed) (see Table 2 and Table 3 respectively). The median 1.40% was selected as the threshold of normal and elevated Th22 frequency. In the sub-cohort of metabolically health subjects(n = 58), the odds ratio was up to 54.47 ($*P<0.0001$). And in obese people who had an elevated Th22, diabetes might occur 8.636 times as often as in those with normal Th22 frequency($*P = 0.0148$), indicating an potential value of Th22 in predicating obese outcomes. However, since Th22 frequency is a continuous variable and there is currently no wide-accepted categorical threshold, we could only make artificial definition according to our data. Moreover, statistical values should be for reference only since the cases of participants in our study did not represent disease prevalence in the natural population.

Besides, there was also a significant increase of Th1 frequency in T2D patients (median, 9.06%; range, 6.01%–14.02%; n = 89) as compared with MHO patients (median, 9.06%; range, 6.01%–14.02%; n = 30) ($*P<0.0001$) and CTLs (median, 9.06%; range, 6.01%–14.02%; n = 28) (Fig. 2B). No significant difference was found in Th1 frequency between MHO patients and CTLs. Consistent with a previous study, Th17 cells were increased in the peripheral blood of MHO (median, 9.06%; range, 6.01%–14.02%; n = 30) and T2D patients (median, 9.06%; range, 6.01%–14.02%; n = 89) as compared with CTLs (median, 9.06%; range, 6.01%–14.02%; n = 28) ($*P<0.0001$). However, our findings failed to demonstrate a significant difference in Th17 frequency between T2D and MHO patients (Fig. 2C).

As preliminary exploration of the interactions between the three pro-inflammatory helper T subsets, inter-subset correlation was evaluated. There was a significantly positive correlation between the frequencies of peripheral Th22 and Th1 cells ($r = 0.2378$, $*P = 0.0037$, n = 147, Spearman analysis; Fig. 2D), Th22 and Th17 cells ($r = 0.3549$, $*P<0.0001$, n = 147, Spearman analysis; Fig. 2E), and Th17 and Th1 cells ($r = 0.4387$, $*P<0.0001$, n = 147, Spearman analysis; Fig. 2F).

Plasma levels of IL-22, IFNγ, and IL-17 were elevated in non-stimulated peripheral blood from MHO and T2D patients

To test the hyperactivity of the pro-inflammatory $CD4^+$ helper T subsets in non-stimulated fresh peripheral blood from MHO (n = 22) and T2D patients (n = 45), plasma levels of the corresponding predominant cytokines IL-22, IFN-γ, and IL-17 were measured by using ELISA. As shown in Figure 3A, there was a notable increase in plasma IL-22 from T2D patients (median, 47.56 pg/mL; range, 30.55–76.89 pg/mL) as compared with MHO patients (median, 36.65 pg/mL; range, 29.52–55.70 pg/mL; $*P<0.0001$) and CTLs (median, 36.33 pg/mL; range, 31.93–40.62 pg/mL; n = 16; $*P<0.0001$). However, there was no significant difference between MHO and CTLs ($P>0.05$). Similarly, the concentrations of plasma IL-17 from our blood donors were consistent (Fig. 3B). There were significantly higher concentrations of IL-17 in T2D patients (median, 3.84 pg/mL; range, 0.81–7.78 pg/mL) as compared with CTLs (median, 2.06 pg/mL; range, 0.81–3.04 pg/mL; $*P<0.0001$) and MHO patients (median, 1.91 pg/mL; range, 0.89–5.11 pg/mL; $*P<0.0001$). There was no significant difference between MHO patients and CTLs ($P>0.05$). There were also significantly higher concentrations of IFN-γ in MHO (median, 1.76 pg/mL; range, 0.33–4.10 pg/mL; $*P<0.0001$) and T2D patients (median, 1.08 pg/mL; range, 0.36–3.43 pg/mL; $*P<0.05$) as compared to CTLs (median, 0.48 pg/mL; range, lower limit to 2.64 pg/mL). No significant difference was found between MHO and T2D patients ($P>0.05$) (Fig. 3C).

For further analysis of the correlation between elevated helper T-cell frequencies and their predominantly secreted cytokines, a correlation study was performed in all plasma donor sub-cohorts (n = 81). As shown in Figure 3A and 3C, there was a significant positive correlation between Th22 frequency and IL-22 concentration ($r = 0.4904$, $*P<0.0001$, Pearson analysis) as well as between Th17 frequency and IL-17 concentration ($r = 0.2412$, $*P = 0.0300$, Spearman analysis). However, there was no statistical correlation between peripheral Th1 cells and non-stimulated circulating levels of IFN-γ ($r = 0.0838$, $P = 0.4657$, Spearman analysis) (Fig. 3B).

Elevated plasma levels of IL-6 and TNF-α in MHO and T2D patients promoted Th22 polarization

TNF-α and IL-6 have been reported as major drivers of Th22 polarization[18,20]. In the present study, we also quantified

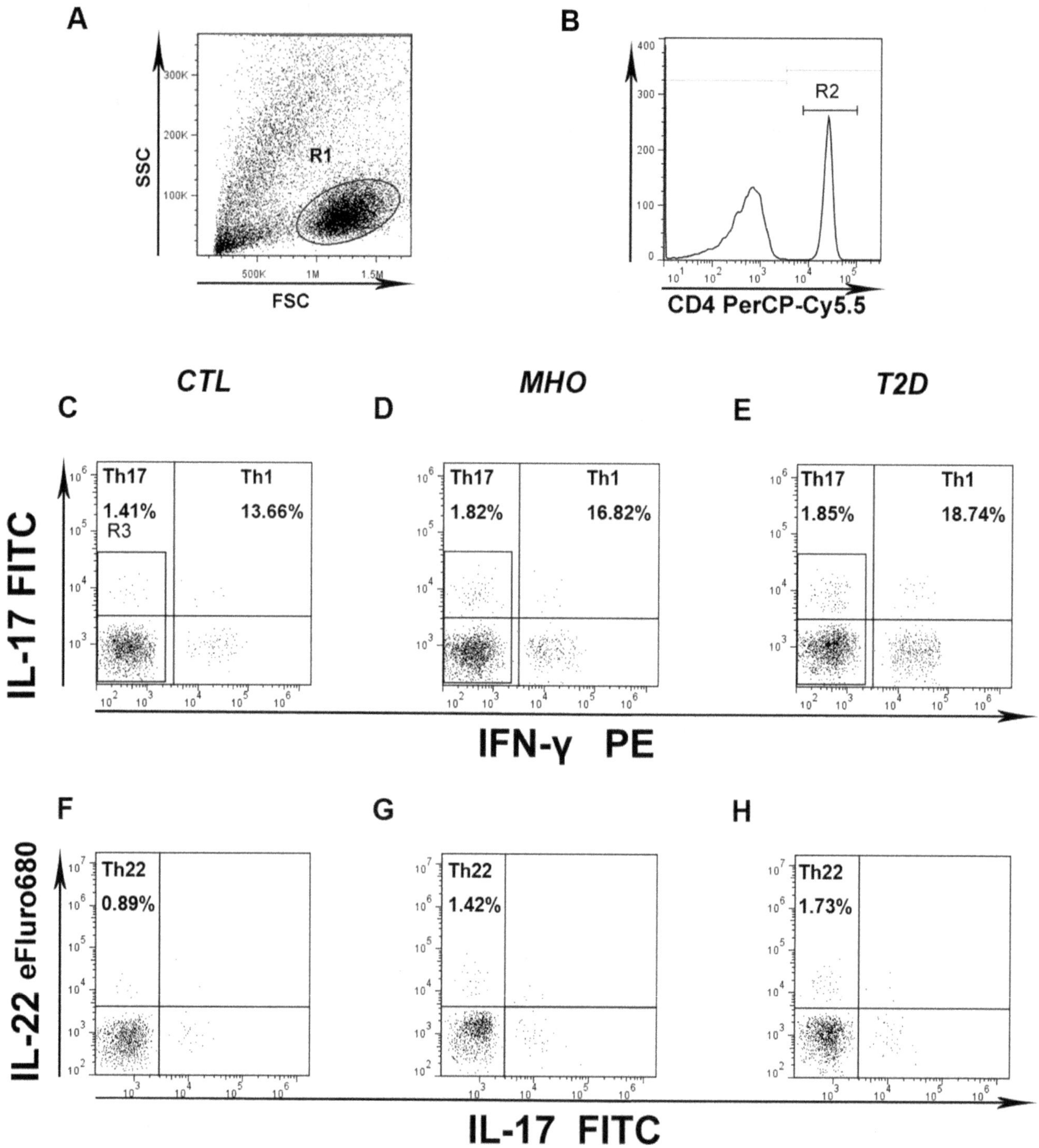

Figure 1. Gating strategy and representative dot plots for flow cytometry analysis. $CD4^+$ T cells (B) were gated from lymphocytes (A) for further phenotyping. (C, D, E) Representative dot plots of peripheral Th1 ($CD4^+$ $IFN\gamma^+$; UR plus LR quadrant) and Th17 frequencies ($CD4^+$ $IFN\gamma^-IL\text{-}17^+$; UL quadrant) from CTLs, MHO, and T2D patients. (F, G, H) Representative FCM dot plots of peripheral Th22 cells ($CD4^+$ $IFN\gamma^-IL\text{-}17^-IL\text{-}22^+$; UL quadrant) from CTLs, MHO, and T2D patients. Numbers in each plot denote the percentages of the indicated helper T subset in the total $CD4^+$ T-cell population.

plasma concentrations of TNF-α and IL-6 by using ELISA. Concordant with previous studies, there were significantly elevated TNF-α levels in MHO (median, 18.15 pg/mL; range, 10.08–49.81 pg/mL; $^*P<0.01$) and T2D patients (median, 46.98 pg/mL; range, 11.07–118.1 pg/mL; $^*P<0.0001$) as compared with CTLs (median, 5.28 pg/mL; range, lower limit to 23.36 pg/mL). There were also significantly higher concentrations of TNF-α in T2D patients as compared to MHO patients ($^*P<0.0001$) (Fig. 3D). While significantly elevated IL-6 levels were observed in T2D patients (median, 11.21 pg/mL; range, 3.09–47.24 pg/mL) as compared to CTLs (median, 7.53 pg/mL; range, 0.79–22.24 pg/mL; $^*P<0.05$), we found no significant difference between MHO

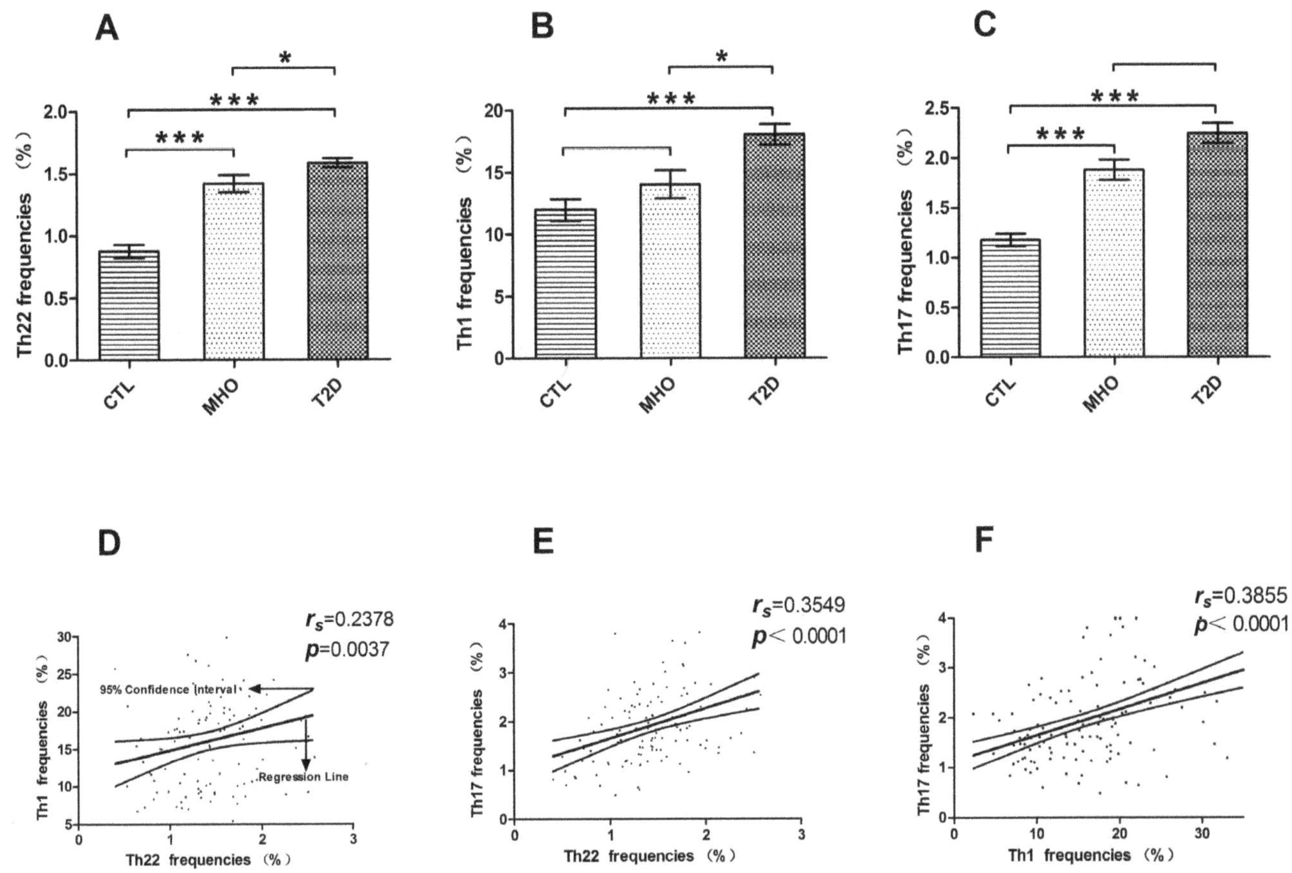

Figure 2. Increased percentages of Th22 cells in peripheral blood from MHO and T2D patients and their correlation with Th1/Th17 frequencies. Circulating percentages of Th22, Th1, and Th17 cells from CTLs, MHO, and T2D patients. (A) Significantly increased percentages of Th22 cells in MHO (1.88±0.10%) and T2D patients (2.247±0.10%) as compared to CTLs (1.18±0.06%) (*P<0.0001). Increased percentages of Th22 cells were also found in MHO patients as compared to T2D patients (*P<0.05). (B) Significant increases in Th1 cells were observed in T2D patients (median, 17.73%; range, 4.652%–42.52%) as compared to CTLs (median, 11.17%; range, 4.724%–25.70%; *P<0.0001) and MHO patients (median, 15.23%; range, 2.297%–27.56%; *P<0.05). There was no significant difference between MHO patients and CTLs. (C) Significantly elevated percentages of Th17 cells were found in T2D (median, 2.08%; range, 0.48%–5.25%; *P<0.0001) and MHO patients (median, 1.815%; range, 1.10%–3.21%; *P<0.0001) as compared to CTLs (median, 1.18%; range, 0.60%–1.80%). There was no significant difference between MHO and T2D patients. (D, E, F) Correlation between the percentages of Th22, Th1, and Th17 cells from all blood donors. There was a positive correlation among all three subsets of helper T cells. Bars represent SEM. Numbers in each figure denote Spearman r and P values.

patients (median, 7.85 pg/mL; range, 3.16–40.12 pg/mL) and CTLs as well as T2D patients (P>0.05) (Fig. 3E). Moreover, correlation analysis revealed the significant relevance of TNF-α (r = 0.6318, *P<0.0001, Spearman analysis) and IL-6 levels (r = 0.2396, *P = 0.0312, Spearman analysis) to Th22 frequency.

Elevated Th22 frequency was bound with insulin resistance in MHO and newly diagnosed T2D patients

As our study revealed an expanded Th22 population in patients with MHO and T2D, we further studied the potential role of this hyperactive phenotype in the development of impaired insulin sensitivity. The homeostasis model of assessment for insulin resistance index (HOMA-IR) has been widely accepted as a good indicator of insulin resistance, especially in patients with comparatively well preserved islet β-cell functions, e.g., MHO patients, prediabetic individuals (impaired glucose tolerance or impaired fasting glucose), and some early-diagnosed T2D patients [26]. Its natural logarithmic value, ln(HOMA-IR), is an even more reliable parameter. In our study, correlation analysis of Th22 frequency and the ln(HOMA-IR) value in a sub-cohort (n = 50) of MHO and

Table 2. Peripheral Th22 frequency and prevalence of obesity in the subset of metabolically healthy participants.

Group	Health	Obesity	Total
Normal	28	19	47
Elevated	0	11	11
Total	28	30	58

Table 3. Peripheral Th22 frequency and prevalence of T2D in the subset of obese participants.

Group	MHO	T2D	Total
Normal	19	2	21
Elevated	11	10	21
Total	30	12	42

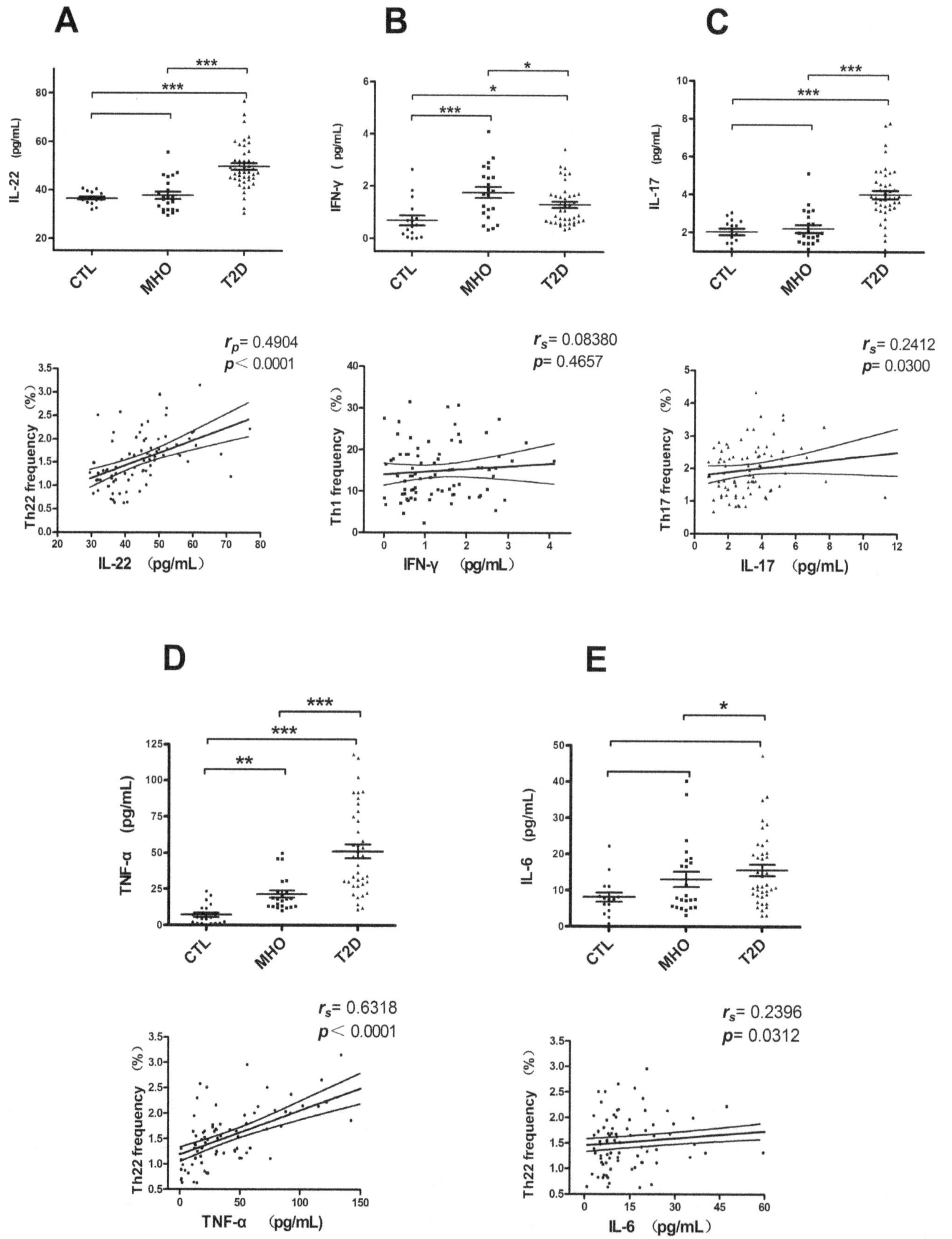
A
B
C
IL-22 (pg/mL)
IFN-γ (pg/mL)
IL-17 (pg/mL)
CTL
MHO
T2D
***
*
r_p= 0.4904
p< 0.0001
r_s= 0.08380
p= 0.4657
r_s= 0.2412
p= 0.0300
Th22 frequency (%)
Th1 frequency (%)
Th17 frequency (%)
IL-22 (pg/mL)
IFN-γ (pg/mL)
IL-17 (pg/mL)
D
E
TNF-α (pg/mL)
IL-6 (pg/mL)
**
r_s= 0.6318
p< 0.0001
r_s= 0.2396
p= 0.0312
Th22 frequency (%)
TNF-α (pg/mL)
IL-6 (pg/mL)

Figure 3. Concentrations of related plasma cytokines in non-stimulated peripheral blood. Concentrations of IL-22, IFN-γ, IL-17, TNF-α, and IL-6 in plasma from CTLs, MHO, and T2D patients. (A) Significantly higher concentrations of IL-22 were observed in T2D patients (median, 47.56 pg/mL; range, 30.55–76.89 pg/mL) as compared to CTLs (median, 36.33 pg/mL; range, 31.93–40.62 pg/mL; $*P<0.0001$) and MHO patients (median, 36.65 pg/mL; range, 29.52–55.70 pg/mL; $*P<0.0001$). There was no significant difference in IL-22 between MHO patients and CTLs ($P>0.05$). (B) Significantly higher concentrations of IFN-γ were found in MHO (median, 1.76 pg/mL; range, 0.33–4.10 pg/mL; $*P<0.0001$) and T2D patients (median, 1.08 pg/mL; range, 0.36–3.43 pg/mL; $*P<0.05$) as compared to CTLs (median, 0.48 pg/mL; range, lower limit to 2.64 pg/mL). No significant difference was found between MHO and T2D patients. (C) Significantly higher concentrations of IL-17 were found in T2D patients (median, 3.84 pg/mL; range, 0.81–7.78 pg/mL) as compared to CTLs (median, 2.06 pg/mL; range, 0.81–3.04 pg/mL; $*P<0.0001$) and MHO patients (median, 1.91 pg/mL; range, 0.89–5.11 pg/mL; $*P<0.0001$). There was no significant difference between MHO patients and CTLs ($P>0.05$). (D) Significantly elevated TNF-α levels were found in MHO (median, 18.15 pg/mL; range, 10.08–49.81 pg/mL; $*P<0.01$) and T2D patients (median, 46.98 pg/mL; range, 11.07–118.1 pg/mL; $*P<0.0001$) as compared with CTLs (median, 5.28 pg/ml; range, lower limit to 23.36 pg/mL). Higher concentrations of TNF-α were also observed in T2D patients compared with MHO patients ($*P<0.0001$). (E) Significantly elevated IL-6 levels were observed in T2D patients (median, 11.21 pg/mL; range, 3.09–47.24 pg/mL) as compared to CTLs (median, 7.53 pg/mL; range, 0.79–22.24 pg/mL; $*P<0.05$). There was no significant difference between MHO patients (median, 7.85 pg/mL; range, 3.16–40.12 pg/mL) and CTLs and T2D patients ($P>0.05$). Correlation analyses between the indicated helper T-cell frequencies and corresponding plasma cytokine levels from each sub-cohort. There was a positive correlation between Th22 frequency and IL-22 concentration (A) and between Th17 and IL-17 (C). There was also a significant positive correlation between Th22 frequency and plasma TNF-α (D) ($*P<0.0001$) and IL-6 (E) ($*P=0.0312$) levels. Bars represent SEM. Numbers in each figure denote Spearman or Pearson r and P values, respectively.

newly diagnosed T2D patients revealed the notable relevance of the expanded Th22 population to increased insulin resistance ($r=0.6771$, $*P<0.0001$, Pearson analysis) (Fig. 4A). However, neither Th1 (Fig. 4B) nor Th17 cells (Fig. 4C), previously described pro-inflammatory $CD4^+$ helper T subsets, had a significant correlation with the ln(HOMA-IR) index. Further, partial correlation analysis in female (n = 22) and male (n = 28) was conducted with the confounding effects of age and sex removed. Significant correlationship between Th22 frequencies and ln(HOMA-IR) values was still present in both male ($r=0.713$, $*P<0.0001$) and female ($r=0.487$, $*P=0.03$) subsets of participants.

Hyperactive Th22 phenotype negatively correlates with residual islet β-cell function in late-stage T2D

As an even more significant expansion of the Th22 population and elevated IL-22 secretion was observed in T2D patients, we investigated the idea of whether the hyperactive Th22 phenotype correlated with the decompensation of β-cell function. The HOMA for β-cell function (HOMA-β) was introduced as a parameter of the residual basal insulin-secreting function of β cells in patients with later-stage T2D [26]. There was an obvious β-cell function loss in this sub-cohort of T2D patients (n = 33), characterized by exhausted insulin secretion. Our findings revealed a remarkable negative correlation between Th22 frequencies and ln(HOMA-β) values ($r=-0.7264$, $*P<0.0001$, Pearson analysis) (Fig. 4D). There was no significant correlation between ln(HOMA-β) values and Th1 or Th17 frequencies (Fig. 4E, 4F). Correlationship between Th22 frequencies and ln(HOMA-β) values remained statistically significant with age controlled by partial correlation analysis in male ($r=0.607$, $*P=0.013$, n = 17) and female ($r=0.850$, $*P<0.0001$, n = 16) subsets of participants respectively.

Discussion

Along with T2D, obesity shares a common pathological process of insulin resistance. It has been proven that insulin resistance is the core initiating and persisting factor in T2D and obesity-associated metabolic syndrome, while the steady loss of β-cell function results in the aggravation of hyperglycemia and development of diabetic complications [2]. In the past two decades, obesity and T2D have been linked to chronic low-grade systemic inflammation, which is postulated to be causal throughout the development of insulin resistance and progression to diabetic complications [3]. Obesity is continually reported with predisposition to autoimmune disorders [6–8]. Moreover, a growing body of evidence published in recent years suggests a substantially increased risk for developing malignancies in patients with T2D [27]. These epidemiologic clues also indicate a plausible link from metabolic pressures to immunologic disturbance and inflammation. However, the specific immunologic sensors triggered in response to metabolic dysfunction to produce a state of inflammation have not been identified. Recent progress in the interaction between immune cell subsets, particularly extension of the knowledge on reciprocal regulation and counterbalance between helper T-cell subsets, sheds some light on the puzzle. Previous studies in rodent obesity/T2D models and patients identified a skewed pro-inflammatory T-cell compartment characterized by elevated Th1 and Th17 cells and decreased Treg cells [11,12,15–17]. Correlation analysis between pro-inflammatory T-cell frequencies and metabolic indicators also implied that the imbalance between T-cell subsets is responsible for the development of obesity and T2D in humans [17].

Compared with the well-known Th1, Th2, Th17, and Treg subsets, Th22 is a newly identified helper T-cell subset with a specific phenotype and distinct function. Th22 cells possess a specific cytokine profile that includes IL-22 and TNF-α, both frequently reported to play important roles in chronic inflammation and tumorigenesis [28,29]. Unlike other cytokines, IL-22 receptors are absent on immune cells, being restricted to tissues instead, thus providing signal directionality from the immune system to tissues [21]. IL-22 regulates cell activity via JAK-STAT3 pathway[21,30]. Though the direct effects of IL-22 on metabolism were poorly reported, there were ermerging studies involving the JAK-STAT3 regulation on metabolism. Chronic activatated JAK-STAT3 pathway has been summarized to contribute to obesity [31] and peripheral insulin resistance[32,33] as well as leptin resistance[33].On the other hand, TNF-α is one of the best described causative factors in obesity-associated insulin resistance and the pathogenesis of T2D [34]. This raises the possibility that Th22 cells might play an independent role in the development of obesity and T2D.

To study whether the Th22 subset is involved in the process of obesity and T2D, the percentages of peripheral Th22 cells in each participant were determined by using flow cytometry. Our study first identified a notably expanded peripheral Th22 population (defined as $CD4^+$ $IFN\text{-}\gamma^-IL\text{-}17^-IL\text{-}22^+$) in both obesity and T2D patients as compared with healthy donors. The increased Th22 population could even aid in distinguishing MHO patients from T2D patients. The increase in Th22 cells was more significant in comparison with Th1 and Th17 cells, the previously described pro-inflammatory subsets in obesity and T2D. There were also

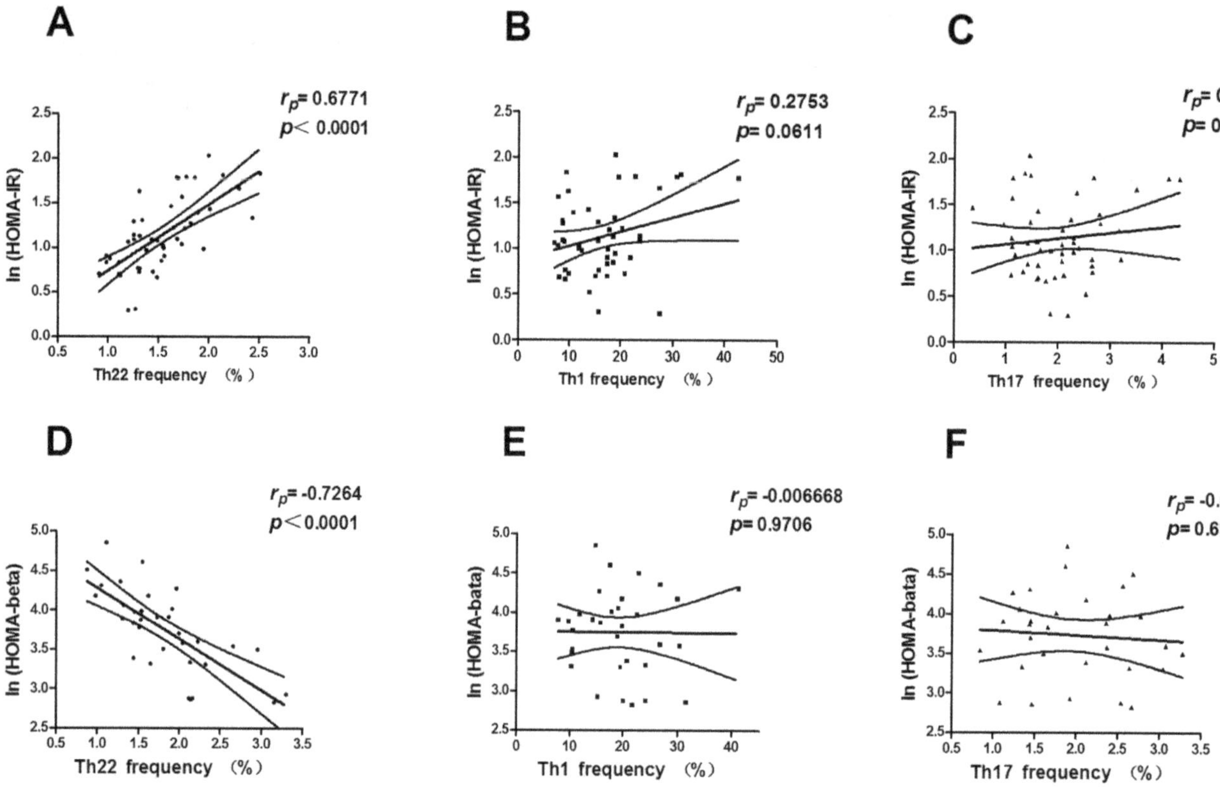

Figure 4. Correlation of peripheral helper T subset percentages with HOMA-IR and HOMA-β. There was a significantly positive correlation of Th22 frequency with ln(HOMA-IR) in MHO and newly diagnosed T2D patients (*P<0.0001) (A) and with ln(HOMA-β) (*P<0.0001) (D) in later-stage T2D patients. (B, C, E, F) The correlation of ln(HOMA-IR) or ln(HOMA-β) value with Th1 or Th17 frequency was not statistically significant. Numbers in each figure denote Pearson r and P values, respectively.

consistently increased levels of IL-22 in both MHO and T2D patients, which was in concert with the previously described inflammatory cytokines. These results indicate that Th22 cells might play a greater role in the immunologic disturbance contributing to disease progression.

As our study revealed an expanded Th22 population in patients with MHO and T2D, we evaluated the potential role of Th22 cells in disease progression. The remarkable positive correlation of ln(HOMA-IR) values with Th22 but not Th1 or Th17 frequencies indicates that Th22 cells may contribute greatly to insulin resistance in both MHO and T2D patients. As we observed an even more hyperactive Th22 phenotype in T2D patients, we further investigated whether Th22 cells exerted a negative effect on islet β-cell function. Again, there was a strong negative correlation of Th22 cells with the clinical indicator of basal β-cell function, ln(HOMA-β). This finding preliminarily demonstrates a causative or even determinant role of Th22 cells in the progressive loss of β-cell function. However, the underlying mechanisms have yet to be discussed.

To explore the sources of the expanded Th22 population, we determined the plasma levels of TNF-α and IL-6, which have been identified as major drivers of Th22 lineage commitment [20]. Consistent with previous studies [35,36], plasma TNF-α levels were elevated in patients with MHO and T2D. In T2D patients, there were even higher TNF-α concentrations accompanied by increased IL-6 levels. In a positive feedback manner, Th22 cells are also a major source of TNF-α. Interestingly, TNF-α has long been established as an important mediator of insulin resistance [34,36–39] and β-cell apoptosis [40]. However, despite its pro-diabetic role being clarified, neutralizing TNF-α in T2D patients was insufficient for reversing the metabolic disturbance [34]. Moreover, without affecting insulin receptor-mediated signal transduction, TNF-α can induce insulin resistance in adipocytes, characterized by loss of insulin receptor substrate-1 and GLUT4 expression [37]. Taken altogether, we hypothesize that apart from its direct influence on adipose tissue and β cells, TNF-α might contribute to the pathogenesis of obesity and T2D in a Th22-dependent manner. Once over-activated by TNF-α and IL-6, Th22 cells exacerbate insulin resistance and aggravate β-cell injuries, thus promoting disease progression.

The study of how metabolic pressures affect the modulation of immune homeostasis [41] and how immune imbalance leads to chronic inflammation in return [42] are now subjects of intensive investigation. While the basic mechanisms governing inflammatory status in the context of metabolic and immunologic disturbance remain to be elucidated, clinical observations provide more clues for further exploration that might be indispensable. Collectively, we identified for the first time a significant elevation of Th22 frequency from the peripheral blood of MHO and T2D patients. An even more hyperactive phenotype of Th22 cells was identified in T2D patients, which renders it of potential value in predicating obese outcomes and evaluating the intervention effect in individuals. Preliminarily, our data suggest that Th22 cells might play a dual role in both the development of insulin resistance and β-cell dysfunction. However, as a single-centered cross-sectional research, our study was exploratory and could not confirm the cause-effect relationship. Further prospective studies with larger sample sizes, animal models as well as in vitro experiments are warranted to validate the potentially causative role of increased Th22 in disease progression of obesity and type 2 diabetes.

Acknowledgments

The authors are especially grateful to their colleagues at the Research Center for Cell Therapy, Key Laboratory of Cardiovascular Remodeling and Function Research, Qilu Hospital, Shandong University, for the technical support.

Author Contributions

Conceived and designed the experiments: RZ LC LS. Performed the experiments: RZ WL CW YL XH JS PL. Analyzed the data: RZ LC LS DT SY. Wrote the paper: RZ LC LS.

References

1. Flier JS (2004) Obesity wars: molecular progress confronts an expanding epidemic. Cell 116: 337–350.
2. Prentki M, Nolan CJ (2006) Islet beta cell failure in type 2 diabetes. J Clin Invest 116: 1802–1812.
3. Hotamisligil GS (2006) Inflammation and metabolic disorders. Nature 444: 860–867.
4. Festa A, D'Agostino R, Jr., Williams K, Karter AJ, Mayer-Davis EJ, et al. (2001) The relation of body fat mass and distribution to markers of chronic inflammation. Int J Obes Relat Metab Disord 25: 1407–1415.
5. Xu H, Barnes GT, Yang Q, Tan G, Yang D, et al. (2003) Chronic inflammation in fat plays a crucial role in the development of obesity-related insulin resistance. J Clin Invest 112: 1821–1830.
6. Boulet LP (2008) Influence of obesity on the prevalence and clinical features of asthma. Clin Invest Med 31: E386–390.
7. Hannan MT (2013) Introduction to special theme section: obesity and the rheumatic diseases. Arthritis Care Res (Hoboken) 65: 4.
8. Fink C, Karagiannides I, Bakirtzi K, Pothoulakis C (2012) Adipose tissue and inflammatory bowel disease pathogenesis. Inflamm Bowel Dis 18: 1550–1557.
9. Weisberg SP, McCann D, Desai M, Rosenbaum M, Leibel RL, et al. (2003) Obesity is associated with macrophage accumulation in adipose tissue. J Clin Invest 112: 1796–1808.
10. Lumeng CN, Bodzin JL, Saltiel AR (2007) Obesity induces a phenotypic switch in adipose tissue macrophage polarization. J Clin Invest 117: 175–184.
11. Wu H, Ghosh S, Perrard XD, Feng L, Garcia GE, et al. (2007) T-cell accumulation and regulated on activation, normal T cell expressed and secreted upregulation in adipose tissue in obesity. Circulation 115: 1029–1038.
12. Kintscher U, Hartge M, Hess K, Foryst-Ludwig A, Clemenz M, et al. (2008) T-lymphocyte infiltration in visceral adipose tissue: a primary event in adipose tissue inflammation and the development of obesity-mediated insulin resistance. Arterioscler Thromb Vasc Biol 28: 1304–1310.
13. Nishimura S, Manabe I, Nagasaki M, Eto K, Yamashita H, et al. (2009) CD8+ effector T cells contribute to macrophage recruitment and adipose tissue inflammation in obesity. Nat Med 15: 914–920.
14. Winer S, Chan Y, Paltser G, Truong D, Tsui H, et al. (2009) Normalization of obesity-associated insulin resistance through immunotherapy. Nat Med 15: 921–929.
15. Feuerer M, Herrero L, Cipolletta D, Naaz A, Wong J, et al. (2009) Lean, but not obese, fat is enriched for a unique population of regulatory T cells that affect metabolic parameters. Nat Med 15: 930–939.
16. Jagannathan-Bogdan M, McDonnell ME, Shin H, Rehman Q, Hasturk H, et al. (2011) Elevated proinflammatory cytokine production by a skewed T cell compartment requires monocytes and promotes inflammation in type 2 diabetes. J Immunol 186: 1162–1172.
17. Zeng C, Shi X, Zhang B, Liu H, Zhang L, et al. (2012) The imbalance of Th17/Th1/Tregs in patients with type 2 diabetes: relationship with metabolic factors and complications. J Mol Med (Berl) 90: 175–186.
18. Trifari S, Kaplan CD, Tran EH, Crellin NK, Spits H (2009) Identification of a human helper T cell population that has abundant production of interleukin 22 and is distinct from T(H)-17, T(H)1 and T(H)2 cells. Nat Immunol 10: 864–871.
19. Eyerich S, Eyerich K, Pennino D, Carbone T, Nasorri F, et al. (2009) Th22 cells represent a distinct human T cell subset involved in epidermal immunity and remodeling. J Clin Invest 119: 3573–3585.
20. Ramirez JM, Brembilla NC, Sorg O, Chicheportiche R, Matthes T, et al. (2010) Activation of the aryl hydrocarbon receptor reveals distinct requirements for IL-22 and IL-17 production by human T helper cells. Eur J Immunol 40: 2450–2459.
21. Zenewicz LA, Flavell RA (2008) IL-22 and inflammation: leukin' through a glass onion. Eur J Immunol 38: 3265–3268.
22. Zhang L, Li YG, Li YH, Qi L, Liu XG, et al. (2012) Increased frequencies of Th22 cells as well as Th17 cells in the peripheral blood of patients with ankylosing spondylitis and rheumatoid arthritis. PLoS One 7: e31000.
23. Hu Y, Li H, Zhang L, Shan B, Xu X, et al. (2012) Elevated profiles of Th22 cells and correlations with Th17 cells in patients with immune thrombocytopenia. Hum Immunol 73: 629–635.
24. Zhang N, Pan HF, Ye DQ (2011) Th22 in inflammatory and autoimmune disease: prospects for therapeutic intervention. Mol Cell Biochem 353: 41–46.
25. Peng D, Xu B, Wang Y, Guo H, Jiang Y (2013) A high frequency of circulating th22 and th17 cells in patients with new onset graves' disease. PLoS One 8: e68446.
26. Haffner SM, Miettinen H, Stern MP (1997) The homeostasis model in the San Antonio Heart Study. Diabetes Care 20: 1087–1092.
27. Habib SL, Rojna M (2013) Diabetes and risk of cancer. ISRN Oncol 2013: 583786.
28. Tian T, Yu S, Ma D (2013) Th22 and related cytokines in inflammatory and autoimmune diseases. Expert Opin Ther Targets 17: 113–125.
29. Shao LL, Zhang L, Hou Y, Yu S, Liu XG, et al. (2012) Th22 cells as well as Th17 cells expand differentially in patients with early-stage and late-stage myelodysplastic syndrome. PLoS One 7: e51339.
30. Duhen T, Geiger R, Jarrossay D, Lanzavecchia A, Sallusto F (2009) Production of interleukin 22 but not interleukin 17 by a subset of human skin-homing memory T cells. Nat Immunol 10: 857–863.
31. Kang HJ, Seo HA, Go Y, Oh CJ, Jeoung NH, et al. (2013) Dimethylfumarate suppresses adipogenic differentiation in 3T3-L1 preadipocytes through inhibition of STAT3 activity. PLoS One 8: e61411.
32. Mashili F, Chibalin AV, Krook A, Zierath JR (2013) Constitutive STAT3 phosphorylation contributes to skeletal muscle insulin resistance in type 2 diabetes. Diabetes 62: 457–465.
33. Wunderlich CM, Hovelmeyer N, Wunderlich FT (2013) Mechanisms of chronic JAK-STAT3-SOCS3 signaling in obesity. JAKSTAT 2: e23878.
34. Moller DE (2000) Potential role of TNF-alpha in the pathogenesis of insulin resistance and type 2 diabetes. Trends Endocrinol Metab 11: 212–217.
35. Katsuki A, Sumida Y, Murashima S, Murata K, Takarada Y, et al. (1998) Serum levels of tumor necrosis factor-alpha are increased in obese patients with noninsulin-dependent diabetes mellitus. J Clin Endocrinol Metab 83: 859–862.
36. Panagiotakos DB, Pitsavos C, Yannakoulia M, Chrysohoou C, Stefanadis C (2005) The implication of obesity and central fat on markers of chronic inflammation: The ATTICA study. Atherosclerosis 183: 308–315.
37. Stephens JM, Lee J, Pilch PF (1997) Tumor necrosis factor-alpha-induced insulin resistance in 3T3-L1 adipocytes is accompanied by a loss of insulin receptor substrate-1 and GLUT4 expression without a loss of insulin receptor-mediated signal transduction. J Biol Chem 272: 971–976.
38. Uysal KT, Wiesbrock SM, Marino MW, Hotamisligil GS (1997) Protection from obesity-induced insulin resistance in mice lacking TNF-alpha function. Nature 389: 610–614.
39. Zinman B, Hanley AJ, Harris SB, Kwan J, Fantus IG (1999) Circulating tumor necrosis factor-alpha concentrations in a native Canadian population with high rates of type 2 diabetes mellitus. J Clin Endocrinol Metab 84: 272–278.
40. Ortis F, Pirot P, Naamane N, Kreins AY, Rasschaert J, et al. (2008) Induction of nuclear factor-kappaB and its downstream genes by TNF-alpha and IL-1beta has a pro-apoptotic role in pancreatic beta cells. Diabetologia 51: 1213–1225.
41. Carbo A, Hontecillas R, Kronsteiner B, Viladomiu M, Pedragosa M, et al. (2013) Systems modeling of molecular mechanisms controlling cytokine-driven CD4+ T cell differentiation and phenotype plasticity. PLoS Comput Biol 9: e1003027.
42. Tang T, Zhang J, Yin J, Staszkiewicz J, Gawronska-Kozak B, et al. (2010) Uncoupling of inflammation and insulin resistance by NF-kappaB in transgenic mice through elevated energy expenditure. J Biol Chem 285: 4637–4644.

6

Increased Risk of Acute Coronary Syndrome among Patients with Urinary Stone Disease

Shun-Fa Hung[1,2¶], Chao-Yuan Huang[3¶], Cheng-Li Lin[4,5], Shiu-Dong Chung[6,7,8], Chi-Jung Chung[9,10], Chia-Hung Kao[11,12*], Chao-Hsiang Chang[5,13*]

1 Division of Urology, Department of Surgery, Far Eastern Memorial Hospital, Ban Ciao, Taipei, Taiwan, **2** Graduate Institute of Clinical Medicine, College of Medicine, Fu-Jen Catholic University, New Taipei, Taiwan, **3** Department of Urology, National Taiwan University Hospital, Taipei, Taiwan, **4** Management Office for Health Data, China Medical University Hospital, Taichung, Taiwan, **5** College of Medicine, China Medical University, Taichung, Taiwan, **6** Division of Urology, Department of Surgery, Far Eastern Memorial Hospital, New Taipei, Taiwan, **7** School of Medicine, College of Medicine, Fu Jen Catholic University, Taipei, Taiwan, **8** Department of Urology, Buddhist Tzu Chi General Hospital and Tzu Chi University, Hualien, Taiwan, **9** Department of Health Risk Management, College of Public Health, China Medical University, Taichung, Taiwan, **10** Department of Medical Research, China Medical University Hospital, Taichung, Taiwan, **11** Graduate Institute of Clinical Medical Science and School of Medicine, College of Medicine, China Medical University, Taichung, Taiwan, **12** Department of Nuclear Medicine and PET Center, China Medical University Hospital, Taichung, Taiwan, **13** Department of Urology, China Medical University and Hospital, Taichung, Taiwan

Abstract

Background/Objectives: Urinary stones (US) are associated with systemic metabolic and endocrine disorders that share risk factors typically associated with acute coronary syndrome (ACS).

Methods: For this investigation, 30 142 patients with US were set as the research group, and 121 768 randomly selected patients were set as the comparison group through frequency matching by age, sex, and index year. Each patient was individually tracked to identify those who developed ACS during the follow-up period. Cox proportional hazards regression and the Kaplan-Meier method were adopted to calculate the hazard ratios of ACS risk and plot the survival curve.

Results: Overall, 275 (13.4 per 10 000 person-y) and 736 events (9.1 per 10 000 person-y) were observed among patients in the research and comparison cohorts, respectively. The patients with US had a substantially lower ACS-free survival rate compared with that of the patients in the comparison cohort ($P<.001$). After adjusting for potential risk factors, the patients with US were observed to have a 1.22-fold higher risk of ACS compared with patients in the comparison cohort (95% confidence interval = 1.05–1.40, $P<.001$), particularly among younger patients.

Conclusions: The results indicate that US is associated with increased risk of developing ACS, particularly among young (≤ 49 years) and male adults. Future studies should examine the possible mechanisms of US-related ACS morbidity by conducting multicenter recruitment and measurements of laboratory data.

Editor: Carmine Pizzi, University of Bologna, Italy

Funding: This study was supported by grants from China Medical University Hospital (DMR-103-012 and DMR-103-018); Taiwan Ministry of Health and Welfare Clinical Trial and Research Center of Excellence (MOHW103-TDU-B-212-113002); Health and welfare surcharge of tobacco products, China Medical University Hospital Cancer Research Center of Excellence (MOHW103-TD-B-111-03, Taiwan); and the International Research-Intensive Centers of Excellence, Taiwan (NSC101-2911-I-002-303). The funders had no role in study design, data collection and analysis, decision to publish, or preparation of the manuscript.

Competing Interests: The authors have declared that no competing interests exist.

* Email: d10040@mail.cmuh.org.tw (C-HK); urology8395@yahoo.com.tw (C-HC)

¶ These authors contributed equally to this work.

¶ These authors also contributed equally to this work.

Introduction

Acute coronary syndrome (ACS) includes ST-segment elevation myocardial infarction (STEMI), non-STEMI (NSTEMI), or unstable angina [1]. The pathomechanism is typically associated with rupture of an atherosclerotic plaque, and partial or complete thrombosis of the infarct-related artery [2]. Previous research has estimated that more than 1 million hospital admissions in the United States are due to ACS [3]. Because of the high mortality and reinfarction rates, ACS is considered a major public health concern [4]. Relevant evidence indicates that the prevalence of ACS increases with age, and is associated with risk factors such as hypertension, diabetes mellitus, hyperlipidemia, and smoking [5–8].

Urinary stone (US) disease is a relatively prevalent disease in western countries [9]. Increasing epidemiological evidence supports an association between urinary tract calculus and obesity, diabetes mellitus, and hypertension [10–15]. These associated chronic medical disorders are major characteristics of the metabolic syndrome (MS), which results specifically from insulin resistance and increases the risk of ACS [16,17]. The high prevalence of US-diagnosed patients with MS indicates that insulin resistance might be involved in the pathophysiology of stone disease [18,19]. Collectively, both US and ACS are recognized as systemic diseases and associated with insulin resistance and metabolic disorders. However, research on the relationship between ACS and US is scarce. Therefore, using a nationwide population-based dataset, we examined the influence of US on the incidence of ACS.

Materials and Methods

Data source

Taiwan launched a single-payer National Health Insurance program in March 1995 that was set up by the Bureau of National Health Insurance (http://www.nhi.gov.tw/english/index.aspx). Since 2000, the National Health Insurance Research Databases (NHIRDs) have been established and managed by the National Health Research Institutes (NHRI) in Taiwan. The NHIRDs, a medical claims database (included inpatient and outpatient claim records, medical treatment and etc.) and personal information (included gender, birthday, residential area and etc.), has been released for research purposes. Longitudinal Health Insurance Database 2000 (LHID2000) is composed of historical claims data for one million patients who are randomly selected from NHIRDs. The NHRI encrypts personal identification numbers to ensure privacy protection and provides researchers with anonymous identification numbers by linking claims data. Disease was defined according to the International Classification of Diseases, 9th Revision, Clinical Modification (ICD-9-CM) in the database. The NHRID encrypts the patients' personal information for privacy protection and provides researchers with anonymous identification numbers associated with the relevant claim information, which includes the patient's sex, date of birth, registry of medical services, and medication prescriptions. Patient consent is not required for accessing the NHIRD.

Data Availability Statement

All data and related metadata are deposited in an appropriate public repository: The study population's data were from Taiwan NHIRD (http://w3.nhri.org.tw/nhird//date_01.html) are maintained by Taiwan National Health Research Institutes (http://nhird.nhri.org.tw/) [20]. The National Health Research Institutes (NHRI) is a non-profit foundation established by the government.

Ethics statement

Because identification numbers of patients had been encrypted, patient consent was not required for this study. This study was approved by the Research Ethic Committee at China Medical University (CMU-REC-101-012). The committee waived the requirement for consent.

Study participants

The section criteria for inclusion in this study are as follows: (1) patients aged more than or equal to 20 years; and (2) newly diagnosed urinary stones (US) (ICD-9-CM codes 592.0, 592.1, 594.0 and 594.1). Patients with previous acute coronary syndrome (ACS) (ICD-9-CM code 410 and 411.1) or incomplete information were excluded. We identified 30,442 patients as a US cohort and used the date of diagnosed US as the index date. Four controls were randomly selected from insured people without US and ACS history before the index date, and they were excluded with the same criteria of the US cohort. The non-US cohort was matched with US cohort based on age category (every 5 years each), sex, and the year of index date. The non-US cohort included 121,768 patients.

Outcome definition

Both cohorts were followed until ACS was diagnosed or censored because of death, loss to follow-up, termination of insurance, or the end of 2010. The comorbidities that might associate with ACS to be included in this study were hypertension (ICD-9-CM codes 401–405), diabetes (ICD-9-CM codes 250), hyperlipidemia (ICD-9-CM codes 272), cerebrovascular disease (CVA) (ICD-9-CM codes 430–438), chronic obstructive pulmonary disease (COPD) (ICD-9-CM codes 490–496), end-stage renal disease (ESRD) (ICD-9-CM code 585), and urinary tract infection (UTI) (ICD-9-CM codes 590 and 595), identified at the baseline.

Statistical analysis

The Chi-square test and t test were used to test the differences in categorical variables included age (≤49, 50–64 and >64 years), sex, income less than New Taiwan Dollar [(NTD) 15,000, 15,000–19,999, and more than 20,000/per month], occupation (white collar, blue collar and other), comorbidities and continuous variables contained age between two cohorts, respectively. The sex-, age-, income- and occupation-specific incidence densities of ACS were estimated in both cohorts. Crude and adjusted hazards ratios (HRs) and 95% confidence intervals (CIs) for ACS in the US cohort compared with the non-US cohort were estimated using univariable and multivariable Cox proportional hazard regression models. The multivariable models were simultaneously adjusted for demographic characteristics, monthly income (NTD), occupation and co-morbidities. Further, the Cox model was also used to estimate the HR of ACS associated with the cumulative frequency of medical visits by US, compared to the non-US cohort. The ACS-free survival rates were estimated using the Kaplan-Meier method, and the difference between the US cohort and non-US cohort was compared using log-rank test. Data were analyzed using SAS statistical software for Windows (version 9.2; SAS Institute Inc, Cary, NC), and the significance level was set at 0.05.

Results

In this study, 30,442 diagnosed US patients at baseline were included and matched to 121,768 controls. Of the 152,210 sampled patients, the mean age was 48.3 and 48.8 for US patients and controls, respectively. Demographic characteristic data are shown in Table 1. The US cohort included more men than women (68.7%) and, because the cohorts were matched on sex, so too did the control cohort. Approximately 56% of participants were ≤49 years of age. Patients with US had a higher prevalence of all baseline comorbidities ($P<0.0001$) except ESRD, which is higher in non-US group ($P<0.001$). The US patients were more likely to have comorbidities of hyperlipidemia (20.3% vs. 13.3%, $p<0.001$), diabetes (12.9% vs. 9.6%, $p<0.001$), hypertension (43.0% vs. 30.8%, $p<0.001$), CVA (7.7% vs. 6.4%, $p<0.001$), COPD (26.0% vs. 19.8%, $p<0.001$), UTI (18.7% vs. 7.5%, $p<0.001$) and less to have ESRD (0.11% vs. 0.32%, $p<0.001$) than controls. In addition, non-US patients had a greater tendency to

Table 1. Comparison of demographics and comorbidity between urinary stones patients and non- urinary stones controls.

	Urinary stones				
	No (N = 121768)		Yes (N = 30442)		
	n	%	n	%	p-value
Age, year					
≤49	68236	56.0	17059	56.0	0.99
50–64	35188	28.9	8797	28.9	
>64	18344	15.1	4586	15.1	
Mean (SD)[†]	48.3	14.8	48.8	14.3	
Sex					
Female	38100	31.3	9525	31.3	0.99
Male	83668	68.7	20917	68.7	
Monthly Income (NTD)					
<15,000	26202	21.5	5746	18.9	<0.0001
15,000–19,999	55175	45.3	14406	47.3	
≥20,000	40391	33.2	10290	33.8	
Occupation					
White collar	64827	53.2	15569	51.1	<0.0001
Blue collar	40406	33.2	11109	36.5	
Others[#]	16535	13.6	3764	12.4	
Comorbidity					
Diabetes	11632	9.55	3929	12.9	<0.0001
Hypertension	26346	21.6	9277	30.5	<0.0001
Hyperlipidemia	16148	13.3	6166	20.3	<0.0001
CVA	7730	6.35	2341	7.69	<0.0001
COPD	24057	19.8	7927	26.0	<0.0001
UTI	9119	7.49	5684	18.7	<0.0001
ESRD	387	0.32	34	0.11	<0.0001

Chi-square test;
[†]T-test.
[#]Other occupations included primarily retired, unemployed, or low income populations.

have monthly income ≤ NT$15,000 ($p<0.001$) and be employed as white collar occupation ($p<0.001$) compared to US patients.

Table 2 shows the incidence rate of ACS and adjusted hazard ratio (HR) among the US cohort and the comparison cohort. The overall incidence rate of ACS was 1.47-fold higher in the US cohort than in the comparison cohort (13.4 vs. 9.12 per 1000 person-years). Kaplan–Meier survival analysis showed that patients with US had significantly higher rates of developing ACS than their comparative cohorts (log-rank test $p<0.001$; Figure 1). After adjusting for patients' monthly income, occupation, hypertension, diabetes, CVA, ESRD, COPD, UTI and hyperlipidemia, the HR in US patients are at higher risk to develop subsequent ACS was 1.22 (95% CI 1.05–1.40) (Table 2). The sex-specific analysis shows the incidence of ACS was greater in men in both cohorts and men in the US cohorts had the greater HR than men in the non-US cohort (adjusted HR = 1.25, 95% CI = 1.06–1.47). Table 2 also shows the further analyses of the association of US with ACS according to age group. It shows that the HRs of ACS between US patients and controls were higher in younger groups. In the age group <49, the adjusted HR was as high as 1.76 (95% CI, 1.33–2.33; $p<0.001$), for those with US compared to controls. However, among the age groups 50–64 and >64, there was no statistical difference in the proportion of ACS between US patients and controls. In addition, US patients with white collar occupation had the highest adjusted HR of 1.28 (95% CI = 1.02–1.59).

Table 3 shows the further analyses of the association of US with ACS according to medical visit frequency for US. It shows that the HRs of ACS between study patients and controls were higher in those who visited for US more than 3 times per year. The adjusted HR was as high as 3.91 (95% CI, 3.14–4.87; $p<0.001$), for those with high visit frequency for US compared to controls.

Discussion

In this investigation, data of 30 442 US-diagnosed patients and 121 768 patients selected as the comparison cohort were analyzed. After adjusting for age, sex, and other potential risk factors, we observed that the risk of developing ACS during a 10-year follow-up period was 1.22-fold higher for the US-diagnosed cohort. Furthermore, we analyzed the association for various age groups, and identified significant associations between US and ACS, particularly among younger adults. To our knowledge, this is the first investigation to report an association between US and ACS based on a nationwide population-based survey, and the first to

Table 2. Incidence and adjusted hazard ratio of ACS stratified by sex, and age compared between with urinary stones and without urinary stones.

	Urinary stones						Compared to non-US	
	No			Yes				
Variables	Event	PY	Rate#	Event	PY	Rate#	Crude HR* (95% CI)	Adjusted HR† (95% CI)
All	736	807017	9.12	275	205894	13.4	1.47(1.28, 1.68)***	1.22(1.05, 1.40)**
Sex								
Female	185	255790	7.23	67	64526	10.4	1.44(1.09, 1.90)*	1.13(0.85, 1.51)
Male	551	551228	10.0	208	141368	14.7	1.47(1.25, 1.73)***	1.25(1.06, 1.47)**
Age								
≤49	139	478225	2.91	82	122156	6.71	2.30(1.75, 3.02)***	1.76(1.33, 2.33)***
50–64	307	226582	13.6	116	57183	20.3	1.50(1.21, 1.85)***	1.17(0.94, 1.46)
>64	290	102210	28.4	77	26556	29.0	1.03(0.80, 1.32)	0.91(0.71, 1.18)
Monthly Income (NTD)								
<15,000	177	163514	10.8	53	36969	14.3	1.32(0.97, 1.80)	1.12(0.82, 1.53)
15,000–19,999	354	365604	9.68	141	97767	14.4	1.49(1.23, 1.81)***	1.20(0.99, 1.47)
≥20,000	205	277899	7.38	81	71158	11.4	1.54(1.19, 2.00)***	1.29(1.00, 1.68)
Occupation								
White collar	308	427597	7.20	114	104247	10.9	1.52(1.23, 1.88)***	1.28(1.02, 1.59)*
Blue collar	307	272019	11.3	129	76366	16.9	1.50(1.22, 1.84)***	1.24(1.00, 1.53)*
Others#	121	107402	11.3	32	25281	12.7	1.13(0.76, 1.66)	0.94(0.63, 1.40)

Rate#, incidence rate, per 10,000 person-years; Crude HR*, related hazard ratio; Adjusted HR†: multivariable analysis including age, sex, monthly income (NTD), occupation and co-morbidities; *$p<0.05$, **$p<0.01$, ***$p<0.0001$.

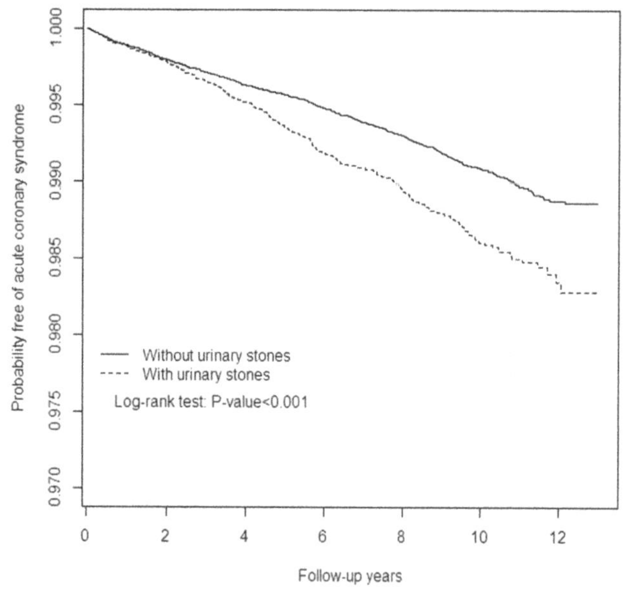

Figure 1. Probability free of acute coronary syndrome for patients with (dashed line) or without (solid line) urinary stones.

suggest that a higher frequency of medical visits related to US is associated with a higher risk of ACS.

US disease is common in the United States, affecting approximately 10.6% of men and 7.1% of women, and its prevalence continues to increase [9]. Numerous studies have indicated an association between stone disease various cardiovascular (CV) risk factors, including hypertension, diabetes, and metabolic syndrome [10–15,21]. According to the CARDIA study, Reiner et al reported a relatively higher prevalence of subclinical atherosclerosis among young adults with a history of kidney stone disease [22], which is supported by the findings of this research. Specifically, we observed that young adults with US are at increased risk of developing subsequent ACS.

According to the National Cholesterol Education Program Adult Treatment Panel III, the metabolic syndrome (MS) comprises criteria related to obesity, hyperglycemia, dyslipidemia, and hypertension (HTN) [17]. Previous research has estimated that the prevalence of MS in the United States is approximately 25%, and increasing [16]. In addition to diabetes and cardiovascular risks, MS has been associated with US disease in recent studies [21,23]. Kohjimoto et al reported that the probability of recurring or multiple stones among patients with 4 MS traits was up to 1.8-fold greater than that for patients without MS traits [24]. Their findings indicated that the clustering of MS traits is associated with increased risk of kidney stone formation. Epidemiological and basic studies have also provided strong indications regarding the association between MS and ACS. The primary features of MS, including hyperglycemia and insulin resistance resulting in systemic chronic inflammation, can lead to endothelial damage and atherosclerosis. In this investigation, the incidence of diabetes in the US-diagnosed cohort was considerably higher than that in the control group. A recent study reported an association between diabetic severity measured according to HbA1c and nephrolithiasis [25]. Weinberg et al estimated that over one million episodes of kidney stones in the United States might be attributable to type 2 diabetes, particularly among patients with poor glucose control [25]. Hyperglycemia and glucosuria might alter renal handling of calcium, phosphorus, and uric acid. Among patients with diabetes, hypercalciuria can be noted. In addition, insulin resistance is associated with abnormality in renal ammonium production, increased urinary acidification, hypocitraturia, and hypercalciuria. Previous studies have suggested insulin resistance as a potential cause of tubular calcium resorption, which leads to hypercalciuria [26–28]. Insulin resistance has also been associated with endogenous oxalate synthesis, which is a mechanism of stone formation [26–28].

These metabolic findings are associated with the development of uric acid and calcium stones. Consequently, both hyperoxaluria and hypercalciuria resulting from poor glycemic control could lead to the formation of calcium oxalate stones. Additionally, uric acid has been reported to be the main component of stones in a considerably high proportion of patients with diabetes [18]. Several studies have shown that uric acid excretion increased in the presence of hyperglycemia and glycosuria, a mechanism that might explain the increased formation of uric acid stones among diabetic patients [29,30]. Rendina et al reported that MS patients are twice as likely to develop renal stones [31]. The Third National Health and Nutrition Examination Survey analysis showed that the probability of self-reported US disease is approximately twice as high among patients with MS than those without [21]. Consistent with the findings of Kohjimoto et al [24], a high number of MS components are associated with an increased risk of developing stone disease [21]. A plausible explanation for the association between MS and nephrolithiasis is that MS is associated with lower urine pH, which is an established characteristic of uric acid urolithiasis and a high risk factor for nephrolithiasis [32–34].

Several epidemiological studies have identified a link between urolithiasis and coronary heart disease. Domingos et al evaluated 23 346 patients and reported a statistically significant association between a self-reported history of kidney stones and myocardial infarction (odds ratio [OR] = 1.34; 95% CI = 1.00–1.79) and

Table 3. The risk of ACS among frequency for medical visits of stones in Cox proportional hazard regression.

Frequency for medical visit, per 1 years	Event	PY	Rate#	Crude HR* (95% CI)	Adjusted HR† (95% CI)
None- urinary stones	736	807017	9.12	1.00	1.00
≤3	183	189711	9.65	1.06(0.90, 1.24)	0.92(0.78, 1.08)
>3	92	16183	56.9	6.23(5.01, 7.75)***	3.91(3.14, 4.87)***
p for trend					<0.0001

Rate#, incidence rate, per 10,000 person-years; Crude HR*, related hazard ratio; Adjusted HR†: multivariable analysis including age, sex, and co-morbidities; *p<0.05, **p<0.01, ***p<0.0001.

stroke (OR = 1.33; 95% CI = 1.02–1.74) after adjusting for age and body mass index (BMI) [35]. However, following multivariable adjustment, only myocardial infarction was significantly associated with US in women. Another study, using the cohort of Olmstead County in Minnesota, enrolled 4564 patients with kidney stones or ureter stones at the baseline who had not previously sustained a myocardial infarction [36]. Compared with 14 144 matched nonstone formers after a mean follow-up period of 9 years, the HR for experiencing a myocardial infarction was 1.31 for stone formers after adjusting for age and sex. The ratio increased to 1.35 after adjusting for other comorbidities related to coronary heart disease, including hypertension, diabetes, obesity, chronic kidney disease, gout, dyslipidemia, and tobacco use [36]. A case-control study conducted by Aydin et al indicated that patients with calcium oxalate nephrolithiasis exhibited a higher Framingham and Systemic Coronary Risk Evaluation (SCORE) scores compared with the age- and sex-matched controls [37]. They suggested that patients with calcium oxalate urolithiasis were at a higher risk of cardiovascular disease and mortality. However, the significant relationship is inconsistent with the findings of other studies. Tang et al examined the relationship between kidney stone disease, all-cause mortality, and CV mortality among US-diagnosed adults by analyzing data from the Third National Health and Nutrition Examination Survey for 1988–1994. However, no independent association of prevalent kidney stone disease with all-cause and CV mortality was identified [38]. A recent large-scale prospective study conducted in the United States employed data from patients (45 748 men, 196 357 women) with no history of CHD at the baseline. These patients had participated in the Health Professionals Follow-up Study, Nurses' Health Study I (NHS I) (90 235 women, age = 30–55 y; follow-up period from 1992 to 2010), and Nurses' Health Study II (NHS II) (106 122 women, age = 25–42 y; follow-up period from 1991 to 2009) to examine the association between a history of kidney stones and the risk of coronary artery disease. After adjusting for potential confounders, the women with a reported history of kidney stones exhibited an increased risk of CHD compared with those with no history in the NHS I (IR = 754 vs 514 per 100 000 person-y; multivariable HR = 1.18; 95% CI = 1.08–1.28) and NHS II (IR = 144 vs 55 per 100 000 person-y; multivariable HR = 1.48; 95% CI = 1.23–1.78). No significant association was observed for men (IR = 1355 vs 1022 per 100 000 person-y; multivariable HR = 1.06; 95% CI = 0.99–1.13) [39]. The results suggested that compared with men, women had a higher probability of being exposed to unknown factors that could increase their risk of cardiovascular disease and kidney stones [39]. However, their study had some limitations, including the majority of the participants being Caucasian, and the information on stone composition was limited to the cohort.

The pathomechanisms observed in patients with MS regarding the development of endocrine, vasogenic, and renal disarrangement are speculated to be involved in the pathology of ACS and US. After adjusting for medical co-morbidities related to MS, US remains an independent risk factor for subsequent ACS; thus, we hypothesized that traditional herbal medicine consumed by patients with US might contribute to stone formation. Stoller et al hypothesized that the pathogenesis of stones might be vascular injury to the vasa recta near the renal papilla [40]. They asserted that repairing damaged vessel walls could involve an atherosclerotic-like reaction that results in calcification of the endothelial wall, which then erodes into the papillary interstitium and the collecting ducts, contributing to stone formation [40]. The findings of this investigation present a potential relationship between US and ACS, which has not yet been thoroughly examined. Unlike previous studies, we examined not only nephrolithiasis, but also other stone diseases of the ureter and bladder. We believe that these results support the findings of other clinical or basic studies, and recommend further investigation to understand the underling mechanisms.

Although the population-based design is a major strength of this research, several limitations require consideration. First, the diagnoses of US and ACS relied on administrative claims data reported by physicians and hospitals. These might be less accurate than diagnoses made according to standardized criteria. Second, information on the lifestyle or behavior of patients is lacking in the NHIRD; thus, it was impossible to adjust for health- and behavior-related factors such as smoking, alcohol consumption, dietary habits, exercise, and BMI, which are known risk factors for ACS. These behaviors are also indicated to be independent but modifiable risk factors for ACS. However, we lacked information on the chewing of betel quid, which has been reported to increase the incidence of hypercalciuria and hypocitraturia. Third, treatment information is not included in the database, and preventive medication for US-diagnosed patients might interfere with the possible relationship between US and ACS. Finally, this investigation might have been subject to surveillance bias because patients with US typically visit physicians more frequently than other patients do. Thus, their increased exposure to the medical care system could lead to early detection of ACS. This would also contribute to an ascertainment bias, in which patients without US might have been less likely to be included as ACS cases than patients with US were. Despite our meticulous research design and adequate control of confounding factors, a crucial limitation was that biases might have remained because of potential unmeasured or unknown confounders. Overall, our results indicate that patients with US have a comparatively higher risk of developing ACS.

In conclusion, we provide large-scale data evaluating the relationship between US and the risk of developing ACS, particularly among young (≤49 years) and male adults. Future studies should examine age differences as a possible mechanism of US-related ACS morbidity by conducting multicenter recruitment and measurements of laboratory data.

Author Contributions

Conceived and designed the experiments: S-FH C-YH C-LL S-DC C-JC C-HK C-HC. Performed the experiments: S-FH C-YH C-LL S-DC C-JC C-HK C-HC. Analyzed the data: C-JC C-HK. Contributed reagents/materials/analysis tools: S-FH C-YH C-LL S-DC C-JC C-HK C-HC. Wrote the manuscript: S-FH C-YH C-LL S-DC C-JC C-HK C-HC.

References

1. Findlay IN, Cunningham AD (2005) Definition of acute coronary syndrome. Heart 91: 857–9.
2. Libby P (2013) Mechanisms of acute coronary syndromes and their implications for therapy. The New England journal of medicine 368: 2004–13.
3. Gumina RJ (2007) New trials and therapies for acute myocardial infarction. The Medical clinics of North America 91: 729–49; xii.
4. Smith SC, Jr., Feldman TE, Hirshfeld JW Jr., Jacobs AK, Kern MJ, et al. (2006) ACC/AHA/SCAI 2005 guideline update for percutaneous coronary intervention: a report of the American College of Cardiology/American Heart Association Task Force on Practice Guidelines (ACC/AHA/SCAI Writing Committee to Update the 2001 Guidelines for Percutaneous Coronary Intervention). Journal of the American College of Cardiology 47: e1–121.
5. Meigs JB (2003) Epidemiology of cardiovascular complications in type 2 diabetes mellitus. Acta diabetologica 40 Suppl 2: S358–61.

6. Stamler J, Vaccaro O, Neaton JD, Wentworth D (1993) Diabetes, other risk factors, and 12-yr cardiovascular mortality for men screened in the Multiple Risk Factor Intervention Trial. Diabetes care 16: 434–44.
7. Teo KK, Ounpuu S, Hawken S, Pandey MR, Valentin V, et al. (2006) Tobacco use and risk of myocardial infarction in 52 countries in the INTERHEART study: a case-control study. Lancet 368: 647–58.
8. Verschuren WM, Jacobs DR, Bloemberg BP, Kromhout D, Menotti A, et al. (1995) Serum total cholesterol and long-term coronary heart disease mortality in different cultures. Twenty-five-year follow-up of the seven countries study. JAMA: the journal of the American Medical Association 274: 131–6.
9. Scales CD, Jr., Smith AC, Hanley JM, Saigal CS, Urologic Diseases in America P (2012) Prevalence of kidney stones in the United States. European urology 62: 160–5.
10. Borghi L, Meschi T, Guerra A, Briganti A, Schianchi T, et al. (1999) Essential arterial hypertension and stone disease. Kidney international 55: 2397–406.
11. Cappuccio FP, Strazzullo P, Mancini M (1990) Kidney stones and hypertension: population based study of an independent clinical association. Bmj 300: 1234–6.
12. Chung SD, Chen YK, Lin HC (2011) Increased risk of diabetes in patients with urinary calculi: a 5-year followup study. The Journal of urology 186: 1888–93.
13. Gillen DL, Coe FL, Worcester EM (2005) Nephrolithiasis and increased blood pressure among females with high body mass index. American journal of kidney diseases: the official journal of the National Kidney Foundation 46: 263–9.
14. Sakhaee K, Capolongo G, Maalouf NM, Pasch A, Moe OW, et al. (2012) Metabolic syndrome and the risk of calcium stones. Nephrology, dialysis, transplantation: official publication of the European Dialysis and Transplant Association - European Renal Association 27: 3201–9.
15. Taylor EN, Stampfer MJ, Curhan GC (2005) Diabetes mellitus and the risk of nephrolithiasis. Kidney international 68: 1230–5.
16. Ford ES, Giles WH, Mokdad AH (2004) Increasing prevalence of the metabolic syndrome among u.s. Adults. Diabetes care 27: 2444–9.
17. Huang PL (2009) A comprehensive definition for metabolic syndrome. Disease models & mechanisms 2: 231–7.
18. Pak CY, Sakhaee K, Moe O, Preminger GM, Poindexter JR, et al. (2003) Biochemical profile of stone-forming patients with diabetes mellitus. Urology 61: 523–7.
19. Sakhaee K, Adams-Huet B, Moe OW, Pak CY (2002) Pathophysiologic basis for normouricosuric uric acid nephrolithiasis. Kidney international 62: 971–9.
20. National Health Insurance Research Database (2010) Introduction to the National Health Insurance Research Database (NHIRD), Taiwan. http://w3.nhri.org.tw/nhird//date_01.html.
21. West B, Luke A, Durazo-Arvizu RA, Cao G, Shoham D, et al. (2008) Metabolic syndrome and self-reported history of kidney stones: the National Health and Nutrition Examination Survey (NHANES III) 1988–1994. American journal of kidney diseases: the official journal of the National Kidney Foundation 51: 741–7.
22. Reiner AP, Kahn A, Eisner BH, Pletcher MJ, Sadetsky N, et al. (2011) Kidney stones and subclinical atherosclerosis in young adults: the CARDIA study. The Journal of urology 185: 920–5.
23. Jeong IG, Kang T, Bang JK, Park J, Kim W, et al. (2011) Association between metabolic syndrome and the presence of kidney stones in a screened population. American journal of kidney diseases: the official journal of the National Kidney Foundation 58: 383–8.
24. Kohjimoto Y, Sasaki Y, Iguchi M, Matsumura N, Inagaki T, et al. (2013) Association of metabolic syndrome traits and severity of kidney stones: results from a nationwide survey on urolithiasis in Japan. American journal of kidney diseases: the official journal of the National Kidney Foundation 61: 923–9.
25. Weinberg AE, Patel CJ, Chertow GM, Leppert JT (2014) Diabetic severity and risk of kidney stone disease. European urology 65: 242–7.
26. Gorbachinsky I, Akpinar H, Assimos DG (2010) Metabolic syndrome and urologic diseases. Reviews in urology 12: e157–80.
27. Sakhaee K (2008) Nephrolithiasis as a systemic disorder. Current opinion in nephrology and hypertension 17: 304–9.
28. Worcester EM, Gillen DL, Evan AP, Parks JH, Wright K, et al. (2007) Evidence that postprandial reduction of renal calcium reabsorption mediates hypercalciuria of patients with calcium nephrolithiasis. American journal of physiology Renal physiology 292: F66–75.
29. Cameron MA, Maalouf NM, Adams-Huet B, Moe OW, Sakhaee K (2006) Urine composition in type 2 diabetes: predisposition to uric acid nephrolithiasis. Journal of the American Society of Nephrology: JASN 17: 1422–8.
30. Daudon M, Traxer O, Conort P, Lacour B, Jungers P (2006) Type 2 diabetes increases the risk for uric acid stones. Journal of the American Society of Nephrology: JASN 17: 2026–33.
31. Rendina D, Mossetti G, De Filippo G, Benvenuto D, Vivona CL, et al. (2009) Association between metabolic syndrome and nephrolithiasis in an inpatient population in southern Italy: role of gender, hypertension and abdominal obesity. Nephrology, dialysis, transplantation: official publication of the European Dialysis and Transplant Association - European Renal Association 24: 900–6.
32. Maalouf NM, Cameron MA, Moe OW, Adams-Huet B, Sakhaee K (2007) Low urine pH: a novel feature of the metabolic syndrome. Clinical journal of the American Society of Nephrology: CJASN 2: 883–8.
33. Eisner BH, Porten SP, Bechis SK, Stoller ML (2010) Diabetic kidney stone formers excrete more oxalate and have lower urine pH than nondiabetic stone formers. The Journal of urology 183: 2244–8.
34. Abate N, Chandalia M, Cabo-Chan AV, Jr., Moe OW, Sakhaee K (2004) The metabolic syndrome and uric acid nephrolithiasis: novel features of renal manifestation of insulin resistance. Kidney international 65: 386–92.
35. Domingos F, Serra A (2011) Nephrolithiasis is associated with an increased prevalence of cardiovascular disease. Nephrology, dialysis, transplantation: official publication of the European Dialysis and Transplant Association - European Renal Association 26: 864–8.
36. Rule AD, Roger VL, Melton LJ, 3rd, Bergstralh EJ, Li X, et al. (2010) Kidney stones associate with increased risk for myocardial infarction. Journal of the American Society of Nephrology: JASN 21: 1641–4.
37. Aydin H, Yencilek F, Erihan IB, Okan B, Sarica K (2011) Increased 10-year cardiovascular disease and mortality risk scores in asymptomatic patients with calcium oxalate urolithiasis. Urological research 39: 451–8.
38. Tang J, Mettler P, McFann K, Chonchol M (2013) The association of prevalent kidney stone disease with mortality in US adults: the National Health and Nutrition Examination Survey III, 1988–1994. American journal of nephrology 37: 501–6.
39. Ferraro PM, Taylor EN, Eisner BH, Gambaro G, Rimm EB, et al. (2013) History of kidney stones and the risk of coronary heart disease. JAMA: the journal of the American Medical Association 310: 408–15.
40. Stoller ML, Meng MV, Abrahams HM, Kane JP (2004) The primary stone event: a new hypothesis involving a vascular etiology. The Journal of urology 171: 1920–4.

7

Insulin Dynamics in Young Women with Polycystic Ovary Syndrome and Normal Glucose Tolerance across Categories of Body Mass Index

Melania Manco[1]*, Lidia Castagneto-Gissey[2], Eugenio Arrighi[2], Annamaria Carnicelli[2], Claudia Brufani[1], Rosa Luciano[1], Geltrude Mingrone[2]

1 Research Unit for Multi-factorial Diseases, Obesity and Diabetes, Scientific Directorate, Bambino Gesù Children Hospital, Rome, Italy, **2** Department of Internal Medicine, Catholic University, School of Medicine, Rome, Italy

Abstract

Background: Evidence favours insulin resistance and compensatory hyperinsulinemia as the predominant, perhaps primary, defects in polycystic ovary syndrome (PCOS). The aim of the present study was to evaluate insulin metabolism in young women with PCOS but normal glucose tolerance as compared with age, body mass index and insulin resistance-matched controls to answer the question whether women with PCOS hypersecrete insulin in comparison to appropriately insulin resistance-matched controls.

Research Design and Methods: Sixty-nine cases were divided according to their body mass index (BMI) in normal-weight (N = 29), overweight (N = 24) and obese patients (N = 16). Controls were 479 healthy women (age 16–49 y). Whole body Insulin Sensitivity (WBISI), fasting, and total insulin secretion were estimated following an oral glucose tolerance test (C-peptide deconvolution method).

Results: Across classes of BMI, PCOS patients had greater insulin resistance than matched controls ($p<0.0001$ for all the comparisons), but they showed higher fasting and total insulin secretion than their age, BMI and insulin resistance-matched peers ($p<0.0001$ for all the comparisons).

Conclusion: Women with PCOS show higher insulin resistance but also larger insulin secretion to maintain normal glucose homeostasis than age-, BMI- and insulin resistance-matched controls.

Editor: Franco Folli, University of Texas Health Science Center at San Antonio, United States of America

Funding: Melania Manco received funds from the Italian Ministry of Health (RF-OPG-2008-1142374; GR-2010 2304957) and from the European Community (FP7-ICT-2012-600932 MD PAEDIGREE; FP7-ICT-2012-610440 DAPHNE). The funders had no role in study design, data collection and analysis, decision to publish, or preparation of the manuscript.

* E-mail: melania.manco@opbg.net

Introduction

Polycystic ovary syndrome (PCOS) occurs in about 10% of women of reproductive age, thus representing one of the commonest endocrine disorders in women [1]. The syndrome is defined, after excluding other disorders which might present in a similar fashion, by occurrence of two of the following three features: i) oligo- or anovulation, ii) clinical and/or biochemical signs of hyperandrogenism, and iii) polycystic ovaries [2].

Severe insulin resistance characterises up to 90% of women with PCOS beyond that predicted by their body mass index (BMI) [2–4]. Indeed, even lean women with PCOS have elevated insulin resistance compared with BMI-matched controls [5].

As a consequence of highly common severe insulin resistance, the risk of impaired glucose tolerance (IGT) and type 2 diabetes mellitus (T2DM) in patients with PCOS significantly exceeds estimates of diabetes in the normal population [6]. Nevertheless, progression from insulin resistance to diabetes requires impaired β-cell function.

As regards insulin secretion, many studies have examined β-cell function in PCOS, but thus far, the results are equivocal. Studies have shown that there is a defect in the glucose-stimulated insulin secretion [7–9], but other studies have found that insulin response is enhanced in women with PCOS, likely as compensation for the peripheral insulin resistance [10–12].

Excess body weight in women with PCOS may accelerate progression toward diabetes by exacerbating both insulin resistance and inappropriate insulin-response. In a longitudinal study of 25 women with PCOS, the BMI of those whose glucose tolerance deteriorated was significantly higher than that of the group whose glucose tolerance improved or remained stable [13].

It is, thus, likely that obesity acts in concert with the intrinsic and apparently distinctive defects in insulin action of women with PCOS to enhance the risk of diabetes. However, no data have been provided on the effect of BMI on the compensatory insulin response, particularly in patients with a normal body weight.

Aim of the present investigation was to assess insulin resistance and compensatory insulin secretion by means of the oral glucose tolerance test (OGTT) in a sample of young PCOS women as compared to a large sample of age and body mass index matched controls. All cases and controls had normal glucose tolerance (NGT) and their BMI ranged from normality to severe obesity.

Methods

A total of 69 women with clinical and hormonal evidence of PCOS were recruited at the Department of Internal Medicine, Catholic School of Medicine in Rome. All women had a standard oral glucose tolerance test (OGTT) with measurement of glucose, insulin and c-peptide levels at every 30 min time-point. They had normal fasting glucose (<5.6 mmol/l) and glucose tolerance (≤ 7.8 mmol/l at 2 h) [14].

PCOS was diagnosed in presence of at least two out of the three diagnostic criteria established by the revised 2003 Rotterdam European Society for Human Reproduction/American Society of Reproductive Medicine PCOS Consensus Workshop Group: i) oligo- and/or anovulation, ii) clinical and/or biochemical signs of hyperandrogenism, and iii) polycystic ovaries [2].

A pregnancy test was ordered on all subjects and none was found to be pregnant. The amount of excess terminal hair growth was first assessed using the modified Ferriman-Gallwey (mF-G) method, scoring the presence of terminal hairs over nine body areas (*i.e.* upper lip, chin, chest, upper and lower abdomen, thighs, upper and lower back, and upper arms) from 0 to 4. To maximize the accuracy of hirsutism scoring, subjects were examined by two physicians (EA & GM). Hirsutism was diagnosed by the presence of mF-G score ≥6 [15].

The presence of acne was also recorded, although no specific scoring system was used.

The study was performed in the early follicular phase (*i.e.* between d 2 and 5 after the last menstrual period). In oligo- or amenorrheic patients, the last menstrual period was either spontaneous or induced by the administration of didrogesterone (10 mg/d for 7 d).

Other endocrinopathies were ruled out by measuring thyroid stimulating hormone, basal serum 17-hydroxyprogesterone, prolactin, and 24 hour urine free cortisol levels. Exclusion criteria included age>50y, known cardiovascular disease, immune and non immune thyroid disease, neoplasm, current smoking, impaired glucose tolerance or diabetes, hypertension (blood pressure, BP, >135/85 mmHg), liver dysfunction, and renal impairment. None of the patients had taken any of the following medications for at least 6 months prior to enrolment in the study: hormonal contraceptives, glucocorticoids, ovulation induction agents, antidiabetic or antiobesity drugs, estrogenic, antiandrogenic, or antihypertensive medications.

Healthy normal-weight volunteers were recruited among medical students, young physicians, and nurses as normal-weight controls. Overweight/obese subjects with no evidence PCOS were recruited from those at their first referral to the Department of Internal Medicine at the Catholic University or the Research Unit for Multifactorial Disease at the Bambino Gesù Hospital for overweight/obesity. They were all free of medication despite severe obesity.

Most of the controls have been enrolled in previous studies [16–19] and were women aged 16–49 y on free diet, with regular menses, no clinical signs of hyperandrogenism (either hirsutism, acne or alopecia) or ultrasound evidence of polycystic ovaries; no systemic/endocrine disease including thyroid disease, no use of medication (including lipid lowering drugs, antihypertensive and insulin sensitizer agents or any medication able to interfere with glucose metabolism), no impaired fasting glucose or glucose intolerance. In all cases and controls, overweight was defined as a BMI ≥25.0 kg/m^2 and obesity as a BMI ≥30 kg/m^2.

The study was approved by the Institutional Review Board at the Catholic School of Medicine. It was conducted in accordance with the Declaration of Helsinki for research in human beings. All patients provided written informed consent prior to study participation. For adolescent girls, written full informed consent was obtained from parents/tutors and written assent absence from patient.

Oral Glucose Tolerance Test and Insulin Metabolism

Blood samples were obtained at baseline and at 30-min intervals for 2 h for measurement of glucose, insulin and c-peptide after ingestion of the glucose load. Insulin resistance was estimated by the homeostasis model of insulin resistance (HOMA-IR; www.dtu.ox.ac.uk/homa) and the Whole-Body Insulin Sensitivity Index (WBISI) [20]. Area under the glucose and the insulin curves were calculated by using the trapezoidal curve. The insulin secretion-sensitivity index-2 (ISSI-2) was calculated as the ratio of the area-under-the-insulin-curve to the area-under-the-glucose curve, multiplied by the Matsuda index [21]. β-cell function was assessed from the OGTT using the C-peptide deconvolution method [22] which provides estimation of both fasting and total insulin secretion and normalized for the body surface area. Total insulin secretion was normalized for a value of WBISI of 5 in order to allow the comparison of insulin secretion between cases and controls with different degree of insulin sensitivity.

Analytical Methods

Serum concentrations of FSH, LH, estradiol (E2), testosteron (T), androstenedione (A), dehydroepiandrosterone sulphate (DHEAS), 17-hydroxyprogesterone (17-OHP), and Sex Hormone Binding Globulin (SHBG) were all assayed by commercially available radioimmunoassays (RIA; Radim, Pomezia, and Ares Serono, Milan, Italy). Samples were immediately processed in a refrigerated centrifuge and stored at −20°C until assay. The intra-assay and inter-assay coefficients of variation obtained were ≤9% for all variables. The free androgen index (FAI) was calculated by the formula: (total T/SHBG)×100. Serum AMH concentrations were determined by enzyme immunoassay (Immunotech–Beckman-Coulter, Fullerton, CA).

Serum glucose, insulin and c-peptide were analyzed at the Catholic University in all subjects. Glucose was measured by the glucose oxidase method (Beckman, Fullerton, CA). Insulin was assayed by microparticle enzyme immunoassay (MEIA; Abbott, Pasadena, CA) with a sensitivity of 1 μU/ml and an intra-assay coefficient of variation (CV) of 6.6%. C-peptide was assayed by radioimmunoassay (MYRIA; Technogenetics, Milan, Italy); this assay has a minimal detectable concentration of 17 pmol/l and intra-assay and interassay CVs of 3.3–5.7 and 4.6–5.3, respectively. Triglycerides, total and high-density lipoprotein (HDL) cholesterol were measured by using commercial methods (ADVIA 2400 Chemistry System, Siemens Healthcare Diagnostic, and Deerfield, IL).

Statistical Analysis and Data Analysis

Continuous data are reported as means and standard deviations, with categorical data as counts and percentages. The Mann Whitney U-test and the nonparametric Spearman correlation coefficient were used for comparisons and correlations. The

Table 1. Anthropometrics, laboratory and insulin metabolism related parameters of controls and PCOS patients according to the obesity status.

	Normal weight women			Overweight women			Obese women		
	Controls	PCOS	P	Controls	PCOS	p	Controls	PCOS	p
N	271	29		151	24		57	16	
Age (years)	25.8±3.4	25.2±4.7	0.09	25.5±3.52	25.1±6.21	0.2	25.3±5.13	28.75±8.5	0.1
BMI (kg/m^2)	21.5±1.8	21.1±1.8	0.3	26.5±1.7	26.6±1.7	0.8	34.3±4.3	37.4±6.6	0.06
Waist circumference (cm)	70.6±6.7	73.1±6.9	0.2	85.2±8.6	90.4±9.6	0.08	97.6±8.6	107.5±12.4	0.01
Total cholesterol (mmol/l)	4.23±0.6	4.53±0.8	0.03	4.44±0.8	4.61±0.8	0.3	4.66±0.83	4.82±0.93	0.6
HDL-cholesterol (mmol/l)	1.67±0.37	1.64±0.28	0.7	1.47±0.33	1.44±0.39	0.9	1.36±0.34	1.24±0.21	0.3
LDL-cholesterol (mmol/l)	2.32±0.63	2.5±0.72	0.2	2.72±0.76	2.53±0.82	0.3	2.89±0.86	3.09±0.86	0.2
Triglycerides (mmol/l)	0.62±0.35	0.78±0.34	<0.0001	0.93±0.47	1.03±0.73	0.9	1.03±0.45	1.22±0.63	0.3
Fasting glucose (mmol/l)	4.73±0.51	4.8±0.36	0.7	4.94±0.48	4.91±0.47	0.7	4.90±0.45	5.13±0.59	0.4
Fasting Insulin (μUI/ml)	4.38±2.23	9.41±4.08	<0.0001	6.59±6.58	11.13±3.67	<0.0001	12.26±8.25	20.63±9.61	<0.0001
2 hour glucose (mmol/l)	5.11±0.96	5.22±1.15	0.6	5.37±1.05	5.36±1.17	0.9	5.79±1.21	5.84±1.14	0.9
HOMA-IR	0.91±0.49	2.01±0.89	<0.0001	1.36±0.65	2.43±0.86	<0.0001	2.19±1.09	4.77±2.62	<0.0001
WBISI	12.8±5.9	6.8±2.95	<0.0001	9.09±4.16	5.31±1.80	<0.0001	5.73±3.24	3.14±1.76	<0.0001
Fasting insulin secretion (pmol min^{-1}m^{-2})	61.55±22.2	82.1±26.8	<0.0001	74.29±25.7	94.92±28.0	0.001	114.9±37.7	157.8±51.2	<0.0001
Total insulin secretion (nmol m^{-2})	37.9±12.1	60±23.6	<0.0001	39.1±11.8	53.95±14	<0.0001	52±16.5	69.8±21.6	<0.0001
AUC insulin (μUI/ml min^{-1})	50.6±36.9	197±109.1	<0.0001	54.9±22.3	240.5±116.9	<0.0001	96.15±62.3	381±227.6	<0.0001
Total Insulin Secretion@5WBISI (nmol m^{-2})	0.80±0.72	2.48±2.45	<0.0001	1.14±0.85	2.36±1.16	<0.0001	2.44±1.68	6.08±4.04	<0.0001
ISSI-2	2.71±1.1	2.37±1	0.4	2.36±1.03	2.14±0.70	0.3	1.98±0.79	1.82±0.63	0.7

Data are expressed as mean ± SD. *P* refers to statistical significance at the Mann-Whitney U test within groups of normal-weight, overweight and obese women. BMI, body Mass Index; HDL, High density lipoprotein; HOMA-IR, Homeostasis Model Assessment of Insulin Resistance; LDL, Low density lipoprotein; WBISI, Whole Body Insulin Sensitivity Index; ISSI-2, Insulin Secretion-Sensitivity Index-2; Total Insulin, Total insulin secretion at a WBISI of 5.

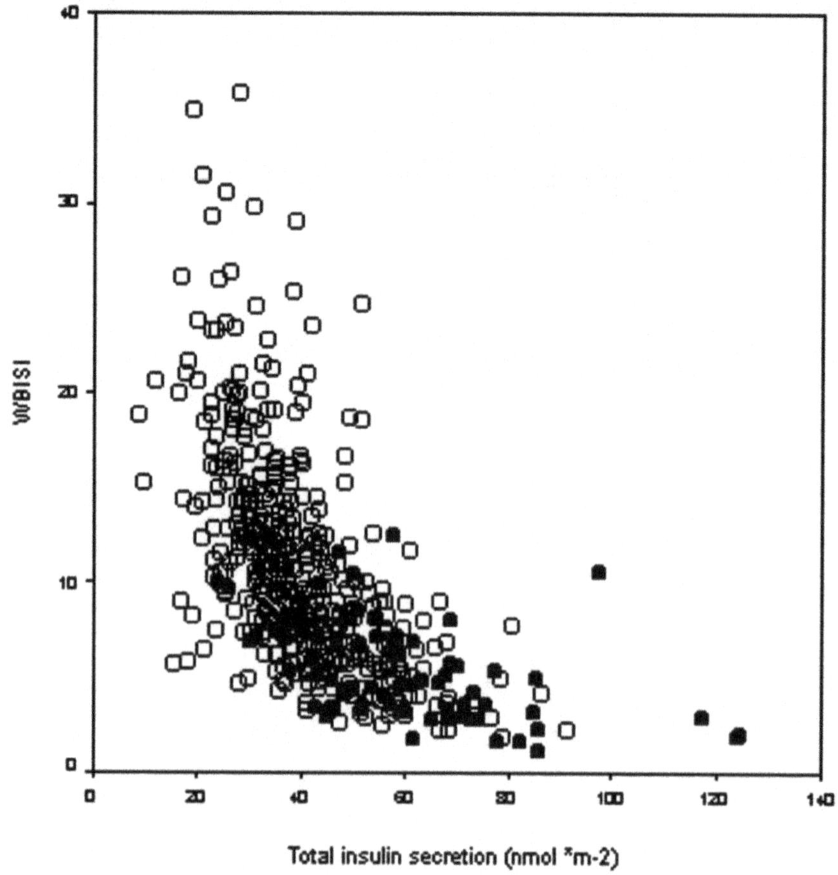

Figure 1. Relationship between insulin sensitivity and secretion in cases and controls. Scatter plot of the relationship between whole body insulin sensitivity (WBISI) and Total insulin secretion in controls (empty circles) and patients with PCOS (filled circles).

ANOVA analysis was used for comparisons among normal-weight, overweight and obese cases.

The *p* value was set as statistically significant at $p<0.05$.

Data analysis was performed by using SPSS statistical software (SPSS V17.0, Inc., Chicago, IL).

Results

Patients were 69 young women (age 16–49 y, BMI 16.1–53.3 kg/m^2); controls were 479 women of matched age (25.7±3.7 y). Among cases, 29 women were normal-weight, 24 overweight and 16 were obese patients. Controls were 271 normal-weight, 151 overweight and 57 obese women. **Tables 1** illustrates anthropometrics, laboratory parameters, and values of insulin metabolism in cases and controls according to their obesity status. In PCOS patients, HOMA-IR, WBISI, fasting and total insulin secretion, ISSI-2 were all statistically different respect with values observed in controls belonging to the different BMI groups.

Regards cases, 66 patients (95.6%) presented with hirsutism, which was equally distributed across classes of BMI; 38 (55%) had acne and 7 (10%) alopecia. The mean m-FG was 14.2±5.3. Oligo/anovulation was diagnosed in 48 cases (69.6%) and ultrasound evidence of polycystic ovaries was observed in 39 cases (56.3%). At the ANOVA, obese cases were the oldest ($p=0.02$), presented with the highest concentrations of SHBG ($p=0.012$); fasting insulin ($p<0.0001$), FAI ($p=0.023$); the worst lipid profile (HDL cholesterol, $p<0.0001$; LDL-cholesterol, $p=0.007$; and triglycerides, $p=0.009$), insulin action (HOMA-IR and WBISI, $p<0.00001$ for both); and the highest fasting insulin secretion ($p<0.0001$).

Figure 1 shows the relationship between WBISI and total insulin secretion in cases and controls.

To further assess whether insulin hypersecretion in PCOS patients results from increased insulin resistance, control and PCOS women were successively defined as insulin sensitive or resistant by using tertiles of both HOMA-IR and WBISI in controls (insulin resistance as HOMA-IR≥1.26 and WBISI<7.91). Accordingly, 98.6% of PCOS patients were resistant having HOMA-IR≥1.26 and 81.2% with WBISI <7.91. **Figure 2** shows in control and PCOS women values of fasting and total insulin secretion in the groups of women insulin resistant according to the HOMA-IR index (panel A); in insulin sensitive (panel B) and insulin resistant women (panel C) according to the values of WBISI.

Mean concentrations of androgens and sex hormones were as it follows: A_4 227.4±36.2 ng/dl; AMH 7.40±3.2 ng/ml; T 6.65±4.43 ng/dl; DHEAs 249.7±113.4 μg/dl; E_2 99.4±68.3 pg/ml; FAI 6.65±7.4 ng/100 ml; LH 5.4±3.08 IU/l; FSH 4.45±1.78 IU/l; LH/FSH 1.24±0.56; SHBG 45.15±36.2 nmol/l.

Correlation Analysis

In cases, fasting insulin secretion and WBISI were significantly correlated with BMI ($r_o=0.571$; $p<0.0001$ and $r_o=-0.520$; $p<0.0001$, respectively) and waist circumference ($r_o=0.687$; $p<0.0001$, and $r_o=-0.590$; $p<0.0001$). **Table 2** reports correlation

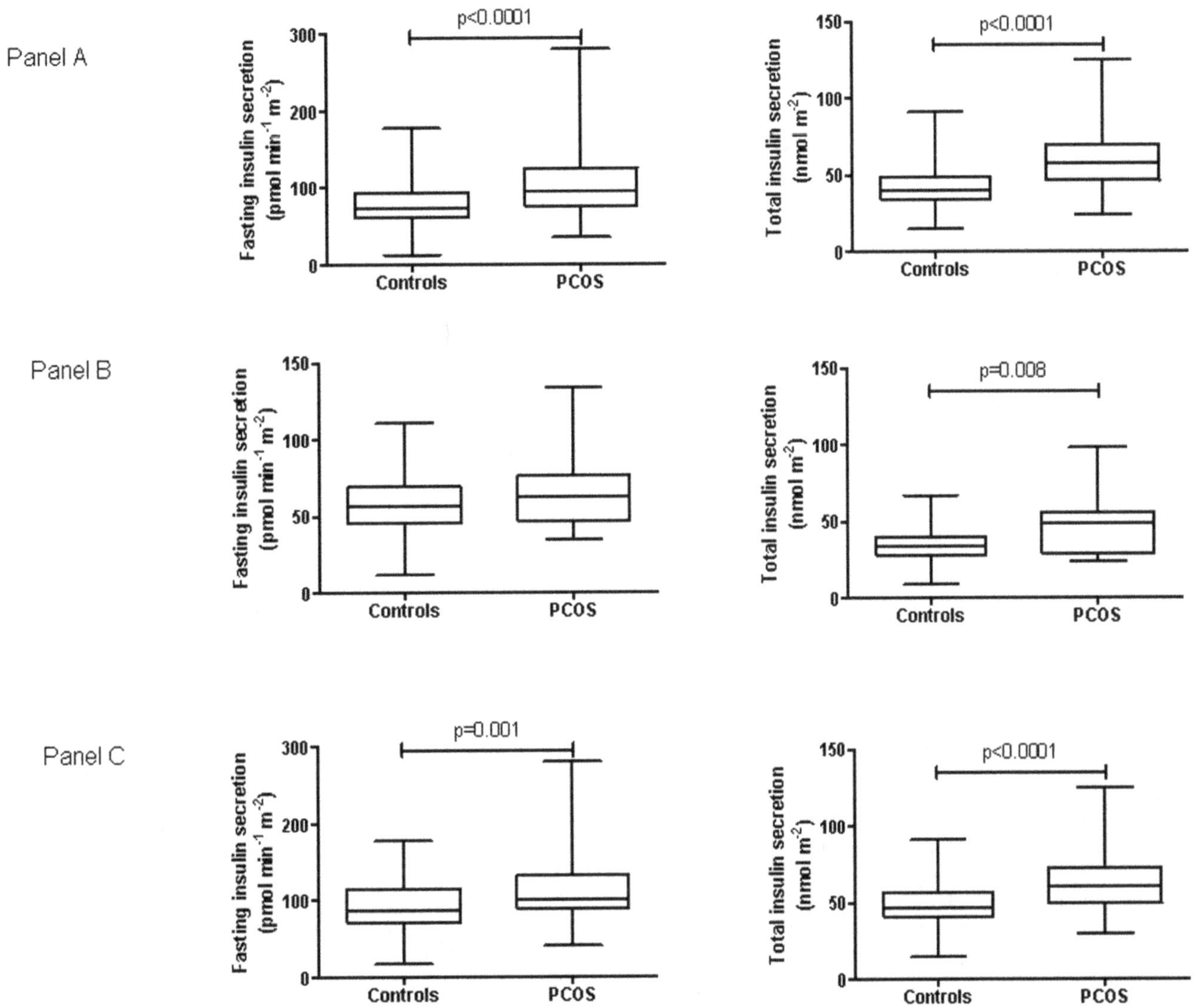

Figure 2. Insulin secretion in insulin sensitive and resistant cases and controls. Fasting and total insulin secretion (box and whiskers, min to max) in control and PCOS women having insulin resistance defined as HOMA-IR ≥1.26 (panel A); insulin sensitivity defined as WBISI ≥7.91 (panel B) and insulin resistance as WBISI<7.91 (panel C).

coefficients of androgens and sex hormone with BMI, HOMA-IR, WBISI, fasting and total insulin secretion, ISSI-2.

In controls, fasting and total insulin secretion were significantly correlated with BMI ($r_o = 0.443$; $p<0.0001$; $r_o = 0.230$; $p<0.0001$) and waist circumference ($r_o = 0.429$; $p<0.0001$; $r_o = 0.175$; $p<0.0001$). WBISI was correlated with BMI ($r_o = -0.482$; $p<0.0001$) and waist ($r_o = 0.477$; $p<0.0001$). ISSI-2 was correlated with waist ($r_o = 0.776$; $p<0.0001$).

Furthermore, multivariate analysis was performed. Fasting secretion was predicted ($r^2 = 0.46$; $p<0.0001$) by having PCOS (coefficient 17; 95%CI 10.5–2.35), being obese (coefficient 15.7; 95%CI 12.3–19), and insulin resistant (coefficient 26.9; 95%CI 22–31.8); total insulin secretion by having PCOS (coefficient 14; 95%CI 10.8–17.4), and being insulin resistant. (coefficient 13.6; 95%CI 11.1–16).

Discussion

Young women with polycystic ovary syndrome but normal glucose tolerance are able to compensate for severe insulin resistance with enhanced β-cell function. They are less insulin sensitive but able to release much more insulin following the glucose ingestion than age and BMI matched controls **(Figure 1)**. Indeed, insulin secretion was normalized for a fixed value of WBISI to take into account differences in insulin sensitivity between PCOS patients and controls and the former hyper-secreted insulin in comparison with insulin-resistance matched control women.

Among the three groups of patients with PCOS differing by the obesity status, lipid profile and insulin action worsened and β-cell insulin release increased significantly with the increasing BMI (**Table 1**). In our series, the use of a glucose disposition index (the ISSI-2) provides an estimate of β-cell functionality relative to the prevailing level of insulin resistance. Moreover, we normalised total insulin secretion by the fixed value of insulin sensitivity of 5 to compare secretion among cases and controls with different BMI. Furthermore, when control and PCOS women were divided as insulin sensitive or resistant according to tertiles of HOMA-IR or

Table 2. Coefficients of correlation in patients with PCOS.

	Body weight	HOMA-IR	WBISI	Fasting insulin secretion	Total Insulin secretion	ISSI-2
A_4	0.131 $P=0.302$	**0.377 $p=0.006$**	**−0.395 $p=0.001$**	**0.252 $p=0.045$**	0.208 $p=0.09$	0.006 $p=0.962$
AMH	−0.231 $P=0.1$	−0.137 $p=0.334$	0.142 $p=0.317$	−0.157 $p=0.266$	−0.055 $p=0.701$	0.006 $p=0.966$
DHEAS	0.183 $p=0.13$	0.168 $p=0.174$	**−0.256 $p=0.037$**	0.122 $p=0.325$	0.189 $p=125$	0.140 $p=0.259$
E_2	−0.037 $p=0.771$	−0.106 $p=0.399$	0.022 $p=0.859$	−0.90 $p=0.473$	0.084 $p=0.504$	−0.10 $p=0.934$
FAI	**0.472 $P<0.0001$**	**0.503 $p<0.0001$**	**−0.606 $p<0.0001$**	**0.494 $p<0.0001$**	**0.459 $p<0.0001$**	−0.075 $p=0.546$
FSH	−0.068 $p=0.623$	**0.269 $p=0.047$**	−0.257 $p=0.06$	0.150 $p=0.447$	0.004 $p=0.974$	−0.281 $p=0.083$
LH	0.122 $p=0.623$	**0.322 $p=0.016$**	**−0.298 $p=0.03$**	**0.378 $p=0.004$**	0.244 $p=0.07$	−0.234 $p=0.03$
LH/FSH	0.124 $p=0.377$	0.173 $p=0.216$	−0.175 $p=0.209$	**0.273 $p=0.048$**	**0.366 $p=0.007$**	−0.109 $p=0.439$
SHBG	**−0.546 $P<0.0001$**	**−0.555 $p<0.0001$**	**0.566 $p<0.0001$**	**−0.574 $p<0.0001$**	**−0.359 $p=0.003$**	0.034 $p=0.784$
T	**0.472 $P<0.0001$**	**0.503 $p<0.0001$**	**−0.606 $p<0.0001$**	**0.494 $p<0.0001$**	**0.459 $p<0.0001$**	−0.75 $p=0.546$

A4, Androstenedione; AMH, Anti-Mullerian Hormone; BMI, body Mass Index;
CBG, Cortisol Binding Globulin; DHEAS, Dehydroepiandrosterone sulfate; E2, 17β-estradiol;
HOMA-IR, Homeostasis Model Assessment of Insulin Resistance; LH, Luteinizing Hormone;
FAI, Free androgen index; FSH, follicle-stimulating hormone; T, testosterone; WBISI, Whole Body Insulin Sensitivity Index; ISSI-2, Insulin.

WBISI, PCOS patients showed still higher fasting and total insulin secretion (**Figure 2**).

Past studies that investigated either insulin action by using the euglycemic hyperinsulinemic clamp, which is considered the gold-standard technique to estimate insulin sensitivity, or the intravenous glucose tolerance test (IVGTT) and β-cell function by the c-peptide deconvolution method, provided divergent results.

Indeed, about half of the past clamp studies found preserved insulin sensitivity in normal-weight women with PCOS when compared with weight-matched controls [10–11,23–26], but some other studies reported some degree of insulin resistance [4,13,27–28]. By using the IVGTT, Gennarelli *et al* [25] found in women with PCOS a significant reduction of the glucose effectiveness, *i.e.* the proportion of glucose uptake independent from insulin activity, while insulin sensitivity, i.e. the proportion of glucose uptake dependent of insulin was normal. As reminded by the authors, the clamp cannot discriminate between insulin dependent and insulin independent glucose uptake, but in normal individuals between 30 and 50% of glucose disposal after an oral glucose load depends on glucose effectiveness [29] which represents the major contributor to glucose disappearance in states of severe insulin resistance [30]. Hence, reduced glucose effectiveness in patients with PCOS would support lower insulin sensitivity following the glucose load as we observed in the present investigation.

Some studies that carefully assessed β-cell function have claimed dysfunctional insulin secretion [7,31–32]. Our data do not support dysfunctional insulin secretion, at least in glucose normotolerant cases, as the latter women release much more insulin than age, BMI and insulin resistance-matched controls following the glucose load. Findings from our study are in keeping with results of a previous study which found in PCOS women higher basal and 24 h insulin concentration, reduced insulin clearance and increased secretion by analysis of 24 hour profiles of insulin and c-peptide and hyperglycaemic clamp [31]. While basal insulin secretion was significantly increased as compared to secretion in controls, their incremental insulin response to a meal was significantly reduced. The reduction in the post-meal response resulted from a reduction in the relative amplitude of meal-related secretory pulses rather than from a reduction in the number of pulses [31]. In our series we did not estimate secretory pulses, but both absolute under the insulin curve and incremental areas were significantly greater in patients with PCOS (**Table 1**). At the IVGTT, Hermann *et al* [32] found that the ability of the β-cell to respond to oscillations in plasma glucose is impaired in women with PCOS. Arslanian *et al* [8] studied NGT and IGT PCOS adolescents. They observed not only reduced insulin sensitivity at the euglycemic clamp, but reduced first phase insulin secretion and glucose disposition index and increased hepatic glucose production by the hyperglycaemic clamp but limited to IGT patients. On the contrary, Gennarelli *et al* [25] and Holte *et al* [10]˙ found no significant difference in the acute ("first-phase") insulin response to intravenous glucose administration.

On purpose, we excluded from our investigation women with IGT, who, for sure would present with increased insulin resistance, defective β-cell function and, therefore, reduced glucose disposition index to focus, on the contrary, on NGT women with various BMI, from normal weight to excess weight, to answer the question whether β-cell function is dysfunctional or, conversely, women with PCOS have insulin hypersecretion and to look at the impact of excessive body weight on insulin secretion.

Major drawbacks of our study are due to the cross-sectional design of the study, the small size-sample of cases, the lack of information on body composition and family history on diabetes as it is well accepted that the presence of family history of T2DM in women with PCOS increases the likelihood of inappropriate β-cell compensation for the degree of insulin resistance [32].

If the enrolment exclusively of cases with normal glucose tolerance in our series does not allow comparing our findings with other researchers' results as they enrolled mostly women with altered glucose tolerance, this choice, however, represents the strength of our study. The lesson from PCOS patients with normal glucose tolerance when considering their high risk of diabetes may be that the β-cell of a woman with PCOS is very early challenged by enhanced insulin resistance and obesity exacerbates this load. The β-cell response to such a challenge may result defective in the long-term in those women who are genetically prone to diabetes, but in women who maintain a normal glucose tolerance it seems to be significantly increased.

Regards to the role of excessive androgens in the natural progression from NGT to diabetes in women with PCOS, our findings are confirmatory of the association between A4, free testosterone and SHBG with enhanced insulin resistance [32], but they also suggest that hyperandrogenemia may affect also insulin secretion as FAI and concentration of SHBG were correlated with insulin secretion (**Table 2**). Unfortunately, as the cross-sectional nature of the present study, we could not rule out whether such effect is direct on the β-cell or indirect through increased insulin resistance and whether β-cell becomes impaired with aging.

In conclusion, PCOS patients with normal glucose tolerance are more insulin resistant than controls, their insulin secretion increases in parallel with raised insulin secretion, but, more importantly, they are able to secrete much more insulin than insulin sensitivity matched peers. As expected, increasing BMI exerts a major effect on both insulin resistance and β-cell insulin response, but high levels of androgens seem to affect both sites, i.e. insulin action and insulin secretion, of the glucose metabolism.

Author Contributions

Conceived and designed the experiments: GM. Performed the experiments: LCG EA AMC CB. Analyzed the data: MM. Contributed reagents/materials/analysis tools: RL. Wrote the paper: MM.

References

1. Randeva HS, Tan BK, Weickert MO, Lois K, Nestler JE, et al. (2012) Cardiometabolic Aspects of the Polycystic Ovary Syndrome. Endocr Rev. Oct;33(5): 812–41.
2. The Rotterdam ESHRE/ASRM-Sponsored PCOS consensus workshop group Revised 2003 consensus on diagnostic criteria and long-term health risks related to polycystic ovary syndrome (PCOS) (2003) Human Reproduction. 19: 41–47.
3. Carmina E, Lobo RA (1999) Polycystic ovary syndrome (PCOS): arguably the most common endocrinopathy is associated with significant morbidity in women. JClin Endocrinol Metab. 84: 1897–1899.
4. Dunaif A, Segal KR, Futterweit W, Dobrjansky A (1989) Profound peripheral insulin resistance, independent of obesity, in polycystic ovary syndrome. Diabetes. 38: 1165–1174.
5. Dunaif A (1999) Insulin action in the polycystic ovary syndrome. Endocrinol Metab Clin North Am. 28: 341–359.
6. Legro RS, Kunselman AR, Dunaif A (2001) Prevalence and predictors of dyslipidemia in women with polycystic ovary syndrome. Am J Med. 111: 607–613.
7. Dunaif A, Finegood DT (1996) Beta-cell dysfunction independent of obesity and glucose intolerance in the polycystic ovary syndrome. J Clin Endocrinol Metab. 81: 942–947.
8. Arslanian SA, Lewy VD, Danadian K (2001) Glucose intolerance in obese adolescents with polycystic ovary syndrome: roles of insulin resistance and beta-cell dysfunction and risk of cardiovascular disease. J Clin Endocrinol Metab. 86: 66–71.
9. Ehrmann DA, Barnes RB, Rosenfield RL, Cavaghan MK, Imperial J (1999) Prevalence of impaired glucose tolerance and diabetes in women with polycystic ovary syndrome. Diabetes Care. 22: 141–146.
10. Holte J, Bergh T, Berne C, Wide L, Lithell H (1995) Restored insulin sensitivity but persistently increased early insulin secretion after weight loss in obese women with polycystic ovary syndrome. J Clin Endocrinol Metab. 80: 2586–2593.
11. Morin-Papunen LC, Vauhkonen I, Koivunen RM, Ruokonen A, Tapanainen JS (2000) Insulin sensitivity, insulin secretion, and metabolic and hormonal parameters in healthy women and women with polycystic ovarian syndrome. Hum Reprod. 15: 1266–1274.
12. Vrbikova J, Grimmichova T, Dvorakova K, Hill M, Stanicka S, et al. (2008) Family history of diabetes mellitus determines insulin sensitivity and beta cell function in polycystic ovary syndrome. Physiol Res. 57: 547–553.
13. Dunaif A, Segal KR, Shelley DR, Green G, Dobrjansky A, et al. (1992) Evidence for distinctive and intrinsic defects in insulin action in polycystic ovary syndrome. Diabetes. 41: 1257–1266.
14. American Diabetes Association (2004) Diagnosis and classification of diabetes mellitus. Diabetes Care. 27 Suppl 1: S5–S10.
15. Ferriman DM, Gallwey JD (1961) Clinical assessment of body hair growth in women. J Clin Endocrinol. 21: 1440–1447.
16. Mingrone G, Manco M, Mora ME, Guidone C, Iaconelli A, et al. (2008) Influence of maternal obesity on insulin sensitivity and secretion in offspring. Diabetes Care. Sep;31(9): 1872–6.
17. Manco M, Panunzi S, Macfarlane DP, Golay A, Melander O, et al. (2010) Relationship between Insulin Sensitivity and Cardiovascular Risk (RISC) Consortium. One-hour plasma glucose identifies insulin resistance and beta-cell dysfunction in individuals with normal glucose tolerance: cross-sectional data from the Relationship between Insulin Sensitivity and Cardiovascular Risk (RISC) study. Diabetes Care. 33(9): 2090–7.
18. Nolfe G, Spreghini MR, Sforza RW, Morino G, Manco M (2012). Beyond the morphology of the glucose curve following an oral glucose tolerance test in obese youth. Eur J Endocrinol. 166(1): 107–14.
19. Manco M, Miraglia Del Giudice E, Spreghini MR, Cappa M, Perrone L, et al. (2012) 1-Hour plasma glucose in obese youth. 49(6): 435–43.
20. Matsuda M, DeFronzo RA (1999) Insulin sensitivity indices obtained from oral glucose tolerance testing: comparison with the euglycemic insulin clamp. Diabetes Care 22 1462–1470.
21. Retnakaran R, Qi Y, Goran MI, Hamilton JK (2011) Evaluation of proposed oral disposition index measures in relation to the actual disposition index. Eur J Endocrinol. Aug;165(2): 323–30.
22. Van Cauter E, Mestrez F, Sturis J, Polonsky KS (1992) Estimation of insulin secretion rates from C-peptide levels. Comparison of individual and standard kinetic parameters for C-peptide clearance. Diabetes. Mar;41(3): 368–77.
23. Ovesen P, Moller J, Ingerslev HJ, Jorgensen JO, Mengel A, et al. (1993) Normal basal and insulin-stimulated fuel metabolism in lean women with the polycystic ovary syndrome. J Clin Endocrinol Metab. 77: 1636–1640.
24. Ciampelli M, Fulghesu AM, Cucinelli F, Pavone V, Caruso A, et al. (1997) Heterogeneity in β cell activity, hepatic insulin clearance and peripheral insulin sensitivity in women with polycystic ovary syndrome. Hum Reprod. 12: 1897–1901.
25. Gennarelli G, Holte J, Berglund L, Berne C, Massobrio M, et al. (2000) Prediction models for insulin resistance in the polycystic ovary syndrome. Hum Reprod. 15: 2098–2102.
26. Cibula D, Sindelka G, Hill M, Fanta M, Skrha J, et al. (2002) Insulin sensitivity in non-obese women with polycystic ovary syndrome during treatment with oral with oral contraceptives containing low-androgenic progestin. Human Reprod. Jan;17(1): 76–82.
27. Toprak S, Yonem A, Cakir B, Guler S, Azal O, et al. (2001) Insulin resistance in nonobese patients with polycystic ovary syndrome. Horm Res. 55: 65–70.
28. Diamanti Kandarakis E, Mitrakou A, Hennes MM, Platanissiotis D, Kaklas N, et al. (1995) Insulin sensitivity and antiandrogenic therapy in women with polycystic ovary syndrome. Metabolism. 44: 525–531.
29. Best JD, Kahn SE, Ader M, Watanabe RM, Ta-Chen N, et al. (1996) Role of glucose effectiveness in the determination of glucose tolerance. Diabetes Care. 19: 1018–1030.
30. Ahrèn B, Pacini G (1998) Age-related reduction in glucose elimination is accompanied by reduced glucose effectiveness and increased hepatic insulin extraction in man. J Clin Endocrinol Metab. 83: 3350–3356.
31. O'Meara NM, Blackman JD, Ehrmann DA, Barnes RB, Jaspan JB, et al. (1993) Defects in beta-cell function in functional ovarian hyperandrogenism. J Clin Endocrinol Metab. 76(5): 1241–7.
32. Ehrmann DA, Sturis J, Byrne MM, Karrison T, Rosenfield RL, et al. (1995) Insulin secretory defects in polycystic ovary syndrome. Relationship to insulin sensitivity and family history of non-insulin-dependent diabetes mellitus. J Clin Invest. 96: 520–527.

8

A Calcium-Deficient Diet in Rat Dams during Gestation and Nursing Affects Hepatic *11β-hydroxysteroid dehydrogenase-1* Expression in the Offspring

Junji Takaya*, Sohsaku Yamanouchi, Kazunari Kaneko

Department of Pediatrics, Kansai Medical University, Moriguchi, Osaka, Japan

Abstract

Background: Prenatal malnutrition can affect the phenotype of offspring by changing epigenetic regulation of specific genes. Several lines of evidence demonstrate that calcium (Ca) plays an important role in the pathogenesis of insulin resistance syndrome. We hypothesized that pregnant female rats fed a Ca-deficient diet would have offspring with altered hepatic glucocorticoid-related gene expression and that lactation would modify these alterations.

Methodology: We determined the effects of Ca deficiency during pregnancy and/or lactation on hepatic *11β-hydroxysteroid dehydrogenase-1* (*Hsd11b1*) expression in offspring. Female Wistar rats consumed either a Ca-deficient (D: 0.008% Ca) or control (C: 0.90% Ca) diet *ad libitum* from 3 weeks preconception to 21 days postparturition. On postnatal day 1, pups were cross-fostered to the same or opposite dams and divided into the following four groups: CC, DD, CD, and DC (first letter: original mother's diet; second letter: nursing mother's diet). All offspring were fed a control diet beginning at weaning (day 21) and were killed on day 200±7. Serum insulin and adipokines in offspring were measured using ELISA kits.

Principal Findings: In males, mean levels of insulin, glucose, and Homeostasis Model Assessment of Insulin Resistance (HOMA-IR) were higher in the DD and DC groups than in the CC group. We found no difference in HOMA-IR between the CC and CD groups in either males or females. Expression of *Hsd11b1* was lower in male DD rats than in CC rats. *Hsd11b1* expression in male offspring nursed by cross-fostered dams was higher than that in those nursed by dams fed the same diet; CC vs. CD and DD vs. DC. In females, *Hsd11b1* expression in DC rats was higher than that in CC rats.

Conclusions: These findings indicated that maternal Ca restriction during pregnancy and/or lactation alters postnatal growth, *Hsd11b1* expression, and insulin resistance in a sex-specific manner.

Editor: Nick Ashton, The University of Manchester, United Kingdom

Funding: This study was supported in part by the Mami Mizutani Foundation and by a Grant-in-Aid for Scientific research (C) from the Japanese Society for the Promotion of Science (No. 24591614). The funders had no role in study design, data collection and analysis, decision to publish, or preparation of the manuscript.

Competing Interests: The authors have declared that no competing interests.

* E-mail: takaya@takii.kmu.ac.jp

Introduction

Calcium (Ca) plays an important role in the pathogenesis of insulin resistance syndrome and obesity, suggesting that hypocalcemia is a risk factor for developing these conditions [1,2]. Several reports have shown an inverse relationship between Ca intake and body fat mass [2,3,4,5]. The Coronary Artery Risk Development in Young Adults Study suggests an intriguing and exciting negative relationship between Ca intake or dairy consumption and obesity and insulin resistance syndrome in young adults [6]. Maternal malnutrition and the resulting low birth weight predispose offspring to various diseases, including adult-onset insulin resistance syndrome [7,8,9,10]. Some experimental and observational findings from humans and animals indicate an association between maternal Ca intake during pregnancy and blood pressure in offspring [11,12], but others do not [13]. Morley *et al.* reported that children whose mothers took Ca supplements during pregnancy had a better lipid profile at 9 years of age compared to children whose mothers did not take Ca supplements [14].

Glucocorticoids such as cortisol are important mediators in the regulation of cardiovascular and metabolic functions. Through activation of glucocorticoid or mineralocorticoid receptors, glucocorticoids impact vascular, adipose, liver, and kidney functions [15,16]. 11β-hydroxysteroid dehydrogenase-1 (11β-HSD1, *Hsd11b1*) affects local cortisol production [17,18]. 11β-HSD1 preferentially catalyzes the conversion of inactive 11-keto-glucocorticoids (cortisone in humans and 11-dehydrocorticosterone in rodents) into active 11β-hydroxyglucocorticoids (cortisol in humans and corticosterone in rodents), and by this mechanism, 11β-HSD1 modulates cell-specific glucocorticoid action [19,20]. 11β-HSD1 activity has been shown to be elevated in obese humans with type 2 diabetes mellitus and metabolic syndrome [21,22].

We previously reported that a low Ca diet alters glucocorticoid metabolism, leading to hepatic up-regulation of *Hsd11b1* in rats [23]. We also reported that feeding a Ca-restricted diet to pregnant rats results in hypomethylation and decreased expression from the *Hsd11b1* promoter in the liver of offspring at day 21 [24].

These findings show that maternal Ca deficiency during pregnancy can affect regulation of non-imprinted genes by altering epigenetic regulation of gene expression, thereby inducing different metabolic phenotypes. The epigenome is an important target of environmental modification. Dietary modification can have a profound effect on DNA methylation and genomic imprinting [25,26]. A remarkable example of an environmental effect on the epigenome is the modification of glucocorticoid receptor methylation seen in the hippocampus of rat pups in response to maternal grooming [27]. Recently Yuen et al. reported that most fetal tissue-specific differentially methylated regions seem to reflect transient DNA methylation changes during development rather than permanent epigenetic signatures [28].

In this context, Ca can be seen as a strong candidate for a modulator of programming effects. We hypothesized that rat dams fed a diet lacking in Ca would produce offspring with altered expression of genes involved in hepatic glucocorticoid metabolism and that lactation would modify these alterations. The early nurturing environment has persistent influences on developmental programming of inter-individual differences in metabolic and endocrine function. Thus, the purpose of this study was to identify the effect of lactation by dams fed different Ca-containing diets on offspring, which were already programmed prenatally [29].

Regulation of hepatic 11β-HSD1 by the fetus or during lactation and its contribution to insulin resistance in the offspring are currently unknown. In this study, we fed pregnant rats a Ca-deficient diet and investigated the effect on insulin-related parameters and mRNA expression of *Hsd11b1* in the liver of offspring. In addition, we used a cross-fostering strategy to assess whether postnatal lactation by Ca-deficient dams contributed to the development of insulin resistance.

Materials and Methods

Animal procedures

Twelve-week-old female Wistar rats obtained from Shimizu Laboratories (Kyoto, Japan) were used. All rats were maintained on a 12-hour light/12-hour dark cycle. Virgin Wistar rats were divided into two dietary groups of five rats each and fed either a control diet (C: 0.90% Ca) or a Ca-deficient diet (D: 0.008% Ca) *ad libitum* for 3 wk. Experimental diets, the compositions of which are presented in Table 1, were prepared weekly in the laboratory. Rats were fed loose pellets in small metal dishes and were given free access to water. After 3 wk, the rats were mated with males who were fed a normal, control diet. The pregnant rats continued consuming their respective diets throughout the gestation and lactation periods.

In all litters, both to obviate the reported effects of litter size on metabolic function and to parallel commonly adopted protocols in the developmental programming literature, larger litters were reduced to six pups at 24 hours postpartum, maintaining equal sex ratios when possible. The fostering was done within 24 hours of birth (usually within 12 hours), and the animals were then disturbed as little as possible for the first 4–5 days after fostering. The following four groups were then established: CC (n = 18), in which offspring of control-diet dams were nursed by control dams (n = 3); DD (n = 18), in which offspring of Ca-deficient-diet dams were nursed by Ca-deficient-diet dams (n = 3); CD (n = 12), in which offspring of control-diet dams were nursed by Ca-deficient-diet dams (n = 2); and DC (n = 12), in which offspring of Ca-deficient-diet dams were nursed by control dams (n = 2). No pups remained with their original birth mother; the pups in all groups came from different litters. No pups were lost subsequent to cross-fostering. On day 21, six female and six male offspring were selected from the CC and DD groups by random removal. Six male and six female pups from each nutritional group were used for the study. The remaining 12 pups were not used. All offspring were weaned at 21 days onto on a control diet (0.90% Ca, supplied by CLEA Japan, Inc., Tokyo, Japan) and maintained on this diet until day 200±7. All 48 pups survived until day 200±7. Blood pressure and heart rate of conscious rats were measured with the tail-cuff method using a blood pressure monitor (Model MK-2000, Muromachi Kikai Co., Ltd., Tokyo, Japan) on the day before sacrifice. Animals were warmed to 35°C, and the mean of at least 10 measurements was taken. Body weight of offspring was measured every week from day 21 to day 200. No measurement of pup weight was made at birth because we did not wish to compromise the success of the cross-fostering by disturbing the pups. After fasting for 12 hours, the rats were decapitated with a guillotine, and blood samples were taken from the trunk. Livers were excised immediately, frozen in liquid nitrogen, and stored at −80°C. This study was carried out in strict accordance with the recommendations in the Guide for the Care and Use of Laboratory Animals of the National Institutes of Health. The protocol was approved by the Committee on the Ethics of Animal Experiments of Kansai Medical University (Permit Number: 11-012). All efforts were made to minimize suffering.

Table 1. Ingredient composition of each diet fed to rats.

Ingredients	Control (g/100g diet)	Calcium deficient (g/100g diet)
Milk casein	24.50	24.50
Corn starch	45.50	45.50
Granulated sugar	10.00	10.00
Corn oil	6.00	6.00
Cellulose powder	5.00	5.00
α-Starch	1.00	1.00
Vitamin mix[1)]	1.00	1.00
Mineral mix[2)]	7.00	7.00
(Calcium)	(0.90)	(0.008)
Total	100.00	100.00

1), 2) refer Table S1 and Table S2.

Analysis of *Hsd11b1* and *cyclophilin* (*Ppia*) mRNA expression

Expression of mRNA in six offspring of each group was measured using real-time PCR. Total RNA was isolated from hepatic tissue samples using an RNeasy Mini Kit (QIAGEN Science, Germantown, MD) according to the manufacturer's instructions and quantified spectrophotometrically at an optical density of 260 nm. Details regarding the oligonucleotide primers for *Hsd11b1* and *Ppia* are listed in Table 2. Real-time PCR amplification of mRNA was performed in a total volume of 25 μl with a One Step SYBR PrimeScript RT-PCR Kit II (Takara Bio Inc., Tokyo, Japan) according to the manufacturer's recommendations. The amplification of mRNA was quantified using relative standard curve methods. To confirm the amplification of specific transcripts, melting curve profiles were produced at the end of each run. Samples were analyzed in duplicate, and expression of the individual transcripts was normalized [30] to expression of *Ppia* (QuantiTect assay QT00177394) [31], which did not differ among groups of offspring.

Table 2. Primer sequences used to amplify mRNA with real-time RT-PCR.

Gene		Primer(5′-3′)
Hsd11b1	Forward	TCATAGACACAGAAACAGCTTTGAAA
	Reverse	CTCCAGGGCGCATTCCT
Ppia	Forward	TTGGGTCGCGTCTGCTTCGA
	Reverse	GCCAGGACCTGTATGCTTCA

Hsd11b1, 11β-hydroxysteroid dehydrogenase 1; *Ppia*, Cyclophilin

Serum measurements

Serum 11β-HSD1 and corticosterone levels. Whole blood from fasting rats was collected from the offspring of the four groups (n = six males and six females in each group). Serum was separated by centrifugation. Serum 11β-HSD1 levels were detected using the Rat Corticosteroid 11-beta-dehydrogenase isozyme 1(HSD11B1) ELISA kit (CUSABIO, Wuhan, China). The lower limit of detection was 3.12 pg/ml. Serum corticosterone levels were detected using the Rat Corticosterone Enzyme Immunoassay Kit (Yanaihara Inc., Shizuoka, Japan). The lower limit of detection was 0.21 ng/ml.

Serum adipokine levels. Concentrations of leptin, insulin, and adiponectin were determined in serum from fasting rats using rat-specific ELISA kits (Morinaga, Yokohama, Japan (leptin and insulin); Otsuka Pharmaceutical, Tokyo, Japan (adiponectin)). The lower limit of detection was 0.4 ng/ml for leptin, 0.1 ng/ml for insulin, and 0.25 ng/ml for adiponectin. Glucose concentrations were measured using a glucose oxidase system (Arkray, Kyoto, Japan). Homeostasis Model Assessment of Insulin Resistance (HOMA-IR) is the product of fasting plasma glucose (mM) and the insulin concentration (ng/mL). Because no rat international unit has been established, the insulin units were converted to the human type for convenience. The equation used for this calculation is: 1 mg = 23.1 IU.

HOMA-IR = [Glucose] × [Insulin]/22.5 and was used as a measure of insulin resistance [32]. HOMA-β = 20× [Insulin]/([Glucose] - 3.5)% and was used as a measure of β-cell function [33].

Serum ionized calcium levels. Serum ionized calcium levels were measured with an automatic ion selective electrode analyzer, Stat Profile pHOx Ultra (NOVA, Newton, MA), which provides results for ionized calcium in a measurement range of 0.10-2.70 mmol/l. The normalized ionized Ca represents the ionized Ca concentration at pH 7.40. The equation used for this calculation is as follows:

$$\log[Ca^{2+}]_{7.4} = \log[Ca^{2+}]_X - 0.24(7.4 - X)$$

where X = measured pH of the sample

$[Ca^{2+}]_X$ = ionized Ca concentration in the sample at the measured pH

$[Ca^{2+}]_{7.4}$ = normalized concentration of ionized Ca at pH 7.40

Statistical analyses

Statistical analyses were performed using JMP 6 software (SAS Institute Inc., Cary, NC). Results are expressed as the means ± standard error (SE). Statistically significant differences among the groups were determined with two-way analysis of variance (ANOVA) with diet and sex as the main factors. If interactions were found, the data were split, and a one-way ANOVA was performed. A standard power calculation was performed on the results using JMP 6 software. Acceptable study power was agreed a priori to be ≥80% (type-I error of ≤0.20). $P<0.05$ was considered statistically significant.

Results

Dams: No significant differences in body weight gain were found between Wistar female rats in the Ca-deficiency (n = 5) group and the control group (n = 5) at the mating. However, ionized Ca concentrations in plasma samples were lower ($P<0.05$) in the Ca-deficient group (1.31±0.05 mmol/l, n = 5) than in the controls (1.39±0.05 mmol/l, n = 5).

Pups: The litter size of six pups was uniform from postnatal day 1 until postnatal day 21. No significant differences in body weight were found at day 21 among the groups. The body weight of female DC offspring was higher than that in CC offspring at day 200±7 ($P<0.05$, Table 3). The body weight of male DC offspring was significantly higher than that in the other groups both on day 100 ($P<0.05$) and on day 200 ($P<0.01$, Table 4). No significant differences were observed among the groups for heart rate or systolic blood pressure.

HOMA-IR and serum adipokine levels

In males, the mean levels of insulin, glucose, and HOMA-IR in DD and DC offspring were higher than those in CC pups (Table 4). Thus, male offspring from Ca-deficient dams developed insulin resistance. In females, the mean insulin levels in DC pups were higher than those in CC offspring (Table 3). In males, mean HOMA-β levels in DC offspring were lower than those in CC pups (Table 4). Thus, lactation from cross-fostered Ca-deficient dams affected insulin secretion in offspring. No significant difference was found among the groups in serum 11β-HSD1 levels (Tables 3 and 4).

In male offspring, mean adiponectin levels from CD, DD, and DC offspring were higher than levels in CC pups. No significant differences were found in serum ionized Ca, corticosterone, or leptin levels in offspring (Tables 3 and 4). Serum ionized Ca showed a pronounced sexual dimorphism, with higher levels in females ($P<0.05$).

Maternal dietary calcium deficiency alters offspring mRNA expression of *Hsd11b1* in the liver

We found a significant effect of sex ($P<0.0001$) on *Hsd11b1* mRNA expression, which was lower in females. *Hsd11b1* mRNA expression was significantly lower in male DD offspring than in the other male groups (Figure 1). In males, *Hsd11b1* mRNA expression in cross-fostered offspring was higher than that in offspring nursed by dams fed the same diet: in males, *Hsd11b1* mRNA expression in CD pups was higher than that in CC pups, and expression in DC offspring was higher than that in DD offspring. In addition, the *Hsd11b1* mRNA expression in female DC offspring was higher than that in CC pups (Figure 1).

Discussion

This study shows that male offspring developed insulin resistance after nursing from Ca-deficient dams. Recently, epigenetic regulation has been shown to contribute to differences in fetal gene expression [31]. For example, we reported hypomethylation but decreased mRNA expression of hepatic *Hsd11b1* in offspring of dams fed a Ca-deficient diet during pregnancy [24]. Serum corticosterone levels of male pups from the Ca-deficient dams were higher than that from the control on day

Table 3. Profile of female offspring on day 200.

	CC	CD	DD	DC
	n=6	**n=6**	**n=6**	**n=6**
Body weight (g) day 21	30±2	26±1	29±4	28±4
day 100	242±5	235±4	226±7	238±10
day 200	254±7	294±11	268±11	304±9*
Heart rate (bpm)	443±7	430±10	427±11	440±21
Systolic BP (mmHg)	106±4	96±3	93±6	108±5
11β-HSD1 (pg/ml)	19.1±7.7	2.0±1.2	28.3±7.3	22.4±14.1
Adiponectin (μg/ml)	7.06±0.31	7.46±0.73	7.83±0.34	7.19±0.79
Leptin (ng/ml)	4.42±0.55	4.77±0.67	4.31±0.32	3.74±0.39
Corticosterone (ng/ml)	795±45	796±78	861±28	789±70
Insulin (ng/ml)	1.69±0.13	2.05±0.21	1.99±0.20	2.61±0.11**
Glucose (mmol/L)	8.1±0.7	10.5±1.3	9.7±0.9	10.2±1.3
HOMA-IR	14.1±0.1	22.1±0. 3	19.8±0.2	27.3±0.1
HOMA-β (%)	170±25	135±32	148±20	180±29
iCa (mmol/L)	1.44±0.02	1.51±0.02	1.47±0.02	1.50±0.03

CC in which offspring of control-diet dams were nursed by control dams; DD in which offspring of Ca-deficient-diet dams were nursed by Ca-deficient-diet dams; CD in which offspring of control-diet dams were nursed by Ca-deficient-diet dams; and DC in which offspring of Ca-deficient-diet dams were nursed by control dams. No pups remained with their original birth mother; the pups in all groups came from different litters. BP: blood pressure
Statistically significant differences among the groups were determined with two-way analysis of variance (ANOVA) with diet and sex as the main factors. If interactions were found, the data were split, and a one-way ANOVA was performed. $^{*}P<0.05$, $^{**}P<0.01$ vs. CC.
Values are represented as means ± SE.

21. These data indicate that maternal Ca deficiency in rats may have contributed to prenatal programming of insulin resistance. Previous reports have shown that the epigenetic effect induced by intrauterine growth restriction is gender specific [34,35,36]. Testosterone may affect epigenetic regulation; however, further investigation is necessary. Serum ionized Ca showed pronounced

Table 4. Profile of male offspring on day 200.

	CC	CD	DD	DC
	n=6	**n=6**	**n=6**	**n=6**
Body weight (g) day 21	36±6	31±6	31±3	32±3
day 100	389±21	363±13	389±17	448±8*
day 200	418±7	419±15	430±12	472±18**
Heart rate (bpm)	400±15	401±12	394±10	384±12
Systolic BP (mmHg)	115±5	110±3	113±4	112±7
11β-HSD1 (pg/ml)	30.3±12.3	49.6±9.3	34.7±9.4	48.3±15.6
Adiponectin (μg/ml)	5.62±0.72	7.58±0.34*	7.30±0.45*	7.28±0.54*
Leptin (ng/ml)	6.36±0.72	6.90±0.47	7.38±0.45	7.93±0.52
Corticosterone (ng/ml)	580±26	556±24	628±18	615±23
Insulin (ng/ml)	2.21±0.10	2.46±0.20	3.02±0.20**	2.90±0.19*
Glucose (mmol/L)	9.1±0.7	9.9±0.6	12.6±1.8*	15.6±2.7**
HOMA-IR	20.6±0.1	25.0±0.1	39.1±0.4**	46.4±0.5**
HOMA-β (%)	182±26	178±20	153±22	111±26*
iCa (mmol/L)	1.39±0.02	1.33±0.03	1.37±0.03	1.38±0.04

CC in which offspring of control-diet dams were nursed by control dams; DD in which offspring of Ca-deficient-diet dams were nursed by Ca-deficient-diet dams; CD in which offspring of control-diet dams were nursed by Ca-deficient-diet dams; and DC in which offspring of Ca-deficient-diet dams were nursed by control dams. No pups remained with their original birth mother; the pups in all groups came from different litters. BP: blood pressure
Statistically significant differences among the groups were determined with two-way analysis of variance (ANOVA) with diet and sex as the main factors. If interactions were found, the data were split, and a one-way ANOVA was performed. $^{*}P<0.05$, $^{**}P<0.01$ vs. CC.
Values are represented as means ± SE.

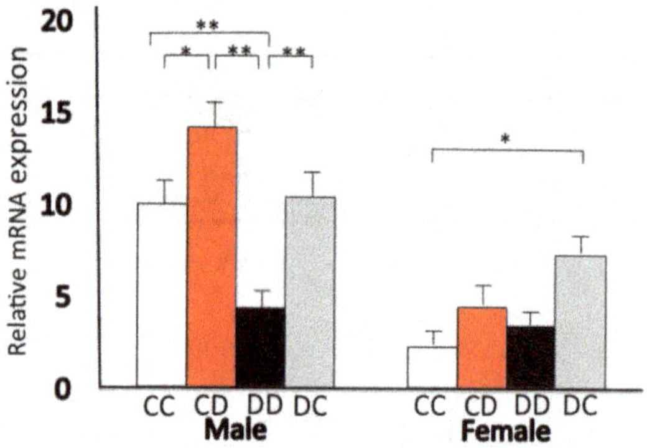

Figure 1. Hepatic mRNA expression levels of *Hsd11b1*. After delivery, foster mothers fed the same or different diets: CC, DD, CD, and DC (first letter: diet of original mother; second letter: diet of nursing mother). Data are represented as the means ± standard error. Statistically significant differences among the groups were determined with two-way analysis of variance (ANOVA), with diet and sex as the main factors. If interactions were found, the data were split and analyzed with one-way ANOVA. *P<0.05, **P<0.01.

sexual dimorphism, with higher levels in females (P<0.05). 11β-HSD1 also shows pronounced sexual dimorphism in the liver, with lower levels in females [37]. In addition, the phenotype in males resulting from fostering is exaggerated compared with that of females, particularly in relation to adiposity and blood pressure [38]. It should be denied that the cross-fostering does not affect this result due to the role of non-maternal nutrition.

We previously reported that *Hsd11b1* expression in the liver increases in response to a Ca-deficient diet in adult rats for 2 wk [23]. In our current study, however, the expression of *Hsd11b1* mRNA in male offspring (DD) from Ca-deficient dams was lower than that in male offspring (CC) from control dams. Down-regulation of *Hsd11b1* suggests that a compensatory mechanism may diminish cortisol production in the liver. Reduced hepatic glucocorticoid exposure also represents a compensatory mechanism that limits the metabolic complications of insulin resistance. No significant difference was found among the groups in serum 11β-HSD1 levels; however, this may have been due to tissue-specific differences between serum and liver. Whether glucocorticoids modulate *Hsd11b1* expression is unknown; hepatic *Hsd11b1* expression is very different from that in other tissues [43,44,46]. Mice that overexpress *Hsd11b1* in adipose tissue develop visceral obesity and insulin resistance [39]. Obese rodents exhibit tissue-specific dysregulation of 11β-HSD1, usually with up-regulation in adipose tissue and down-regulation in liver [40,41]. In both obese Zucker rats and obese humans, 11β-HSD1 activity is high in adipose tissue, but low in liver [42,43,44]. In adipose tissue and smooth muscle cells, glucocorticoid induces *Hsd11b1* mRNA expression, but controversial results have been obtained in the liver [42,43]. Whether such tissue-specific dysregulation occurs in obese patients with type 2 diabetes is uncertain. Down-regulation of 11β-HSD1 in the liver in euglycemic obesity can be viewed as an adaptive process to decrease intra-hepatic glucocorticoid concentrations [45]; failure to decrease 11β-HSD1 in type 2 diabetes may result in increased intrahepatic cortisol levels, which exacerbates the adverse metabolic phenotype.

Our data show that metabolic programming effects are modified by nutrition in the immediate postnatal period. Hepatic *Hsd11b1* expression in cross-fostered male offspring (DC and CD) was higher than that in offspring (DD and CC) nursed by dams fed the same diet. Mismatched nutrition after birth, i.e., cross-fostered nursing, disrupts the adaptation that has been programmed in the fetus. Although hepatic expression of *Hsd11b1* in offspring from Ca-deficient dams may have been originally up-regulated by epigenetic mechanisms, *Hsd11b1* was likely down-regulated by other mechanisms during the early postnatal period. If the nutritional environment established before birth is mismatched after birth, the balance established by this compensation collapses. Metabolic programming effects translate into an adverse intra-uterine environment during pregnancy. Altered mismatched nutritional experience during the suckling period can impact adult health in the offspring [47,48]. These findings lead to the hypothesis that factors present in breast milk may regulate the epigenetics of pups. In addition, our data showed that cross-fostered lactation induced higher body weight. These early adaptations in the liver (expression levels of *Hsd11b1*) and hypothalamus (supporting hyperphagia and increased body weight gain) persist in the post-weaning period. Thus, nutrition during the prenatal period and/or lactation may affect epigenetic mechanisms in the offspring. Although the precise mechanisms that support metabolic programming effects due to altered nutritional experiences in the immediate postnatal period are not well understood, altered *Hsd11b1* mRNA expression has been implicated in this process [49].

We conclude that maternal Ca restriction during pregnancy alters postnatal growth, *Hsd11b1* expression, and insulin resistance in a sex-specific manner. The present study provides further support for the hypothesis that early postnatal lactation plays a sexually divergent role in programming the phenotype later in life.

Acknowledgments

The authors wish to thank Dr. Yukihiro Okihana for technical assistance.

Author Contributions

Conceived and designed the experiments: JT KK. Performed the experiments: JT SY. Analyzed the data: JT. Contributed reagents/materials/analysis tools: JT. Wrote the paper: JT.

References

1. Drouillet P, Balkau B, Charies MA, Vol S, Bedouel M, et al. (2007) Calcium consumption and insulin resistance syndrome parameters. Data from the epidemiological study on the insulin resistance syndrome (DESIR). Nutr Metab Cardiovasc Dis 17: 486–492.
2. Zemel MB, Shi H, Greer B, Dirienzo D, Zemel PC (2000) Regulation of adiposity by dietary calcium. FASEB J 14: 1132–1138.
3. Davis KM, Heaney RP, Recker RR, Lappe JM, Barger-Lux MJ, et al. (2000) Calcium intake and body weight. J Clin Endocrinol Metab 85:4635–4638.
4. Heaney RP, Davies KM, Barger-Lux MJ (2002) Calcium and weight: clinical studies. J Am Coll Nutr 21:152S–155S.
5. Lin YC, Lyle RM, McCabe LD, McCabe GP, Weaver CM, et al. (2000) Dairy calcium is related to changes in body composition during a two-year exercise intervention in young women. J Am Coll Nutr 19:754–760.
6. Pereira MA, Jacobs DR, Van Horn L, Slattery ML, Kartashov AI, et al. (2002) Dairy consumption, obesity, and the insulin resistance syndrome in young adults. The CARDIA Study. J Am Med Assoc 287:2081–2089.

7. Valdez R, Athens MA, Thompson GH, Bradshaw BS. Stem MP (1994) Birthweight and adult health outcomes in a biethnic population in the USA. Diabetologia 37: 624–631.
8. Warner MJ, Ozanne SE (2010) Mechanisms involved in the developmental programming of adulthood disease. Biochem J 427: 333–347.
9. Bateson P, Barker D, Clutton-Brock T, Deb D, D'Udine B, et al. (2004) Developmental plasticity and human health. Nature 430: 419–421.
10. Peixoto-Silva N, Frantz ED, Mandarim-de-Lacerda CA, Pinheiro-Mulder A (2011) Maternal protein restriction in mice causes adverse metabolic and hypothalamic effects in the F1 and F2 generations. Br J Nutr 106: 1364–1373
11. Belizan JM, Gillman MW, Rifas-Shiman SL, Kleinman KP, Rich-Edwards JW, et al. (2004) Maternal Calcium Intake and Offspring Blood Pressure. Circulation 110: 1990–1995.
12. Bergel E, Belizan JM (2002) A deficient maternal calcium intake during pregnancy increases blood pressure of the offspring in adult rats. BJOG 109:540–545.
13. Bakker R, Rifas-Shiman SL, Kleinman KP, Lipshultz SE, Gillman MW (2008) Maternal Calcium Intake During Pregnancy and Blood Pressure in the Offspring at Age 3 Years: A Follow-up Analysis of the Project Viva Cohort. Am J Epidemiol 168:1374–1380.
14. Morley R, Carlin JB, Dwyer T (2004) Maternal calcium supplementation and cardiovascular risk factors in twin offspring. Int J Epidemiol 33:1304–1309.
15. Walker BR (2007) Glucocorticoids and cardiovascular disease. Eur J Endocrinol 157:545–559.
16. Goodwin JE, Geller DS (2012) Glucocorticoid-induced hypertension. Pediatr Nephrol 27:1059–1066.
17. Seckl JR, Walker BR (2011) Minireview: 11β-hydroxysteroid dehydrogenase type 1-A tissue-specific amplifier of glucocorticoid action. Endocrinoligy 142: 1371–1376.
18. Draper N, Stewart PM (2005) 11β-hydroxysteroid dehydrogenase and the pre-receptor regulation of corticosteroid hormone action. J Endocrinol 186: 251–271.
19. Low SC, Chapman KE, Edwards CRW, Seckl JR (1994) 'Liver-type' 11 beta-hydroxysteroid dehydrogenase cDNA encodes reductase but not dehydrogenase activity in intact mammalian COS-7 cells. J. Mol. Endocrinol 13:167–174.
20. Voice M, Seckl JR, Edwards CRW, Chapman KE (1996) 11 beta-hydroxysteroid dehydrogenase type 1 expression in 2S FAZA hepatoma cells is hormonally regulated: a model system for the study of hepatic glucocorticoid metabolism. Biochem J 317:621–625.
21. Stimson RH, Andrew R, McAvoy NC, Tripathi D, Hayes PC, et al. (2011) Increased Whole-Body and Sustained Liver Cortisol Regeneration by 11β-Hydroxysteroid Dehydrogenase Type 1 in Obese Men With Type 2 Diabetes Provides a Target for Enzyme Inhibition. Diabetes 60:720–725.
22. Torrecilla E, Fernández-Vázquez G, Vicent D, Sánchez-Franco F, Barabash A, et al. (2012) Liver upregulation of genes involved in cortisol production and action is associated with metabolic syndrome in morbidly obese patients. Obes Surg 22:478–486.
23. Takaya J, Iharada A, Okihana H, Kaneko K (2011) Upregulation of hepatic 11β-hydroxysteroid dehydrogenase-1 expression in calcium-deficient rats. Ann Nutr Metab 59: 73–78.
24. Takaya J, Iharada A, Okihana H, Kaneko K (2013) A calcium-deficient diet in pregnant, nursing rats induces hypomethylation of specific cytosines in the *11β-hydroxysteroid dehydrogenase-1* promoter within pup liver. Nutr Res 33: 961–970.
25. Waterland RA, Lin JR, Smith CA, Jirtle RL (2006) Post-weaning diet affects genomic imprinting at the insulin-like growth factor2 (Igf2) locus. Hum Mol Genet 15: 705–716.
26. Waterland RA, Jirtle RL (2003) Transposable elements: targets for early nutritional effects on epigenetic gene regulation. Mol Cell Biol 23:5293–5300.
27. Weaver IC, Cervoni N, Champagne FA, D'Alessio AC, Schrma S, et al. (2004) Epigenetic programming by maternal behavior. Nature Neurosci 7:847–854.
28. Yuen RK, Neumann SM, Fok AK, Penaherrera MS, McFadden DE, et al. (2011) Extensive epigenetic reprogramming in human somatic tissues between fetus and adult. Epigenetics Chromatin 5;4:7. doi: 10.1186/1756-8935-4-7.
29. Weaver IC (2009) Epigenetic effects of glucocorticoids. Semin Fetal Neonatal Med 14:143–150.
30. Bustin SA (2000) Absolute quantification of mRNA using real-time reverse transcription polymerase chain reaction assays. J Mol Endocrinol 25: 169–193
31. Lillycrop KA, Phillips ES, Jackson AA, Hanson MA, Burdge GC (2005) Dietary protein restriction of pregnant rats induces and folic acid supplementation prevents epigenetic modification of hepatic gene expression in the offspring. J Nutr 135:1382–1386
32. Matthews DR, Hosker JP, Rudenski AS, Naylor BA, Treacher DF, et al. (1985) Homeostasis model assessment: insulin resistance and beta-cell function from fasting plasma glucose and insulin concentrations in man. Diabetologia 28:412–419.
33. Hermans MP, Levy JC, Morris RJ, Turner RC (1999) Comparison of tests of beta-cell function across a range of glucose tolerance from normal to diabetes. Diabetes 48:1779–1786.
34. Fu Q, Yu X, Callaway CW, Lane RH, McKnight RA (2009) Epigenetics: intrauterine growth retardation (IUGR) modifies the histone code along the rat hepatic IGF-1 gene. FASEB J 23:2438–2449.
35. Gong L, Pan YX, Chen H (2010) Gestational low protein diet in the rat mediates Igf2 gene expression in male offspring via altered hepatic DNA methylation. Epigenetics 5:619–626.
36. Ng SF, Lin RC, Laybutt DR, Barres R, Owens JA, et al. (2010) Chronic high-fat diet in fathers programs β-cell dysfunction in female rat offspring. Nature 467:963–966.
37. Lax ER, Ghraf R, Schriefers H (1978) The hormonal regulation of hepatic microsomal 11beta-hydroxtsteroid dehydrogenase activity in the rat. Acta Endocrinologica 89:352–357.
38. Matthews PA, Samuelsson AM, Seed P, Pombo J, Oben JA, et al. (2011) Fostering in mice induces cardiovascular and metabolic dysfunction in adulthood. J Physiol 589:3969–3981.
39. Masuzaki H, Paterson J, Shinyama H, Morton NM, Mullins JJ, et al. (2001) A transgenic model of visceral obesity and the metabolic syndrome. Science 294: 2166–2170.
40. Hemanowski-Vosatka A, Balkovec JM, Cheng K, Chen HY, Hernandez M, et al. (2005) 11beta-HSD1 inhibition ameliorates metabolic syndrome and prevents progression of atherosclerosis in mice. J Exp Med 202:517–27.
41. Liu Y, Nakagawa Y, Wang Y, Li R, Li X, et al. (2003) Leptin activation of corticosterone production in hepatocytes may contribute to the reversal of obesity and hyperglycemia in leptin-deficient ob/ob mice. Diabetes 52: 1409–1416.
42. Livingstone DE, Jones GC, Smith K, Jamieson PM, Andrew R, et al. (2000) Understanding the role of glucocorticoids in obesity: tissue-specific alterations of corticosterone metabolism in obese Zucker rats. Endocrinology 141: 560–563.
43. Rask E, Olsson T, Sodenberg S, Andrew R, Livingstone DE, et al. (2001) Tissue-specific dysregulation of cortisol metabolism in human obesity. J Clin Endocrinol Metab 86: 1418–1421.
44. Paulmyer-Lacrox O, Boullu S, Oliver C, Alessi MC, Grino M (2002) Expression of the mRNA coding for 11beta-hydroxysteroid dehydrogenase type 1 in adipose tissue from obese patients: an in situ hybridization study. J Clin Endocrinol Metab 87: 2701–2705.
45. Valsamakis G, Anwar A, Tomlinson JW, Shackleton CH, McTernan PG, et al. (2004) 11beta-hydroxysteroid dehydrogenase type 1 activity in lean and obese males with type 2 diabetes mellitus. J Clin Endocrinol Metab 89:4755–4761.
46. Lindsay RS, Wake DJ, Nair S, Bunt J, Livingstone DE, et al. (2003) Subcutaneous adipose 11 beta-hydroxysteroid dehydrogenase type 1 activity and messenger ribonucleic acid levels are associated with adiposity and insulinemia in Pima Indians and Caucasians. J Clin Endocrinol Metab 88:2738–2744.
47. Patel MS, Srinivasan M (2011) Metabolic programming in the immediate postnatal life. Ann Nutr Metab 58 Suppl 2:18–28. doi: 10.1159/000328040.
48. Srinivasan M, Mahmood S, Patel MS (2013) Metabolic programming effects initiated in the suckling period predisposing for adult-onset obesity cannot be reversed by calorie restriction. Am J Physiol Endocrinol Metab 304:E486–94. doi: 10.1152/ajpendo.00519.2012.
49. Boullu-Ciocca S, Dutour A, Guillaume V, Achard V, Oliver C, et al. (2005) Postnatal diet-induced obesity in rats upregulates systemic and adipose tissue glucocorticoid metabolism during development and in adulthood: its relationship with the metabolic syndrome. Diabetes 54:197–203.

9

Left Ventricular Hypertrophy and Insulin Resistance in Adults from an Urban Community in the Gambia

Bernard Cudjoe Nkum[1]*, Frank Botsi Micah[1], Theophilus C. Ankrah[1], Ousman Nyan[2]

1 Department of Medicine, School of Medical Sciences, Kwame Nkrumah University of Science and Technology, Kumasi, Ghana, **2** Department of Medicine, Royal Victoria Teaching Hospital, Banjul, The Gambia

Abstract

Objective: To determine the association between left ventricular hypertrophy and insulin resistance in Gambians.

Design: Cross-sectional study.

Setting: Outpatient clinics of Royal Victoria Teaching Hospital and Medical Research Council Laboratories in Banjul.

Participants: Three hundred and sixteen consecutive patients were enrolled from outpatient clinics. The data of 275 participants (89 males) were included in the analysis with a mean (± standard deviation) age of 53.7 (±11.9) years.

Interventions: A questionnaire was filled and anthropometric measurements were taken. 2-D guided M-mode echocardiography, standard 12-1ead electrocardiogram, fasting insulin and the oral glucose tolerance test were performed.

Main Outcome Measures: The Penn formula was used to determine the left ventricular mass index, 125 g/m^2 in males and 110 g/m^2 in females as the cut-off for left ventricular hypertrophy. Using the fasting insulin and fasting glucose levels, the insulin resistance was estimated by the homeostatic model assessment formula. Logistic regression analysis was used to determine the association between left ventricular hypertrophy and insulin resistance.

Results: The mean Penn left ventricular mass index was 119.5 (±54.3) and the prevalence of Penn left ventricular mass index left ventricular hypertrophy was 41%. The mean fasting glucose was 5.6 (±2.5) mmol/l, fasting insulin was 6.39 (±5.49) µU/ml and insulin resistance was 1.58 (±1.45). There was no association between Penn left ventricular mass index left ventricular hypertrophy and log of insulin resistance in univariate (OR = 0.98, 95% CI = 0.80 - 1.19, p = 0.819) and multivariate logistic regression (OR = 0.93, 95% CI = 0.76–1.15, p = 0.516) analysis.

Conclusion: No association was found in this study between left ventricular hypertrophy and insulin resistance in Gambians and this does not support the suggestion that insulin is an independent determinant of left ventricular hypertrophy in hypertensives.

Editor: Maria Eugenia Saez, CAEBi, Spain

Funding: This study was funded by the Medical Research Council (MRC), UK. The funder had no role in study design, data collection and analysis, decision to publish, or preparation of the manuscript.

Competing Interests: The authors have declared that no competing interests exist.

* E-mail: bcnkum@yahoo.co.uk

Introduction

Left ventricular hypertrophy (LVH) and insulin resistance (IR) are both strong adverse factors for cardiovascular disease. The co-existence of LVH and IR is a clinical finding, which must be taken seriously, even in the absence of blood pressure levels above the usual limits for initiating drug therapy because it is a predictor of adverse risk for mortality and morbidity.

The association of hypertension and IR has been studied extensively as part of the metabolic syndrome [1]. The association between hypertension and LVH is also well established with hypertension being one of the leading causes of LVH [2–4]. Answers to whether IR plays any role in the pathogenesis of LVH from the various studies have been variable, with some showing a clear relationship while others have demonstrated no association between IR and LVH.

In a study of 40, otherwise healthy, non-diabetic, normotensive obese subjects Sasson et al demonstrated that IR was strongly associated with LVH and that this association was independent of blood pressure and body mass index (BMI) [5]. Lind et al., found LVH to be closely associated with IR and in multiple regression analysis IR accounted for 47% of the variability of left ventricular mass [6].

IR was found to have no influence on left ventricular mass index in a study of 29 non-obese hypertensive patients [7]. Another study of 50 non-diabetic participants revealed that after controlling for blood pressure and BMI, insulin concentration, secretion and action was not an independent determinant of LVH [8].

The prevalence and relevance LVH and IR in Gambians are unknown. The aim and objective of this study are to determine the association between LVH and IR in Gambians.

Materials and Methods

Ethics Statement

The study was approved by The Gambia Government/MRC Ethical Committee. All the participants signed or thumb printed an informed consent form after careful consideration and explanation.

This was a cross sectional study conducted at the Royal Victoria Teaching Hospital, Banjul and the Medical Research Council (MRC) Laboratories, Fajara, The Gambia. Patients with hypertension attending the Royal Victoria Teaching Hospital hypertension clinic were recruited consecutively. The non-hypertensive patients were recruited from the Gate Clinic of the MRC Laboratories, Fajara. These were patients who reported with minor infections and were not diabetic and had no cardiovascular disease. The recruitment of participants was conducted from January to May 2000.

Patients with morbid obesity (BMI>35 kg/m^2), systemic or metabolic diseases, severe inter-current illnesses; known diabetes mellitus, cardiovascular disease (excluding hypertension) or labile hypertension (labile hypertension is when the blood pressure is sometimes above or sometimes below 140/90 mmHg), [9] were excluded from the study. Patients who were not known diabetes mellitus patients but who were found to be so after oral glucose tolerance test (OGTT) were included.

A questionnaire was administered by a field worker using the appropriate local language and a physical examination was done by one physician. The weight of participants was measured (to the nearest 0.1 kg) on electric scales (Secca r 770, CMS London), with subjects wearing light clothes and without footwear. The height was measured to the nearest 0.5 cm without footwear or head gear using standardised stadiometers. Hip and waist circumferences were measured using a plastic tape measure and recorded to the nearest 0.5 cm. The blood pressure was measured on the left arm using digital blood pressure machines (Omron r HOM – 705 CP, Japan) [10] and these were calibrated to the standard mercury sphygmomanometer every two weeks. Three readings were taken and the mean of the later two readings was used in the analysis [11].

A 3.5 MHz transducer on Hitachi EUB – 405 ultrasound scanner was used in performing 2-dimensional M-mode guided echocardiography on participants. The subjects were studied most commonly in the left lateral or partial left lateral position. The posterior left ventricular wall thickness was measured from the endocardial echo to the edge of the acoustic epicardial echo while the inter-ventricular septum was measured between its endocardial echoes [12].

The left ventricular end-diastolic diameter (LVEDD) was measured from the leading edge of the anterior endocardium to the leading edge of the posterior wall endocardium at end-diastole. The left ventricular end-systolic diameter (LVESD) was measured from inner edge of the anterior endocardium to the inner edge of the posterior wall endocardium of the left ventricle at end-systole. Polaroid paper were used to record all the distances, time and heart rate during the procedure.

An OGTT was carried out on participants during which, insulin levels were measured. The OGTT was performed using 75 g anhydrous glucose in 300–350 ml of water. A Haemocue analyser (Haemocue AB, Sweden) was used to immediately determine glucose level on fasting, 30 min and 120 min samples. The detailed results of the OGTT are presented in another article which is in print. However the information was used in classifying participants as DM in this study. Insulin level of a fasting sample was measured in the MRC NCD Laboratory with the Abbott IMx Immunoassay Analyser, which utilises a Micro-particle Enzyme Immunoassay (MEIA).

Using the fasting insulin and fasting glucose levels, the IR was estimated by the homeostatic model assessment (HOMA) formula.

The following definitions were adopted for this study.

1. Hypertension is systolic blood pressure≥140 and/or diastolic blood pressure≥90.mmHg in subjects who are not taking antihypertensive medication.
2. Overall Obesity is Body Mass Index (BMI)≥30 kg/m^2.
3. Central Obesity or High Waist Hip Ratio (WHR) is WHR>0.9 for males and>0.8 for females.
4. Diabetes. World Health Organisation Study Group on Diabetes Mellitus (1998). Fasting venous blood glucose>7.0 mmol/L and or 2 h post glucose capillary whole blood≥11.1 mmol/L [13].
5. Insulin Resistance (IR) = $\text{FastingVenousInsulin} \div 22.5e^{-\text{lnFastingVenousGlucose}}$ (The homeostasis model assessment formula).
6. Echocardiographic LVH Criteria

Penn convention/Formula: Left ventricular mass (PLVM) (g) = 1.04 {(IVSTD + LVPWTD + LVEDD) 3 – LVEDD3} – 13.6

Penn left ventricular mass indexed to body surface area (PLVMI) (g/m^2)

Body Surface Area (m^2) = $\sqrt{\{Weight(kg) \times Height(cm)\} \div 3600}$

Penn left ventricular mass index (PLVMI) = PLVM/BSA

Penn left ventricular echocardiographic LVH (PLVMILVH) defined by:

PLVMI>125 g/m^2 in males and PLVMI>110 g/m^2 in females [14].

7. Smoking was defined as "ever smoked" as compared to non-smoking which was defined as "never smoked".

The data was analysed using Stata version 8.0. The mean and standard deviation (sd) were used for continuous variables, and were compared using standard t-test. Discrete variables were analysed using Pearson chi squared test. The results of OGTT and IR were not normally distributed so a logarithmic transformation was done and this was used in all further analysis. Univariate and multivariate linear regression was used to analyse the association between log of IR and variables such as sex, smoking, hypertension, DM, BMI≥30, high WHR, antihypertensive treatment, age, BMI, WHR, SBP, DBP and fasting glucose. The association between PLVMILVH and log of IR was analysed using univariate and multivariate logistic regression controlling for various confounding variables. P-values of less than 0.050 were taken as statistically significant.

Results

Two hundred and eight consecutive patients (70 males) with hypertension on treatment and 108 non-hypertensive patients (39 males) were enrolled from outpatient clinics for our initial study [15]. However the data of 275 participants (89 males) were included in this analysis and results. Those excluded had missing variables especially of IR or echocardiographic LVH.

The mean (± sd) age of participants was 53.7 (±11.9) years and the age range was 27–85 (Tables 1 and 2). The males were older

Table 1. The clinical characteristics of participants by sex.

	Male (n = 89)	Female (n = 186)	All (n = 275)	P
	Mean (SD)	Mean (SD)	Mean (SD)	(t test)
Age (years)	55.7 (10.0)	52.7 (12.6)	53.7 (11.9)	0.051
Weight (kg)	70.8 (15.4)	71.1 (15.8)	70.8 (15.6)	0.591
Height (m)	1.70 (0.07)	1.61 (0.06)	1.64 (0.08)	<0.0001
BMI (kg/m^2)	24.1 (5.2)	27.5 (6.1)	26.4 (6.0)	<0.0001
WHR	0.89 (0.06)	0.88 (0.07)	0.88 (0.06)	0.066
SBP (mmHg)	140 (26)	134 (27)	136 (27)	0.134
DBP (mmHg)	83 (13)	83 (14)	83 (14)	0.678

t = Two sample t test with equal variance.
P = Statistical significance of difference.
n = Number.
SD = Standard deviation.
BMI = Body Mass Index BMI ≥ 30 (kg/m^2) = General obesity.
WHR = Waist hip ratio = Central obesity.
SBP = Systolic Blood Pressure.
DBP = Diastolic Blood Pressure.

than the females ($p = 0.051$). Weight was similar in both males and females but because the males were significantly taller their BMI was significantly lower than the females ($p<0.0001$). Prevalence of general obesity was 26% and this was significantly higher in the females ($p<0.0001$). The prevalence of central obesity was much higher (73%) and this was also higher in the females ($p<0.0001$). Mean systolic blood pressure (SBP) (136 mmHg), mean diastolic blood pressure (DBP) (83 mmHg), prevalence of hypertension (65%) and undiagnosed diabetes mellitus (DM) (15%) were similar in both the males and females. Smoking was more common in the male participants ($p<0.001$).

There were 166 (60.4%) participants (55 males) on antihypertensive drugs and all of them were hypertension patients. However 13 hypertensives were not on drug treatment and none of the nonhypertensives were on antihypertensive treatment. There were 28 participants on a combination of 3 drugs, 94 on a 2 drug combination and 44 on monotherapy. The majority (137 participants) were on bendrofluazide and this was followed by methyldopa, propranolol, nifedipine, hydralazine, hydrochlorothiazide and atenolol in that order. There was a patient each on amlodipine and captopril.

The echocardiographic characteristics of participants were all significantly higher in the males than the females except LVEDD which was similar in both sexes (Table 3). The mean (± sd) PLVMI was 135.3 (±56.2) for the males, 111.9 (±51.8) for the females and 119.5 (±54.3) for all the participants. The prevalence of echocardiographic LVH, PLVMILVH was 49% in males, 37% in females and 41% for both males and females.

There were no statistically significant sex differences in the biochemical characteristics of the participants (Table 4). The mean (± sd) fasting glucose was 5.6 (±2.5) mmol/l, the mean fasting insulin was 6.39 (±5.49) μU/ml and the mean IR (HOMA score) was 1.58 (±1.45).

In univariate logistic regression analysis with PLVMILVH as the outcome variable there were significant association between PLVMILVH and sex ($p = 0.052$), hypertension ($p = 0.008$), antihypertension treatment ($p = 0.028$), age ($p = 0.002$), WHR ($p = 0.021$) and SBP ($p = 0.001$)(Table 5). However there was no association between PLVMILVH and DM ($p = 0.771$), smoking ($p = 0.082$), log of fasting glucose ($p = 0.885$), high WHR ($p = 0.382$), BMI ($p = 0.284$), DBP ($p = 0.056$) and BMI > 30 ($p = 0.234$).

With log of IR as the outcome variable there were significant association between log of IR and DM ($p<0.001$), high WHR ($p = 0.038$), WHR ($p = 0.006$), BMI ($p<0.001$) and log of fasting glucose ($p<0.001$) (Table 6). There was no association between log of IR and sex ($p = 0.667$), smoking ($p = 0.229$), hypertension ($p = 0.272$), antihypertension treatment ($p = 0.202$), BMI > 30 ($p = 0.080$), age ($p = 0.971$), SBP ($p = 0.723$) and DBP ($p = 0.999$).

More importantly there was no association between PLVMILVH and log of IR in univariate logistic regression analysis (OR = 0.98, $p = 0.819$) (Table 5).

From the results of the univariate analysis WHR was the only variable which was associated with both PLVMILVH and log of IR. Therefore in a multiple logistic regression analysis we modeled with PLVMILVH as the outcome variable and WHR and log of IR as the explanatory variables. There was no significant association between PLVMILVH and log of IR (OR = 0.93, $p = 0.516$). WHR was however still associated with both PLVMILVH and log of IR (OR = 2.01, $p = 0.017$). There was

Table 2. The clinical characteristics of participants by sex.

	Male (n = 89)	Female (n = 186)	All (n = 275)	P
	Number (%)	Number (%)	Number (%)	(χ^2 test)
Age Range (yr)	32–80	27–85	27–85	
Smoking	46 (51.7)	15 (8.1)	61 (22.2)	< 0.001
Hypertension	60 (67.4)	119 (64.0)	179 (65.1)	0.576
Diabetes	12 (13.5)	29 (15.6)	41 (14.9)	0.646
BMI≥30	9 (10.1)	61 (32.8)	70 (25.5)	<0.001
HIGH WHR	37 (41.6)	163 (87.6)	200 (72.7)	<0.001
Antihypertensive Treatment	55 (61.8)	111 (59.7)	166 (60.4)	0.737

χ^2 = Pearson chi squared test.
P = statistical significance of difference.
n = Number.
BMI≥30 (kg/m^2) = General obesity.
WHR = Waist hip ratio = Central obesity.
HIGH WHR = WHR>0.9 for males and>0.8 for females.

Table 3. The echocardiographic characteristics of participants by sex.

	Male (n = 89)	Female (n = 186)	All (n = 275)	P
	Mean (SD)	Mean (SD)	Mean (SD)	(t test)
LVPWTD (mm)	1.2 (0.3)	1.1 (0.3)	1.1 (0.3)	0.003
IVSTD (mm)	1.3 (0.4)	1.2 (0.3)	1.2 (0.4)	0.002
LVEDD (mm)	4.3 (0.6)	4.2 (0.7)	4.2 (0.7)	0.121
LVESD (mm)	28.6 (6.4)	26.7 (6.8)	27.3 (6.8)	0.032
PLVM (g)	245.5 (102.1)	198.0 (93.0)	213.4 (98.4)	<0.001
PLVMI (g/m^2)	135.3 (56.2)	111.9 (51.8)	119.5 (54.3)	<0.001
*PLVMILVH (%)	44 (49.4)	69 (37.1)	113 (41.1)	0.052 ((χ^2)

t = Two sample t test with equal variance.
χ^2 = Pearson chi squared test.
P = statistical significance of difference.
n = Number.
SD = Standard deviation.
* Number.

still no significant association between PLVMILVH and log of IR in other models with PLVMILVH as the outcome variable and controlling for different variables. In further multivariate analysis with PLVMILVH as the outcome variable and controlling for various variables which were associated PLVMILVH in univariate analysis, the following variables were found to be associated with PLVMILVH, age (OR = 1.03, p = 0.018) and SBP (OR = 1.01, p = 0.006). When multiple regression analysis was done with log of IR as the outcome variable and the variable which were associated with log of IR in univariate analysis were included, BMI (r = 0.05, p<0.001) and log of fasting glucose (r = 0.98, p<0.001) were found to be the variables which were significantly associated with log of IR.

Further subgroup univariate logistic regression analysis with PLVMILVH as the outcome variable and log of IR as the explanatory variables was carried out for the various categorical variables. There was no association between PLVMILVH and log of IR in males, females, smokers, non-smokers, hypertensives, non-hypertensives, DM, non-DM, BMI ≥ 30, BMI < 30, high WHR and normal WHR (Table 7).

Discussion

In this study the relationship between LVH and IR was investigated using fasting blood glucose, fasting insulin and the HOMA formula for estimating IR and PLVMI. There was no statistical significant association between PLVMILVH and IR in these participants in univariate and multivariate regression analysis after controlling for various variables. Also in subgroup analysis using univariate logistic regression analysis there was no significant association between these two variables. Therefore, IR may not play a role in the development of LVH in this population of Gambians.

The most significant risk factors for LVH were the older the age of the subject and the higher the SBP rather than IR. On the other hand the significant risk factors for IR were high BMI and high fasting blood glucose. WHR which was a common significant variable to both LVH and IR was still significant in the multiple regression model but after adjusting for this variable there was still no significant association between LVH and IR.

Several mechanisms have been proposed to explain why there should be a direct relationship between IR and LVH. To date the best indirect evidence is the fact that angiotensin II receptor blockers correct both IR and LVH [16]. Angiotensin II type 1 receptors activity and numbers are up-regulated by the presence of IR [17]. LVH on the other hand is promoted by the mitogenic effect of angiotensin II on the angiotensin II type 1 receptors on smooth muscle cell of blood vessels. This eventually leads to hypertrophy of arterial wall and increased vascular resistance [18]. The effect of angiotensin II via angiotensin II type 1 receptors on the myocytes of the heart also directly promotes LVH [19]. This stimulation of LVH may partly be explained by an increased oxidative stress of the myocardium caused by angiotensin II [20].

Other direct and indirect mechanisms have been proposed for the contribution of IR in the development of LVH. These include the disordered and increased re-adsorption of sodium in the kidneys [21,22], the increased activation of the sympathetic nervous system [23] and the production of insulin growth factor-1 [24]. Others are the direct action of increased levels of insulin on the myocytes of the heart resulting in cardiac hypertrophy and remodeling, the promotion of the growth of vascular smooth muscle cells and lipotoxicity. These mechanisms also stimulate LVH further through the promotion of arteriosclerosis and increased arterial wall stiffness [22,25]. IR results in compensatory hyperinsulinemia which is considered to be a crucial factor in the development of the metabolic syndrome [26,27].

The association between LVH and IR from the published literature has been variable. There have been several studies reporting a positive relationship while there are not too few papers

Table 4. The biochemical characteristics of participants by sex.

	Male (n = 89)	Female (n = 186)	All (n = 275)	P
	Mean (SD)	Mean (SD)	Mean (SD)	(t test)
Fasting Glucose (mmol/l)	5.9 (3.4)	5.5 (1.8)	5.6 (2.5)	0.240
Fasting Insulin (μU/ml)	6.04 (5.34)	6.55 (5.57)	6.39 (5.49)	0.470
Insulin Resistance (HOMA score)	1.50 (1.42)	1.62 (1.46)	1.58 (1.45)	0.516

t = Two sample t test with equal variance.
P = statistical significance of difference.
n = Number.
SD = Standard deviation.

Table 5. Univariate analysis of variables with PVLMILVH as the outcome variable.

	OR	CI	P
Sex	0.60	0.36–1.00	0.052
Smoking	1.66	0.94–2.95	0.082
Hypertension	2.04	1.21–3.45	0.008
Diabetes	0.90	0.46–1.78	0.771
BMI≥30	1.39	0.81–2.41	0.234
HIGH WHR	0.79	0.46–1.35	0.382
Age	1.03	1.01–1.06	0.002
Weight	1.01	1.00–1.03	0.164
Height	1.83	0.09–35.36	0.689
BMI	1.02	0.98–1.06	0.284
WHR	1.97	1.01–2.02	0.021
SBP	1.02	1.01–1.03	0.001
DBP	1.02	1.00–1.04	0.056
Log of Fasting Glucose	1.07	0.42–2.75	0.885
Log of Insulin Resistance	0.98	0.80–1.19	0.819
Antihypertensive Treatment	0.57	0.34–0.94	0.028

P = Statistical test of significance of association.
CI = Confidence Interval.
OR = Odds Ratio.
BMI = Body Mass Index BMI≥30 (kg/m^2) = General obesity.
WHR = Waist hip ratio = Central obesity.
SBP = Systolic Blood Pressure.
DBP = Diastolic Blood Pressure.
HIGH WHR = WHR>0.9 for males and >0.8 for females.

Table 6. Univariate analysis of variables with log of Insulin Resistance as the outcome variable.

	R	CI	P
Sex	0.07	−0.24–0.37	0.667
Smoking	−0.21	−0.55–0.13	0.229
Hypertension	0.17	−0.13–0.46	0.272
Diabetes	0.72	0.33–1.11	<0.001
BMI≥30	0.29	−0.04–0.62	0.080
HIGH WHR	0.34	0.02–0.65	0.038
Age	0.0002	−0.01–0.10	0.971
Weight	0.02	0.01–0.03	<0.001
Height	0.64	−1.11–2.40	0.472
BMI	0.05	0.02–0.07	<0.001
WHR	3.08	0.91–5.26	0.006
SBP	−0.001	−0.01–0.004	0.723
DBP	−0.001	−0.01–0.01	0.999
Log of Fasting Glucose	0.98	0.43–1.53	<0.001
PLVMILVH	0.03	−0. 32–0.26	0.820
Antihypertensive Treatment	−0.19	−0.48–0.10	0.202

P = Statistical test of significance of association.
CI = Confidence Interval.
R = Regression Coefficient.
BMI = Body Mass Index BMI≥30 (kg/m^2) = General obesity.
WHR = Waist hip ratio = Central obesity.
SBP = Systolic Blood Pressure.
DBP = Diastolic Blood Pressure.
HIGH WHR = WHR>0.9 for males and >0.8 for females.

which have established that there is no relationship between LVH and IR. Significant associations between IR and LVH have been demonstrated in hypertensive patients as well as obese subjects [5,28–30]. The Framingham Heart Study showed a positive correlation of IR to LVH in female participants, but not in male subjects. However this correlation in females was attenuated after adjusting for BMI [31]. Our study did not show a significant association between LVH and IR before and after adjusting for hypertension, sex, general or central obesity. Further there was no significant association between LVH and IR in males nor females, hypertensives nor obese particiapants.

Other studies however have shown only weak association between LVH and IR [32] or no correlation at all after adjustments for other variables [7,8,33,34]. In a study of 107 males aged 50 years and over, no relationships were observed between IR and LVH [35]. Top *et al* demonstrated in 70 diabetic patients that there was no statistically significant correlation between LVH and HOMA derived IR [36]. In our study we excluded all previously diagnosed DM patients but included 41 previously undiagnosed DM patients who were diagnosed from OGTT. Among this subgroup there was no significant association between LVH and IR, a finding similar to the Top *et al* study. IR and fasting insulin has also been shown not to be associated with LVH in healthy people, independent of obesity. This was in a cross-sectional relational study carried out in 153 healthy subjects, comprising 76 men and 77 women who were normotensive, had a normal oral glucose tolerance test, no cardiovascular disease and none were on any medication [37]. Sherif *et al* investigated the relationship between left ventricular mass index (using cube function indexed to height in 52 premenopausal African American

Table 7. Multivariate analysis of variables with PVLMILVH as the outcome variable and log of Insulin Resistance as the explanatory variable.

	OR	CI	P
Male	1.14	0.80–1.63	0.475
Female	0.91	0.71–1.17	0.471
Smoking	1.07	0.74–1.55	0.735
No smoking	0.96	0.75–1.22	0.732
Hypertension	0.89	0.71–1.13	0.335
No hypertension	1.23	0.79–1.93	0.363
Diabetes	1.01	0.54–1.90	0.981
No diabetes	0.98	0.79–1.22	0.851
BMI≥30	1.33	0.89–1.98	0.160
BMI<30	0.85	0.66–1.08	0.174
HIGH WHR	0.95	0.75–1.20	0.645
Normal WHR	1.11	0.75–1.65	0.602
Antihypertensive Treatment	0.94	0.74–1.19	0.603
No Antihypertensive Treatment	1.01	0.70–1.47	0.950

P = Statistical test of significance of association.
CI = Confidence Interval.
R = Regression Coefficient.
BMI = Body Mass Index BMI≥30 (kg/m^2) = General obesity.
WHR = Waist hip ratio = Central obesity.
HIGH WHR = WHR>0.9 for males and >0.8 for females.

women) and cardiovascular risk factors [38]. They used the oral glucose tolerance test and the euglycaemic clamp. Left ventricular mass index was not associated with IR [38]. These findings are similar to our study where there was no significant association between LVH and IR before and after controlling for diabetes, fasting glucose and BMI.

This study is one of the few cardiovascular studies which have been undertaken in The Gambia. To date there has not been any published data on LVH nor IR from this small West African country. This is the major strength of this pioneering study. The finding of no association between LVH and IR therefore raises the question as to whether this is an observation peculiar to this community or part of the world. The main weakness of the study was the fact that it was a hospital based study which was fraught with various biases including selection and proximity biases. Another potential limitation of this study was the fact that the insulin levels were measured only in the fasting state but not after the glucose load was administered. Some studies have demonstrated a positive association between LVH and postload insulin levels [30]. Further as a cross sectional study the findings needs to be further confirmed by bigger studies of different and better study designs such as longitudinal cohort studies. Consequently there is the urgent need for more cardiovascular studies generally in The Gambia and specifically to explore the relationship between LVH and IR. These surveys should be larger community based studies as well as in participants with specific risk factors like obesity, metabolic syndrome, hypertension and DM.

Conclusion

There was no significant association between echocardiographic LVH and IR in this population of Gambians. Our findings do not support the suggestion that insulin is an independent determinant of LVH in hypertensives.

Acknowledgments

We are grateful to Dr. Hilton Whittle, Prof. J. W. Acheampong, Dr.T. Corrah, Dr. S. Allen, Dr. K. McAdam, Dr. Alieu Gaye, Mr. Winston Banya and Mr. Ben Sam.

Author Contributions

Conceived and designed the experiments: BCN ON TCA. Performed the experiments: BCN. Analyzed the data: FBM BCN TCA ON. Contributed reagents/materials/analysis tools: BCN ON. Wrote the paper: FBM BCN TCA ON.

References

1. Alberti KG, Zimmet P, Shaw J (2006) Metabolic syndrome—a new world-wide definition. A Consensus Statement from the International Diabetes Federation. Diabet Med. 23(5):469–80.
2. Kahan T (1998) The importance of left ventricular hypertrophy in human hypertension. J Hypertens Suppl. 16(7):S23–9.
3. Agabiti-Rosei E, Muiesan ML, Salvetti M (2006) Evaluation of subclinical target organ damage for risk assessment and treatment in the hypertensive patients: left ventricular hypertrophy. J Am Soc Nephrol. 17(4 Suppl 2):S104–8.
4. Ruilope LM, Schmieder RE (2008) Left ventricular hypertrophy and clinical outcomes in hypertensive patients. Am J Hypertens. 21(5):500–8. Epub 2008 Mar 13.
5. Sasson Z, Rasool Y, Bhesania T, Rasooly I (1993) Insulin resistance is an important determinant of left ventricular mass in the obese. Circulation. 88(4 Pt1):1431–6.
6. Lind L, Andersson PE, Andrén B, Hänni A, Lithell HO (1995) Left ventricular hypertrophy in hypertension is associated with the insulin resistance metabolic syndrome. J Hypertens. 13(4):433–8.
7. Costa CH, Batista MC, Moises VA, Kohlmann NB, Ribeiro AB, et al. (1995) Serum insulin levels, 24-hour blood pressure profile, and left ventricular mass in nonobese hypertensive patients. Hypertension. 26(6 Pt 2):1085–8.
8. Galvan AQ, Galetta F, Natali A, Muscelli E, Sironi AM, et al. (2000) Insulin resistance and hyperinsulinemia: No independent relation to left ventricular mass in humans. Circulation. 102(18):2233–8.
9. Expert Committee on Arterial Hypertension and Ischaemic Heart Disease. Arterial hypertension and ischaemic heart disease: preventive aspects; Report of an expert committee. Wld Hlth Org. techn. Rep. Ser. No. 231. 1962; 28.
10. Hammond IW, Devereux RB, Alderman MH, Lutas EM, Spitzer MC, et al. (1986) The prevalence and correlates of echocardiographic left ventricular hypertrophy among employed patients with uncomplicated hypertension. J Am Coll Cardiol. 7: 639–650.
11. Mayet J, Shahi M, Foale RA, Poulter NR, Sever PS, et al. (1994) Racial differences in cardiac structure and function in essential hypertension. Br Med J. 308:1011–1014.
12. Attah EB, Falase AO (1977) Large flabby hearts in hypertension. Am Heart J. 94: 189–195.
13. Rydén L, Standl E, Bartnik M, Van den Berghe G, Betteridge J, et al. (2007) Task Force on Diabetes and Cardiovascular Diseases of the European Society of Cardiology (ESC); European Association for the Study of Diabetes (EASD). Guidelines on diabetes, pre-diabetes, and cardiovascular diseases: executive summary. The Task Force on Diabetes and Cardiovascular Diseases of the European Society of Cardiology (ESC) and of the European Association for the Study of Diabetes (EASD). Eur Heart J. 28(1):88–136.
14. (2007) Compendium of European Society of Cardiology Guidelines 2007. Pp 19.
15. Nkum BC, Nyan O, Corrah T, Ankrah TC, Allen S, et al. (2009) Resting electrocardiographic and echocardiographic findings in an urban community in the Gambia. Journal of Science and Technology. 29:130–140.
16. Okada K, Hirano T, Ran J, Adachi M (2004) Olmesartan medoxomil, an angiotensin II receptor blocker ameliorates insulin resistance and decreases triglyceride production in fructose-fed rats. Hypertens Res. 27(4):293–9.
17. Nickenig G, Röling J, Strehlow K, Schnabel P, Böhm M (1998) Insulin induces upregulation of vascular AT1 receptor gene expression by posttranscriptional mechanisms. Circulation. 98(22):2453–60.
18. Daemen MJ, Lombardi DM, Bosman FT, Schwartz SM (1991) Angiotensin II induces smooth muscle cell proliferation in the normal and injured rat arterial wall. Circ Res. 68(2):450–6.
19. Homcy CJ (1998) Signaling hypertrophy: how many switches, how many wires. Circulation. 97(19):1890–2.
20. Whaley-Connell A, Govindarajan G, Habibi J, Hayden MR, Cooper SA, et al. (2007) Angiotensin II-mediated oxidative stress promotes myocardial tissue remodeling in the transgenic (mRen2) 27 Ren2 rat. Am J Physiol Endocrinol Metab. 293(1):E355–63. Epub 2007 Apr 17.
21. Rocchini AP, Katch V, Kveselis D, Moorehead C, Martin M, et al. (1989) Insulin and renal sodium retention in obese adolescents. Hypertension. 14(4):367–74.
22. Poornima IG, Parikh P, Shannon RP (2006) Diabetic cardiomyopathy: the search for a unifying hypothesis. Circ Res. 98(5):596–605.
23. Scherrer U, Sartori C (1997) Insulin as a vascular and sympathoexcitatory hormone: implications for blood pressure regulation, insulin sensitivity, and cardiovascular morbidity. Circulation. 96(11):4104–13.
24. Ito H, Hiroe M, Hirata Y, Tsujino M, Adachi S, et al. (1993) Insulin-like growth factor-I induces hypertrophy with enhanced expression of muscle specific genes in cultured rat cardiomyocytes. Circulation. 87(5):1715–21.
25. Hsueh WA, Law RE (1999) Insulin signaling in the arterial wall. Am J Cardiol. 84(1A):21J–24J.
26. Ferrannini E, Haffner SM, Mitchell BD, Stern MP (1991) Hyperinsulinaemia: the key feature of a cardiovascular and metabolic syndrome. Diabetologia. 34(6):416–22.
27. Grundy SM (1998) Hypertriglyceridemia, atherogenic dyslipidemia, and the metabolic syndrome. Am J Cardiol. 81(4A):18B–25B.
28. Urbina EM, Gidding SS, Bao W, Elkasabany A, Berenson GS (1999) Association of fasting blood sugar level, insulin level, and obesity with left ventricular mass in healthy children and adolescents: The Bogalusa Heart Study. Am Heart J. 138(1 Pt 1):122–7.
29. Sharp SD, Williams RR (1992) Fasting insulin and left ventricular mass in hypertensives and normotensive controls. Cardiology. 81(4–5):207–12.
30. Verdecchia P, Reboldi G, Schillaci G, Borgioni C, Ciucci A, et al. (1999) Circulating insulin and insulin growth factor-1 are independent determinants of left ventricular mass and geometry in essential hypertension. Circulation. 100(17):1802–7.
31. Rutter MK, Parise H, Benjamin EJ, Levy D, Larson MG, et al. (2003) Impact of glucose intolerance and insulin resistance on cardiac structure and function: sex-related differences in the Framingham Heart Study. Circulation. 107(3):448–54.
32. Ilercil A, Devereux RB, Roman MJ, Paranicas M, O'Grady MJ, et al. (2002) Associations of insulin levels with left ventricular structure and function in American Indians: the strong heart study. Diabetes. 51(5):1543–7.
33. Rheeder P, Stolk RP, Mosterd A, Pols HA, Hofman A, et al. (1999) Insulin resistance syndrome and left ventricular mass in an elderly population (The Rotterdam Study). Am J Cardiol. 84(2):233–6, A9.

34. Malmqvist K, Isaksson H, Ostergren J, Kahan T (2001) Left ventricular mass is not related to insulin sensitivity in never-treated primary hypertension. J Hypertens. 19(2):311–7.
35. Barud W, Makaruk B, Myśliński W, Palusiński R, Hanzlik J (2004) Hypertension, and not sex hormones or insulin resistance affects left ventricular mass in aging men. Ann Univ Mariae Curie Sklodowska [Med]. 59(1):232–6.
36. Top C, Sahan B, Onde ME (2007) The relationship between left ventricular mass index and insulin sensitivity, postprandial glycaemia, and fasting serum triglyceride and adiponection levels in patients with type 2 diabetes. J Int Med Res. 35(6):909–16.
37. Ebinç H, Ebinç FA, Ozkurt ZN, Doğru T, Yilmaz M (2006) Relationship of left ventricular mass to insulin sensitivity and body mass index in healthy individuals. Acta Cardiol. 61(4):398–405.
38. Sherif K, Barrett M, Kushner H, Falkner B (2000) The association of left ventricular mass with cardiovascular risk factors in African American women. Am J Med Sci. 320(1):13–7.

10

CD44 Plays a Critical Role in Regulating Diet-Induced Adipose Inflammation, Hepatic Steatosis, and Insulin Resistance

Hong Soon Kang[1], Grace Liao[1], Laura M. DeGraff[1], Kevin Gerrish[2], Carl D. Bortner[3], Stavros Garantziotis[4], Anton M. Jetten[1]*

1 Cell Biology Section, National Institutes of Health, Research Triangle Park, North Carolina, United States of America, **2** Microarray Group, National Institutes of Health, Research Triangle Park, North Carolina, United States of America, **3** Laboratory of Signal Transduction, Division of Intramural Research, National Institute of Environmental Health Sciences, National Institutes of Health, Research Triangle Park, North Carolina, United States of America, **4** Matrix Biology Section, LRB, National Institutes of Health, Research Triangle Park, North Carolina, United States of America

Abstract

CD44 is a multifunctional membrane receptor implicated in the regulation of several biological processes, including inflammation. CD44 expression is elevated in liver and white adipose tissue (WAT) during obesity suggesting a possible regulatory role for CD44 in metabolic syndrome. To study this hypothesis, we examined the effect of the loss of CD44 expression on the development of various features of metabolic syndrome using CD44 null mice. Our study demonstrates that CD44-deficient mice (CD44KO) exhibit a significantly reduced susceptibility to the development of high fat-diet (HFD)-induced hepatic steatosis, WAT-associated inflammation, and insulin resistance. The decreased expression of genes involved in fatty acid synthesis and transport (Fasn and Cd36), *de novo* triglyceride synthesis (Mogat1), and triglyceride accumulation (Cidea, Cidec) appears in part responsible for the reduced hepatic lipid accumulation in CD44KO(HFD) mice. In addition, the expression of various inflammatory and cell matrix genes, including several chemokines and its receptors, osteopontin, and several matrix metalloproteinases and collagen genes was greatly diminished in CD44KO(HFD) liver consistent with reduced inflammation and fibrogenesis. In contrast, lipid accumulation was significantly increased in CD44KO(HFD) WAT, whereas inflammation as indicated by the reduced infiltration of macrophages and expression of macrophage marker genes, was significantly diminished in WAT of CD44KO(HFD) mice compared to WT(HFD) mice. CD44KO(HFD) mice remained considerably more insulin sensitive and glucose tolerant than WT(HFD) mice and exhibited lower blood insulin levels. Our study indicates that CD44 plays a critical role in regulating several aspects of metabolic syndrome and may provide a new therapeutic target in the management of insulin resistance.

Editor: Lorraine Brennan, University College Dublin, Ireland

Funding: This research was supported by the Intramural Research Program of the NIEHS, NIH (Z01-ES-101586). The funders had no role in study design, data collection and analysis, decision to publish, or preparation of the manuscript.

Competing Interests: The authors have declared that no competing interests exist.

* E-mail: jetten@niehs.nih.gov

Introduction

Obesity is a major health-care concern in many Westernized countries. In the United States 30% of the population is considered obese, while more than 66% of adults and almost 17% of children and adolescents are overweight [1,2]. Obesity highly increases the risk of several pathologies, including type 2 diabetes, cardiovascular disease, and nonalcoholic fatty liver disease (NAFLD). Underlying the etiology of these pathologies is a disruption of the integrated control of lipid and glucose homeostasis in several tissues, including, the liver, adipose tissue, muscle, and pancreas. Several mechanisms have been implicated in the development of insulin resistance. Abnormal accumulation of lipids in the liver has been reported to cause hepatic steatosis and accelerate the progression of insulin resistance [3,4,5]. This is supported by findings showing that deficiencies in a number lipid transport, lipogenic or lipolytic genes promote or inhibit the development of hepatic steatosis and insulin resistance. It is well recognized that obesity is associated with systemic low-grade inflammation and that this is an important contributory factor in the development of insulin resistance [4,6,7,8]. Increased infiltration of proinflammatory M1 macrophages and other immune cells, including T lymphocytes, in adipose tissue and the subsequent release of proinflammatory cytokines, has been shown to play a critical role in this enhanced inflammatory state [9,10,11].

CD44 is a multifunctional cell membrane protein that can act as a receptor for hyaluronan and osteopontin (Opn; also named secreted phosphoprotein 1 or Spp1) [12,13]. CD44 is expressed by most cells, including macrophages and hepatocytes, and has been implicated in many biological processes, including development, cancer metastasis, and cell adhesion [12,14,15]. CD44 has been reported to regulate a variety of inflammatory responses, including the induction of proinflammatory cytokines and the migration of macrophages and neutrophils [16,17]. Binding of hyaluronan to CD44 can promote the interaction with a number of other cell surface proteins, for instance Tlr4 and EGFR, and influence the activity a variety of downstream protein kinase signaling pathways, including the MAP kinase and Akt pathways [13,18]. A recent study reported an alternative mechanism of action that involved proteolytic cleavage of CD44, translocation of its intracytoplasmic domain to the nucleus, where it subsequently regulated the expression of the matrix metalloproteinase 9 gene (*MMP-9*) by interacting with DNA within its promoter region [19].

Recent studies showed that obesity-induced hepatic steatosis and WAT-associated inflammation are accompanied with increased CD44 expression and opened the possibility that CD44 might play a regulatory role in obesity and associated pathologies [20,21]. To obtain further insights into the function of CD44 in metabolic syndrome, we compared the development of diet-induced hepatic steatosis, WAT-associated inflammation, and type 2 diabetes between wild type (WT) mice and mice deficient in CD44 expression (CD44KO). Our study demonstrates that CD44KO mice fed a high fat diet (HFD) are significantly less susceptible to developing hepatic steatosis, inflammation, and fibrogenesis. In addition, adipose tissue-associated accumulation of pro-inflammatory M1 macrophages was considerably less in CD44KO(HFD) compared to WT(HFD) mice and CD44KO(HFD) mice display greater insulin sensitivity and glucose tolerance. Taken together, our results suggest that CD44 may play a critical role in linking obesity to the development of insulin resistance by promoting hepatic steatosis and the infiltration of macrophages in adipose tissue. Because CD44 functions as a receptor, it might provide a convenient therapeutic target in the management of type 2 diabetes.

Materials and Methods

Experimental Animals

CD44-deficient mice were obtained from T. Mak [22] and backcrossed onto C57BL/6J for >10 generations. Male mice were supplied *ad libitum* with a normal chow NIH-A31 diet (ND). For diet induced-obesity (DIO) studies, 8–12 week-old male mice were fed a high fat diet (HFD: D12492, Research Diets Inc., New Brunswick, NJ) for 21 weeks, unless indicated otherwise. Adiposity was determined with a PIXImus densitometer (Lunar Corp., Madison, WI). All animal protocols followed the guidelines outlined by the NIH Guide for the Care and Use of Laboratory Animals and were approved by the Institutional Animal Care and Use Committee at the NIEHS.

Histology and Immunohistochemistry

Liver, white and brown adipose tissue specimens (n = 4–6) were fixed in 10% neutralized buffered formalin (NBF), and embedded in paraffin. Five microns (5 μm) of tissue sections were stained with hematoxylin-eosin. In order to detect macrophages, sections of white adipose tissue (WAT) were stained with an F4/80 antibody (Santa Cruz, CA) and avidin-biotin-peroxidase detection system.

Lipid and Glucose Analysis

Blood levels of glucose, cholesterol, triglycerides, and high-density lipoprotein (HDL) were analyzed as described previously [23] using the Cobas Mira Classic Chemistry System (Roche Diagnostics Systems Inc., Montclair, NJ). Serum insulin levels were analyzed with an insulin ELISA kit (Millipore, St. Charles, MO). To measure liver triglyceride and cholesterol contents, livers were homogenized and lipids extracted as previously reported [24]. Triglyceride and cholesterol levels were measured with Stanbio assay kits (Stanbio Laboratory, Boerne, TX).

Microarray Analysis

Microarray analysis was performed using the Agilent 1-color protocol as described in previously [25] with RNA isolated from liver and WAT of WT(HFD) and CD44KO(HFD) mice (n = 5). The microarray data discussed in this report have been deposited in NCBIs Gene Expression Omnibus at http://www.ncbi.nlm.nih.gov/geo #GSE43104.

RNA Isolation and Quantitative Real-time PCR (QRT-PCR)

Total RNA was isolated from liver and WAT with an RNeasy Mini kit from Qiagen (Valencia, CA). QRT-PCR analyses were performed as described previously [26]. QRT-PCR reactions were carried out in triplicate with StepOnePlus Real Time PCR system (Applied Biosystems). The sequences of primers and probes are listed in **Table S1**. All results were normalized relatively to the 18S or GAPDH transcripts. Student's t-test was used to calculate the p-value.

Western Blot Analysis

Protein lysates were prepared from WAT of mice fed a HFD using RIPA lysis buffer. Proteins were subsequently examined by Western blot analysis using antibodies against phosphorylated p38 MAP kinase (p-p38), phosphorylated JNK (p-JNK), and total p38 MAP kinase (p38) (Cell Signaling Technology).

Isolation of the Stromal-vascular Fraction (SVF) and Flow Cytometry Analysis

The isolation of the SVF from epididymal WAT (eWAT) was carried out as described [23]. Macrophage and T lymphocyte populations were stained with fluorescent-conjugated monoclonal antibodies against F4/80, CD11b, CD11c, and CD206, or CD3, CD4, and CD8, respectively, and subsequently analyzed with a BD LSR II Flow cytometer (Becton Dickinson) using FACSDiVa software.

Glucose Tolerance Test (GTT), Insulin Tolerance Test (ITT) and Adiponectin Elisa

After an overnight fast, WT and CD44 KO mice were injected intraperitoneally with glucose (2 g/kg) or insulin (0.75 U/kg) (Eli Lilly, Indianapolis, IN) and blood glucose levels determined to analyze GTT and ITT, respectively. A glucometer and glucose test strips (Nova Biomedical, Waltham, MA) were used to measure blood glucose. Circulating adiponectin levels were determined with an Elisa kit from R&D systems (Minneapolis, MN).

Results

Total Body Weight and Tissue Mass of CD44KO(HFD) Mice

Recent studies showed a correlation between the level of CD44 expression and hepatic steatosis in obese patients [20]. Studies from our own laboratory revealed that CD44 was expressed at significantly higher levels in WAT of WT mice fed a HFD (**Fig. 1A**) and was also elevated in liver of 7 months old mice or mice fed a HFD compared to 2 months old mice. A similar correlation between CD44 expression and obesity was observed in WAT of WT mice and mice deficient in the nuclear receptor TAK1 (also called TR4) mice that are resistant to HFD-induced obesity (**Figure S1**) [23]. The association of obesity and increased expression of CD44 in liver and WAT suggested that CD44 might have a role in regulating certain aspects of metabolic syndrome.

To obtain further insights into the potential role of CD44 in metabolic syndrome, we monitored the development of diet-

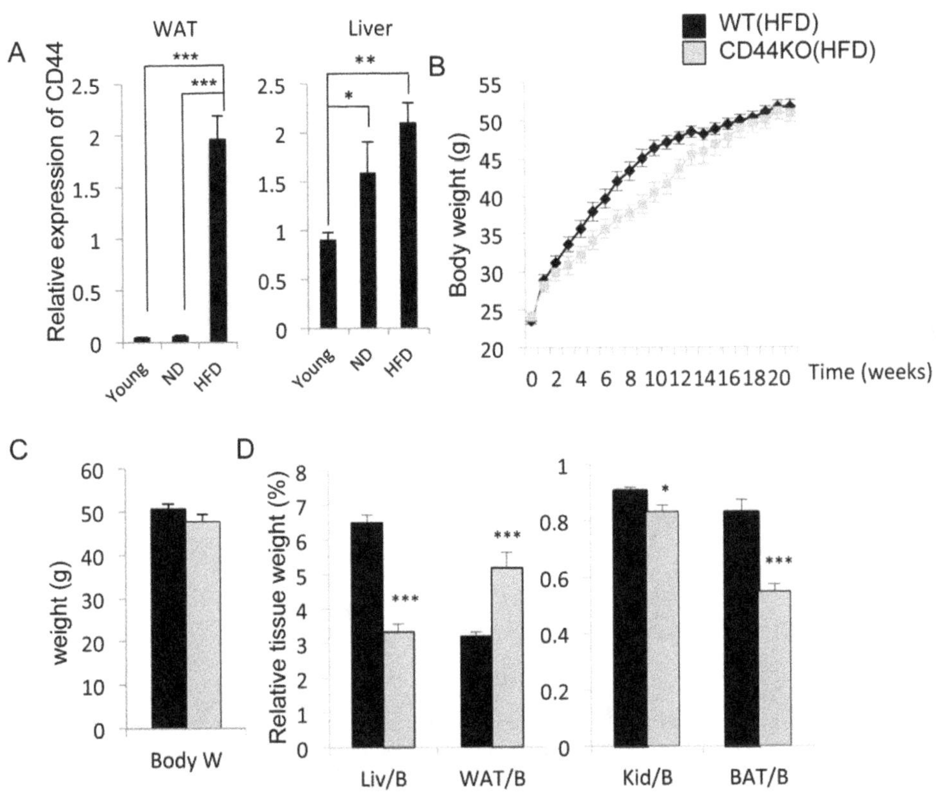

Figure 1. Comparison of total body mass and the relative tissue weight in CD44KO(HFD) and WT(HFD) mice. A) The expression of CD44 mRNA was analyzed in liver and WAT from 2 month-old WT (n = 6) or 7 month-old (n = 5) mice or mice fed a normal (ND) or HFD by QRT-PCR. B) Twelve week-old male mice (WT, n = 8; CD44KO, n = 8) were fed an HFD for 21 weeks and weight gain monitored. (C) Total body weight of mice fed an HFD for 21 weeks was plotted (WT, n = 8; CD44KO, n = 8). (D) Comparison of the relative weights of liver, WAT, kidneys, and BAT after 21 weeks on an HFD. Data present mean±SEM, *p<0.05, **p<0.01, ***p<0.001.

induced hepatic steatosis, adipose-associated inflammation, and type 2 diabetes in WT and CD44KO mice fed with a HFD ((WT(HFD) and CD44KO(HFD), respectively) for 21 weeks. CD44KO mice did not gain as much body weight as WT mice during the first 14 weeks on a HFD, while after 18 weeks the total body weights of WT and CD44KO mice were not significantly different (**Fig. 1B, C**). At 21 weeks, the relative weight of liver and brown adipose tissue (BAT) from CD44KO(HFD) mice was lower compared to WT(HFD) mice. In contrast, the relative weight of WAT was significantly higher (60%) compared to that of WT(HFD) mice, while the relative kidney weight was slightly decreased in CD44KO(HFD) mice (**Fig. 1D**). No significant difference in total body weight or the relative weight of WAT, kidney, and BAT was observed between 2 months old WT and CD44KO mice fed a normal diet, while the relative liver weight was slightly higher for CD44KO mice (**Figure S2**).

CD44KO Mice are Protected against Diet-induced Hepatic Steatosis

We next examined whether CD44-deficiency had any affect on the development of HFD-induced hepatic steatosis. Examination of histological sections of liver from WT(HFD) and CD44KO(HFD) showed a significant decrease in lipid accumulation in CD44KO(HFD) liver compared to WT(HFD) liver (**Fig. 2A, B**), while little difference was observed between livers of WT and CD44KO mice fed a normal diet (**Fig. 2C, D**). Lipid analysis indicated that hepatic cholesterol levels were increased to a similar degree in CD44KO(HFD) as in WT(HFD) mice (**Fig. 2E**). Although hepatic triglyceride levels were enhanced in both WT(HFD) and CD44KO(HFD) mice, this increase was about 50% less in CD44KO(HFD) consistent with the reduced fat accumulation observed in histological sections (**Fig. 2E**). The decrease in triglyceride accumulation in CD44KO(HFD) indicated that these mice were more resistant to the development of diet-induced hepatic steatosis.

The reduced accumulation of triglycerides is controlled at multiple levels, including fatty acid uptake, synthesis and storage of triglycerides, fatty acid oxidation, and lipolysis [4,27]. To obtain greater insight into the mechanisms by which CD44KO mice are resistant to the development of hepatosteatosis, we compared the hepatic gene expression profiles between WT(HFD) and CD44KO(HFD) mice by microarray analysis (http://www.ncbi.nlm.nih.gov/geo; accession number GSE43104). Loss of CD44 function affected the expression of many genes that are implicated in lipid metabolism (**Table 1**). This analysis showed that several lipogenic genes, including Mogat1 and 2, Cd36, and Fasn, were expressed at significantly lower levels in CD44KO liver than in WT liver (**Table 1**). QRT-PCR analysis confirmed that the expression of Cd36, encoding a fatty acid transporter, and monoacylglycerol O-acyltransferase 1 (Mogat1), which is part of an alternative pathway of triglyceride synthesis, were expressed at 50–70% lower levels in CD44KO(HFD) liver than in WT(HFD) liver (**Fig. 2F**). The expression of Fasn, which is involved in *de novo* fatty acid synthesis, was also expressed at lower levels in CD44KO(HFD) liver. The expression of several other acyltransferases involved in triglyceride synthesis, including glycerol-3-

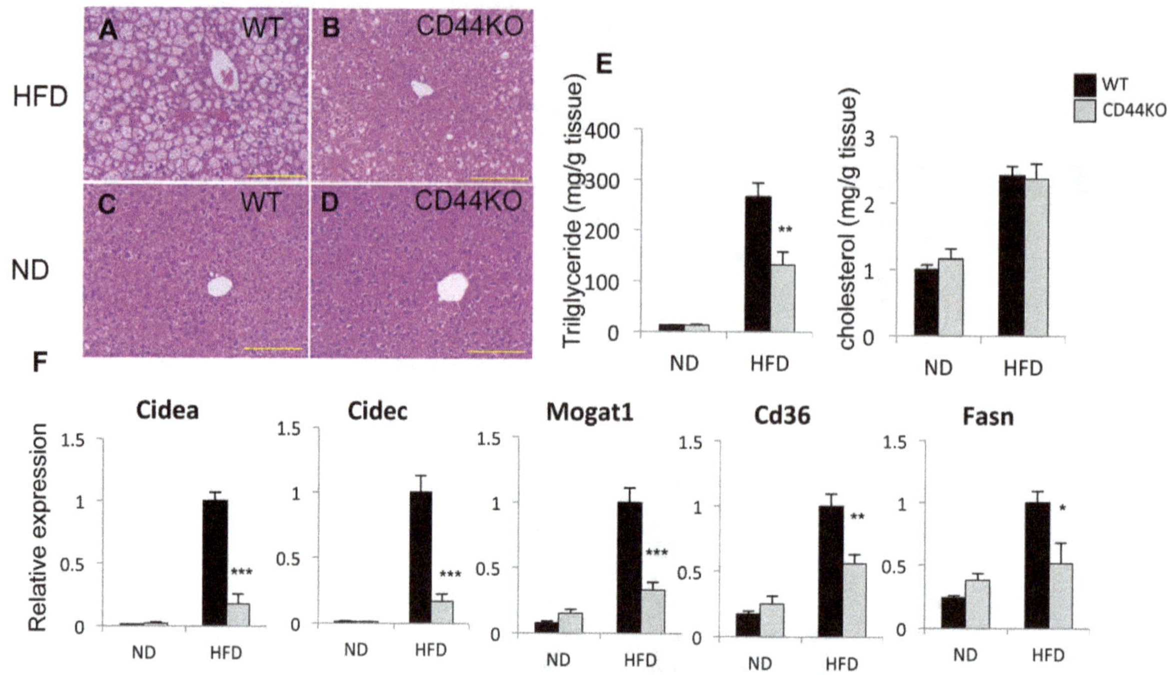

Figure 2. Hepatic steatosis was dramatically decreased in CD44KO(HFD). A–D) Representative H&E stained sections of liver were presented. Scale bar indicates 200 μm. E) Comparison of hepatic triglyceride and cholesterol levels. F) Comparison of gene expression in the livers of WT or CD44KO mice fed a normal diet (ND) or a high fat diet (HFD) (n = 5–6 mice per each group). Data present mean±SEM, *p<0.05, **p<0.01, ***p<0.001.

phosphate acyltransferase (Gpat), acyl-glycerol-3-phosphate acyltransferases (Agpats), and diacylglycerol acyltransferase 1 and 2 (Dgat1 and Dgat2), was not significantly different between WT(HFD) and CD44KO(HFD) (**Figure S3A**). A dramatic decrease was observed in the induction of the cell death-inducing DFFA-like effectors a and c (*Cidea* and *Cidec*) in CD44KO(HFD) liver compared to WT(HFD) liver. Cidea and Cidec function as important regulators of energy homeostasis with roles in lipid storage and lipolysis [28]. Additional genes that are associated with triglyceride synthesis and were decreased in CD44KO(HFD) liver, included elongation of long chain fatty acids 5 and 7 (Elovl5 and -7), apolipoprotein a4 (Apoa4), perilipin 4 (Plin4), and lipin1 (Lpin1) (**Table 1**). No significant change was observed in the expression of several genes involved in lipid oxidation (Cpt-1α and Pparα), lipolysis (Hsl and Atgl), and gluconeogenesis (G6pase and Foxo1) (**Figure S3B**). These results indicated that the reduced hepatic steatosis in CD44KO mice is at least in part related to a diminished expression of a number of genes critically involved in the regulation of the uptake, synthesis, and accumulation of triglycerides rather than increased lipid oxidation, lipolysis, or increased gluconeogenesis.

Biochemical analysis of sera from WT and CD44KO mice fed a ND or HFD showed that CD44KO(HFD) mice exhibited significantly lower serum cholesterol levels, while triglyceride levels were higher compared to WT(HFD) mice (**Fig. 3A, B**). The blood levels of high-density lipoprotein (HDL) and low-density lipoprotein (LDL) were increased under HFD conditions, but little difference was observed between the two genotypes (**Fig. 3C, D**).

CD44KO Mice Display Reduced Hepatic Inflammation

Abnormal accumulation of lipids leads to NAFLD that encompasses various levels of severity of inflammation, hepatotoxicity, and fibrogenesis [29]. Analysis of blood levels of alanine aminotransferase (ALT) and aspartate aminotransferase (AST), biomarkers of hepatotoxicity, showed that their levels were dramatically increased in WT(HFD) mice compared to WT(ND), but were not significantly enhanced in CD44KO(HFD) mice (**Fig. 3E, F**). These data suggest that CD44KO(HFD) mice were considerably protected against the development of hepatotoxicity compared to WT(HFD) mice.

Our gene expression profiling further revealed that many genes encoding chemokines and their receptors were decreased in liver of CD44KO mice (**Table 1**). These included the chemokine (C-C motif) ligands Ccl4, 5, and 7, the chemokine (C-X3-C) receptor 1 (Cx3cr1), and the chemokine (C-C motif) receptors Ccr2 and Ccr7. The expression of several other genes associated with immune responses and inflammation, including the lymphocyte antigen 6 complex, locus D and C1 (Ly6d and Ly6c1), the interleukin receptor 1 type 2 (Il1r2), and the CD8 antigens α and β1 (Cd8a and Cd8b1), were decreased in CD44KO(HFD) liver (**Table 1**). QRT-PCR analysis confirmed that the expression of Ccl2, Ccl7, Ccr2, and Ccr5 were decreased in liver of CD44KO mice fed a HFD (**Fig. 4**). QRT-PCR analysis further confirmed the decreased expression of Ly6d in liver of CD44KO(HFD) mice compared to WT(HFD) mice consistent with a report showing that Ly6d expression positively correlates with hepatosteatosis (**Fig. 4**) [30]. The expression of the pro-inflammatory cytokine, osteopontin (Opn) and its receptor CD44, was also considerably induced in WT(HFD) liver in agreement with previous observations [20,31,32]. The induction of Opn was significantly diminished in CD44KO liver (**Fig. 4**). Together, these observations are consistent with the conclusion that CD44 deficiency in mice protects against hepatosteatosis-associated inflammation.

Inflammation and fibrogenesis are closely related during the progression of NAFLD [33]. Microarray analysis showed that a number of cellular matrix genes that are associated with increased

Table 1. Partial list of genes reduced or increased in liver of CD44KO(HFD) mice compared to WT(HFD) mice.

Functional Category	GeneBank Accession #	Gene Symbol	Gene description	Fold Change (KO/WT)
Inflammation associated genes				
Chemokine				
	NM_013654	Ccl7	chemokine (C-C motif) ligand 7	-5.23
	NM_009987	Cx3cr1	chemokine (C-X3-C) receptor 1	−5.21
	NM_013653	Ccl5	chemokine (C-C motif) ligand 5	−4.30
	NM_009915	Ccr2	chemokine (C-C motif) receptor 2	−3.50
	NM_013652	Ccl4	chemokine (C-C motif) ligand 4	−3.35
	NM_008510	Xcl1	chemokine (C motif) ligand 1	−2.68
	NM_009142	Cx3cl1	chemokine (C-X3-C motif) ligand 1	−2.42
	NM_011888	Ccl19	chemokine (C-C motif) ligand 19	−2.32
	NM_008599	Cxcl9	chemokine (C-X-C motif) ligand 9	−2.12
	NM_007719	Ccr7	chemokine (C-C motif) receptor 7	−2.10
	NM_009917	Ccr5	chemokine (C-C motif) receptor 5	−1.99
	NM_007722	Cxcr7	chemokine (C-X-C motif) receptor 7	−1.98
	NM_009141	Cxcl5	chemokine (C-X-C motif) ligand 5	−1.95
	NM_001025192	Cxadr	coxsackie virus and adenovirus receptor	−1.68
	NM_009910	Cxcr3	chemokine (C-X-C motif) receptor 3	−1.53
	NM_018866	Cxcl13	chemokine (C-X-C motif) ligand 13	15.44
Immune response				
	NM_009851	Cd44	CD44 antigen	−18.50
	NM_010742	Ly6d	lymphocyte antigen 6 complex, locus D	−17.13
	NM_001081110	Cd8a	CD8 antigen, alpha chain	−8.94
	M17534	CD8b1	CD8 antigen, beta chan 1	−3.39
	NM_001042580	Cd63	CD63 antigen	−3.19
	NM_010555	Il1r2	interleukin receptor 1, type II	−1.71
	NM_010741	Ly6c1	lymphocyte antigen 6 complex, locus C1	−1.65
	NM_019408	Nfkb2	nuclear factor of κ light polypept. enhancer B cells	−1.55
Matrix				
	NM_008607	Mmp13	matrix metallopeptidase 13	−11.90
	NM_010809	Mmp3	matrix metallopeptidase 3	−4.54
	NM_007742	Col1a1	collagen, type I, alpha 1	−4.37
	NM_021334	Itgax	integrin alpha X	−4.03
	NM_008605	Mmp12	matrix metallopeptidase 12	−3.62
	NM_007737	Col5a2	collagen, type V, alpha 2	−3.06
	NM_145467	Itgbl1	integrin, beta-like 1	−3.05
	NM_009930	Col3a1	collagen, type III, alpha 1	−3.03
	NM_020008	Clec7a	C-type lectin domain family 7, member a	−3.27
	NM_011580	Thbs1	thrombospondin 1	−3.21
	NM_007403	Adam8	a disintegrin and metallopeptidase domain 8	−3.19
Functional Category	GeneBank Accession #	Gene Symbol	Gene description	Fold Change (KO/WT)
	NM_001038604	Clec5a	C-type lectin domain family 5, member a	−3.08
	NM_033612	Cela1	chymotrypsin-like elastase family, member 1	−2.68
	NM_010705	Lgals3	lectin, galactose binding, soluble 3 (Mac-2)	−2.51
	NM_008495	Lgals1	lectin, galactose binding, soluble 1	−2.35
	NM_011693	Vcam1	vascular cell adhesion molecule 1	−2.24
	NM_011581	Thbs2	thrombospondin 2	−2.12
	AK037794	Itga4	integrin alpha 4	−2.05
	NM_010810	Mmp7	matrix metallopeptidase 7	−1.70

Table 1. Cont.

Functional Category	GeneBank Accession #	Gene Symbol	Gene description	Fold Change (KO/WT)
	NM_008611	Mmp8	matrix metallopeptidase 8	−1.62
	AF026509	Itgb3	integrin beta 3	2.94
	NM_010766	Marco	macrophage receptor with collagenous structure	7.73
Transcription				
	NM_007498	Atf3	activating transcription factor 3	−2.80
	NM_008091	Gata3	GATA binding protein 3	−1.69
	NM_009283	Stat1	signal transducer and activator of transcription 1	−1.57
	NM_011487	Stat4	signal transducer and activator of transcription 4	−1.57
	NM_011756	Zfp36	zinc finger protein 36	1.89
Lipid accumulation associated genes				
	NM_029001	Elovl7	elongation of long chain fatty acids, member 7	−9.83
	NM_007468	Apoa4	apolipoprotein A-IV	−5.20
	NM_007702	Cidea	cell death-inducing DFFA-like effector a	−4.42
	NM_178373	Cidec	cell death-inducing DFFA-like effector c	−4.34
	NM_027881	Osbpl3	oxysterol binding protein-like 3	−3.7
	NM_020564	Sult5a1	sulfotransferase 5A1	−3.62
	NM_177448	Mogat2	monoacylglycerol O-acyltransferase 2	−3.54
	NM_020568	Plin4	perilipin 4	−2.67
	NM_026713	Mogat1	monoacylglycerol O-acyltransferase 1	−2.39
	NM_001033336	Abcc4	ATP-binding cassette, sub-family C, member 4	−2.00
	NM_015763	Lpin1	lipin 1	−2.00
	NM_007988	Fasn	fatty acid synthase	−1.82
	NM_134255	Elovl5	elongation of long chain fatty acids, member 5	−1.70
	NM_007643	Cd36	Cd36 antigen	−1.55

fibrogenesis, including several collagen genes (Col1a1, 3a1, and 5a2) and matrix metalloproteinases (Mmp3, 12, and 13), were decreased in liver of CD44KO(HFD) mice (**Table 1**). These results suggest that CD44 deficiency in mice protects not only against inflammation, but also against the onset of fibrogenesis.

CD44KO Mice Exhibited Increased Adiposity

Examination of the total body fat percentage measured by PIXImus dual-energy X-ray absorptiometry, indicated that CD44KO(HFD) mice exhibited a significantly higher body fat index than WT(HFD) mice (**Fig. 5A**) consistent with the observed increase in the relative weight of epididymal WAT (**Fig. 1D**). In addition, the average size of CD44KO(HFD) adipocytes was larger than that of WT(HFD) adipocytes suggesting increased accumulation of lipids in CD44KO(HFD) adipocytes (**Fig. 5B, C**). The latter is supported by the increased expression of the lipogenic genes, Cidec and Fasn (**Fig. 5D**). Gene profiling analysis with WAT on WT(HFD) and CD44KO(HFD) mice identified a number of additional lipogenic genes, including Fabp1, Elovl6, and Mogat2, that were increased in CD44KO(HFD) WAT compared to WT(HFD) WAT (**Table S2**) consistent with the observed increased adiposity in CD44KO(HFD) mice. In contrast, no difference in the expression of the lipases, Hsl and Atgl, was observed. Previous studies reported increased expression of several adipokines, including leptin, Il-6, and Ccl2, in adipose tissues of obese mice [7,34]. Similarly, the expression of leptin, Il-6, and Ccl2 was significantly increased in WAT of both WT(HFD) and CD44KO(HFD) mice; however, the increase in leptin and Il-6 expression was significantly greater in CD44KO(HFD) mice (**Fig. 5E**). No change in the level of expression of adiponectin, which plays a critical role in regulating inflammation and lipid metabolism and is down-regulated in obesity [35], was observed between WT(HFD) and CD44KO(HFD) nor in the circulating level of adiponectin (**Figure S4**).

Adipose-associated Inflammation was Reduced in CD44KO Mice Fed with an HFD

Adipose tissue-associated inflammation, including increased infiltration of macrophages and T lymphocytes, has been reported to play a critical role in the development of obesity-linked pathologies, including insulin resistance [9,10,11]. Immunohistochemical analysis showed that compared to WT(HFD) mice, WAT of CD44KO(HFD) mice contained significant fewer crown-like structures (CLS), phagocytic macrophages surrounding dead adipocytes and adipocyte remnants (**Fig. 6A, B**). Moreover, QRT-PCR analysis demonstrated that the level of expression of the macrophage-specific markers, F4/80 (Emr1) and Mac-2, were significantly reduced in CD44KO(HFD) WAT (**Fig. 6C**). In addition, the ratio between alternatively activated (M2) macrophages ($F4/80^+CD11C^-CD206^+$) and classical activated (M1) macrophages ($F4/80^+CD11C^+CD206^-$) in WAT from CD44KO(HFD) mice was about 2:1, compared to 1:1 in WAT from WT(HFD) mice (**Fig. 6D**). The reduction in M1 macrophages was supported by the reduced expression of Cd11c in

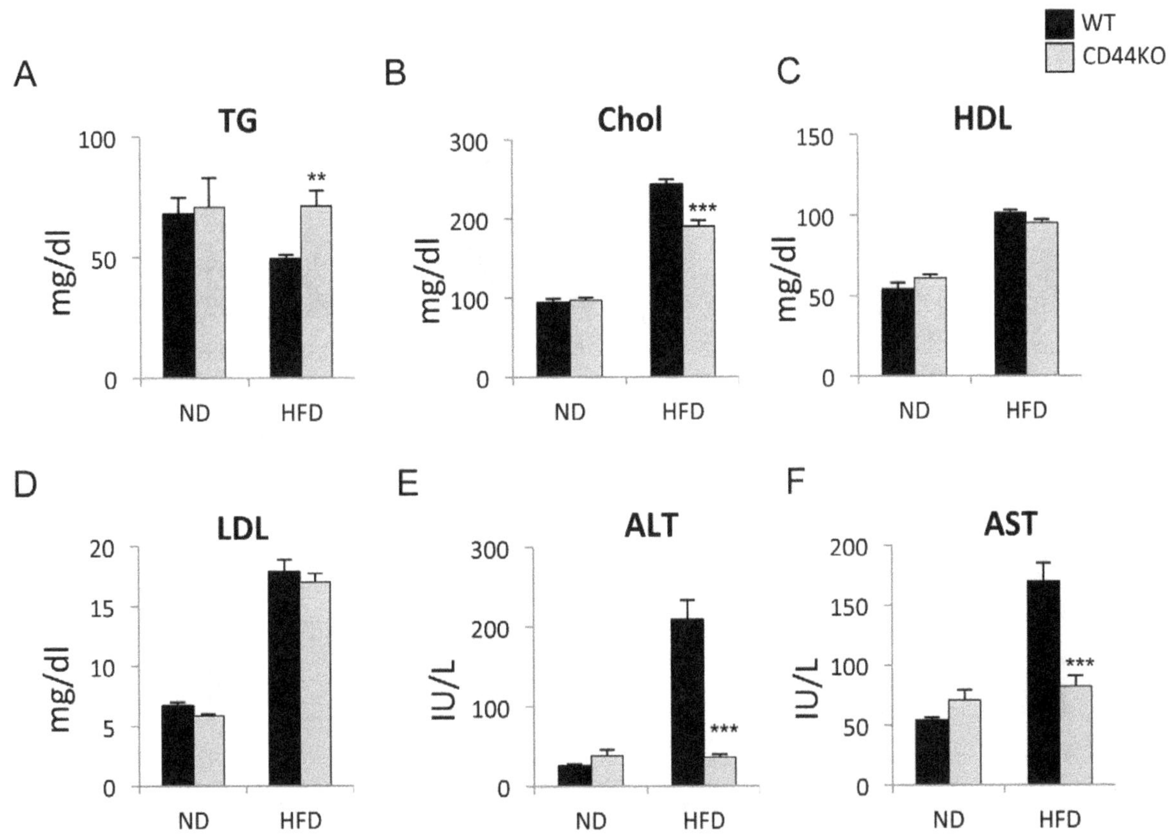

Figure 3. Activity of hepatic injury associated enzymes was decreased in CD44KO(HFD) compared to WT(HFD) mice. Levels of serum lipid (A–D), and alanine aminotransferase (ALT) and aspartate aminotransferase (AST) activity (E–F) were analyzed in WT and CD44KO mice fed a normal diet (ND) or a high fat diet (HFD) (n = 6–8 mice for each group). Data present mean±SEM, $^{**}p<0.01$, $^{***}p<0.001$.

WAT of CD44KO(HFD) mice (**Fig. 6E**). WAT of both WT and CD44KO fed a ND consisted largely (90%) of M2 macrophages (**Figure S5**). To examine differences in immune responsiveness between WT and CD44KO macrophages, the response of peritoneal macrophages to LPS was compared; however, no significant differences were observed between the two genotypes in the induction of several inflammatory genes, including Ccl2 and Ccl5 (not shown).

Comparison of the gene expression profiles between WAT of WT(HFD) and CD44KO(HFD) showed that a number of inflammatory genes, including several cell surface antigens, tryptases and cyto/chemokines and their receptors, were down-regulated in CD44KO(HFD) WAT (**Table S2**). The observed decreased expression of several macrophage-associated genes, including interleukin 1 receptor antagonist (Il1rn), Mmp12, F4/80, Cd11c, Msr1, and Toll-like receptor 8 (Tlr8), supported the reduced macrophage accumulation in WAT of CD44KO(HFD) mice (**Table S2; Fig. 6F**). Although Opn expression was greatly induced in WAT of HFD mice, in contrast to liver no significant difference was observed between the two genotypes (**Fig. 6F**).

Recent studies indicated that the accumulation of $CD8^+$ T lymphocytes also play a critical role in WAT-associated inflammation [9]. **Fig. 7A** shows that the percent $CD3^+$ T lymphocytes and $CD8^+$ T lymphocytes was significantly decreased in WAT of CD44KO(HFD) compared to WT(HFD) mice consistent with reduced adipose-associated inflammation in CD44KO(HFD) mice. The decreased level of Cd3, Cd8a and Cd8b expression identified by microarray analysis (**Table S2**) is consistent with reduced infiltration of $CD3^+$ and $CD8^+$ cells. Together, these observations support the conclusion that adipose-associated inflammation is decreased in WAT of CD44KO(HFD) mice compared to WT(HFD) mice and is in part related to reduced infiltration and activation of M1 macrophages and CD8 lymphocytes.

Adiposity has been shown to be associated with activation of several kinases in WAT, including c-Jun amino-terminal kinases (JNKs) and p38 mitogen-activated protein kinase (p38 MAPK) [36,37,38]. Moreover, stimulation of CD44 signaling has been reported to activate p38 in different cell systems [39,40]. We therefore examined the effect of loss of CD44 expression on the level of activation of these kinases in WAT by Western blot analysis. As shown in Fig. 7B, while phosphorylated JNK (pJNK) was unchanged, the level of phosphorylated p38 was dramatically decreased in WAT of CD44KO(HFD) mice compared to WT(HFD) mice. These results indicate that in WAT loss of CD44 results in a selective inhibition of the activation of p38 MAPK. Opn has been recently reported to activate p38 via CD44 [39], one might therefore speculate that activation of this pathway is impaired in CD44KO WAT.

CD44 Mice are Protected against Diet-induced Insulin Resistance

Nonalcoholic fatty liver disease is almost invariably associated with insulin resistance [27]. To examine whether CD44KO(HFD) mice were less sensitive to the development of type 2 diabetes, glucose tolerance (GTT) and insulin tolerance tests (ITT) were

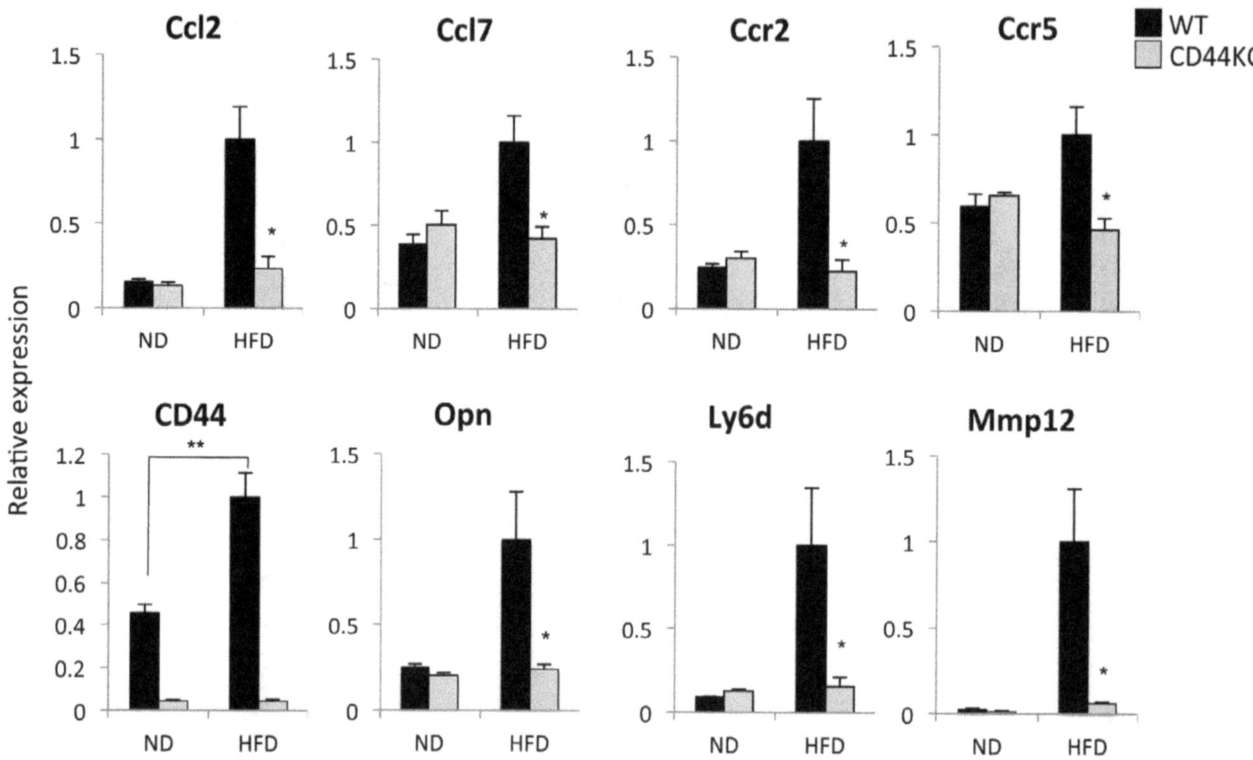

Figure 4. The induction of inflammatory genes was decreased in liver of CD44KO(HFD) compared to WT(HFD) mice. Comparison of gene expression in the liver of WT or CD44KO mice fed a normal diet (ND) or a high fat diet (HFD) (n = 5–6 mice per each group). Data present mean±SEM, *p<0.05, **p<0.01, ***p<0.001.

performed at 6, 12, and 21 weeks of HFD feeding. As shown in **Fig. 8A**, at 6-weeks of HFD CD44KO mice were considerably more glucose tolerant than WT mice, while only a slight difference in insulin sensitivity was observed. At 12 weeks of HFD, CD44KO mice were significantly more glucose tolerant and insulin sensitive than WT mice. By 21 weeks of HFD, CD44KO mice remained considerably less glucose intolerance and insulin sensitive than WT mice (**Fig. 8A**). Insulin resistance often results in increased insulin production in an attempt to compensate for the decreased insulin sensitivity. As shown in **Fig. 8B**, serum insulin levels were significantly lower in CD44KO(HFD) mice than WT(HFD) mice. Together, these results indicate that CD44KO mice were less susceptible to the development of HFD-induced insulin resistance.

Discussion

In this study, we examined the effect of CD44 deficiency on the development of diet-induced obesity and associated pathologies in mice. We demonstrated that CD44KO mice are protected against the development of diet-induced hepatic steatosis as indicated by the lower levels of hepatic triglycerides and reduced hepatotoxicity, inflammation, and fibrogenesis. In addition, our data showed that CD44KO mice are considerably less susceptible to the development of diet-induced adipose inflammation, insulin resistance, and glucose-intolerance.

The accumulation of triglycerides during hepatic steatosis is mediated by several mechanisms, including changes in lipid transport, *de novo* synthesis, storage, fatty acid oxidation, and lipolysis. Our study demonstrated that the diet-induced increase in the expression of several genes implicated in the regulation of lipid metabolism was diminished considerably in the liver of CD44(HFD) mice. Of the genes analyzed, the expression of the cell death-inducing DFF45-like effector (CIDE) genes, Cidea and Cidec, was the most dramatically affected by CD44 deficiency (**Fig. 2**). Both Cidea and Cidec play a critical role in the regulation of lipid storage, lipid droplet formation, and lipolysis [24,41,42]. The expression of CD36, which among other things facilitates the transport of fatty acids into the liver, as well as the expression of several genes involved in fatty acid biosynthesis, including fatty acid synthase (Fasn), and Elovl5 and -7, were also significantly reduced in CD44(HFD) liver compared to WT(HFD) liver. Moreover, the expression of Mogat1, which is part of an alternative pathway of *de novo* triglyceride synthesis, was greatly diminished in CD44(HFD) liver, while the expression of Dgat1 and Dgat2, which are important in the classical *de novo* triglyceride synthesis pathway, was not different between the two genotypes. In addition to their control of lipid metabolism, several of these lipogenic genes, including Cidea, Cidec, and Cd36, play a critical role in regulating the development of hepatic steatosis and insulin sensitivity [24,28,43]. Mice deficient in Cidea or Cidec have been shown to exhibit reduced hepatic lipid accumulation and improved insulin sensitivity, while overexpression of Cidea in mouse liver promoted hepatic steatosis. Cd36 deficiency has been reported to protect mice against diet-induced hepatic steatosis and insulin resistance, while increased expression has the inverse effect [44,45]. The reduced expression of Cidec, Cidea, Cd36, Mogat1, and Fasn, as well as Elovl5 and 7, may provide a mechanism for the diminished hepatic fatty acid uptake and triglyceride synthesis, and the decreased lipid accumulation and be at least in part responsible for the reduced hepatic steatosis and insulin resistance observed in CD44KO mice (Fig. 9).

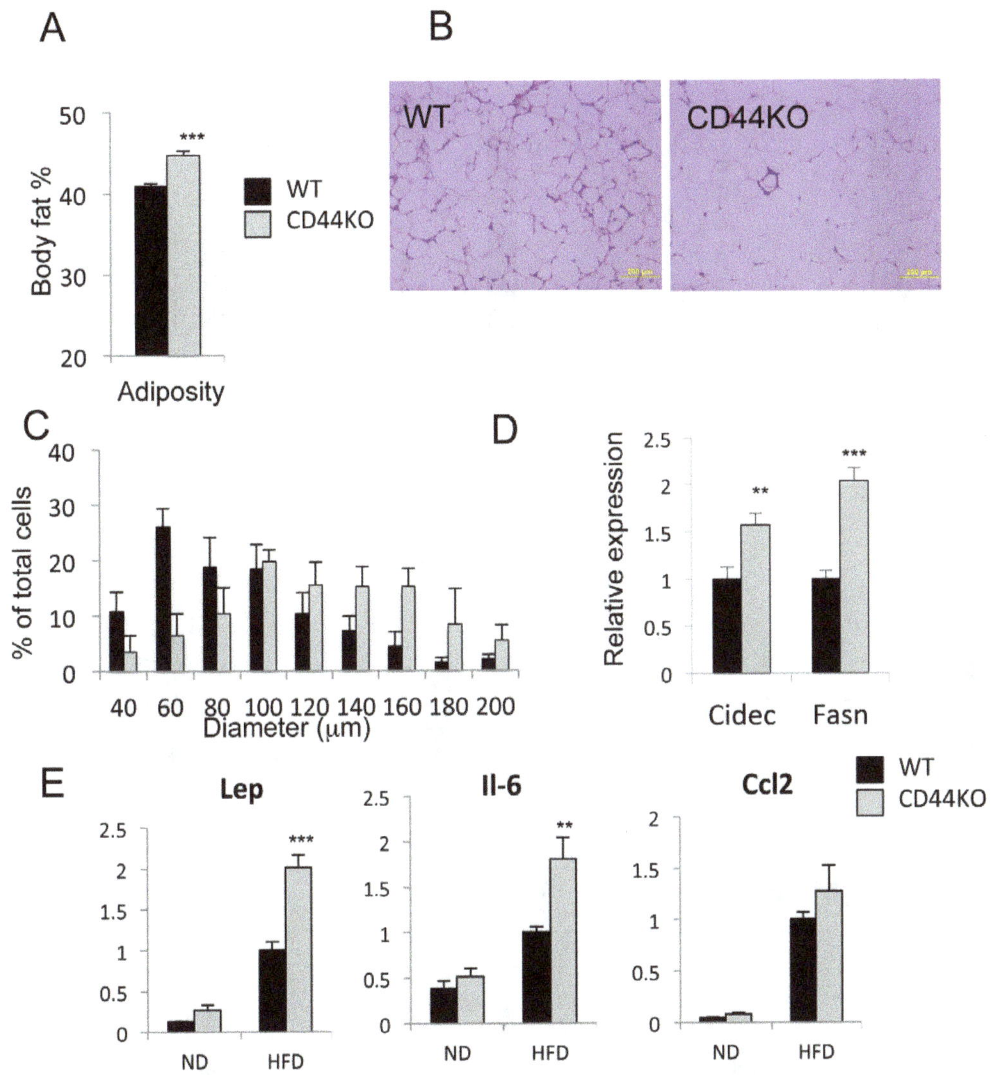

Figure 5. Total body fat was increased in CD44KO(HFD) compared to WT(HFD) mice. A) Total body fat mass from mice fed a HFD for 21 weeks was analyzed by Piximus densitometry. B) Representative H&E stained sections of WAT were presented. Scale bar indicates 200 μm. C) Comparison of the cell size of WAT adipocytes from WT(HFD) and CD44KO(HFD). Cell diameters in sections of WAT from 4 mice in each group were measured and the percentages of the different cell sizes calculated and plotted. D) Increased Cidec and Fasn expression in WAT of CD44KO(HFD) compared to WT(HFD) mice (n = 5–6 mice per each group). E) Comparison of gene expression in WAT of WT or CD44KO mice fed a normal diet (ND) or a high fat diet (HFD) (n = 5–6 mice per each group).

In addition to triglyceride accumulation, inflammation, hepatotoxicity, and fibrogenesis are important features in the progression of NAFLD [33,46,47]. We provided evidence suggesting that hepatotoxicity was greatly reduced in CD44KO(HFD) mice compared to WT(HFD) mice as indicated by the significantly lower blood levels of the biomarkers, ALT and AST. We further observed that the liver of CD44KO(HFD) liver displayed less inflammation than WT(HFD) liver as indicated by gene expression profiling. The expression of a number of proinflammatory cytokines, including several chemokines (Ccl2, Ccl5, Ccl7) and their receptors (Ccr2, Ccr5), metalloproteinases, and Opn, was reduced in CD44KO liver. Several of these genes, including the Ccr2 and Ccr5 signaling pathways, have been implicated in the mobilization of monocytes [48]. These observations are consistent with previous reports showing a link between Opn expression and progression of hepatic injury and inflammation and an association between the level of Ccl2 expression and the severity of hepatosteatosis [20,37,49]. Ccl2 is produced by hepatocytes and hepatic macrophages and functions as a potent chemoattractive mediator for bone marrow-derived macrophages, while both Ccl2 and Opn can function as activators of M1 macrophages [20,32,50]. A strong link has been established between the regulation of inflammation and fibrogenesis [33]. The reduced hepatic expression of matrix metalloproteinases and several collagens in CD44KO(HFD) mice is consistent with the conclusion that these mice are protected against the onset of hepatosteatosis-associated fibrosis. The latter is consistent with recent findings on the role of CD44 in lung fibrosis [51]. Thus, the observed decreased expression of various chemokines and their receptors as well as several cellular matrix genes in CD44KO(HFD) mice might be at least in part responsible for the reduced hepatic inflammation injury, and fibrogenesis, and consequently for its protective effect against hepatosteatosis (Fig. 9).

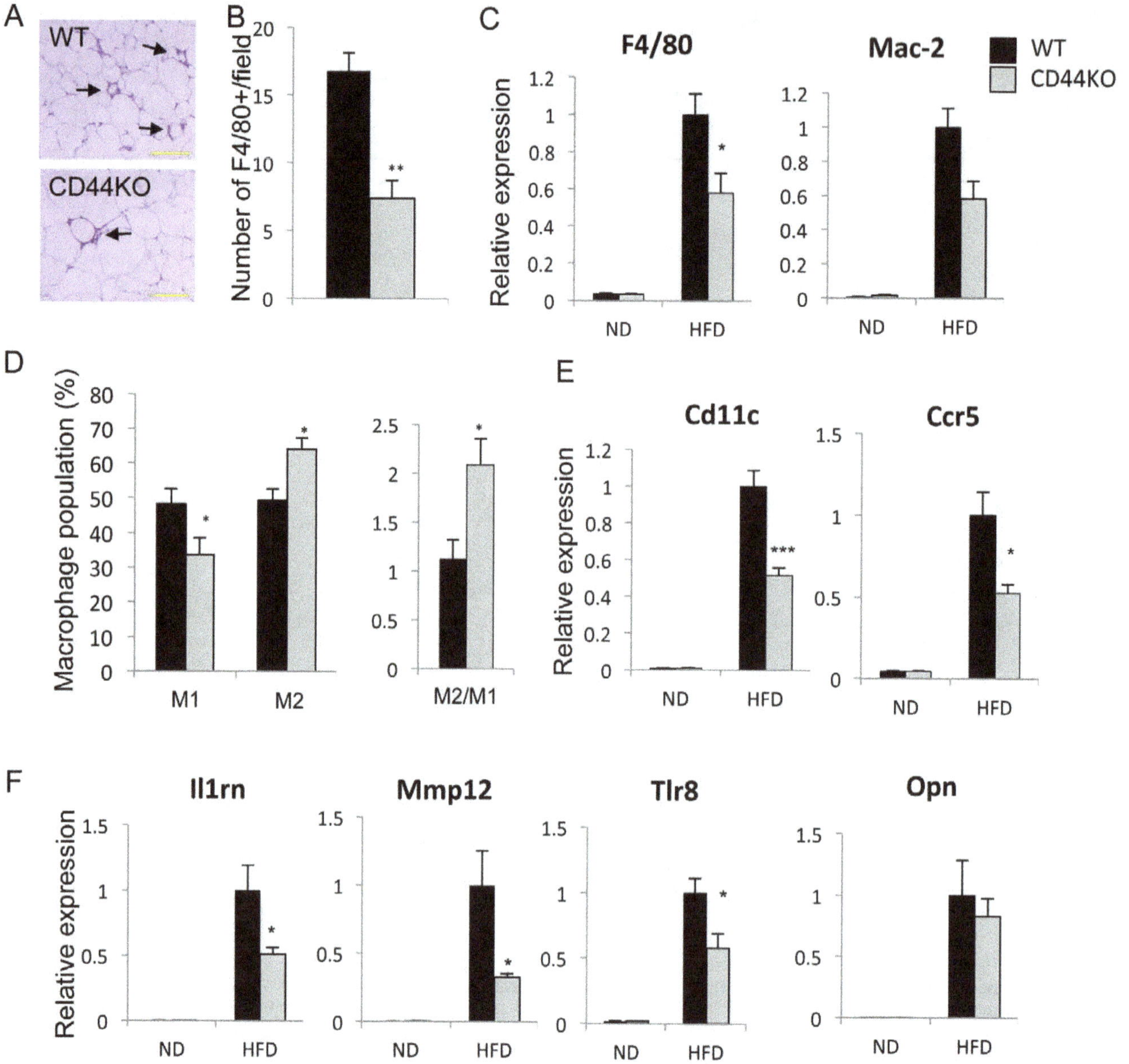

Figure 6. Adipose tissue inflammation was reduced in CD44KO(HFD) compared to WT(HFD) mice. A) Macrophages in crown-like structures (CLS) were identified by immunohistochemical staining with an F4/80 antibody as indicated by arrows. Scale bar indicates 250 μm. B) The number of CLS was decreased in CD44KO(HFD) compared to WT(HFD) mice. F4/80 positive cells in at least 4 randomly selected fields in sections from 4 different mice were counted. C) Comparison of the expression of macrophage markers, F4/80 and Mac-2, in WAT of WT or CD44KO mice fed a normal diet (ND) or a high fat diet (HFD) (n = 5–6 mice per each group). D) SVF cells from WAT of WT(HFD) mice (n = 6) and CD44KO(HFD) mice (n = 8) were examined by FACS analysis with F4/80, CD11b, CD11c, and CD206 antibodies. The percentage and ratio of pro-inflammatory macrophage (M1: F4/80$^+$CD11C$^+$CD206$^-$) and anti-inflammatory macrophage (M2: F4/80$^+$CD11C$^-$CD206$^+$) were determined. Expression of several macrophage markers (E) and inflammatory markers (F) was analyzed in WAT of WT or CD44KO mice fed a normal diet (ND) or a high fat diet (HFD) (n = 5–6 mice per each group).

In most mouse obesity models, the development of hepatic steatosis and increased adiposity are often associated [23]. Unexpectedly however, in contrast to the decrease in hepatic steatosis, lipid accumulation was enhanced in WAT CD44KO(HFD) mice, which appeared to be due to an increase in lipid storage. This may be in part related to the enhanced expression of Fasn, Elovl3 and -6, FABP1, and Cidec, a key factor regulating triglyceride storage and lipid droplet size in WAT [28,41] rather than changes in lipolysis since the expression of the major lipases, Hasl and Atgl, was not significantly different between WAT of WT and CD44KO mice. As the expression of Pparγ was not different between genotype groups, increased lipid storage in CD44KO WAT may not be due to expansion or development of adipocytes (**Figure S4**). Differences in adiposity might involve altered energy intake and expenditure; however, no significant differences in food intake, oxygen consumption, CO_2 production, and heat generation were observed between WT and CD44KO mice (**Figure S6**). Thus, the effects on hepatic steatosis and adiposity appear to be related to an immune-mediated

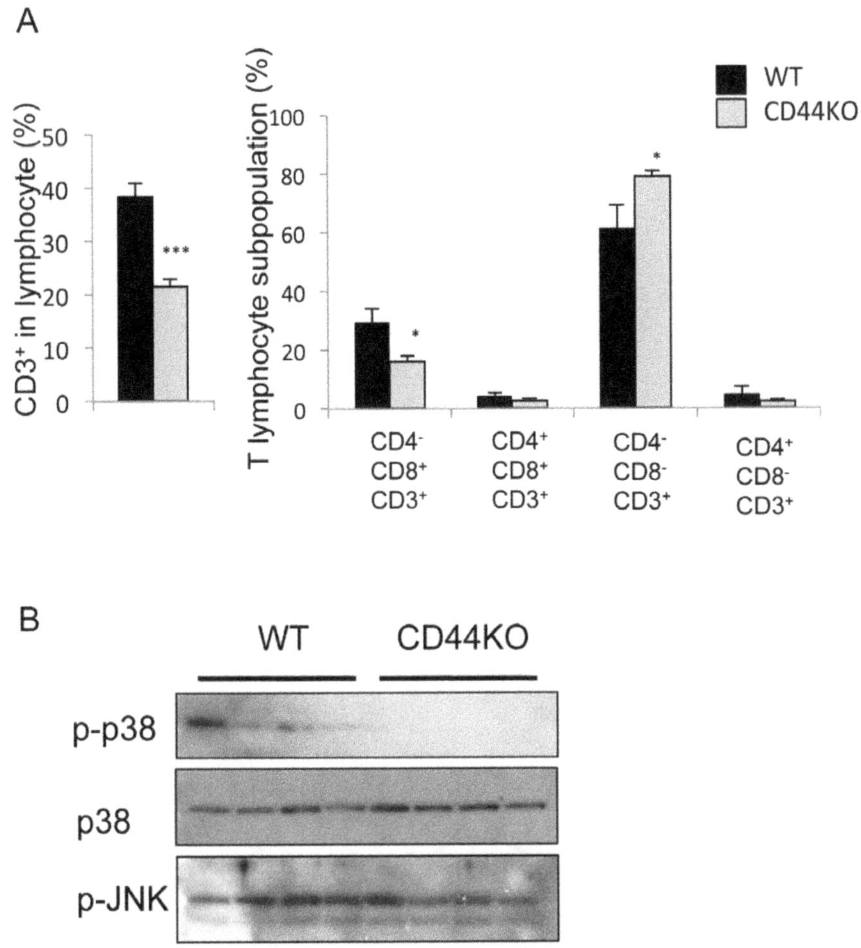

Figure 7. The CD3$^+$ lymphocyte population and level of activated p38 MAPK in WAT of CD44KO(HFD) is reduced compared to WT (HFD) mice. The percentages of different CD4/CD8 cell populations were determined by FACS analysis. The percentage of CD8 single-positive T lymphocytes (CD4$^-$CD8$^+$) was decreased in WAT of CD44KO(HFD) compared to WT (HFD) mice. (n = 5–6 mice per each group). Data represent mean±SEM. *p<0.05, ***p<0.001. (B) Protein lysates were extracted from WAT of WT(HFD) and CD44KO(HFD) mice, and Western blot analysis was performed using phosphorylated or total p38 MAPK antibodies and phosphorylated JNK antibody.

modulation of lipid metabolism, rather than changes in food intake or energy expenditure in CD44KO mice.

In contrast to adiposity, WAT-associated inflammation was significantly reduced in CD44(HFD) mice. This was indicated by gene expression profile analysis showing that a number of inflammatory genes, including Il17a, Il33, Il1rn, Ccrl1, and Ccl6, were significantly reduced in WAT of CD44KO(HFD) mice (**Table** S2). In addition, the number of macrophages associated with WAT of CD44KO(HFD) mice was significantly lower compared to WT(HFD) WAT as indicated by the presence of considerably fewer crown-like structures and significantly lower levels of expression of the macrophage markers, F4/80, Cd11c, and Mac-2. Furthermore, the expression of the cytokine receptor Ccr5, which plays a critical role in the recruitment and activation of WAT macrophages [52], was significantly lower in CD44KO(HFD) WAT than WT(HFD) WAT. Moreover, the ratio of anti-inflammatory M2 macrophages over pro-inflammatory M1 macrophages was significantly higher in CD44KO(HFD) WAT (**Fig. 6**). Together, these observations support the conclusion that chemotaxis as well as the activation of pro-inflammatory macrophages is significantly reduced in CD44KO(HFD) WAT. In addition to the reduction in macrophages, the number of cytotoxic CD8$^+$ T lymphocytes, which play an essential role in the initiation and propagation of adipose inflammation [9], and the expression Cd3 and Cd8 antigens was significantly lower in WAT of CD44KO(HFD) mice suggesting a role for CD44 in regulating the migration and recruitment of these cells as well. It is well recognized that obesity is associated with low-grade systemic inflammation and that WAT-associated inflammation plays a key role in obesity-linked pathologies, including insulin resistance [53,54]. Thus, the reduced inflammation observed in WAT of CD44KO(HFD) mice might be a part of the mechanism that protects these mice against insulin resistance and glucose-intolerance (Fig. 9).

Adipokines produced by adipocytes play a critical role in regulating inflammation, lipid metabolism as well as insulin resistance [35]. Adiponectin plays a protective role against inflammation by reducing expression of proinflammatory cytokines through inhibition of NF-κB signaling pathway [35,55,56] and regulate fatty acid oxidation in liver though activation of PPARα and adenosine monophosphate-activated protein kinase (AMPK). However, the expression of adiponectin in WAT as well as the circulating level of adiponectin were not changed between genotypes (**Figure** S4). This suggests that the protection against adipose-associated inflammation and hepatosteatosis in CD44KO(HFD) mice is not causally related to differences in

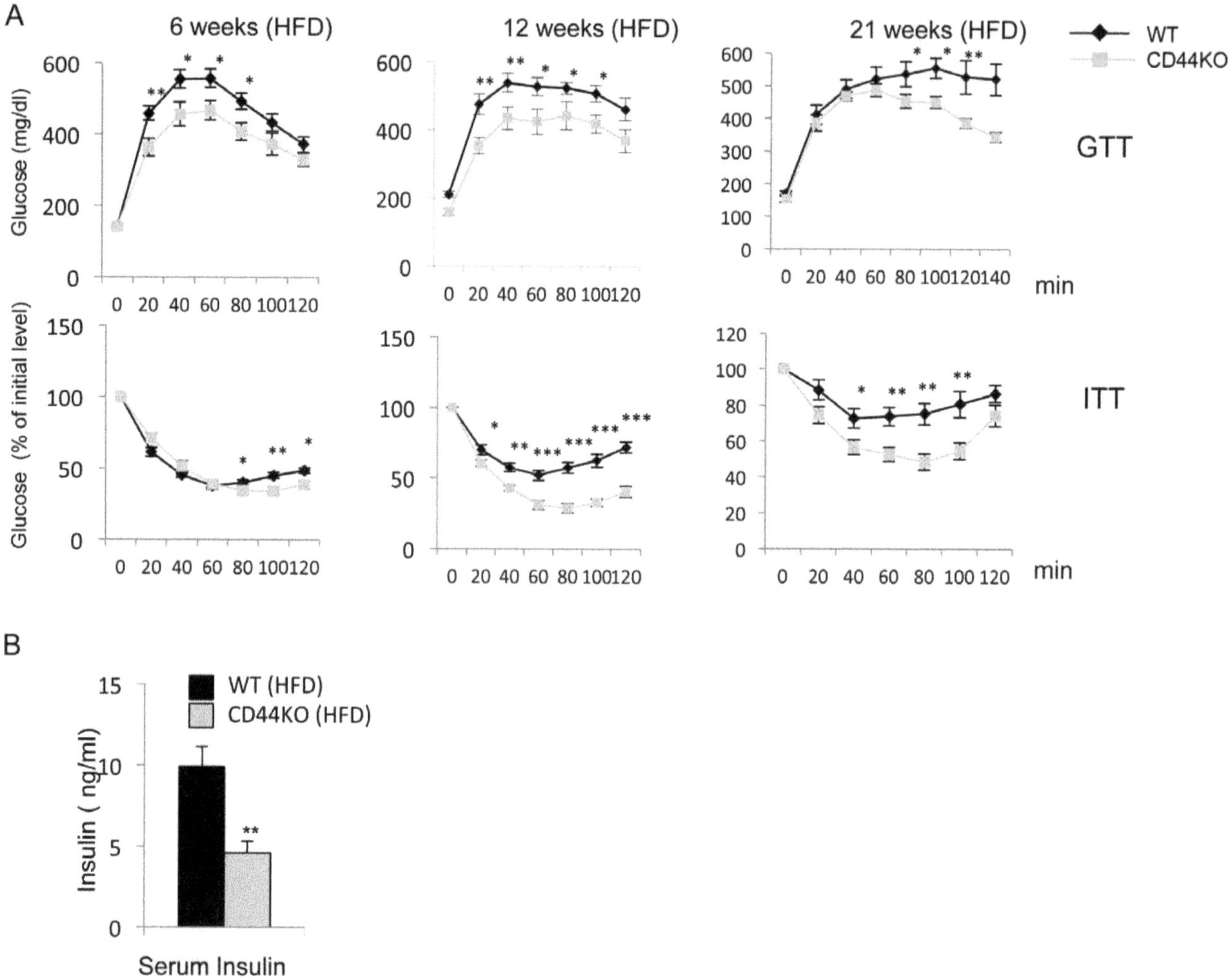

Figure 8. CD44KO mice are protected against HFD-induced insulin resistance and glucose intolerance. A) Glucose tolerance test (GTT) and insulin tolerance test (ITT) were analyzed in WT and CD44KO mice fed an HFD for 6 weeks, 12 weeks, or 21 weeks (n = 6–8 mice for each group). Blood glucose levels were analyzed every 20 min for up to 2 hrs after glucose or insulin injection, for GTT or ITT respectively. B) Blood insulin levels were analyzed in WT and CD44KO mice fed a HFD for 21 weeks (WT, n = 7; CD44KO, n = 8). Data represent mean±SEM. *p<0.05, **p<0.01, ***p<0.001.

adiponectin levels. Our observation that the level of expression of PPARα and genes involved in fatty acid oxidation was not significantly different between WT and in CD44KO liver is consistent with our data that adiponectin levels are unchanged between WT and CD44KO mice.

While this manuscript was in preparation, an expression-based genome-wide association (eGWAS) study linked *CD44* to type 2 diabetes in humans and reported that CD44-deficiency ameliorates insulin resistance in mice and humans [21]. Our study showing that CD44KO mice are protected against the development of diet-induced adipose inflammation and insulin resistance, is consistent with that report. However, our study provides additional insights into the crucial role of CD44 in diet-induced hepatic steatosis, inflammation, and fibrogenesis, and WAT- and liver-associated inflammation and suggests that migration and activation of inflammatory cells may be critical elements affected by the absence of CD44 (Fig. 9).

The precise mechanism by which this multi-functional protein regulates diet-induced inflammation and insulin resistance needs further study. CD44 might regulate the expression of certain lipogenic and inflammatory genes by a direct mechanism involving the interaction of its intracellular domain with respective promoter regions as recently reported for *MMP-9* [19]. It is intriguing that the pro-inflammatory cytokine Opn, which interacts with CD44, has also been reported to play a role in cell migration, macrophage activation, and inflammation in obesity [32,57,58]. Like CD44KO mice, Opn-deficient mice are protected against the development of HFD-induced hepatic steatosis, WAT-associated inflammation, and insulin resistance, while lipid storage in WAT is increased [31,37]. Although Opn acts through several receptor mechanisms, one might hypothesize that the decreased susceptibility observed in both knockout mouse models might be due in part to disruption of the Opn-CD44 signaling pathway. This hypothesis is consistent with recent reports showing that Opn mediates obesity-induced migration and infiltration of macrophages in WAT [32,59,60] and this modulation appears to involve the CD44 pathway [61]. Therefore, one might hypothesize that the reduced hepatic steatosis and WAT-associated inflammation in CD44KO mice might be due in part to the inability of Opn to activate the CD44 pathway. It is interesting

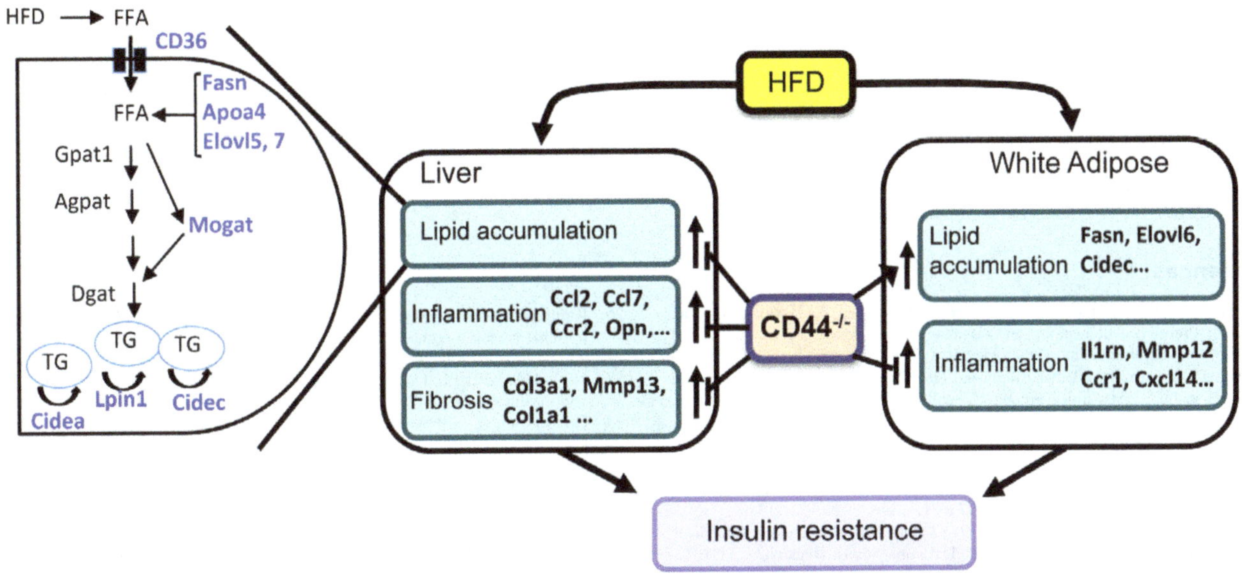

Figure 9. Schematic view of the links between CD44 deficiency and the development of diet-induced hepatic steatosis, inflammation, and fibrogenesis, adipose-associated inflammation, and insulin resistance. In liver, HFD induces the expression of many lipogenic genes, including Cd36, Fasn, Elovl, Apoa4, Mogat and Cidec and Cidea, which enhance the transport, synthesis, and accumulation of triglycerides. In addition, the expression of several inflammatory genes, such as Ccl2, Ccl7, Ccr2, and Opn, and fibrotic genes, including Col3a1, Mmp13, and Col1a1, are elevated and related to the observed increase in hepatic inflammation and the onset of hepatic fibrogenesis. In adipose tissue, HFD induces expression of several lipogenic genes and inflammatory genes (e.g., Il1rn, Mmp12, Ccr1, Cxcl14). The induction of these genes is in part responsible for the increased lipid accumulation and inflammation in WAT. Hepatosteatosis and WAT-associated inflammation subsequently promote the development of insulin resistance and glucose intolerance. The reduced expression of lipogenic, inflammatory, and fibrogenic genes in CD44-deficient mice is linked to their resistance to develop diet-induced hepatosteatosis. The inhibition of inflammatory genes and of the infiltration of macrophages and $CD8^+$ lymphocytes in WAT of CD44KO mice results in reduced WAT-associated inflammation, while elevated expression of lipogenic genes is at least in part related to the observed increase in adiposity. The inhibition of hepatosteatosis and WAT-associated inflammation protects CD44-deficient mice against the development of insulin-resistance and glucose intolerance.

to note that obesity in humans and mice is associated with increased expression of Opn in both liver and WAT [20]. Our study shows that the expression of Opn was greatly repressed in liver of CD44KO(HFD) mice, but not in WAT. Thus, suppression of Opn expression in liver may provide an additional mechanism for the reduced susceptibility CD44KO(HFD) mice to hepatic steatosis and insulin resistance.

In summary, our study demonstrates that mice deficient in CD44 are considerably resistant to diet-induced hepatic steatosis, fibrogenesis, and inflammation, adipose-associated infiltration of M1 macrophages, glucose intolerance, and insulin resistance (Fig. 9). These observations suggest that CD44 provides a critical link between metabolic changes and the development of inflammation and insulin resistance. Because CD44 functions as a receptor, it may provide a convenient therapeutic target in the management of lipid dysregulation in diet-induced liver disease and type 2 diabetes.

Supporting Information

Figure S1 The expression of CD44 mRNA was analyzed in WAT from WT (n = 6) or orphan nuclear receptor TAK1 knockout (TAK1$^{-/-}$) (n = 6) mice fed a HFD by QRT-PCR.

Figure S2 Comparison of the relative weights of liver, WAT, kidneys, and BAT of WT or CD44KO mice fed a normal diet (ND). (WT, n = 6; CD44KO, n = 6). Data present mean±SEM, $^*p<0.05$, $^{**}p<0.01$, $^{***}p<0.001$.

Figure S3 (A) The expression of genes involved in classical pathway of triglyceride synthesis Dgat1 and Dgat2 was not different in liver between WT(HFD) and CD44(HFD) mice. (B) Comparison of gene expression in liver of WT or CD44KO mice fed a ND or an HFD. (n = 5–6 mice per each group). Data present mean±SEM, $^*p<0.05$, $^{**}p<0.01$, $^{***}p<0.001$.

Figure S4 (A) Expression of adiponectin in WAT of WT or CD44KO mice fed a normal diet (ND) or a high fat diet (HFD) (n = 5–6 mice per each group) was analyzed by QRT-PCR. (B) Circulating levels of adiponectin from sera were analyzed by an Elisa kit (R&D systems).

Figure S5 Macrophage populations of SVF cells from WAT of WT(ND) and CD44KO(ND) mice (n = 6 mice per each group) were examined by FACS. No difference was observed in the percentage of M1 and M2 macrophages between WT and CD44KO mice before HFD.

Figure S6 Oxygen consumption, CO_2 production, Heat generation, and respiratory exchange ratio (RER) were analyzed in WT(HFD) and CD44KO(HFD) mice (n = 6 mice per each group) with a LabMaster system (TSE systems INC, Chesterfield, MO).

Table S1 List of QRT-PCR primers.

Table S2 Partial list of genes reduced or increased in WAT of CD44KO(HFD) mice compared to WT(HFD) mice.

Acknowledgments

The authors would like to thank Dr. Xiaoling Li and Dr. Kristin Lichti-Kaiser, NIEHS, for their valuable comments on the manuscript.

Author Contributions

Conceived and designed the experiments: HSK SG AMJ. Performed the experiments: HSK GL LMD KG CDB. Analyzed the data: KG HSK AMJ. Contributed reagents/materials/analysis tools: SG CDB. Wrote the paper: HSK SG AMJ.

References

1. Browning JD, Szczepaniak LS, Dobbins R, Nuremberg P, Horton JD, et al. (2004) Prevalence of hepatic steatosis in an urban population in the United States: impact of ethnicity. Hepatology 40: 1387–1395.
2. Ogden CL, Carroll MD, Kit BK, Flegal KM (2012) Prevalence of obesity and trends in body mass index among US children and adolescents, 1999–2010. JAMA 307: 483–490.
3. Hebbard L, George J (2011) Animal models of nonalcoholic fatty liver disease. Nat Rev Gastroenterol Hepatol 8: 35–44.
4. Samuel VT, Shulman GI (2012) Mechanisms for insulin resistance: common threads and missing links. Cell 148: 852–871.
5. Fabbrini E, Sullivan S, Klein S (2010) Obesity and nonalcoholic fatty liver disease: biochemical, metabolic, and clinical implications. Hepatology 51: 679–689.
6. Gregor MF, Hotamisligil GS (2011) Inflammatory mechanisms in obesity. Annu Rev Immunol 29: 415–445.
7. Donath MY, Shoelson SE (2011) Type 2 diabetes as an inflammatory disease. Nat Rev Immunol 11: 98–107.
8. Lumeng CN, Saltiel AR (2011) Inflammatory links between obesity and metabolic disease. J Clin Invest 121: 2111–2117.
9. Nishimura S, Manabe I, Nagasaki M, Eto K, Yamashita H, et al. (2009) CD8+ effector T cells contribute to macrophage recruitment and adipose tissue inflammation in obesity. Nat Med 15: 914–920.
10. Odegaard JI, Ricardo-Gonzalez RR, Red Eagle A, Vats D, Morel CR, et al. (2008) Alternative M2 activation of Kupffer cells by PPARdelta ameliorates obesity-induced insulin resistance. Cell Metab 7: 496–507.
11. Weisberg SP, McCann D, Desai M, Rosenbaum M, Leibel RL, et al. (2003) Obesity is associated with macrophage accumulation in adipose tissue. J Clin Invest 112: 1796–1808.
12. Johnson P, Ruffell B (2009) CD44 and its role in inflammation and inflammatory diseases. Inflamm Allergy Drug Targets 8: 208–220.
13. Toole BP (2009) Hyaluronan-CD44 Interactions in Cancer: Paradoxes and Possibilities. Clin Cancer Res 15: 7462–7468.
14. Zoller M (2011) CD44: can a cancer-initiating cell profit from an abundantly expressed molecule? Nat Rev Cancer 11: 254–267.
15. Jiang D, Liang J, Noble PW (2011) Hyaluronan as an immune regulator in human diseases. Physiol Rev 91: 221–264.
16. McKee CM, Penno MB, Cowman M, Burdick MD, Strieter RM, et al. (1996) Hyaluronan (HA) fragments induce chemokine gene expression in alveolar macrophages. The role of HA size and CD44. J Clin Invest 98: 2403–2413.
17. Hollingsworth JW, Li Z, Brass DM, Garantziotis S, Timberlake SH, et al. (2007) CD44 regulates macrophage recruitment to the lung in lipopolysaccharide-induced airway disease. Am J Respir Cell Mol Biol 37: 248–253.
18. Solis MA, Chen YH, Wong TY, Bittencourt VZ, Lin YC, et al. (2012) Hyaluronan regulates cell behavior: a potential niche matrix for stem cells. Biochem Res Int 2012: 346972.
19. Miletti-Gonzalez KE, Murphy K, Kumaran MN, Ravindranath AK, Wernyj RP, et al. (2012) Identification of Function for CD44 Intracytoplasmic Domain (CD44-ICD): MODULATION OF MATRIX METALLOPROTEINASE 9 (MMP-9) TRANSCRIPTION VIA NOVEL PROMOTER RESPONSE ELEMENT. J Biol Chem 287: 18995–19007.
20. Bertola A, Deveaux V, Bonnafous S, Rousseau D, Anty R, et al. (2009) Elevated expression of osteopontin may be related to adipose tissue macrophage accumulation and liver steatosis in morbid obesity. Diabetes 58: 125–133.
21. Kodama K, Horikoshi M, Toda K, Yamada S, Hara K, et al. (2012) Expression-based genome-wide association study links the receptor CD44 in adipose tissue with type 2 diabetes. Proc Natl Acad Sci U S A.
22. Schmits R, Filmus J, Gerwin N, Senaldi G, Kiefer F, et al. (1997) CD44 regulates hematopoietic progenitor distribution, granuloma formation, and tumorigenicity. Blood 90: 2217–2233.
23. Kang HS, Okamoto K, Kim YS, Takeda Y, Bortner CD, et al. (2011) Nuclear orphan receptor TAK1/TR4-deficient mice are protected against obesity-linked inflammation, hepatic steatosis, and insulin resistance. Diabetes 60: 177–188.
24. Zhou Z, Yon Toh S, Chen Z, Guo K, Ng CP, et al. (2003) Cidea-deficient mice have lean phenotype and are resistant to obesity. Nat Genet 35: 49–56.
25. Kang HS, Okamoto K, Takeda Y, Beak JY, Gerrish K, et al. (2011) Transcriptional profiling reveals a role for RORalpha in regulating gene expression in obesity-associated inflammation and hepatic steatosis. Physiol Genomics 43: 818–828.
26. Kang HS, Angers M, Beak JY, Wu X, Gimble JM, et al. (2007) Gene expression profiling reveals a regulatory role for ROR alpha and ROR gamma in phase I and phase II metabolism. Physiol Genomics 31: 281–294.
27. Nagle CA, Klett EL, Coleman RA (2009) Hepatic triacylglycerol accumulation and insulin resistance. J Lipid Res 50 Suppl: S74–79.
28. Gong J, Sun Z, Li P (2009) CIDE proteins and metabolic disorders. Curr Opin Lipidol 20: 121–126.
29. Wouters K, van Gorp PJ, Bieghs V, Gijbels MJ, Duimel H, et al. (2008) Dietary cholesterol, rather than liver steatosis, leads to hepatic inflammation in hyperlipidemic mouse models of nonalcoholic steatohepatitis. Hepatology 48: 474–486.
30. Guillen N, Navarro MA, Arnal C, Noone E, Arbones-Mainar JM, et al. (2009) Microarray analysis of hepatic gene expression identifies new genes involved in steatotic liver. Physiol Genomics 37: 187–198.
31. Chapman J, Miles PD, Ofrecio JM, Neels JG, Yu JG, et al. (2010) Osteopontin is required for the early onset of high fat diet-induced insulin resistance in mice. PLoS One 5: e13959.
32. Zeyda M, Gollinger K, Todoric J, Kiefer FW, Keck M, et al. (2011) Osteopontin is an activator of human adipose tissue macrophages and directly affects adipocyte function. Endocrinology 152: 2219–2227.
33. Fujii H, Kawada N (2012) Inflammation and fibrogenesis in steatohepatitis. Journal of gastroenterology 47: 215–225.
34. Ouchi N, Parker JL, Lugus JJ, Walsh K (2011) Adipokines in inflammation and metabolic disease. Nat Rev Immunol 11: 85–97.
35. Buechler C, Wanninger J, Neumeier M (2011) Adiponectin, a key adipokine in obesity related liver diseases. World journal of gastroenterology : WJG 17: 2801–2811.
36. Hirosumi J, Tuncman G, Chang L, Gorgun CZ, Uysal KT, et al. (2002) A central role for JNK in obesity and insulin resistance. Nature 420: 333–336.
37. Kiefer FW, Neschen S, Pfau B, Legerer B, Neuhofer A, et al. (2011) Osteopontin deficiency protects against obesity-induced hepatic steatosis and attenuates glucose production in mice. Diabetologia 54: 2132–2142.
38. Wan Z, Frier BC, Williams DB, Wright DC (2012) Epinephrine induces PDK4 mRNA expression in adipose tissue from obese, insulin resistant rats. Obesity (Silver Spring) 20: 453–456.
39. Zheng YH, Tian C, Meng Y, Qin YW, Du YH, et al. (2012) Osteopontin stimulates autophagy via integrin/CD44 and p38 MAPK signaling pathways in vascular smooth muscle cells. Journal of cellular physiology 227: 127–135.
40. Pivetta E, Scapolan M, Wassermann B, Steffan A, Colombatti A, et al. (2011) Blood-derived human osteoclast resorption activity is impaired by Hyaluronan-CD44 engagement via a p38-dependent mechanism. Journal of cellular physiology 226: 769–779.
41. Nishino N, Tamori Y, Tateya S, Kawaguchi T, Shibakusa T, et al. (2008) FSP27 contributes to efficient energy storage in murine white adipocytes by promoting the formation of unilocular lipid droplets. J Clin Invest 118: 2808–2821.
42. Keller P, Petrie JT, De Rose P, Gerin I, Wright WS, et al. (2008) Fat-specific protein 27 regulates storage of triacylglycerol. J Biol Chem 283: 14355–14365.
43. Zhou L, Xu L, Ye J, Li D, Wang W, et al. (2012) Cidea promotes hepatic steatosis by sensing dietary fatty acids. Hepatology 56: 95–107.
44. Hajri T, Han XX, Bonen A, Abumrad NA (2002) Defective fatty acid uptake modulates insulin responsiveness and metabolic responses to diet in CD36-null mice. J Clin Invest 109: 1381–1389.
45. Nicholls HT, Kowalski G, Kennedy DJ, Risis S, Zaffino LA, et al. (2011) Hematopoietic cell-restricted deletion of CD36 reduces high-fat diet-induced macrophage infiltration and improves insulin signaling in adipose tissue. Diabetes 60: 1100–1110.
46. Consolo M, Amoroso A, Spandidos DA, Mazzarino MC (2009) Matrix metalloproteinases and their inhibitors as markers of inflammation and fibrosis in chronic liver disease (Review). Int J Mol Med 24: 143–152.
47. Hemmann S, Graf J, Roderfeld M, Roeb E (2007) Expression of MMPs and TIMPs in liver fibrosis - a systematic review with special emphasis on anti-fibrotic strategies. J Hepatol 46: 955–975.
48. Tsou CL, Peters W, Si Y, Slaymaker S, Aslanian AM, et al. (2007) Critical roles for CCR2 and MCP-3 in monocyte mobilization from bone marrow and recruitment to inflammatory sites. J Clin Invest 117: 902–909.
49. Mandrekar P, Ambade A, Lim A, Szabo G, Catalano D (2011) An essential role for monocyte chemoattractant protein-1 in alcoholic liver injury: regulation of proinflammatory cytokines and hepatic steatosis in mice. Hepatology 54: 2185–2197.

50. Nio Y, Yamauchi T, Iwabu M, Okada-Iwabu M, Funata M, et al. (2012) Monocyte chemoattractant protein-1 (MCP-1) deficiency enhances alternatively activated M2 macrophages and ameliorates insulin resistance and fatty liver in lipoatrophic diabetic A-ZIP transgenic mice. Diabetologia.

51. Li Y, Jiang D, Liang J, Meltzer EB, Gray A, et al. (2011) Severe lung fibrosis requires an invasive fibroblast phenotype regulated by hyaluronan and CD44. The Journal of experimental medicine 208: 1459–1471.

52. Kitade H, Sawamoto K, Nagashimada M, Inoue H, Yamamoto Y, et al. (2012) CCR5 Plays a Critical Role in Obesity-Induced Adipose Tissue Inflammation and Insulin Resistance by Regulating Both Macrophage Recruitment and M1/ M2 Status. Diabetes.

53. Hotamisligil GS (2006) Inflammation and metabolic disorders. Nature 444: 860–867.

54. Schenk S, Saberi M, Olefsky JM (2008) Insulin sensitivity: modulation by nutrients and inflammation. J Clin Invest 118: 2992–3002.

55. Hursting SD, Hursting MJ (2012) Growth signals, inflammation, and vascular perturbations: mechanistic links between obesity, metabolic syndrome, and cancer. Arterioscler Thromb Vasc Biol 32: 1766–1770.

56. Li L, Wu LL (2012) Adiponectin and interleukin-6 in inflammation-associated disease. Vitam Horm 90: 375–395.

57. Shevde LA, Das S, Clark DW, Samant RS (2010) Osteopontin: an effector and an effect of tumor metastasis. Curr Mol Med 10: 71–81.

58. Morimoto J, Kon S, Matsui Y, Uede T (2010) Osteopontin; as a target molecule for the treatment of inflammatory diseases. Curr Drug Targets 11: 494–505.

59. Nakamachi T, Nomiyama T, Gizard F, Heywood EB, Jones KL, et al. (2007) PPARalpha agonists suppress osteopontin expression in macrophages and decrease plasma levels in patients with type 2 diabetes. Diabetes 56: 1662–1670.

60. Nystrom T, Duner P, Hultgardh-Nilsson A (2007) A constitutive endogenous osteopontin production is important for macrophage function and differentiation. Exp Cell Res 313: 1149–1160.

61. Zhu B, Suzuki K, Goldberg HA, Rittling SR, Denhardt DT, et al. (2004) Osteopontin modulates CD44-dependent chemotaxis of peritoneal macrophages through G-protein-coupled receptors: evidence of a role for an intracellular form of osteopontin. J Cell Physiol 198: 155–167.

11

The Characterization of Obese Polycystic Ovary Syndrome Rat Model Suitable for Exercise Intervention

Chuyan Wu[§], **Feng Lin**[§], **Shuwei Qiu, Zhongli Jiang***

Department of Rehabilitation Medicine, The First Affiliated Hospital of Nanjing Medical University, Nanjing, China

Abstract

Objective: To develop a new polycystic ovary syndrome (PCOS) rat model suitable for exercise intervention.

Method: Thirty six rats were randomly divided into three experimental groups: PCOS rats with high-fat diet (PF, n = 24), PCOS rats with ordinary diet (PO, n = 6), and control rats with ordinary diet (CO, n = 6). Two kinds of PCOS rat model were made by adjustment diet structure and testosterone injection for 28 days. After a successful animal model, PF model rats were randomly assigned to three groups: exercise with a continuation of high-fat diet (PF-EF, n = 6), sedentary with a continuation of high-fat diet (PF-SF, n = 6), exercise with an ordinary diet (PF-EO, n = 6). Fasting blood glucose (FBG) and insulin (FINS), estrogen (E2), progesterone (P), and testosterone (T) in serum were determined by RIA, and ovarian morphology was evaluated by Image-Pro plus 6.0.

Results: Body weight, Lee index, FINS increased significantly in PF rat model. Serum levels of E_2 and T were significantly higher in PF and PO than in CO. Ovary organ index and ovarian areas were significant lower in PF than in CO. After intervention for 2 weeks, the levels of 1 h postprandial blood glucose (PBG_1), 2 h postprandial blood glucose (PBG_2), FINS and the serum levels of T decreased significantly in PF-EF rats and PF-EO rats. The ratio of FBG/FINS was significant higher in PF-EO rats than in PF-SF rats. Ovarian morphology showed that the numbers of preantral follicles and atretic follicles decreased significantly, and the numbers of antral follicles and corpora lutea increased significantly in the rats of PF-EF and PF-EO.

Conclusion: By combination of high-fat diet and testosterone injection, the obese PCOS rat model is conformable with the lifestyle habits of fatty foods and insufficient exercise, and has metabolic and reproductive characteristics of human PCOS. This model can be applied to study exercise intervention.

Editor: Harpal Singh Randeva, University of Warwick – Medical School, United Kingdom

Funding: This study was supported by National Nature Science Foundation of China (81101452). The support from the Priority Academic Program Development (PAPD) of Jiangsu Higher Education Institutions is also appreciated. The funders had no role in study design, data collection and analysis, decision to publish, or preparation of the manuscript.

Competing Interests: The authors have declared that no competing interests exist.

* E-mail: jiangzh3721@163.com

§ These authors contributed equally to this work.

Introduction

Polycystic ovary syndrome (PCOS) is a heterogeneous syndrome that is characterized by anovulation, clinical and/or biochemical signs of hyperandrogenism, and abnormal ovarian morphology [1]. It is the most common endocrine disorder in women of reproductive age, affecting 5–10% of women in this age group [2].

Various methods have been used to induce PCOS in rodents, including exposure to androgens, estrogens, aromatase inhibitors, antiprogesterone agents, constant light and genetic modifications [3]. Estradiol valerateis often used to make a PCOS rat model, which has several characteristics of acyclicity and polycystic ovarian changes without the typical metabolic disturbances of human PCOS [4–7]. Letrozole, a nonsteroidal aromatase inhibitor, blocks the conversion of testosterone to estradiol and also induces PCOS in 6-week-old female rats. Continuous administration of letrozole, 200 mg/d, to female rats for 90day starting before puberty results in a PCOS model with reproductive and metabolic features of the syndrome [8]. The letrozole model targets the study of aromotase deficiency–induced classic PCOS [3] and can used for studying the mechanism for the complex pathogenesis of PCOS [8]. Continuous exposure to dihydrotestosterone (DHT) can develop an obese PCOS rat model which has typical hormonal disorders and ovarian morphological changes [9]. The DHT model may be suitable for studies of both ovarian and metabolic features of the syndrome. The insulin sensitivity and estrus cyclicity in DHT induced PCOS rat model can be improved by running wheel exercise [10], although circulating sex hormones were not measured. The model by administration of testosterone to immature female rats seeks to incorporate both the morphological changes as well as the hormonal disorders seen in PCOS. It was demonstrated that testosterone administration blocked the ovulatory process in the model of immature rats. After injection of testosterone propionate for up to 28 days, typical high insulin blood levels and the fasting glucose/insulin ratio was dramatically reduced in the animals. Nevertheless, because a large pool of primordial follicles was still well preserved as well as a small fraction of preantral and antral follicles were still remained, this model can lend itself for the therapy of PCOS phenotype [11]. In our previous study, swimming training for 2 weeks improved significantly body weight index, insulin resistance and the androgen level in PCOS rat model induced by testosterone injection [12].

The pathogenesis of PCOS is poorly understood until now. Starting from early life and extending through lifecycle, environmental insults may affect susceptible women who finally demonstrate the clinical phenotype of PCOS. High-fat diet and sedentary lifestyle emerge as the major environmental determinant of PCOS [13]. Many studies have reported that the rats fed with high-fat diet develop insulin resistance which is one of the important features of PCOS [14–16]. Many researchers have demonstrated that the improvement of insulin sensitivity decreased androgen concentration [17–19]. Exercise training can significantly improve insulin resistance, thus reducing serum levels of androstenedione and dehydroepiandrosterone [20]. However, several studies have demonstrated that simple dietary intervention did not improve insulin resistance. A European randomized dietary intervention study for 12 weeks had confirmed that overall reduction of dietary SFA had no effect on insulin sensitivity in weight-stable obese subjects [21]. Rajaie et al also found that compared a calorie-restricted moderately restricted carbohydrate and high fat diet (43%–47% of total calories as carbohydrate and 36%–40% as dietary fats) with a calorie-restricted high-carbohydrate and low fat diet (60%–65% of energy from carbohydrates and 20%–25% from fats), there was not statistically different changes in fasting plasma glucose and insulin [22]. Therefore, in the lifestyle interventions, exercise is used as an important measure and diet is considered as a supporting factor. According to unhealthy lifestyle such as high-fat diet and lack of exercise existing in human PCOS, the purpose of the present study is to develop new animal model to fit exercise intervention. In this present study, obese PCOS rat model manifesting hyperinsulinemia, hyperandrogenemia and morphological feature of polycystic ovaries was successfully created by the combination of high-fat diet and testosterone propionate injection, and then intervened by exercise training with diet structure adjustment. The results indicated that exercise intervention can effectively improve the reproductive endocrine environment of the obese PCOS model rats.

Materials and Methods

Ethics Statement

Thirty-six Wistar female rats (50–70 g, 21 days old) were purchased from Shanghai SLC Co. (Shanghai, China), kept in temperature-controlled rooms (22°C), with light from 08:00 to 20:00 h and dark from 20:00 to 08:00 h and free access to water. The experimental protocols were approved and strictly followed by the Institutional Animal Care and Use Committees of Nanjing Medical University (permit number: NJMU/IACUC_20120210_01) in strict accordance with the Guidelines for the Care and Use of Laboratory Animals (National Research Council of People's Republic of China, 2010).

Study procedure

All rats were randomly divided into three experimental groups (Fig. 1): PCOS model with high-fat diet (PF, n = 24), PCOS model with ordinary diet (PO, n = 6), and control group with ordinary diet (CO, n = 6). PF rats were fed with high-fat diet for 28 days. CO rats were fed with ordinary diet. High-fat diet composed of 22% fat, 48% carbohydrate, and 20%protein with total calorific value 44.3KJ/Kg [23] and ordinary diet composed of 5% fat, 53% carbohydrate, 23% protein, with total calorific value 25KJ/Kg were ordered in Shanghai SLC Co. (Shanghai, China). At the same time, these rats in PF and PO were subcutaneously injected daily at 8:00 for 28 days with testosterone propionate of 1 mg/100 g body weight dissolved in tea oil [11]. The rats in CO were injected daily with the same volume of tea oil alone. At the day after the end of 28 days of injection, total 18 rats from PF, PO and CO with 6 rats in each group were sacrificed by cervical dislocation.

Then, the remaining 18 rats in PF were randomly assigned to three groups (Fig. 1): exercise with high-fat diet (PF-EF, n = 6), exercise with ordinary diet (PF-EO, n = 6), sedentary with high-fat diet (PF-SF, n = 6). The rats in PF-EF and PF-SF continued feeding with high-fat diet, and the rats in PF-EO were fed with ordinary diet for two weeks. The exercise rats in PF-EF and PF-EO were forced to swim simultaneously without a load at with 120 min/d and 6 d/week for two weeks in a barrel filled with water maintained at 33–35°C to a depth of 40–50 cm, in which the area for every rat is enough to swim freely. The non-exercise rats in PF-FS were placed in shallow water at 33–35°C, 120 min, 6 day/week for two weeks of housing [12].All the rats were sacrificed by cervical dislocation between 08:00 and 11:00 AM under fasting condition at24 h after the end of the last training session with 3% pentobarbital abdominal anesthesia. Blood and ovary samples were collected from all animals.

Measurements of body weight, body length and ovary weight

Body weight and length of rats were measured weekly from 21days of age. Body length was defined as the distance from nose to anus of rats. Lee index reflects the body fat as a parameter [LI = body weight (g) $^{1/3}$ ×1000/body length (cm)] [11]. Bilateral ovaries of one rat were weighed, in which the mean values were regarded as the ovary weight. Ovarian organ index = ovary weight/body weight $\times 10^{-3}$ [12].

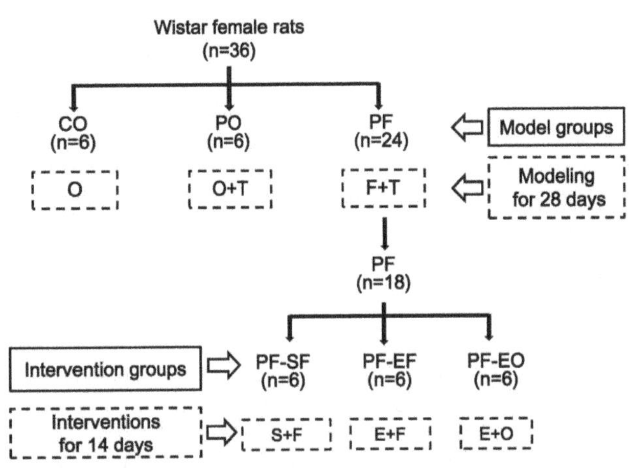

Figure 1. The experiment protocol. O: ordinary diet; F: high fat diet; T: testosterone propionate; CO: control group with ordinary diet; PO: PCOS model with ordinary diet; PF: PCOS model with high-fat diet; S: no exercise; E: exercise; PF-SF: sedentary with high-fat diet in PF rats; PF-EF: exercise with high-fat diet in PF rats; PF-EO: exercise with ordinary diet in PF rats.

Vaginal smears

Vaginal smears were monitored daily to determine the stage of cyclicity from 42 days of age to the end of experiment. In this procedure, smears obtained by vaginal washing were dyed with methylthioninium chloride and then analyzed under a microscope for the predominant cell type in vaginal smears. The estrus cycle experiences four stages of proestrus, estrus, metoestrus, and diestrus. Cycles with duration of 4–5 days were considered as regular [3]. At the beginning of experiment, all rats showed regular cycles.

Oral glucose tolerance test (OGTT)

Before sacrificed, all rats were fasted overnight and infused intragastrically with 2 g glucose per kilogram of body weight. Blood samples were collected at 0 min, 60 min and 120 min after oral glucose used to evaluate fasting blood glucose (FBG), 1 h postprandial blood glucose (PBG_1) and 2 h postprandial blood glucose (PBG_2), respectively [23].

Serum analysis

Blood samples obtained from all rats fasting for 12 h were centrifuged at 2500 *g* for 10 min and stored at −80°C. Fasting serum levels for insulin (FINS), estrogen (E_2), progesterone (P), and testosterone (T) were determined using correspondent commercial RIA kits (Northern biological technical institute, Beijing, P. R. China). Fasting blood glucose (FBG) was analyzed by GOD-PAP. Insulin resistance index is defined as the ratio of FBG/FINS [11].

Ovarian morphology analysis

When rats were sacrificed, the ovaries were dissected from connective tissue, fixed in 10% formalin for 24 h, dehydrated in increasing concentrations of ethanol, followed by immersion in xylene, and embedded in paraffin. The ovaries were longitudinally and serially sectioned at 4 μm from the center. Serial sections were mounted on 3 slides, deparaffinized with xylene, hydrated with successive decreasing concentrations of ethanolin water, and then stained with hematoxylin and eosin (HE). The section with the largest area was chosen for analysis to count the numbers of preantral, antral and atretic follicles, and corporalutea [24]. Atretic follicles were confirmed when one of the following characteristics was observed, such as the presence of pyknosis in the granulose cell, granulosa cells present in the follicular fluid, or theca cell hypertrophy. Sections were photographed with a camera (Olympus BX51, Japan) at ×40, ×100, and ×200 magnifications. The area of the ovary was determined with a calibrated scale tool in the virtual microscope. Then, the areas of the largest section (at ×40 magnification), all corporalutea (at ×100 magnification), and thickness of theca cell layer and granulosa cell layer (from 3 visual fields of follicles at ×200 magnification) were measured with Image-Pro plus 6.0.

Statistical analyses

Data were expressed as means ±SD. Statistical evaluations were performed with SPSS software (version 16.0, SPSS, Chicago, IL, USA). All the data were analyzed by one-way ANOVA, and $p < 0.05$ was considered significant. When the ANOVA revealed significant differences among three experimental groups, post hoc analysis was performed by using Bonferroni's method of multiple comparisons (3 repeated tests; $p < 0.0167$ was considered significant for each test).

Results

Vaginal smears

The vaginal smears were monitored during whole experiment. The vaginas in all rats mostly opened at 40 days old. The regular estrous cycle of 4–5 days was observed in control (Fig. 2). However, there were many white cells, less epithelial cell, and keratinocytein vaginal smears of PO and PF rats, indicating these rats persisted in diestrus and no ovulation happened. After 2 weeks, the rats in PF-EF and PF-EO restored to normal estrous cycles, while the rats in PF-SF still showed persistent diestrus.

Changes of metabolic and endocrine variables in PCOS model induced by high-fat diet and testosterone propionate

The metabolic and endocrine variables were measured on the 28th day of experiment in three groups of CO, PO and PF. Body weight and Lee index in PF significantly increased in comparison with CO and PO. The levels of FBG were significantly lower in PF than in CO. The levels of FINS were significantly higher in PF than in PO and CO, while ratios of FBG/FINS in PF significantly decreased in comparison with other two groups. Serum levels of E_2 and T were significantly higher in PF and PO than in CO (Table 1).

Changes of ovarian morphological parameters in PCOS model induced by high-fat diet and testosterone propionate

Ovarian morphological parameters were measured on the 28th day of experiment in three groups of CO, PO and PF (Fig. 3). Ovary organ index and ovarian areas were significant lower in PF than in CO. Corpora lutea in PF and PO were not observed. In comparison with CO group, thickness of theca layer, numbers of preantral follicle, numbers of atretic follicle, total numbers of follicle and ratios of numbers of atretic follicle to total numbers of follicles significantly increased in PF and PO, while thickness of granular layer significantly decreased in PF and PO (Table 2).

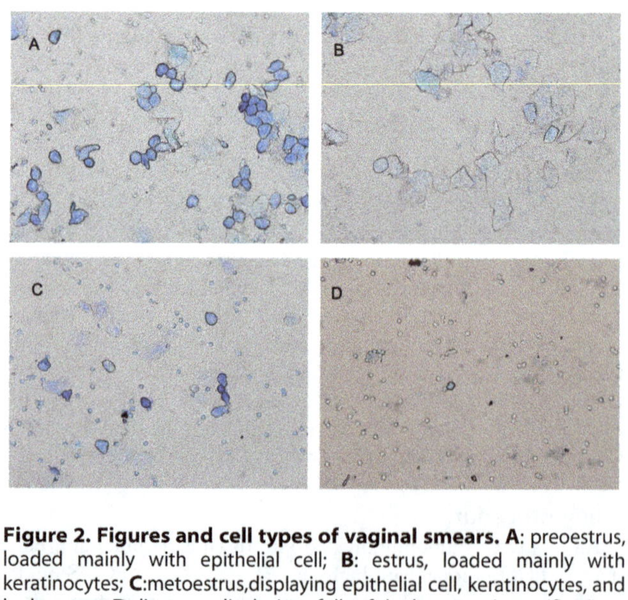

Figure 2. Figures and cell types of vaginal smears. A: preoestrus, loaded mainly with epithelial cell; **B**: estrus, loaded mainly with keratinocytes; **C**:metoestrus,displaying epithelial cell, keratinocytes, and leukocytes; **D**:diestrus, displaying full of leukocytes (magnification ×100).

Table 1. Changes of metabolic and endocrine variables in obese PCOS model induced by high-fat diet.

	CO	PO	PF
Body weight(g)	138.33±10.51	149.83±10.07	172.33±11.52 *#
Body length(cm)	17.22±0.64	17.96±0.64	17.65±0.75
Lee Index	300.35±3.61	295.76±3.90	315.36±8.39 *#
FBG (mmol/l)	5.38±0.55	4.88±0.46	4.38±0.60 *
PBG_1 (mmol/l)	9.15±0.53	8.72±1.35	9.43±0.82
PBG_2 (mmol/l)	6.95±0.61	6.43±0.71	7.53±1.56
FINS (uIU/ml)	21.63±4.02	23.90±4.03	50.58±6.86*#
FBG/FINS	0.26±0.05	0.23±0.09	0.10±0.03 *#
E_2 (ng/ml)	1.60±0.31	2.41±0.56 *	2.61±0.28 *
P (ng/ml)	0.39±0.22	0.31±0.16	0.25±0.06
T (ng/ml)	0.17±0.08	28.32±7.24 *	31.92±6.31 *

Values are means ± SD.
*$p<0.0167$ versus CO by Bonferoni post-hoc test.
#$p<0.0167$ versus PO by Bonferoni post-hoc test.

Effects of exercise and diet on metabolic and endocrine variables in PF rats

The metabolic and endocrine variables were measured at the end of experiment in PF-SF, PF-EF and PF-EO. Body weight was significantly lower in PF-EF and PF-EO than in PF-SF. The levels of FBG were significant higher in PF-EO than in PF-SF. The levels of PBG_1, PBG_2 and FINS were significantly lower in PF-EF and PF-EO than in PF-SF, while the levels of PBG_2 were significantly lower in PF-EO than in PF-EF. In comparison with PF-SF, the ratio of FBG/FINS increased significantly in PF-EO. Serum levels of T were significantly lower in PF-EF and PF-EO than in PF-SF. There were no statistical differences in serum levels of E_2 and P in the three groups of PF-SF, PF-EF and PF-EO (Table 3).

Effects of exercise and diet on ovarian morphologic parameters in PF rats

Ovarian morphological parameters were measured on the end of experiment in PF-SF, PF-EF and PF-EO. In comparison with PF-SF, ovary organ index, ovarian areas, numbers of antral follicle, and numbers of corpora lutea significantly increased, while thickness of theca layer, numbers of preantral follicle, numbers of atretic follicle, total numbers of follicle, and ratio of numbers of atretic follicle to total numbers of follicle significantly decreased in PF-EF and PF-EO. The ratios of numbers of corpora lutea to total numbers of follicles were significantly higher in PF-EF and PF-EO than in PF-SF, and were significantly lower in PF-EF than in PF-EO. Other parameters in corpora lutea areas and thickness of theca layer were significantly higher in PF-EO than in PF-SF (Table 4).

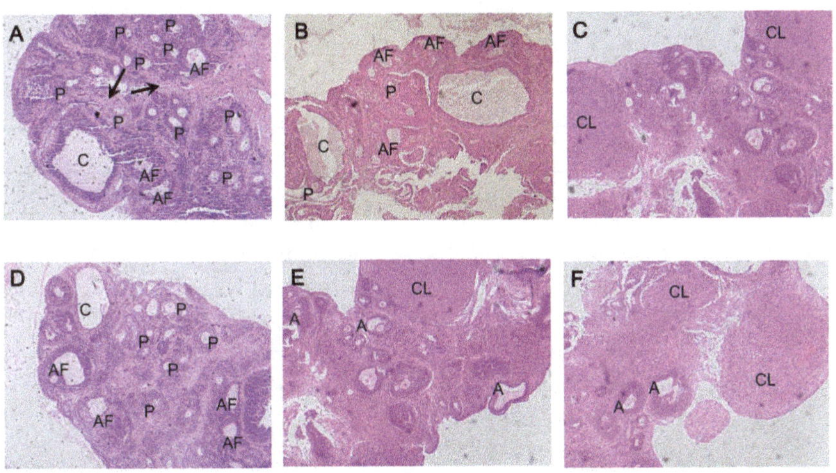

Figure 3. Ovarian morphology of rats from three groups (×100). A: PF. A lot of preantral follicles (P) and atretic follicles (AF) with enlargement of stroma (arrow) and cystic follicles (C) are shown in the section. **B: PO.** A lot of preantral follicles (P), atretic follicles (AF) and cystic follicles(C) are shown in the section. **C: CO.** Various stages of development follicles and some corpora lutea (CL) are shown. **D: PF-SF.** A lot of preantral follicles (P) and atretic follicles (AF), and cystic follicles(C) are shown in the section. **E: PF-EF.** A lot of antral follicles (A) and a bit of corpora lutea (CL) are shown in the section. **F: PF-EO.** A lot of antral follicles (A) and a bit of corpora lutea (CL) are shown in the section.

Table 2. Changes of ovarian morphological parameters in PF.

	CO	PO	PF
Ovary weight(mg)	18.55±3.41	16.09±2.37	15.80±1.79
Ovarian organ index($\times10^{-3}$)	0.14±0.03	0.12±0.02	0.09±0.02 *
Ovarian area(mm^2)	2.79±0.49	1.77±0.88	1.07±0.18 *
Corpora lutea area(mm^2)	1.04±0.48	0.00±0.00 *	0.00±0.00 *
Thickness of granular layer(μm)	35.05±4.63	24.36±5.14 *	24.03±4.91 *
Thickness of theca layer(μm)	14.56±1.28	19.04±2.39 *	19.63±1.94 *
Numbers of preantral follicle	3.67±1.63	7.67±1.86 *	10.20±1.30*
Numbers of antral follicle	2.83±2.40	2.83±1.47	1.80±0.84
Numbers of atretic follicle	1.17±1.17	7.00±1.90*	9.00±3.67 *
Total numbers of follicle	7.67±3.67	17.50±3.94 *	21.00±2.65 *
Numbers of corpora lutea	4.00±1.26	0.00±0.00 *	0.00±0.00 *
Ratio of corpora lutea area to ovarian area	0.37±0.16	0.00±0.00 *	0.00±0.00*
Ratio of numbers of corpora lutea to total numbers of follicle	0.62±0.34	0.00±0.00 *	0.00±0.00 *
Ratio of numbers of atretic follicle to total numbers of follicle	0.13±0.12	0.40±0.08 *	0.42±0.12*

Values are means ± SD.
*p<0.0167 versus CO by Bonferoni post-hoc test.

Microscopic observation of ovarian section

Follicles in various stages of development and atretic follicle in small amounts were observed on sections from PF-EF, PF-EO and CO. A large number of preantral and atretic follicles and some cystic follicles were observed in PO, PF and PF-SF. The pathological characteristics such as thickened ovarian adventitial coat, obvious demixing between theca interna and theca externa, inspissated theca cell layer, and apparent proliferation of ovarian stroma were observed in PO, PF and PF-SF (Fig. 3).

Discussion

In this study, the obese PCOS rats were successfully induced by using high-fat diet and testosterone injection at the same time. The PF rats had endocrine and reproductive characteristics such as hyperandrogenemia, hyperinsulinemia, anovulation, and enlarged ovaries with follicular atresia and multiple cysts in the periphery, which is consistent with human PCOS [25]. A difference of approximately 24% in body weight was observed between PF rats and CO rats. This body weight difference has been assumed in the literature as inferring obesity [26]. Except for body weight, the Lee Index in PF rats displayed a statistically significant difference compared with rats of CO and PO. Therefore, PF rats were considered as an obese PCOS model.

Diet, as the major environmental determinant, plays an important role during early stages of human development from prenatal life to puberty[13].The dietary intake of advanced glycated end products(AGEs) such as lipid and protein-rich foods is increasingly recognized as a determinant of metabolic and cardiovascular morbidity [27,28]. Diamanti-Kandarakis et al. found that the rats with high-fat feeding manifested concurrent increase of testosterone, suggesting an impact of dietary AGEs on

Table 3. Effects of exercise and diet on metabolic and endocrine variables in PF rats.

	PF-SF	PF-EF	PF-EO
Body weight(g)	213.00±9.86	188.50±7.77*	174.33±11.81*
Body length(cm)	19.31±0.61	19.24±0.49	18.69±0.57
Lee Index	309.21±5.85	298.03±8.95	299.01±9.08
FBG(mmol/l)	4.00±0.32	4.20±0.42	4.75±0.31*
PBG_1 (mmol/l)	9.11±0.33	7.70±0.49*	7.01±0.64*
PBG_2 (mmol/l)	9.20±1.42	7.40±0.94*	5.67±0.43*#
FINS(uIU/ml)	21.75±0.73	17.63±1.66*	16.89±1.20*
FBG/FINS	0.18±0.02	0.24±0.04	0.29±0.05*
E_2 (ng/ml)	1.72±0.31	1.36±0.51	1.30±0.28
P (ng/ml)	0.44±0.10	0.54±0.08	0.59±0.18
T (ng/ml)	0.18±0.02	0.08±0.04 *	0.07±0.03*

Values are means ± SD.
*p<0.0167 versus PF-SF by Bonferoni post-hoc test.
#p<0.0167 versus PF-EF by Bonferoni post-hoc test.

Table 4. Effects of exercise and diet on ovarian morphological parameters in obese PCOS rats.

	PF-SF	PF-EF	PF-EO
Ovarian weight(mg)	13.92±1.06	16.02±1.62	16.11±1.57
Ovarian organ index($\times 10^{-3}$)	0.07±0.00	0.09±0.01*	0.09±0.01*
Ovarian area(mm^2)	4.74±0.65	5.73±0.45*	6.17±0.47*
Corpora lutea area(mm^2)	1.18±0.43	1.52±0.52	2.03±0.42*
Thickness of granular layer(μm)	22.59±3.53	26.04±5.03	29.28±3.35*
Thickness of theca layer(μm)	16.76±1.78	13.96±1.61*	13.37±1.53*
Numbers of preantral follicle	9.83±2.79	5.67±1.75*	3.67±1.21*
Numbers of antral follicle	2.33±1.37	6.17±1.47*	7.17±1.17*
Numbers of atretic follicle	5.33±2.16	2.00±0.89*	1.33±1.03*
Total numbers of follicle	17.50±2.07	13.83±2.23*	12.16±1.47*
Numbers of corpora lutea	3.00±1.10	5.67±0.82*	8.33±2.58*
Ratio of corpora lutea area to ovarian area	0.25±0.11	0.26±0.08	0.33±0.08
Ratio of numbers of corpora lutea to total numbers of follicle	0.17±0.06	0.42±0.08*	0.68±0.17*#
Ratio of numbers of atretic follicle to total numbers of follicle	0.31±0.13	0.14±0.05*	0.11±0.09*

Values are means ± SD.
*$p<0.0167$ versus PF-SF by Bonferoni post-hoc test.
#$p<0.0167$ versus PF-EF by Bonferoni post-hoc test.

ovarian tissue [29]. Androgen excess plays an important role in the pathophysiology of PCOS and has been hypothesized to be the final common pathway for the development of the signs and symptoms of this disorder. The majority (80%) of adults with PCOS have hyperandrogenemia [30]. Long-term administration of androgens can induce visceral obesity and consecutive insulin resistance. Abdominal adiposity, insulin resistance and compensatory hyperinsulinemia could trigger androgenization in women [31]. The predominate increase of TP and E_2 in PO and PF was considered to be mostly due to persistent TP injection in this present study. Frankset al. reported that the characteristic feature of polycystic ovaries is an apparent failure to select a dominant follicle and the accumulation of antral follicles 2–8 mm in size. It was assumed that this appearance reflects an androgen-induced arrest in antral follicle development [32]. Several studies on rats have demonstrated that continuous exposure of post pubertal animals to steroid hormones, either via regular s.c. dosing or continuous release pellet implant, produces an anovulatory phenotype in these animals [33]. In this present study, ovarian morphological parameters in both PF and PO rats manifested large, atretic antral follicles, follicular cysts with a thickened theca interna cell layer, a diminished granulosa cell compartment, and few fresh corpora lutea, consistent with the research by Beloosesky et al [11]. Ovarian organ index and ovarian area were significantly less in PF rats than in CO rats. These results suggest that a high-fat diet is more likely to form typical PCOS morphological changes in comparison with ordinary diet.

Sedentary behavior, as assessed by sitting time, is increased in human PCOS and is being increasingly recognized as a contributor both to elevated adiposity and to obesity-associated [34]. In this present study, the obese PCOS rat model induced by high-fat diet and testosterone injection imitated successfully the unhealthy lifestyle habits such as high lipid diet and insufficient exercise of human PCOS. Testosterone administration induces insulin resistance, attributed to effects on glucose transport. Another finding was reduced capillary density in the muscle despite increased muscle weight [9]. Previous studies showed that high fat diet of obese mice and humans could lead to increased FFA influx through the portal vein into the liver, which could result in a state of IR [14]. These PF rats manifested significant metabolic characteristics of insulin resistance (increase of FINS and decrease of FBG/FINS) and overweight or obesity (increase of Lee Index) in comparison with PO rats. Insulin resistance has been recognized to contribute not only to metabolic but also to reproductive aspects of the syndrome [13,35]. Numerous studies also have shown that a high-fat diet can cause insulin resistance in muscles at rest [15]. Although insulin resistance is not enough to become the diagnosis of PCOS, it is present in up to 50% women with PCOS [36]. Overweight or obesity is a common feature of PCOS women [37,38]. The link between PCOS and overweight or obesity also has been confirmed in adolescent PCOS patients [39].

Exercise based lifestyle modifications are successfully employed to treat obese and overweight women with PCOS [2]. Morifuji et al. reported that intake of dietary soya protein and exercise training by swimming for 2 weeks had an additive effect on decreases of insulin resistant and body fat in rats [40]. Our previous study has shown that exercise for 2 weeks increased insulin sensitivity, decreased serum androgen levels, and recovered normal ovarian morphology in PCOS rats without high-fat diet [12]. In this present study, swimming training for 2 weeks, with or without a high-fat diet, significantly decreased PBG_1, PBG_2, FINS and the lever of testosterone, and improved ovarian morphology indexes in PF rats. Lungeret al. suggested the use of FINS as a simple screening test for assessment of insulin resistance in women with PCOS [36]. In this present study, the decrease of FINS after swimming training indicated the improvement of insulin resistance to be associated with exercise rather than diet.

Overweight and obesity impact the clinical reproductive and metabolic features of the syndrome. Long-term complications of obesity such as cardiovascular risk and diabetes, as well as those over the short term in reproductive function, are significantly improved by lifestyle modification. Weight loss decreases significantly hyperinsulinemia and hyperandrogenism in women with PCOS [42]. High-fiber diet and low-fat diets enriched with monounsaturated fats may help to reduce body weight [43].

Several studies have paid close attention to impacting of low carbohydrate and standard dietary intervention regimens on both amount of weight lost as well as specific metabolic and endocrine features of human PCOS [44]. In a short-term crossover trial of human PCOS within 16 days, fasting insulin was lower following a low carbohydrate (43%) diet relative to a standard carbohydrate diet (56% carbohydrate, 31% fat, 16% protein). Fasting glucose, insulin sensitivity, and the circulating concentrations of reproductive hormones were not significantly affected by the intervention [45]. In our present study, the ratio of fasting glucose to fasting insulin in PF-EO rats was significantly higher than that in PF-SF rats, and the levels of PBG2 were significantly lower in PF-EO rats than in PF-EF rats. These results suggested that dietary constitutes had a certain influence on blood glucose.

The appearance of corpora lutea is considered as occurrence of ovulation. In this present study, only a few corpora lutea were observed in PF-SF. Four rats in PF-SF showed persistent diestrus and the other two PF-SF rats showed irregular cycles. Manneras et al. also reported that the PCOS rat model induced by DHT had irregular cycles [9]. Their ovaries had large, atretic antral follicles, follicular cysts with a thickened theca interna cell layer, and few fresh corpora lutea, similar to our present results. In this present study, swimming training for 2 weeks, with or without high-fat diet, increased significantly the numbers of corpora lutea, the ratio of numbers of corpora lutea to total numbers of follicle and numbers of antral follicle, and decreased significantly numbers of preantral follicle and atretic follicle, according with Manni's research [7]. These results suggest that exercise is conducive to promoting follicular maturation and ovulation. The possible explanation for the improvement of cyclicity is that decreased sympathetic activity will have a direct impact on the ovaries and affect the sex steroid synthesis pathways. It has been shown that physical exercise can decrease sympathetic nerve activity, improve menstrual frequency, and decrease the levels of several sex steroids in women with PCOS [10]. In addition, significant increases in thickness of granular layer and corpora lutea area were found in PF-EO rats but not in PF-EF rats. The ratio of numbers of corpora lutea to total numbers of follicle was also significantly higher in PF-EO rats than in PF-EF rats, suggesting that dietary adjustments had an additional role on promotion of ovulation. Lifestyle intervention of human PCOS has been widely accepted. From our research results, exercise training may play a more important role on reproductive/endocrine outcomes.

Different mechanisms of reproductive function improved by exercise may be involved to explain their beneficial effects on glucose/insulin homeostasis. Insulin sensitivity improvement itself is the pivotal factor involved in the restoration of ovarian function. Several reports have demonstrated that loss of body weight is related to increase of insulin sensitivity [46,47]. Exercise could ameliorate insulin sensitivity not only by a large reduction of body weight and visceral fat [48] but also by cellular muscle metabolism enhancement. Skeletal muscle is the main site of glucose deposition implicated in insulin resistance, and it is well known that physical exercise influences the expression and/or activity of proteins involved in insulin signal transduction in skeletal muscle [49] such as the translocation of GLUT-4 glucose transporters to the plasma membrane and transverse tubules [41]. Previous studies demonstrated improvement of insulin resistant induced by exercise was accompanied with the concurrent decrease of hyperandrogenism [12,20]. It is speculated that androgen may be involved in some sections of glucose metabolism, which needs to be confirmed by further studies.

Conclusively, our present study demonstrated that obese PCOS rat model created successfully by a combination of high-fat diet and testosterone injection was conformable with metabolic and reproductive characteristics of human PCOS and can be used for mechanism study of exercise intervention on reproductive/ endocrine outcomes of PCOS.

Author Contributions

Conceived and designed the experiments: FL ZLJ. Performed the experiments: CYW SWQ. Analyzed the data: CYW FL SWQ. Contributed reagents/materials/analysis tools: CYW FL SWQ. Wrote the paper: CYW FL ZLJ.

References

1. Norman RJ, Dewailly D, Legro RS, Hickey TE (2007) Polycystic ovary syndrome. Lancet 370: 685–697.
2. Norman RJ, Wu R, Stankiewicz MT (2004) Polycystic ovary syndrome. Med J Aust 180: 132–137.
3. Shi D, Vine DF (2012) Animal models of polycystic ovary syndrome: a focused review of rodent models in relationship to clinical phenotypes and cardiometabolic risk. Fertil Steril 98: 185–193.
4. Lara HE, Ferruz JL, Luza S, Bustamante DA, Borges Y, et al. (1993) Activation of ovarian sympathetic nerves in polycystic ovary syndrome. Endocrinology 133: 2690–2695.
5. Stener-Victorin E, Lundeberg T, Waldenstrom U, Manni L, Aloe L, et al. (2000) Effects of electro-acupuncture on nerve growth factor and ovarian morphology in rats with experimentally induced polycystic ovaries. Biol Reprod 63: 1497–1503.
6. Stener-Victorin E, Lindholm C (2004) Immunity and beta-endorphin concentrations in hypothalamus and plasma in rats with steroid-induced polycystic ovaries: effect of low-frequency electroacupuncture. Biol Reprod 70: 329–333.
7. Manni L, Cajander S, Lundeberg T, Naylor AS, Aloe L, et al. (2005) Effect of exercise on ovarian morphology and expression of nerve growth factor and alpha(1)- and beta(2)-adrenergic receptors in rats with steroid-induced polycystic ovaries. J Neuroendocrinol 17: 846–858.
8. Maliqueo M, Sun M, Johansson J, Benrick A, Labrie F, et al. (2013) Continuous administration of a P450 aromatase inhibitor induces polycystic ovary syndrome with a metabolic and endocrine phenotype in female rats at adult age. Endocrinology 154: 434–445.
9. Manneras L, Cajander S, Holmang A, Seleskovic Z, Lystig T, et al. (2007) A new rat model exhibiting both ovarian and metabolic characteristics of polycystic ovary syndrome. Endocrinology 148: 3781–3791.
10. Benrick A, Maliqueo M, Miao S, Villanueva JA, Feng Y, et al. (2013) Resveratrol is not as effective as physical exercise for improving reproductive and metabolic functions in rats with dihydrotestosterone-induced polycystic ovary syndrome. Evid Based Complement Alternat Med 2013: 964070.
11. Beloosesky R, Gold R, Almog B, Sasson R, Dantes A, et al. (2004) Induction of polycystic ovary by testosterone in immature female rats: Modulation of apoptosis and attenuation of glucose/insulin ratio. Int J Mol Med 14: 207–215.
12. Qiu S, Wu C, Lin F, Chen L, Huang Z, et al. (2009) Exercise training improved insulin sensitivity and ovarian morphology in rats with polycystic ovary syndrome. Horm Metab Res 41: 880–885.
13. Diamanti-Kandarakis E, Christakou C, Marinakis E (2012) Phenotypes and enviromental factors: their influence in PCOS. Curr Pharm Des 18: 270–282.
14. Zhao S, Chu Y, Zhang C, Lin Y, Xu K, et al. (2008) Diet-induced central obesity and insulin resistance in rabbits. J Anim Physiol Anim Nutr (Berl) 92: 105–111.
15. Tanaka S, Hayashi T, Toyoda T, Hamada T, Shimizu Y, et al. (2007) High-fat diet impairs the effects of a single bout of endurance exercise on glucose transport and insulin sensitivity in rat skeletal muscle. Metabolism 56: 1719–1728.
16. Flanagan AM, Brown JL, Santiago CA, Aad PY, Spicer LJ, et al. (2008) High-fat diets promote insulin resistance through cytokine gene expression in growing female rats. J Nutr Biochem 19: 505–513.
17. Cataldo NA, Abbasi F, McLaughlin TL, Basina M, Fechner PY, et al. (2006) Metabolic and ovarian effects of rosiglitazone treatment for 12 weeks in insulin-resistant women with polycystic ovary syndrome. Hum Reprod 21: 109–120.
18. Khorram O, Helliwell JP, Katz S, Bonpane CM, Jaramillo L (2006) Two weeks of metformin improves clomiphene citrate-induced ovulation and metabolic profiles in women with polycystic ovary syndrome. Fertil Steril 85: 1448–1451.
19. Guzick DS (2007) Ovulation induction management of PCOS. Clin Obstet Gynecol 50: 255–267.
20. Palomba S, Giallauria F, Falbo A, Russo T, Oppedisano R, et al. (2008) Structured exercise training programme versus hypocaloric hyperproteic diet in

obese polycystic ovary syndrome patients with anovulatory infertility: a 24-week pilot study. Hum Reprod 23: 642–650.

21. Tierney AC, McMonagle J, Shaw DI, Gulseth HL, Helal O, et al. (2011) Effects of dietary fat modification on insulin sensitivity and on other risk factors of the metabolic syndrome—LIPGENE: a European randomized dietary intervention study. Int J Obes (Lond) 35: 800–809.
22. Rajaie S, Azadbakht L, Khazaei M, Sherbafchi M, Esmaillzadeh A (2014) Moderate replacement of carbohydrates by dietary fats affects features of metabolic syndrome: A randomized crossover clinical trial. Nutrition 30: 61–68.
23. Zhang M, Lv XY, Li J, Xu ZG, Chen L (2008) The characterization of high-fat diet and multiple low-dose streptozotocin induced type 2 diabetes rat model. Exp Diabetes Res 2008: 704045.
24. Liu G, Shi F, Blas-Machado U, Duong Q, Davis VL, et al. (2005) Ovarian effects of a high lactose diet in the female rat. Reprod Nutr Dev 45: 185–192.
25. Hickey M, Doherty DA, Atkinson H, Sloboda DM, Franks S, et al. (2011) Clinical, ultrasound and biochemical features of polycystic ovary syndrome in adolescents: implications for diagnosis. Hum Reprod 26: 1469–1477.
26. Cavagni J, Wagner TP, Gaio EJ, Rego RO, Torres IL, et al. (2013) Obesity may increase the occurrence of spontaneous periodontal disease in Wistar rats. Arch Oral Biol 58: 1034–1039.
27. Cai W, Gao QD, Zhu L, Peppa M, He C, et al. (2002) Oxidative stress-inducing carbonyl compounds from common foods: novel mediators of cellular dysfunction. Mol Med 8: 337–346.
28. Goldberg T, Cai W, Peppa M, Dardaine V, Baliga BS, et al. (2004) Advanced glycoxidation end products in commonly consumed foods. J Am Diet Assoc 104: 1287–1291.
29. Diamanti-Kandarakis E, Piperi C, Korkolopoulou P, Kandaraki E, Levidou G, et al. (2007) Accumulation of dietary glycotoxins in the reproductive system of normal female rats. J Mol Med (Berl) 85: 1413–1420.
30. Azziz R, Carmina E, Dewailly D, Diamanti-Kandarakis E, Escobar-Morreale HF, et al. (2006) Positions statement: criteria for defining polycystic ovary syndrome as a predominantly hyperandrogenic syndrome: an Androgen Excess Society guideline. J Clin Endocrinol Metab 91: 4237–4245.
31. Schuring AN, Schulte N, Sonntag B, Kiesel L (2008) Androgens and insulin—two key players in polycystic ovary syndrome. Recent concepts in the pathophysiology and genetics of polycystic ovary syndrome. Gynakol Geburtshilfliche Rundsch 48: 9–15.
32. Franks S, Stark J, Hardy K (2008) Follicle dynamics and anovulation in polycystic ovary syndrome. Hum Reprod Update 14: 367–378.
33. Tyndall V, Broyde M, Sharpe R, Welsh M, Drake AJ, et al. (2012) Effect of androgen treatment during foetal and/or neonatal life on ovarian function in prepubertal and adult rats. Reproduction 143: 21–33.
34. Moran LJ, Ranasinha S, Zoungas S, McNaughton SA, Brown WJ, et al. (2013) The contribution of diet, physical activity and sedentary behaviour to body mass index in women with and without polycystic ovary syndrome. Hum Reprod 28: 2276–2283.
35. Dunaif A (1997) Insulin resistance and the polycystic ovary syndrome: mechanism and implications for pathogenesis. Endocr Rev 18: 774–800.
36. Lunger F, Wildt L, Seeber B (2013) Accurate screening for insulin resistance in PCOS women using fasting insulin concentrations. Gynecol Endocrinol 29: 541–544.
37. Norman RJ, Davies MJ, Lord J, Moran LJ (2002) The role of lifestyle modification in polycystic ovary syndrome. Trends Endocrinol Metab 13: 251–257.
38. Yildiz BO, Knochenhauer ES, Azziz R (2008) Impact of obesity on the risk for polycystic ovary syndrome. J Clin Endocrinol Metab 93: 162–168.
39. Coviello AD, Legro RS, Dunaif A (2006) Adolescent girls with polycystic ovary syndrome have an increased risk of the metabolic syndrome associated with increasing androgen levels independent of obesity and insulin resistance. J Clin Endocrinol Metab 91: 492–497.
40. Morifuji M, Sanbongi C, Sugiura K (2006) Dietary soya protein intake and exercise training have an additive effect on skeletal muscle fatty acid oxidation enzyme activities and mRNA levels in rats. Br J Nutr 96: 469–475.
41. Hayashi T, Wojtaszewski JF, Goodyear LJ (1997) Exercise regulation of glucose transport in skeletal muscle. Am J Physiol 273: E1039–1051.
42. Al-Nozha O, Habib F, Mojaddidi M, El-Bab MF (2013) Body weight reduction and metformin: Roles in polycystic ovary syndrome. Pathophysiology 20: 131–137.
43. Vignesh JP, Mohan V (2007) Polycystic ovary syndrome: a component of metabolic syndrome? J Postgrad Med 53: 128–134.
44. Hoeger KM (2007) Obesity and lifestyle management in polycystic ovary syndrome. Clin Obstet Gynecol 50: 277–294.
45. Douglas CC, Gower BA, Darnell BE, Ovalle F, Oster RA, et al. (2006) Role of diet in the treatment of polycystic ovary syndrome. Fertil Steril 85: 679–688.
46. (2004) National Institute for Clinical Excellence. Fertility assessment and treatment for people with fertility problems. A clinical guideline. London: RCOG Press.
47. Hamilton-Fairley D, Kiddy D, Anyaoku V, Koistinen R, Seppala M, et al. (1993) Response of sex hormone binding globulin and insulin-like growth factor binding protein-1 to an oral glucose tolerance test in obese women with polycystic ovary syndrome before and after calorie restriction. Clin Endocrinol (Oxf) 39: 363–367.
48. Lord JM, Norman R (2006) Obesity, polycystic ovary syndrome, infertility treatment: lifestyle modification is paramount. BMJ 332: 609.
49. Hawley JA (2004) Exercise as a therapeutic intervention for the prevention and treatment of insulin resistance. Diabetes Metab Res Rev 20: 383–393.

12

B Lymphocyte Stimulator (BLyS) is Expressed in Human Adipocytes *In Vivo* and is Related to Obesity but not to Insulin Resistance

Nike Müller[1], Dominik M. Schulte[1], Susann Hillebrand[1], Kathrin Türk[1], Jochen Hampe[1], Clemens Schafmayer[2], Mario Brosch[1], Witigo von Schönfels[2], Markus Ahrens[2], Rainald Zeuner[1], Johann O. Schröder[1], Matthias Blüher[3], Christian Gutschow[4], Sandra Freitag-Wolf[5], Marta Stelmach-Mardas[1], Carina Saggau[1], Stefan Schreiber[1], Matthias Laudes[1]*

1 Department I of Internal Medicine, University of Kiel, Kiel, Germany, **2** Department of General, Abdominal, Thoracic and Transplantation Surgery, University of Kiel, Kiel, Germany, **3** Department for Internal Medicine, Clinic for Endocrinology and Nephrology, University of Leipzig, Leipzig, Germany, **4** Department of General, Visceral and Cancer Surgery, University of Cologne, Cologne, Germany, **5** Institute of Medical Informatics and Statistics, University of Kiel, Kiel, Germany

Abstract

Inflammation and metabolism have been shown to be evolutionary linked and increasing evidence exists that pro-inflammatory factors are involved in the pathogenesis of obesity and type 2 diabetes. Until now, most data suggest that within adipose tissue these factors are secreted by cells of the innate immune system, e. g. macrophages. In the present study we demonstrate that *B lymphocyte stimulator* (BLyS) is increased in human obesity. In contrast to several pro-inflammatory factors, we found the source of BLyS in human adipose tissue to be the adipocytes rather than immune cells. In grade 3 obese human subjects, expression of BLyS *in vivo* in adipose tissue is significantly increased ($p<0.001$). Furthermore, BLyS serum levels are elevated in grade 3 human obesity (862.5+222.0 pg/ml vs. 543.7+60.7 pg/ml in lean controls, $p<0.001$) and are positively correlated to the BMI ($r=0.43$, $p<0.0002$). In the present study, bariatric surgery significantly altered serum BLyS concentrations. In contrast, weight loss due to a very-low-calorie-formula-diet (800 kcal/d) had no such effect. To examine metabolic activity of BLyS, in a translational research approach, insulin sensitivity was measured in human subjects *in vivo* before and after treatment with the human recombinant anti-BLyS antibody belimumab. Since BLyS is known to promote B-cell proliferation and immunoglobulin secretion, the present data suggest that adipocytes of grade 3 obese human subjects are able to activate the adaptive immune system, suggesting that in metabolic inflammation in humans both, innate and adaptive immunity, are of pathophysiological relevance.

Editor: Jörg Hermann Fritz, McGill University, Canada

Funding: This work was supported by Deutsche Diabetes Stiftung (319/06/12 to Dominik M. Schulte). The funders had no role in study design, data collection and analysis, decision to publish, or preparation of the manuscript.

Competing Interests: The authors have declared that no competing interests exist.

* E-mail: matthias.laudes@uk-sh.de

Introduction

Obesity is associated with a reduced life-span [1] and represents a fast-growing health problem that is reaching epidemic proportions worldwide [2]. It leads to several chronic co-morbidities including type 2 diabetes, dyslipidemia and atherosclerosis [3]. The risk to develop type 2 diabetes is estimated to be nine fold higher for obese than for lean men [4].

It is already known that the development of insulin resistance and type 2 diabetes is associated with inflammatory mechanisms in adipose tissue [5]. This relationship can be explained by hypertrophic and functionally impaired adipocytes in visceral and subcutaneous fat depots due to a positive energy balance. In this pathophysiological condition various bioactive molecules are being produced and secreted by adipocytes which can activate the infiltration of cells of the innate immune system, e. g. macrophages. [5–7]. These cells are able to inhibit adipogenesis from mesenchymal stem cells via classical pro-inflammatory cytokines and wnt-molecules in a paracrine manner [6–8]. As a consequence, hindered adipogenesis reduce the fat storage capacity of adipose tissue. This results in ectopic lipid accumulation in liver and skeletal muscle leading to insulin resistance of these metabolically important tissues and eventually type 2 diabetes [9,10].

In rodents, *B lymphocyte stimulator* (BLyS) has recently been demonstrated to be secreted by hypertrophic, mature adipocytes [11–13]. BLyS is known to play an important role in activating B-lymphocytes [14,15]. Hence, BLyS is considered as a novel factor that links obesity to inflammation [11]. BLyS, also termed as B cell-activating factor (BAFF), belongs to the TNF ligand family, and has been identified as a factor that promotes B cell proliferation and immunoglobulin secretion [14,15].

Since *in vivo* data in humans on the pathological significance of BLyS in low-grade inflammation of adipose tissue are rare, we intended to clarify whether (1) BLyS is expressed in human adipocytes *in vivo*, (2) BLyS expression in adipose tissue *in vivo* differs between lean and obese +/− insulin resistant human subjects, (3) BLyS serum concentrations are dysregulated in obese +/− insulin resistant patients, (4) BLyS responds to different weight loss therapies in obese humans and (5) inhibition of BLyS in humans *in vivo* by the neutralizing antibody belimumab alters insulin sensitivity.

Materials and Methods

All studies were approved by the local ethics committees (Number: D475/11, University of Kiel, Germany). Written informed consent was obtained from each subject before inclusion into the study.

Study populations

1.) Adipose tissue biopsy study populations. Human subcutaneous adipose tissue biopsies for immunohistology were taken during elective surgical procedures from lean controls (n = 3; 45.3+11.6 years; 66.7% males; body mass index (BMI): 23+1.3 kg/m^2), overweight subjects (n = 3; 48.3+4.2 years; 66.7% males; 27.6+1.7 kg/m^2) and obese individuals with type 2 diabetes (n = 3; 53.7+15.5 years; 33.3% males; 36.8+1.5 kg/m^2). Exclusion criteria for this study have been described earlier [6]. Type 2 diabetes in patients of the third group was sufficiently controlled only by dietary intervention with or without metformin therapy.

For determining BLyS transcript levels in total adipose tissue samples, RNA was isolated from subcutaneous and visceral adipose tissue which was obtained during elective surgical procedures. The RNA study population consisted of lean controls and obese individuals with and without insulin resistance. Lean controls and grade 3 obese subjects +/− type 2 diabetes were equally distributed regarding gender while BMI and age were significantly different (**table 1**).

2.) FoCus cohort study population. As part of the Food Chain Plus (FoCus) project [http://www.focus.uni-kiel.de] a total number of n = 30 serum samples were obtained. The study population was divided into a lean control group, a grade 1+2 obesity group without insulin resistance and a grade 1+2 obesity group with insulin resistance (**table 1**).

3.) Nutritional intervention study population. The nutritional intervention group consisted of n = 16 subjects (45.3+7.4 years, 43.8% males, 42.2+6.2 kg/m^2). This group was treated with a very-low-calorie formula diet (VLCD, Optifast 52 (Nestle Nutrition)) with a total caloric intake of approximately 800 kcal/d for 3 months. Inclusion criteria of this study population have been described earlier [16]. Seven patients suffered from arterial hypertension; one patient each suffered from gastroesophageal reflux, gonarthrose, non-alcoholic steatohepatitis or asthma. Two patients suffered from type 2 diabetes which was being controlled appropriately. One patient received a hormone replacement therapy; two patients took ß-blocker and one patient ACE inhibitors. Antihistamines or gastric acid neutralizing drugs were being taken by one patient each.

4.) Bariatric surgery intervention study population. Sera of 26 patients (42.1+11.8 years, 11.5% males, 48.7+7.4 kg/m^2) were obtained before and 6 months after bariatric surgery. This intervention led to a mean weight reduction of 37.5 kg (140.7+28.8 kg to 103.2+25.4 kg). In the scope of bariatric surgery three patients received gastric bypass whereas all other subjects underwent sleeve gastrectomy. Regarding comorbidities and medications, seven patients suffered from arterial hypertension. One patient each had diabetic neuropathy, hyperuremia, epilepsy, gastroesophageal reflux or bronchial asthma. Thyroid and gallbladder have been removed in one patient. Two patients suffered from efficiently controlled hypothyroidism and three from type 2 diabetes which was controlled by insulin and metformin therapy. Three patients took calcium antagonists; six patients took ACE inhibitors and four patients ß-blocker. Diuretics were being taken by six patients. Nine patients regularly took analgetics; three patients cholesterol-reducing drugs. Nine patients took antidepressants, three patients were on allopurinol, 11 patients took gastric acid neutralizing drugs. Furthermore, four patients took thyroxin.

5.) Belimumab intervention study population. A total number of n = 5 patients with treatment indication for belimumab (Benlysta (Human Genome Sciences and GlaxoSmithKline), approved for the treatment of systemic lupus erythematodes), an anti-BLyS human monoclonal antibody, were treated for 4 weeks. 5 female patients with systemic lupus erythematodes (SLE) were included. BLyS is known to be elevated in patients with autoimmune diseases, such as *systemic lupus erythematosus* (SLE), Sjogren's syndrome, and rheumatoid arthritis [17]. One patient was additionally suffering from rheumatoid arthritis, and one patient had additionally pleuritis. Mean age was 48.4+18.9 years, mean BMI of these females was 26.6+4.3 kg/m^2. All patients showed a response to belimumab treatment in terms of SLE disease activity indicated by improvement in at least one clinical sign (e. g. fatique) or a laboratory measure (e. g. increase in leucocytes). In order to examine the effect on insulin sensitivity the HOMA-IR and the leptin-to-adiponectin-ratio (LAR) were determined before and after treatment as described earlier [8].

Separation of stromal vascular fractions and mature adipocytes from human adipose tissue biopsies

Subcutaneous adipose tissue samples were obtained from obese subjects undergoing elective open abdominal surgery in general anesthesia. All subjects fasted for 6 hrs prior to the operation. Adipose tissue biopsies were taken under sterile conditions and were transported into the laboratory in phosphate buffered saline. After dicing the tissue into 1–2-mm pieces, samples were digested in collagenase buffer (Hanks' balanced salt solution (PAA Laboratories GmbH, Cölbe, Germany), 3 mg/ml type I collagenase (Life Technologies GmbH, Darmstadt, Germany), and 2% bovine serum albumin (biomol GmbH, Hamburg, Germany) at 37°C for 1 h. The digest was filtered through a 260-µm stainless steel mesh and centrifuged at 400× *g* for 5 min. The supernatant containing the floating mature adipocytes was lysed in RIPA buffer (50 mM Tris-HCl, 150 mM NaCl, 0.5% sodium deoxycholate, 0.1% SDS, 1% NP-40, PhosSTOP (Roche, Penzberg, Germany), protease inhibitor cocktail (Sigma)). The cell pellet containing the stromal vascular fraction was treated with red cell lysis buffer (0.154 M NH4Cl, 10 mM KHCO3, 0.1 mM EDTA) for 5 min at room temperature. After several washing steps with red cell lysis buffer the pellet containing the stromal vascular fraction was lysed in RIPA buffer, PhosSTOP and protease inhibitor cocktail. Afterwards, lysed cell extracts were centrifuged at 4°C at 14,000 rpm for 30 min.

Western Blotting

40 µg of protein per sample were added to 4× loading buffer (bromophenol blue and Laemmli buffer), heated to 95°C for 5 min, and separated on a 12% SDS-PAGE. Proteins were transferred to polyvinylidene fluoride membranes (Carl Roth GmbH, Karlsruhe, Germany). The following antibodies were used according to the instructions of the manufacturer: BLyS (ab16081; Abcam, USA), BCMA (ab5972, Abcam, USA). GAPDH (#2118, Cell Signaling, USA) and all secondary antibodies except anti-rat (ab102265, Abcam, USA) were purchased from Cell Signaling Technology (Frankfurt, Germany).

Table 1. Baseline characteristics of the study populations of the BLyS mRNA in human total adipose tissue biopsies of lean, grade 3 obese +/− insulin resistance (IR) and of BLyS measurements in sera of lean, grade 1+2 obese +/− insulin resistance.

mRNA level	*visceral*						
	lean	**obese**	**obese+IR**	**p-value**	t_1	t_2	t_3
male:female	**10:6**	**19:3**	**5:1**	**0.2071**			
BMI (kg/m²)	22.1+2.9	52.9+9.2	50.4+7.2	<0.0001	<0.001	<0.001	ns
age (years)	57.1+5.2	42.7+10.4	47.7+9.0	<0.0001	<0.001	ns	ns
	subcutaneous						
	lean	**obese**	**obese+IR**	**p-value**	t_1	t_2	t_3
male:female	**11:4**	**25:2**	**7:4**	**0.0776**			
BMI (kg/m²)	22.6+1.9	47.2+11.1	47.5+10.5	<0.0001	<0.001	<0.001	ns
age (years)	57.0+5.3	40.6+10.1	52.8+11.8	<0.0001	<0.001	ns	<0.01
serum level							
	lean	**obese**	**obese+IR**	**p-value**	t_1	t_2	t_3
male:female	**2:8**	**2:8**	**2:8**	1.0000			
age (years)	57.7+14.66	56.4+10.7	57.3+4.4	0.9627			
weight (kg)	62.9+9.9	112.9+21.9	111.1+23.5	<0.0001	<0.001	<0.001	ns
BMI (kg/m²)	21.9+2.5	37.9+6.9	38.1+5.0	<0.0001	<0.001	<0.001	ns
glucose (mg/dl)	96.0+11.7	94.3+11.2	103.1+12.2	0.1539			
insulin (µU/ml)	5.1+2.5	7.2+1.3	27.8+8.1	<0.0001	ns	<0.001	<0.001
triglycerides (mg/dl)	91.5+39.3	119.4+57.1	150.8+58.0	0.0550			
CRP (mg/l)	1.1+0.4	4.4+3.8	7.3+8.3	0.0008	<0.01	<0.01	ns
HOMA-IR index	1.2+0.6	1.7+0.2	7.0+1.8	<0.0001	ns	<0.001	<0.001
BLyS (pg/ml)	543.7+63.9	514.1+140.9	600.2+168.6	0.1876			

t_1: lean vs. obese.
t_2: lean vs. obese+IR.
t_3: obese vs. obese+IR.
Shown are means+SD for each group.

RNA isolation and *Taqman* Quantitative Real Time Reverse Transcription-PCR

100 milligrams of frozen total adipose tissue from lean and grade 3 obese +/− type 2 diabetes were ground with 3 mm stainless steel balls using liquid nitrogen cooling (MM301 Mixer Mill, Retsch, Haan, Germany) for 30 sec to a fine powder. RNA was isolated using Trizol (Life Technologies GmbH) following the manufacturer's protocol. cDNA synthesis was further performed using Advantage RT for PCR kit (Clontech Laboratories, Saint-Germain-en-Laye, France) according to the manufacturer's instructions. Expression levels of BLyS and housekeeping gene ß-actin were determined using suitable TaqMan Gene Expression Assay kits (for BLyS: Hs00198106_m1; for ß-actin: Hs99999903_m1; Applied Biosystems, Darmstadt, Germany).

Immunohistology

Immunohistochemistry was performed using BLyS antibody (LS-B2081; LifeSpan BioScience) as described earlier [16].

Enzyme-linked immunosorbent assay (ELISA)

Serum was assayed for BLyS using the Quantikine ELISA Kit (DBLYS0B; R&D Systems, Inc., Wiesbaden, Germany) according to the manufacturer's instructions (according to the manufacturer: Sensitivity: 6.44 pg/ml. Specificity: <0.5% cross-reactivity observed with available related molecules. <50% cross-species reactivity observed with species tested). ELISA for adipokine measurement were purchased from IBL International (Hamburg, Germany) as follows: Adiponectin ELISA (BV51001, analytical-sensitivity: 0.2 µg/ml), Leptin ELISA (RE53151, analytical-sensitivity: 1.0 ng/ml) and were performed according to the instructions of the manufacturer.

Statistical analysis

Statistical analysis was performed using GraphPad Prism 5.01 Software. Associations between categorical variables were assessed by Chi-squared test. If the assumption of normal distribution of the continuous data was not violated Student's t-test or ANOVA was used. In case of not normal distributed data the Mann-Whitney U test or Kruskal-Wallis test was applied. Moreover, regression analysis with BLyS expression as the dependent variable was used in order to avoid an effect of possible confounding factors as age. The significance level was set at 5% and multiple comparisons were done using Bonferroni or Dunn's post test.

Results

BLyS expression in human adipose tissue

Immunohistochemistry of adipose tissue biopsies exhibited BLyS to be present within the cytoplasm of adipocytes *in vivo* in human subjects with obesity with and without type 2 diabetes but to a lesser extend in lean controls (**figure 1A**). The higher magnification shown in **figure 1B** suggests that the major source of BLyS within adipose tissue are mature adipocytes, since no obvious staining was observed in the stromal vascular fraction. In order to further examine whether BLyS is only expressed in mature adipocytes or also in certain cells of the stromal vascular fraction, we next separated mature adipocytes and the stromal vascular fraction of visceral and subcutaneous adipose tissue biopsies from n = 5 obese humans by collagenase digestion and performed western blots for BLyS and the BLyS receptor BCMA. This experiment showed that the major source of BLyS and BCMA in adipose tissue are mature adipocytes (**figure 1C**) while the different cells in the stromal vascular fraction do not contribute to adipose tissue BLyS and BCMA expression in a significant manner. Also, as shown in figure 1C, no significant difference in BLyS expression was found between subcutaneous and visceral mature adipocytes (**figure 1C**).

In order to compare BLyS expression levels between lean controls and obese human subjects with and without type 2 diabetes, we performed real-time RT-PCR using RNA extracted from human visceral and subcutaneous adipose tissue biopsies. These experiments revealed a significant increase in BLyS expression in both adipose tissue depots of obese human subjects compared to lean controls (**figure 2A+B**). However, as shown in **figure 2A+B**, BLyS expression levels did not significantly differ between non-diabetic and diabetic obese human subjects. Further statistical analysis showed that relative BLyS expression was higher in males (n = 77) than in females (n = 20) (1.23+0.09 versus 1.18+0.08, $p<0.05$), higher in subcutaneous (n = 53) than in visceral (n = 44) adipose tissue (1.23+0.09 versus 1.20+0.09, $p<0.05$) and higher in diabetic (n = 17) than in non-diabetic (n = 80) subjects (1.28+0.04 versus 1.20+0.09, $p<0.01$). In addition we found a significant negative correlation with age ($r = -0.48$,

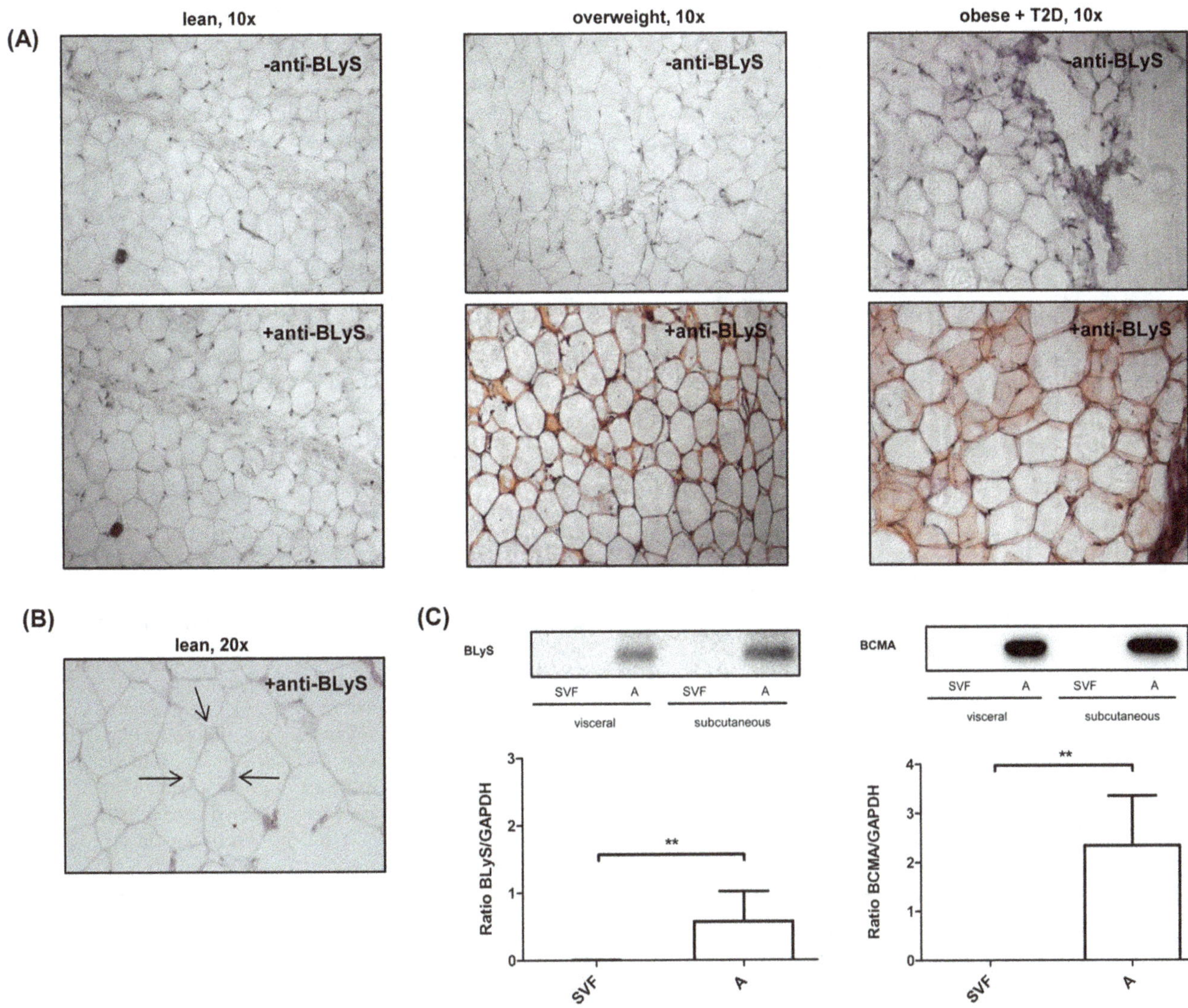

Figure 1. BLyS expression in adipose tissue in humans *in vivo*. (A) BLyS immunohistochemistry (lower panel) and haematoxylin staining (upper panel) of subcutaneous adipose tissue biopsies of lean (left), overweight (middle) and obese+type 2 diabetes (T2D) (right) human subjects (10×). The reddish color represents BLyS-positive mature adipocytes. (B) shows 20× magnification of the immunohistochemistry of a lean adipose tissue biopsy in which the arrows demonstrate the stromal vascular fraction. The lean representative was chosen as BLyS expression was rarely detectable in their adipocytes, thus resulting in a more reliable visual interpretation of the stromal vascular fraction. (C) BLyS and BCMA protein detection revealed that BLyS and BCMA is only expressed in the mature adipocyte [A] fraction but not in the stromal vascular fraction [SVF]. Densitometry graphs data in this figure are shown as means+SEM (n = 5).

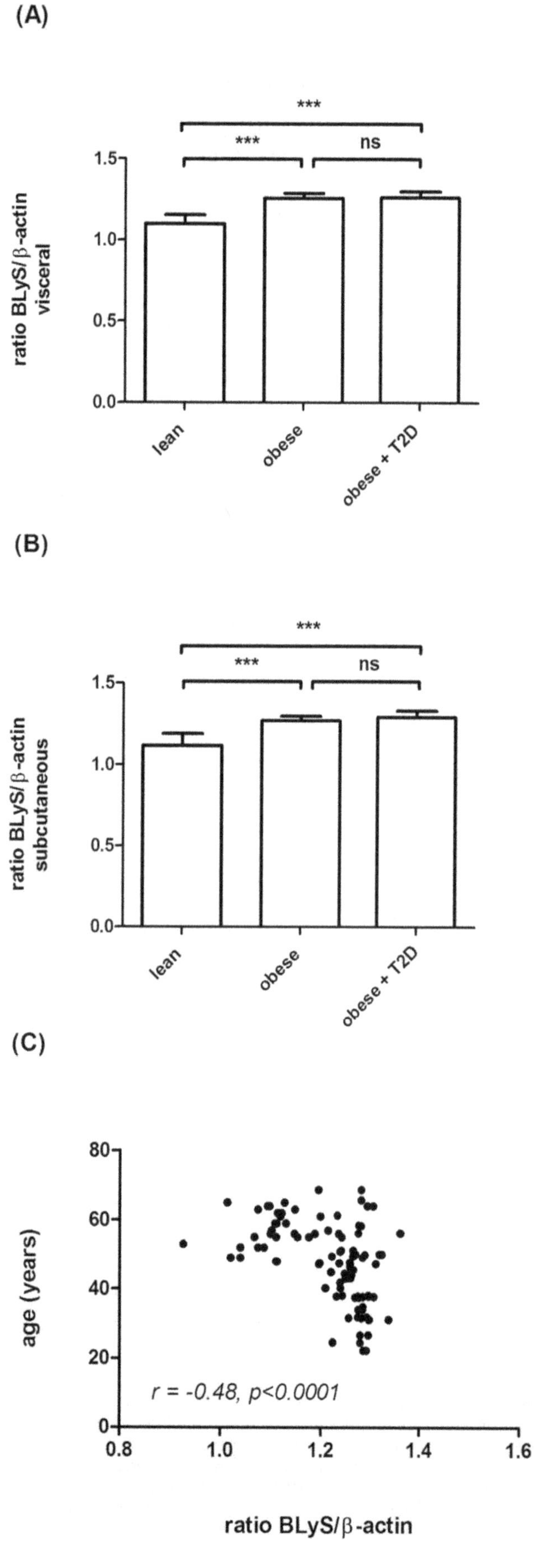

Figure 2. BLyS mRNA level in (A) visceral and (B) subcutaneous adipose tissue of lean control subjects, patients with grade 3 obesity +/− type 2 diabetes (T2D). RNA was isolated from total subcutaneous and visceral adipose tissue biopsies. Data in this figure are shown as means+SD. (C) shows a significant negative correlation between age and BLyS expression ($r = -0.48$, $p<0.0001$) in a combined analysis of all biopsy samples.

$p<0.0001$ (**figure 2**)). Since the mean age was different between the groups, we also performed age-adjusted analysis of the expression levels shown in figure 2. This analysis revealed stable results, indicating that age is not a major confounder of the results obtained.

BLyS serum concentrations in human obesity

In order to investigate whether BLyS serum levels vary between lean controls, grade 1+2 obese individuals (BMI 30–40 kg/m^2) with insulin resistance and grade 1+2 obese individuals (BMI 30–40 kg/m^2) without insulin resistance, we performed ELISA assays in serum samples collected from such subjects. The groups were equally distributed in terms of age and gender (**table 1**). Insulin resistance was estimated by the HOMA-IR index for which values below 2.0 were supposed to be as normal [18]. As shown in **table 1**, in this analysis BLyS serum concentrations ranged from 543.7+63.9 pg/ml to 600.2+168.6 pg/ml and were not significantly different between the groups.

Since we did not find a significant association of BLyS serum levels with grade 1 and 2 obesity (BMI 30–40 kg/m^2), we next aimed to examine whether BLyS serum levels are increased in grade 3 obese subjects (BMI>40 kg/m^2). This experiment showed that serum BLyS concentrations are elevated in grade 3 obesity (mean BMI: 47.5+6.6 kg/m^2, mean BLyS: 862.5+222.0 pg/ml) which was significantly different to lean controls (mean BMI: 21.9+2.5 kg/m^2, mean BLyS: 543.7+60.7 pg/ml) and grade 1+2 obese subjects (mean BMI: 35.4+2.8 kg/m^2, mean BLyS: 627.6+193.2 pg/ml) (**figure 3A**). Correlation analysis of serum BLyS levels with the BMI in the different subjects of our research cohorts ($n = 72$) indicated an overall significant positive correlation ($r = 0.43$, $p<0.0002$) (**figure 3B**).

Effects of VLCD and bariatric surgery on BLyS serum levels

As there is evidence that weight-loss strategies reduce low-grade inflammation in obese human subjects [16,19], we next examined BLyS serum levels before and after different weight loss strategies. In the first study population, 16 obese subjects were treated with a nutritional intervention using a VLCD (approximately 800 kcal/d) for 3 months. Mean weight loss achieved accounted for 17.9 kg (125.2+15.5 kg to 102.5+13.2 kg) corresponding to a BMI reduction from 42.2+6.2 kg/m^2 to 34.6+5.6 kg/m^2. BLyS serum levels were not reduced due to the weight loss achieved and accounted to 934.22+185.8 pg/ml before and 960.72+300.4 pg/ml after 3 months of the nutritional intervention (**figure 4A**). In the second study population, BLyS serum samples were measured in obese human subjects before and 6 months after bariatric surgery. The later time point for blood sampling in the surgical group (6 months versus 3 months in the VLCD) was used, since several weeks after a surgical procedure is performed healing processes including inflammatory reactions can be expected which potentially will also induced BLyS expression. Bariatric surgery induced a mean weight loss of 37.5 kg (140.7+28.8 kg to 103.2+25.4 kg) in a time period of 6 months (BMI before: 48.7+7.4 kg/m^2; BMI after: 35.7+7.2 kg/m^2). Interestingly, as for

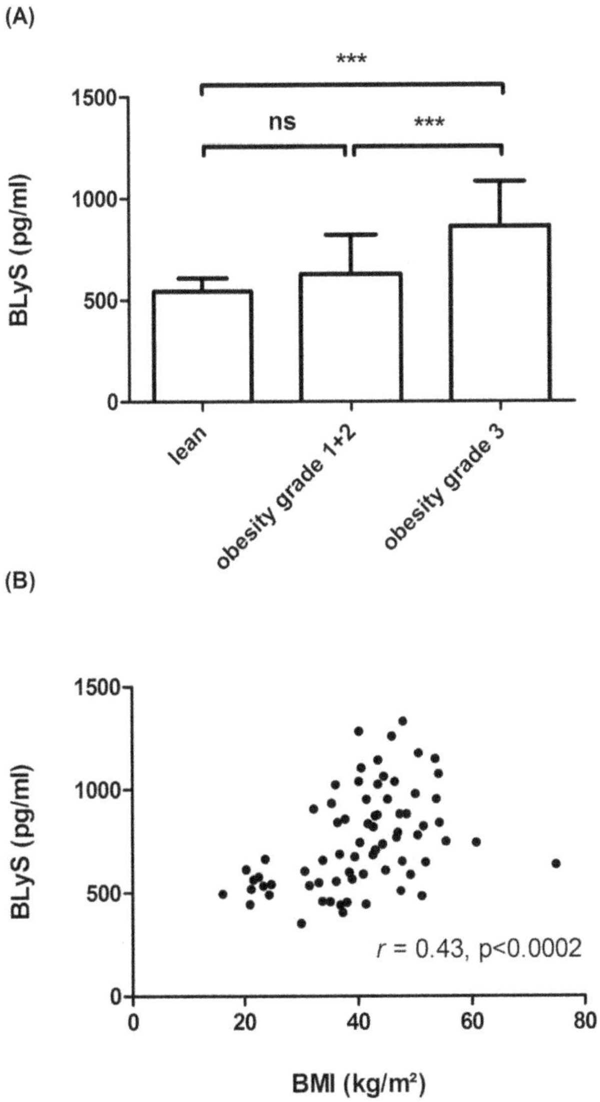

Figure 3. BLyS serum levels in human obesity. (A) represents significant differences between different grades of obesity (grade 1+2 (BMI≥30 to <40 kg/m^2), n = 20 and grade 3 (BMI≥40 kg/m^2), n = 42) and normal-weight ((BMI≤25 kg/m^2), n = 10) human control subjects. (B) shows the correlation (r = 0.43, p<0.0002) between BLyS serum levels and BMI of n = 72 human subjects used in this study. Data in this figure are shown as means+SD.

what was found for the VLCD, BLyS serum levels were not reduced after the surgical intervention. Instead BLyS levels exhibited even a mild but significant increase (BLyS before: 872.5+189.1 pg/ml; BLyS after: 982.0+177.1 pg/ml, p = 0.03) (**figure 4B**).

Effects of BLyS inhibition on insulin sensitivity in human subjects *in vivo*

In order to examine whether BLyS is of functional relevance in terms of development of insulin resistance in humans *in vivo*, the effect of BLyS on human insulin sensitivity was examined in a translational research approach. Therefore, blood samples were drawn before and 4 weeks after treatment of human subjects with the neutralizing monoclonal anti-BLyS antibody belimumab. Subsequently, insulin sensitivity was estimated by HOMA-IR and the leptin-to-adiponectin ratio (LAR). LAR is a very accurate measure for insulin sensitivity with close correlation to hyperinsulinemic-euglycemic clamp data [18]. The study population exhibited reduced insulin sensitivity before administration of belimumab, as indicated by an increased basal HOMA-IR and LAR. As shown in **table 2**, neither HOMA-IR nor LAR was influenced by belimumab treatment.

Discussion

Adipose tissue has long been regarded as a silent and passive organ, storing excess energy as triglycerides and releasing energy as fatty acids. Due to intensive research over the last decades adipose tissue now is also referred to as an endocrine and immune organ secreting a wide variety of metabolic and immune factors. They can initiate and influence inflammation, metabolism, appetite regulation and many other processes [20,21].

BLyS is a TNF ligand family member known to promote B-cell proliferation and immunoglobulin secretion [22,23]. In the present study, we demonstrate that within human adipose tissue BLyS is expressed in mature adipocytes and that expression is increased in obesity in both, visceral and subcutaneous fat depots (**Figure 2**). Further analysis showed that mature adipocytes are the major source of BLyS within adipose tissue, since we did not find a significant expression in the stromal vascular fraction (**figure 1**). This finding also suggests that BLyS is up-regulated during differentiation of preadipocytes (localized within stromal vascular fraction) into mature fat cells, which is in agreement to previously reported findings in the murine 3T3-L1 cell line [11,12].

Significant higher serum levels were found in grade 3 obese patients (BMI≥40 kg/m^2) but not in grade 1+2 obese subjects (**figure 3**) compared to lean controls. In this respect it has to be mentioned, that most factors identified so far in low-grade inflammation of adipose tissue are part of the innate immune system [5]. BLyS on the other hand is known to activate B-lymphocytes and to promote immunoglobulin secretion and thereby serves a marker for the adaptive immune system. Hence, the data presented here suggest that both compartments of the immune system are activated in human obesity, which is in agreement with several recent reports. For example Fabbrini E et al. in 2013 showed an association between adipose tissue CD4$^+$ T-cell populations and insulin resistance in obese human individuals [24].

Factors of the innate immunity induced in low-grade inflammation of adipose tissue are known to be involved in the pathogenesis of insulin resistance. For example, in one of our previous studies we have shown that blockade of IL-6 signaling in humans *in vivo* by the monoclonal antibody tocilizumab increased insulin sensitivity [10]. Using a similar translational approach, in the present study we examined insulin sensitivity in humans treated with belimumab, a monoclonal antibody blocking BLyS activity *in vivo*. In contrast to what was shown for IL-6 inhibition, in that experiment BLyS inhibition did not significantly alter insulin sensitivity (**table 2**). It has to be mentioned that this experiment has to be interpreted carefully, since only 5 human individuals have been examined and all of the subjects were suffering from an immunological disease. However, this finding is in agreement with the data, that in the present study neither BLyS expression levels in human adipose tissue nor BLyS serum levels in obese human subjects are associated with insulin resistance (**figure 2, table 1**).

The data obtained in the present study may even suggest that BLyS might display potential beneficial immune-modulating effects, since we identified BLyS not to be reduced but up-

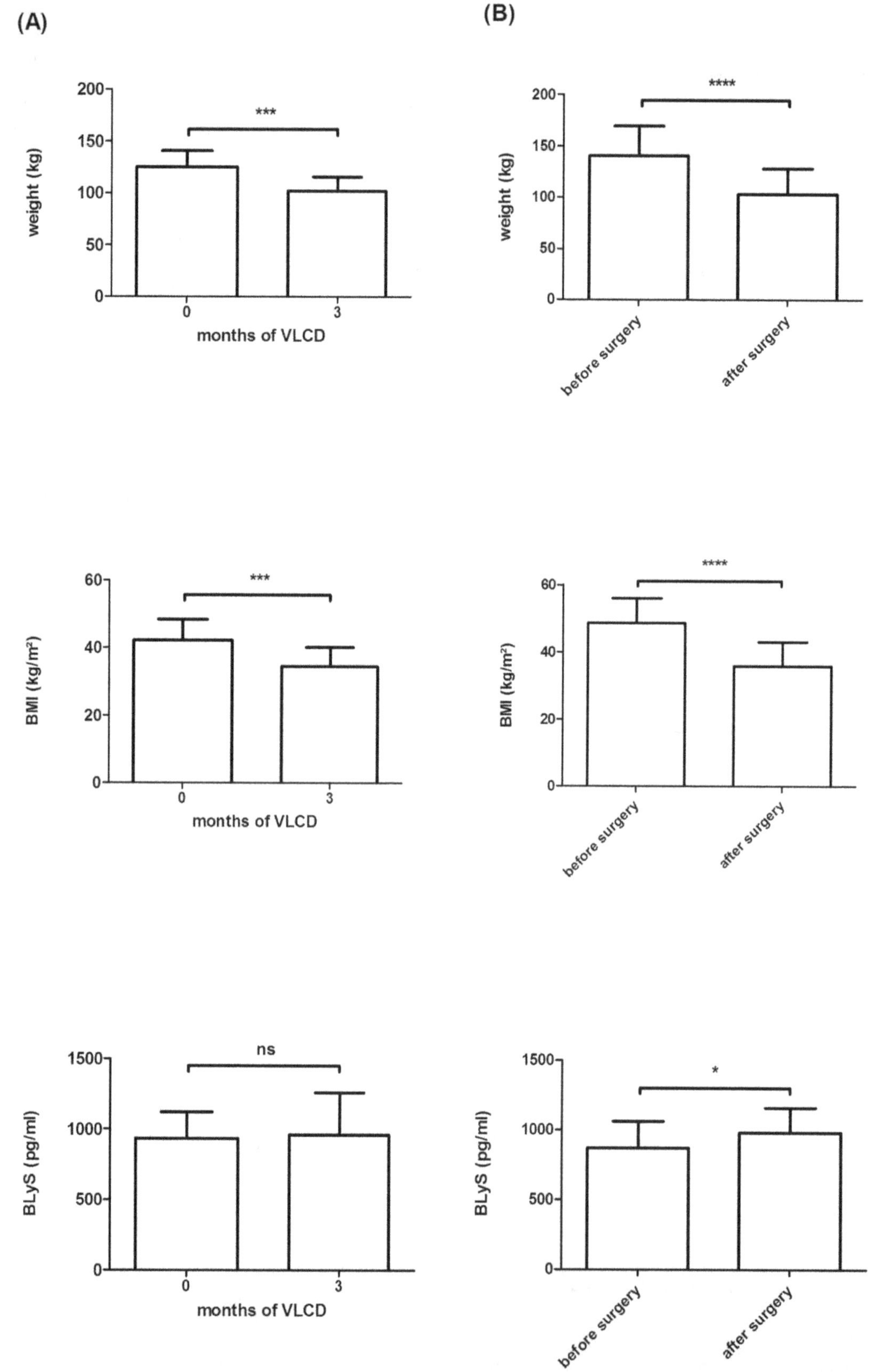

Figure 4. Anthropometric measures and BLyS serum concentrations before and after (3 months) of a very low calorie formula diet (VLCD) (approximately 800 kcal/d) as well as before and after (6 months) bariatric surgery in obese individuals. (A) Significant weight reduction (upper and middle panel) and no change of BLyS serum levels by VLCD (lower panel). Data in this figure are shown as means+SD of n = 16 obese human subjects during a VLCD. (B) Significant weight reduction (upper and middle panel) and significant increase of BLyS serum levels by

Table 2. Insulin resistance before and after belimumab treatment.

	before	after	p-value
insulin (µU/ml)	23.4+19.3	21.5+20.0	0.8857
glucose (mg/dl)	96.5+18.4	85.5+11.1	0.3429
HOMA-IR index	**5.1+3.5**	**4.3+3.7**	**0.4857**
leptin	24.8+8.4	26.8+14.9	0.8031
adiponectin	19.1+10.2	16.2+3-9	0.6180
LAR	**1.4+0.6**	**1.3+0.5**	**0.9687**

Insulin resistance was measured by HOMA-IR and leptin-to-adiponectin-ratio (LAR). Data are given as means+SD of n = 5 patients treated with anti-BLyS antibody belimumab for a time period of 4 weeks.

regulated after bariatric surgery of grade 3 obese subjects (**figure 4B**). Also, a weight loss to a lower extend by a VLCD did not significantly reduce BLyS serum concentrations in the present study (**figure 4A**). This is in contrast to was found for factors of the innate immunity. For example TNF-α and IL-6 have both been shown to be down-regulated during weight loss procedures [25,26].

The hypothesis that BLyS might be a beneficial factor in metabolic inflammation in human obesity is further supported by the data of an independent research group, showing that BLyS expression, like PPAR-γ expression, is induced during 3T3-L1 adipogenesis [13], supposing a positive but not a negative effect in human adipose tissue biology. Thus, taking these findings together it might be speculated that BLyS serves as a balancing immune modulator rather than a classical pro-inflammatory factor in low-grade inflammation of adipose tissue. On the other hand, since the status of B-cells in human adipose tissue at the present time is not so clear as in animal models, BLyS could also play solely a role in adipocyte differentiation rather than playing a potent link with adaptive immunity.

In summary, the present study provides evidence, that BLyS is a novel factor in human adipose tissue biology. Thereby BLyS exerts several important differences compared to most other factors in that field: (1) BLyS is specifically related to grade 3 obesity but not to grade 1+2 obesity, (2) BLyS links the adaptive rather than innate immune system to metabolism, (3) BLyS is not involved in the pathogenesis of human insulin resistance and (4) the increase of BLyS after bariatric surgery might indicate beneficial immune-modulating activity rather than negative effects on adipose tissue biology. Therefore, BLyS will be an interesting research candidate for future studies in the growing field of metabolic inflammation.

Acknowledgments

We are particularly grateful to all of the participants in the conducted studies for their dedication and contribution to the research. We would further like to thank Mrs. Katrin Neumann for her technical assistance.

Author Contributions

Conceived and designed the experiments: JH C. Schafmayer JOS SS ML. Performed the experiments: NM DS SH KT M. Brosch WS MA CG RZ M. Blüher C. Saggau MS. Analyzed the data: NM DS SH JH SFW ML. Contributed reagents/materials/analysis tools: JH C. Schafmayer WS MA M. Blüher CG RZ. Wrote the paper: NM ML.

References

1. Adams KF, Schatzkin A, Harris TB, Kipnis V, Mouw T, et al. (2006) Overweight, obesity, and mortality in a large prospective cohort of persons 50 to 71 years old. N Engl J Med 355: 763–778.
2. James PT, Rigby N, Leach R (2004) The obesity epidemic, metabolic syndrome and future prevention strategies. Eur J Cardiovasc Prev Rehabil 11: 3–8.
3. Van Gaal LF, Mertens IL, De Block CE (2006) Mechanisms linking obesity with cardiovascular disease. Nature 444: 875–880.
4. Weinstein AR, Sesso HD, Lee IM, Cook NR, Manson JE, et al. (2004) Relationship of physical activity vs body mass index with type 2 diabetes in women. JAMA 292: 1188–1194.
5. Tilg H, Moschen AR (2008) Inflammatory mechanisms in the regulation of insulin resistance. Mol Med 14: 222–231.
6. Bilkovski R, Schulte DM, Oberhauser F, Mauer J, Hampel B, et al. (2011) Adipose tissue macrophages inhibit adipogenesis of mesenchymal precursor cells via wnt-5a in humans. Int J Obes (Lond) 35: 1450–1454.
7. Bilkovski R, Schulte DM, Oberhauser F, Gomolka M, Udelhoven M, et al. (2010) Role of WNT-5a in the determination of human mesenchymal stem cells into preadipocytes. J Biol Chem 285: 6170–6178.
8. Schultz O, Oberhauser F, Saech J, Rubbert-Roth A, Hahn M, et al. (2010) Effects of inhibition of interleukin-6 signalling on insulin sensitivity and lipoprotein (a) levels in human subjects with rheumatoid diseases. PLoS One 5: e14328.
9. Wang CP, Chung FM, Shin SJ, Lee YJ (2007) Congenital and environmental factors associated with adipocyte dysregulation as defects of insulin resistance. Rev Diabet Stud 4: 77–84.
10. Virtue S, Vidal-Puig A (2010) Adipose tissue expandability, lipotoxicity and the Metabolic Syndrome–an allostatic perspective. Biochim Biophys Acta 1801: 338–349.
11. Kim YH, Choi BH, Cheon HG, Do MS (2009) B cell activation factor (BAFF) is a novel adipokine that links obesity and inflammation. Exp Mol Med 41: 208–216.
12. Hamada M, Abe M, Miyake T, Kawasaki K, Tada F, et al. (2011) B cell-activating factor controls the production of adipokines and induces insulin resistance. Obesity (Silver Spring) 19: 1915–1922.
13. Pelekanou V, Kampa M, Kafousi M, Darivianaki K, Sanidas E, et al. (2008) Expression of TNF-superfamily members BAFF and APRIL in breast cancer: immunohistochemical study in 52 invasive ductal breast carcinomas. BMC Cancer 8: 76.
14. Moore PA, Belvedere O, Orr A, Pieri K, LaFleur DW, et al. (1999) BLyS: member of the tumor necrosis factor family and B lymphocyte stimulator. Science 285: 260–263.
15. Schneider P, MacKay F, Steiner V, Hofmann K, Bodmer JL, et al. (1999) BAFF, a novel ligand of the tumor necrosis factor family, stimulates B cell growth. J Exp Med 189: 1747–1756.
16. Schulte DM, Muller N, Neumann K, Oberhauser F, Faust M, et al. (2012) Pro-inflammatory wnt5a and anti-inflammatory sFRP5 are differentially regulated by nutritional factors in obese human subjects. PLoS One 7: e32437.
17. Mackay F, Silveira PA, Brink R (2007) B cells and the BAFF/APRIL axis: fast-forward on autoimmunity and signaling. Curr Opin Immunol 19: 327–336.
18. Finucane FM, Luan J, Wareham NJ, Sharp SJ, O'Rahilly S, et al. (2009) Correlation of the leptin:adiponectin ratio with measures of insulin resistance in non-diabetic individuals. Diabetologia 52: 2345–2349.
19. Reaven GM (2003) Importance of identifying the overweight patient who will benefit the most by losing weight. Ann Intern Med 138: 420–423.
20. Schaffler A, Muller-Ladner U, Scholmerich J, Buchler C (2006) Role of adipose tissue as an inflammatory organ in human diseases. Endocr Rev 27: 449–467.
21. Schaffler A, Scholmerich J, Salzberger B (2007) Adipose tissue as an immunological organ: Toll-like receptors, C1q/TNFs and CTRPs. Trends Immunol 28: 393–399.
22. Litinskiy MB, Nardelli B, Hilbert DM, He B, Schaffer A, et al. (2002) DCs induce CD40-independent immunoglobulin class switching through BLyS and APRIL. Nat Immunol 3: 822–829.
23. Nardelli B, Belvedere O, Roschke V, Moore PA, Olsen HS, et al. (2001) Synthesis and release of B-lymphocyte stimulator from myeloid cells. Blood 97: 198–204.
24. Fabbrini E, Cella M, McCartney SA, Fuchs A, Abumrad NA, et al. (2013) Association between specific adipose tissue CD4+ T-cell populations and insulin resistance in obese individuals. Gastroenterology 145: 366–374 e361–363.
25. Kopp HP, Kopp CW, Festa A, Krzyzanowska K, Kriwanek S, et al. (2003) Impact of weight loss on inflammatory proteins and their association with the insulin resistance syndrome in morbidly obese patients. Arterioscler Thromb Vasc Biol 23: 1042–1047.
26. Viana EC, Araujo-Dasilio KL, Miguel GP, Bressan J, Lemos EM, et al. (2013) Gastric bypass and sleeve gastrectomy: the same impact on IL-6 and TNF-alpha. Prospective clinical trial. Obes Surg 23: 1252–1261.

13

Mice Lacking Natural Killer T Cells are More Susceptible to Metabolic Alterations following High Fat Diet Feeding

Brittany V. Martin-Murphy[3]☯, Qiang You[1,2]☯, Hong Wang[4], Becky A. De La Houssaye[5], Timothy P. Reilly[6], Jacob E. Friedman[5], Cynthia Ju[2]*

1 Department of Biotherapy, Second Affiliated Hospital, Nanjing Medical University, Nanjing, Jiangsu, China, **2** Skaggs School of Pharmacy and Pharmaceutical Sciences, University of Colorado Anschutz Medical Campus, Aurora, Colorado, United States of America, **3** Barbara Davis Center for Diabetes, University of Colorado Anschutz Medical Campus, Aurora, Colorado, United States of America, **4** Division of Endocrinology, Diabetes & Metabolism, University of Colorado Anschutz Medical Campus, Aurora, Colorado, United States of America, **5** Department of Pediatrics, University of Colorado Anschutz Medical Campus, Aurora, Colorado, United States of America, **6** Drug Safety Evaluation, Research & Development, Bristol-Myers Squibb Company, Princeton, New Jersey, United States of America

Abstract

Current estimates suggest that over one-third of the adult population has metabolic syndrome and three-fourths of the obese population has non-alcoholic fatty liver disease (NAFLD). Inflammation in metabolic tissues has emerged as a universal feature of obesity and its co-morbidities, including NAFLD. Natural Killer T (NKT) cells are a subset of innate immune cells that abundantly reside within the liver and are readily activated by lipid antigens. There is general consensus that NKT cells are pivotal regulators of inflammation; however, disagreement exists as to whether NKT cells exert pathogenic or suppressive functions in obesity. Here we demonstrate that CD1d$^{-/-}$ mice, which lack NKT cells, were more susceptible to weight gain and fatty liver following high fat diet (HFD) feeding. Compared with their WT counterparts, CD1d$^{-/-}$ mice displayed increased adiposity and greater induction of inflammatory genes in the liver suggestive of the precursors of NAFLD. Calorimetry studies revealed a significant increase in food intake and trends toward decreased metabolic rate and activity in CD1d$^{-/-}$ mice compared with WT mice. Based on these findings, our results suggest that NKT cells play a regulatory role that helps to prevent diet-induced obesity and metabolic dysfunction and may play an important role in mechanisms governing cross-talk between metabolism and the immune system to regulate energy balance and liver health.

Editor: Jianping Ye, Pennington Biomedical Research Center, United States of America

Funding: This work was supported by National Institute of Health grants F31DK082269 (BVM), RO1ES012914 (CJ), R01-DK059767 (JEF) and P30DK048520 to the Colorado Nutrition and Obesity Research Center (NORC). The funders had no role in study design, data collection and analysis, decision to publish, or preparation of the manuscript.

Competing Interests: Timothy P. Reilly is employed by Bristol-Myers Squibb Company. However, there are no patents, products in development or marketed products to declare.

* E-mail: Cynthia.ju@ucdenver.edu

☯ These authors contributed equally to this work.

Introduction

Inflammatory processes in metabolically-active tissues have emerged as a universal feature of obesity and its co-morbidities, including non-alcoholic fatty liver disease (NAFLD). While initial work highlighted the contribution of macrophages to tissue inflammation and insulin resistance [1–4], recent studies demonstrate that adaptive and other innate immune cells also participate in obesity-induced pathogenesis of these conditions [5–7]. However, the molecular and cellular pathways by which the immune system contributes to the control of tissue and systemic metabolism remain poorly understood.

Natural killer T (NKT) cells constitute a unique subset of immune cells that are present in various peripheral organs, such as the liver where they represent 30–50% of total liver lymphocytes [8,9]. NKT cells express a semi-invariant T cell receptor that recognizes glycolipid antigens presented by the MHC class I-like molecule CD1d. Upon activation via the TCR, NKT cells exert their immunoregulatory functions via the production of both Th1 and Th2 cytokines, such as IL-4 and IFN-γ [10,11]. NKT cells have been reported to protect against or contribute to a variety of diseases [12,13]. Although a variety of NKT cell populations have been identified, including Type I, Type II, and NKT-like cells [10,11], Type I represents the vast majority of NKT cells and is the best characterized subset in mouse and human. Type I NKT cells express a TCR composed by rearrangement of the Vα14 gene segment (or Vα24 in human) to the Jα18 segment. The loss of either CD1d or Jα18 impairs NKT cell development in the thymus and yields an NKT cell deficient mouse. Jα18$^{-/-}$ mice are deficient only in Type I NKT cells. In contrast, CD1d$^{-/-}$ mice lack both Type I and Type II NKT cells, as CD1d is required for positive selection of both subsets in the thymus.

Murine models of obesity (*ob/ob* mice and high-fat diet [HFD] feeding) display decreased numbers of NKT cells [14–16] in the liver. Further, when NKT cells are adoptively transferred into *ob/ob* mice, liver steatosis is reduced and glucose sensitivity is markedly improved [14,15,17,18]. When NKT cells are stimulated by glucocerebroside, a decrease in fat accumulation in the liver has been observed [19,20]. Conversely, an increase of NKT cells have been reported in the liver of patients with advanced NAFLD [21]. Recently it was also shown that NKT cell activation in adipose tissue of HFD-fed mice causes impairment of metabolic functions through the release of proinflammatory cytokines and the recruitment of other pathogenic immune cells [22]. Thus, both suppressive and inflammatory functions have been ascribed to NKT cells in an obese state.

The present studies add to the developing knowledge of a role for NKT cells in obesity by showing that $CD1d^{-/-}$ mice, which lack both Type I and Type II NKT cells, are more susceptible to diet-induced obesity and metabolic perturbations. Because studies thus far used $CD1d^{-/-}$ mice on C57Bl/6 background, we chose to study $CD1d^{-/-}$ mice on a Balb/c background to address the impact of genetic background on the results. Notably, Balb/c mice are well known to be resistant to HFD-induced obesity [23], a finding we confirmed in WT mice. However, following high fat feeding in $CD1d^{-/-}$ mice, we observed increased weight gain and adipose-tissue expansion compared to WT mice. Furthermore, NKT cell-deficient mice developed fatty liver, elevated liver enzymes, insulin resistance, and glucose intolerance, associated with increased appetite and an increase in inflammatory mRNA gene expression pattern. These results suggest that NKT cells play an important role in regulating susceptibility to obesity, perhaps through modulating immune cell responses during diet induced obesity.

Materials and Methods

Ethics Statement

All animal procedures were approved by the Institutional Animal Care and Use Committee of the University of Colorado Anschutz Medical Campus.

Animal Care and Maintenance

Female Wild-type (WT) BALB/c and $CD1d^{-/-}$ mice on a BALB/c background (Jackson Laboratories, Bar Harbor, ME), were maintained on a constant 12 hr light: 12 hr dark cycle with free access to water and ad libitum access to standard chow diet or HFD (58 kcal% fat with sucrose Surwit Diet, D12331, Research Diets Inc. New Brunswick, NJ). Animals were maintained under pathogen-free conditions in the Center for Laboratory Animal Care at University of Colorado Anschutz Medical Campus.

Glucose and Insulin Tolerance Tests

All mice were fasted overnight prior to glucose tolerance test and 5 hr prior to insulin tolerance testing. Glucose and insulin tolerance tests were performed by bolus i.p. injection of glucose (1 g/kg) or insulin (0.35 U/kg), respectively. Blood glucose was measured from the tail using a glucometer (OneTouch Ultra Smart) at baseline (0) and 10, 20, 30, 45, 60, 90 and 120 min after injection.

Metabolic Parameters

Body composition was measured on anesthetized mice by dual-energy X-ray absorptiometry using a mouse densitometer (PIXImus2; Lunar, Madison, WI). Blood was collected by retro-orbital bleed. The degree of liver injury was determined by measurement of serum ALT levels using a colorimetric assay (Teco Diagnostics, Anaheim, CA). Serum triglycerides were determined using a triglyceride GPO reagent kit (TECO diagnostics, Anaheim, CA). Extraction of tissue triglycerides was performed using chloroform:methanol at a 2:1 ratio, as previously described [24]. For oil red O staining [25], frozen liver sections were obtained, placed in OTC and snap-frozen in liquid nitrogen for subsequent sectioning.

Indirect Calorimetry and Physical Activity Measurements

An open-ended indirect calorimetry system coupled with Columbus Instruments Opto M3 multichannel activity monitor was used to measured average daily food intake, oxygen consumption (O_2) and Carbon dioxide (CO_2) production in mice as previously described [26]. In brief, animals were placed in 4 individual metabolic chambers for measurements taken over three days with free access to food and water. Respiratory quotient (RQ) and metabolic rate were calculated and stored in a computer configured with data acquisition hardware (Analogic, Wakefield, MA) and software (Labtech, Wilmington, MA). Metabolic rate was normalized to lean body weight.

Quantitative Real Time-PCR

Total RNA was isolated from liver using RNeasy mini kit (Qiagen), as described by the manufacturer. RNA purity and integrity were verified by measuring the ratio of absorbance at 260 and 280 nm (A_{260}/A_{280}). RNA (1 μg) was reverse-transcribed to cDNA using SuperScript II Reverse Transcriptase (Invitrogen, Grand Island, NY). cDNA was used for quantitative real-time PCR in conjunction with the GoTaq Gene Expression System and gene specific primers. mRNA levels were quantified by using a Real-Time PCR 7500 SDS system and software (Applied Biosystems, Carlsbad, CA).

Liver Nonparenchymal Cell (NPC) Isolation and Flow Cytometric Analysis

Hepatic NPCs were isolated at indicated times during HFD feeding, using a previously established method [27] with slight modifications. In brief, mice were anesthetized and liver tissues were perfused *in situ* via the superior vena cava with a perfusion buffer [1X Hank's Balanced Salt Solution (HBSS) followed by *in vitro* digestion with digestion buffer [1X HBSS supplemented with 0.05% collagenase (Type IV, Sigma), 1.25 mM $CaCl_2$, 4 mM $MgSO_4$ and 10 mM HEPES]. Following *in vitro* digestion, the liver was disrupted in ACD solution [1X HBSS supplemented with 0.5% fetal bovine serum (FBS), 0.6% citrate-dextrose solution, 1X penicillin/streptomycin, and 10 mM HEPES] and the cells passed through a 100 μm cell strainer. The cells were centrifuged at 30× g for 3 min to pellet hepatocytes. Cells in the supernatant were then centrifuged at 320× g for 5 min, resuspended in complete RPMI media (RPMI supplemented with 10% FBS, 10 mM HEPES and 1X penicillin/streptomycin) and then fractionated using 30% (w/v) Nycodenz (Axis-Shield) at 1.155 g/mL to yield liver NPCs free of erythrocytes.

To prevent non-specific binding, liver NPCs were blocked with normal rat serum (Sigma) and anti-mouse FcãR II/III (clone 93, eBioscience). Liver NPCs were subsequently characterized by staining with the following antibodies from eBioscience: fluorescein isothiocyanate (FITC) conjugated anti-mouse CD3, phycoerythrin (PE) conjugated anti-mouse Foxp3, PE conjugated anti-mouse IL-17A, and from BioLegend: allophycocyanin (APC) conjugated anti-mouse F480, and PE-cyanine (Cy)7 conjugated anti-mouse CD11b. Seven-aminoactinomycin D (7-AAD) viability staining solution (eBioscience) was used to determine cellular viability. Cells were analyzed on a FACSCalibur cytometer (Becton Dickinson Immunocytometry System) using FlowJo 6.3.3 software (Tree Star, Inc.). For flow cytometric analysis, cells were initially gated on forward scatter (FSC) and side scatter (SSC) and then gated on live cells (7-AAD^{-}).

Immunoblot Analysis

Mice fed with HFD for 20 weeks were sacrificed, and perigonadal white adipose tissues were dissected and homogenized in lysis buffer containing protease inhibitors. Samples (30 μg) were resolved on 12% polyacrylamide gels and transferred to nitrocellulose membranes (Bio-Rad Laboratories Inc., Hercules, CA). Membranes were blocked with 5% fat-free milk and probed with antibodies against total AKT and phospho-AKT Ser 473 (1:1,000, Cell Signaling, Danvers, MA) overnight at 4°C. Membranes were then incubated with horseradish peroxidase-conjugated goat anti-rabbit IgG antibody (1:2,000; Jackson ImmunoResearch Laboratories, Inc. West Grove, PA) for 1 hour at room temperature. Membranes were prepared using Pierce ECL Pierce ECL Plus Western Blot Substrate (Thermo Fisher Scientific Inc. Rockford, IL) and exposed to X-ray film. The scanned bands' intensity was determined by Adobe Photoshop and the ratio of pAKT versus total AKT was calculated.

Statistics

Statistical analysis was performed using the student's t test and one and two-way ANOVA with Bonforroni post-test. Differences in values were considered significant at $P<0.05$.

Results

CD1d$^{-/-}$ Mice Are More Susceptible than WT Mice to HFD-Induced Weight Gain and Fat Accumulation in the Liver and Adipose

We found that even on regular chow diet, CD1d$^{-/-}$ mice (21.34±1.44 g, n = 23) were significantly heavier than WT mice (19.58±1.66, n = 22) at 8 weeks of age. To compare their responses to HFD, WT and CD1d$^{-/-}$ mice were fed a 58% Kcal HFD for 20 weeks, beginning at 8 weeks of age. Body weight of CD1d$^{-/-}$ mice was significantly greater than WT mice, starting at 12 weeks and remaining elevated until sacrifice at 20 weeks (Figure 1).

To determine the reasons for increased body weight, indirect calorimetry characterization of energy balance was carried out following HFD exposure. The CD1d$^{-/-}$ mice displayed a significantly greater average daily food intake (Figure 2A) and a trending decrease in the metabolic rate (Figure 2B) compared to WT. No significant difference was observed in the average respiratory quotient (RQ) between WT and CD1d$^{-/-}$ mice (Figure 2C). Furthermore, CD1d$^{-/-}$ mice displayed a trend for

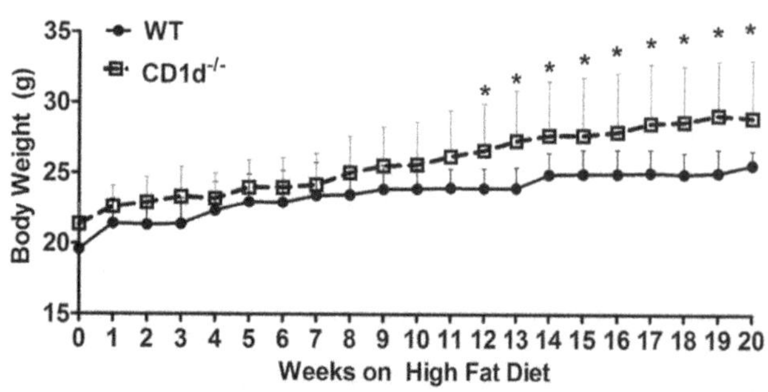

Figure 1. Greater daily food intake and weight gain are observed in CD1d$^{-/-}$ mice compared with WT mice. Balb/c WT and CD1d$^{-/-}$ mice were fed a HFD for the durations indicated and monitored for total body weight gain. * $p<0.05$ versus WT mice. Results from two independent experiments were combined. (n>15 mice per groups).

reduction in physical activity (Figure 2D and 2E). These data suggest that the protective role of NKT cells in obesity could be due to regulation of food intake during HFD-induced obesity.

HFD-fed CD1d$^{-/-}$ mice showed significantly greater serum triglyceride compared to WT mice (Figure 3A) beginning at 8 weeks of age. The amount of liver triglycerides was significantly higher in CD1d$^{-/-}$ mice than WT mice at 20 weeks (Figures 3B and 3C). This result is consistent with previous report of increased hepatic accumulation of triglyceride in NKT-deficient mice [16].

Balb/c mice are well known to be resistant to HFD-induced obesity [23]. Consistent with this, we observed a lack of significant increase in WAT volume in WT mice on HFD (Figure 4A). Remarkably, CD1d$^{-/-}$ mice on a HFD showed a significant increase in adipose tissue mass (Figure 4B, 4C). Dual x-ray lean absorptiometry (DEXA) revealed that CD1d$^{-/-}$ mice had a significantly greater total and percent fat compared to WT mice, while the lean body mass was similar (Figure 4D).

CD1d$^{-/-}$ Mice Are More Susceptible than WT Mice to HFD-Induced Metabolic Alterations

After 20 weeks of HFD feeding, CD1d$^{-/-}$ and WT mice were tested for insulin resistance and glucose tolerance. Fasting glucose levels were increased by 22% in CD1d$^{-/-}$ mice compared with WT mice (Fig. 5A). Insulin tolerance testing (ITT) revealed a significantly greater fasting glucose levels in CD1d$^{-/-}$ mice compared to WT mice (Figure 5C), a common phenotype seen in diabetic animals and patients with insulin resistance. It is noteworthy that serum glucose levels were higher in CD1d$^{-/-}$ mice than WT mice during the first 10 min after an i.p. injection of insulin and also showed a rebound effect at 120 min post-insulin injection. Upon GTT, the CD1d$^{-/-}$ mice displayed a slower rate of glucose clearance, suggesting the development of glucose intolerance (Figure 5B). We then examined insulin signaling and compared the extents of AKT activation in the adipose tissues of WT and CD1d$^{-/-}$ mice. The levels of pAKT and the ratio of pAKT/total AKT are significantly reduced in CD1d$^{-/-}$ mice (Figure 5D). The data suggest that insulin sensitivity is impaired in CD1d$^{-/-}$ mice. Together, these data suggest the possible involvement of both peripheral and hepatic insulin resistance.

Cellular Analysis of Liver and White Adipose Tissue (WAT) in WT and CD1d$^{-/-}$ Mice

Insulin resistance is believed to be initiated by a low grade systemic inflammatory process that occurs in obesity. It is well documented that the number of macrophages within the adipose tissue increases in obesity and that these cells participate in the inflammatory process and pathogenesis of metabolic disorders [1,3,7]. We observed trends of increase in the percentage of macrophages in the liver at 14 and 20 weeks of HFD feeding of CD1d$^{-/-}$ mice compared to WT mice (Figure 6A). However, the number of macrophages did not appear to change in the WAT of either WT or CD1d$^{-/-}$ mice (Figure 6B).

The pro-inflammatory nature of Th17 cells has been implicated in the pathogenesis of metabolic disorders [28–30]. While we did not observe any significant difference in Th17 cells in the liver between WT and CD1d$^{-/-}$ mice at 8, 14 or 20 wks following HFD (Figure 6C), HFD feeding appeared to cause an increase in the percentage of Th17 cells in both WT and CD1d$^{-/-}$ mice compared to the Th17 percentage in standard chow-fed mice (5%, data not shown).

HFD feeding caused a decrease of the percentage of regulatory T cells (Treg) in the liver of both WT and CD1d$^{-/-}$ mice (Treg was 20% in naïve liver). However, there was no significant

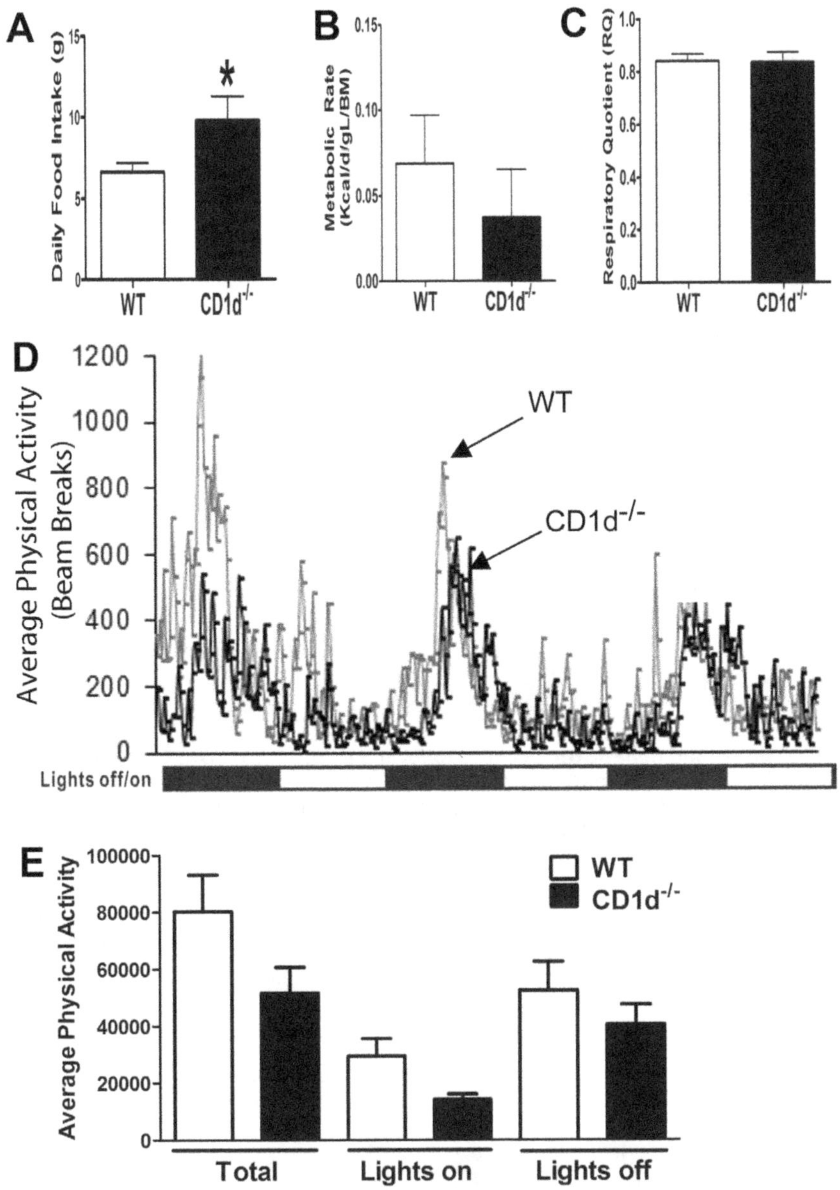

Figure 2. Energy balance is altered in CD1d$^{-/-}$ mice following HFD feeding. WT and CD1d$^{-/-}$ mice were fed HFD for 20 weeks. Average daily food intake (**A**), metabolic rate (**B**) and respiratory quotient (**C**) were measured in an indirect calorimeter. Physical activity was measured as the number of breaks in infrared beams through the 3-day calorimetry experiment (**D, E**). Results represent mean ± SEM of 6 mice per group.

difference in liver Treg between WT and CD1d$^{-/-}$ mice (Figure 6E). In contrast, the percentage of Treg in WAT was significantly lower in CD1d$^{-/-}$ mice than WT mice at 8 weeks following HFD (Figure 6F). This decrease in Treg is consistent with published reports of decreased number of Treg in obese animals and patients [6].

Comparison of Hepatic and WAT Gene Expression in WT and CD1d$^{-/-}$ Mice

To further explore whether an altered inflammatory profile was present in the liver and WAT of CD1d$^{-/-}$ mice following 20 weeks HFD feeding, we examined the gene expression of a variety of cytokines and chemokines. Consistent with our metabolic data showing insulin resistance, the levels of IL-6 in the liver and adipose tissue were higher in CD1d$^{-/-}$ mice than WT mice (Figures 7A, B). We further observed a significant increase in monocyte chemotactic protein (MCP)-1 and macrophage inflammatory protein (MIP)-1 in the liver of CD1d$^{-/-}$ mice (Figure 7A). This data correlates with the trending increase in macrophage infiltration observed in the liver of CD1d$^{-/-}$ mice following 14 and 20 weeks HFD. Markedly greater levels of the anti-inflammatory cytokine IL-10 were also observed in the liver of CD1d$^{-/-}$ mice, which may serve as an adaptive mechanism to suppress inflammation (Figure 7A) [31]. Interestingly, in contrast to the liver, with the exception of IL-6, all inflammatory mediators, such as IFN-γ, MCP-1 and MIP-1 were decreased in the WAT of CD1d$^{-/-}$ mice compared to WT (Figure 7B). This decrease in inflammatory cytokines and chemokines in the WAT of CD1d$^{-/-}$ mice may be an adaptive response. Liver steatosis is characterized by increased hepatic insulin resistance and a shift to increased lipogenesis. As such, we sought to examine the genes

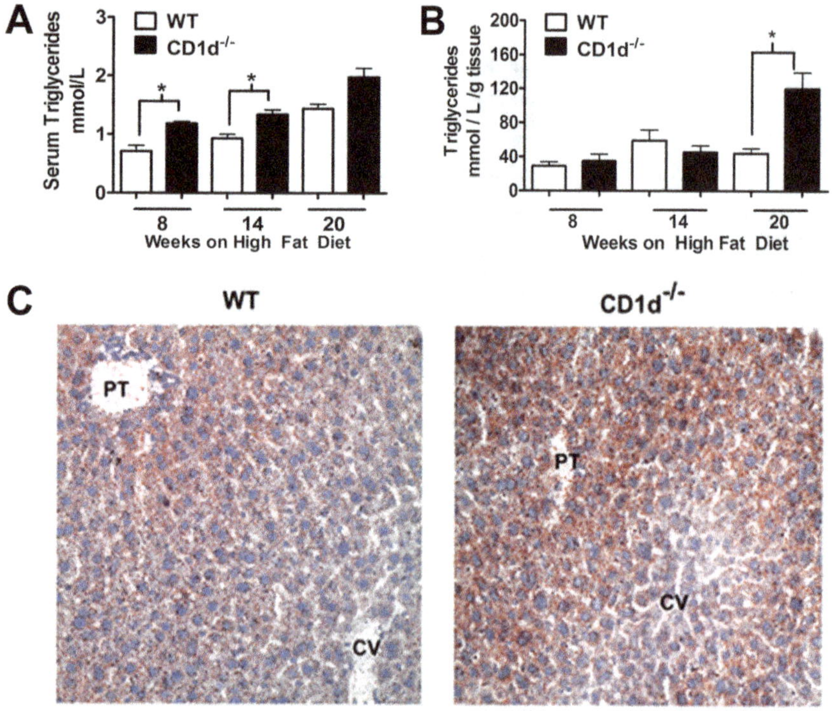

Figure 3. CD1d$^{-/-}$ mice display greater increases of serum and hepatic triglycerides following HFD. WT and CD1d$^{-/-}$ mice were fed a HFD for the durations indicated and monitored for serum (**A**) and liver (**B**) triglycerides. * $p<0.05$ versus WT mice. Results from two independent experiments were combined. (n>15 mice per group). Panel **C**, photomicrograph (400× final magnification) of Oil red O staining of liver sections from WT and CD1d$^{-/-}$ mice following 20 weeks HFD feeding. CV, central vein; PT, Portal Triad.

involving de-novo liver lipogenesis. We observed a significant increase in peroxisome proliferator-activated receptor gamma coactivator (PGC-1) in the liver of CD1d$^{-/-}$ mice compared to WT (Figure 7C). PGC-1 is a transcriptional co-activator important

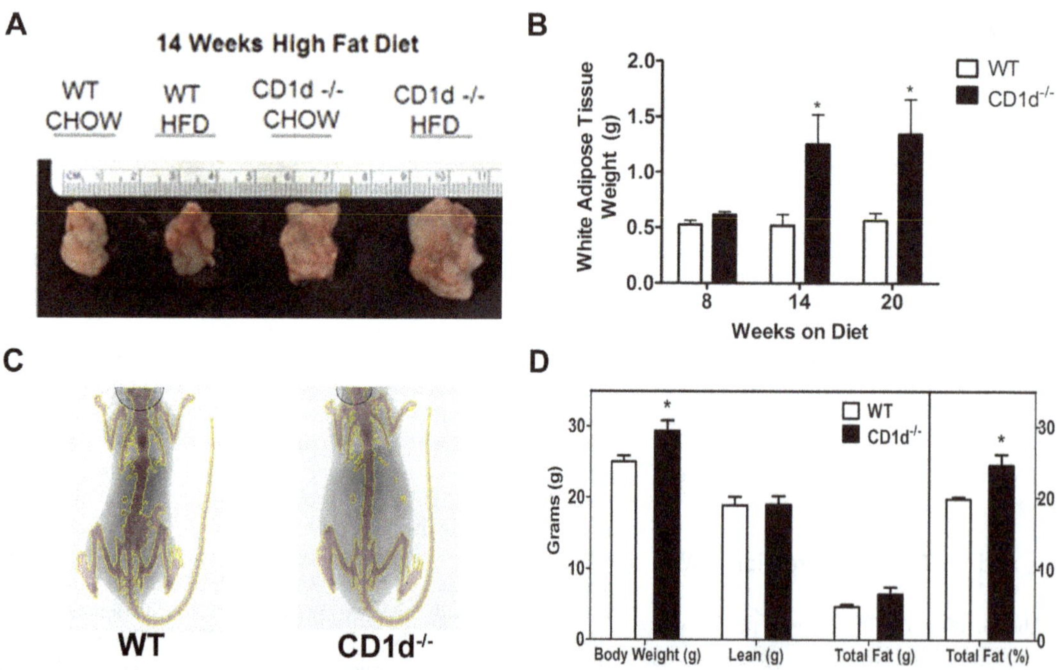

Figure 4. CD1d$^{-/-}$ mice display greater WAT and total percent fat compared to WT mice. WT and CD1d$^{-/-}$ mice were fed HFD for the durations indicated whereupon mice were sacrificed and WAT removed to measure size (**A**) and total tissue weight (**B**). Body composition and fat mass was measured by DEXA following 20 weeks on HFD (**C, D**). * $p<0.05$ versus WT mice. Results represent mean ± SEM of 6 mice per group.

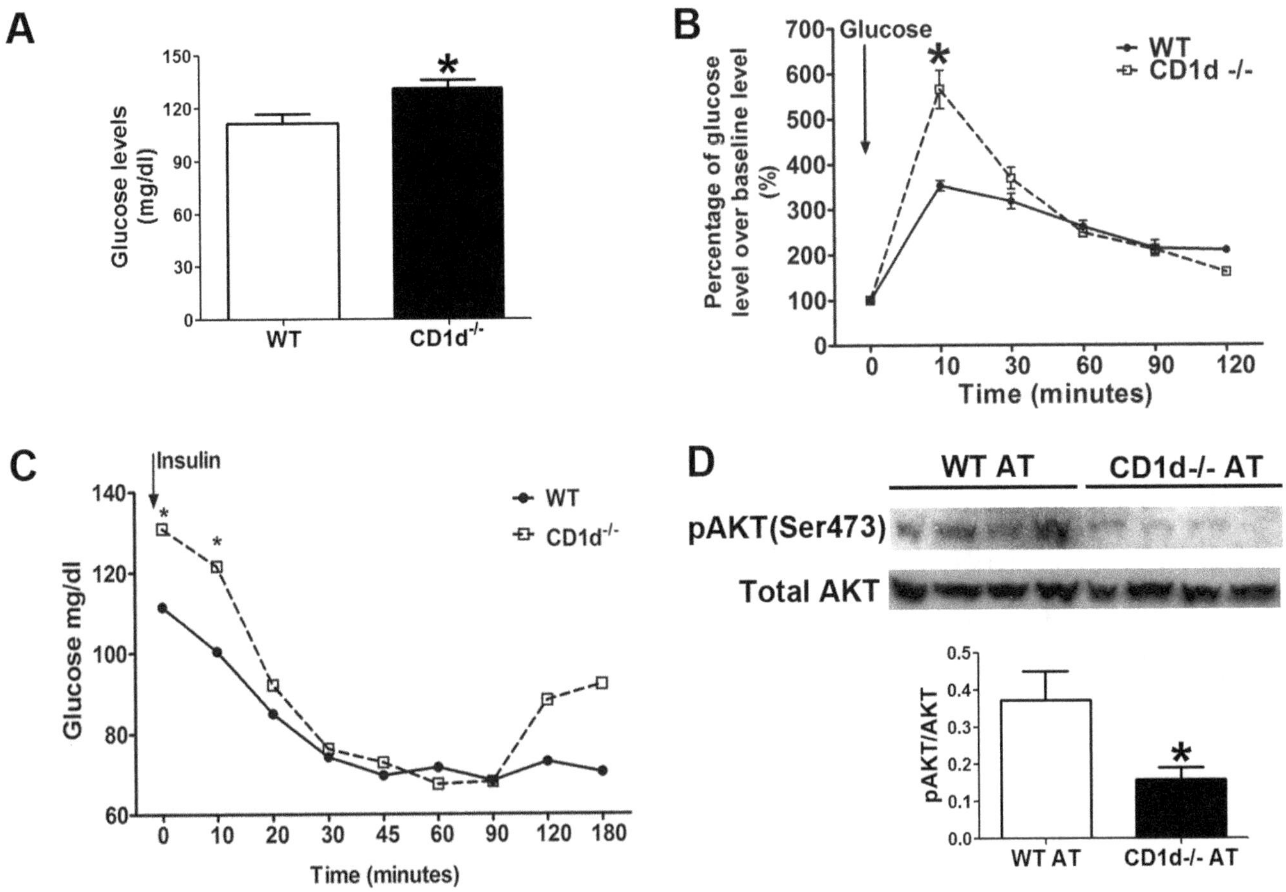

Figure 5. CD1d$^{-/-}$ mice show increased glucose intolerance and insulin resistance compared to WT mice. WT and CD1d$^{-/-}$ mice were fed a HFD for 20 weeks. Fasting glucose levels (A), GTT (**B**) and ITT (**C**) were compared. Results from two independent experiments were combined. (n≥7 mice per group). (**D**) pAKT and total AKT expression levels were determined in white adipose tissues of 4 mice per group by Western blot. The ratio of pAKT/AKT was calculated and compared between WT and CD1d$^{-/-}$ mice. * $p<0.05$ versus WT mice.

in the induction of peroxisome proliferator-activated receptor (PPAR)-α expression and increased mitochondrial β-oxidation, but may also play an important role in gluconeogenesis. We also observed a trend of increase in stearoyl-coenzyme A desaturase 1 (SCD-1) in the liver of CD1d$^{-/-}$ mice compared to WT. SCD-1 is the rate limiting enzyme involved in the conversion of saturated fatty acids to monounsaturated fatty acids (Figure 7C). The increases of PGC-1 and SCD-1 are consistent with an insulin resistant phenotype in the liver [32] and correlate with the more severe insulin resistance observed in CD1d$^{-/-}$ mice following HFD feeding. In contrast to the insulin resistance found in the liver of CD1d$^{-/-}$ mice, the WAT displayed an insulin sensitive phenotype with marked increase in PGC-1 and slight increase in PPAR-α (Figure 7D). Furthermore, a significant decrease in SCD-1 and sterol regulatory binding protein-1 (SREBP-1), a protein indirectly required for cholesterol and fatty acid biosynthesis, was observed in the WAT of CD1d$^{-/-}$ mice (Figure 7D).

Discussion

Our data indicate a regulatory role of NKT cells in preventing diet-induced obesity and its metabolic consequences. Even on an obesity resistant Balb/c background, CD1d$^{-/-}$ mice lacking both Type 1 and Type 2 NKT cells were susceptible to HFD-induced increases in food intake and body weight, WAT accumulation, glucose intolerance and insulin resistance. The animals also demonstrated decreasing trends in metabolic rate and activity. Such observations are suggestive of a role for NKT cells in modulation of appetite regulation and energy balance. The exact mechanisms whereby NKT cells regulate immune responses and energy homeostasis are unknown; however, mounting evidence suggests that HFD affects immune cells in multiple tissues, including the hypothalamus [33] and the microbiota in the gut, with consequences on energy balance [34]. Together with evidence that NKT cell-deficient mice show increased liver inflammatory genes and steatosis, we suggest that NKT cells play a potentially broad role in modulating HFD-induced metabolic disorders, particularly in the liver but perhaps in other tissues as well.

The role of NKT cells in metabolic disease has been examined through the utilization of either CD1d$^{-/-}$, which lack both Type I and Type II NKT cells, or Jα18$^{-/-}$ mice which lack only the Type I NKT cells. However, results from these studies are controversial. Some studies revealed no difference or only marginal differences in lipid accumulation, glucose tolerance and insulin resistance between NKT cell-deficient and WT mice following HFD feeding [16,35]. In contrast, other studies demonstrated increased liver triglyceride content, increased liver injury and inflammation following HFD feeding [18,36]. These discrepancies may be due to the influence of mouse genetic background and susceptibility to metabolic disease, types of diets,

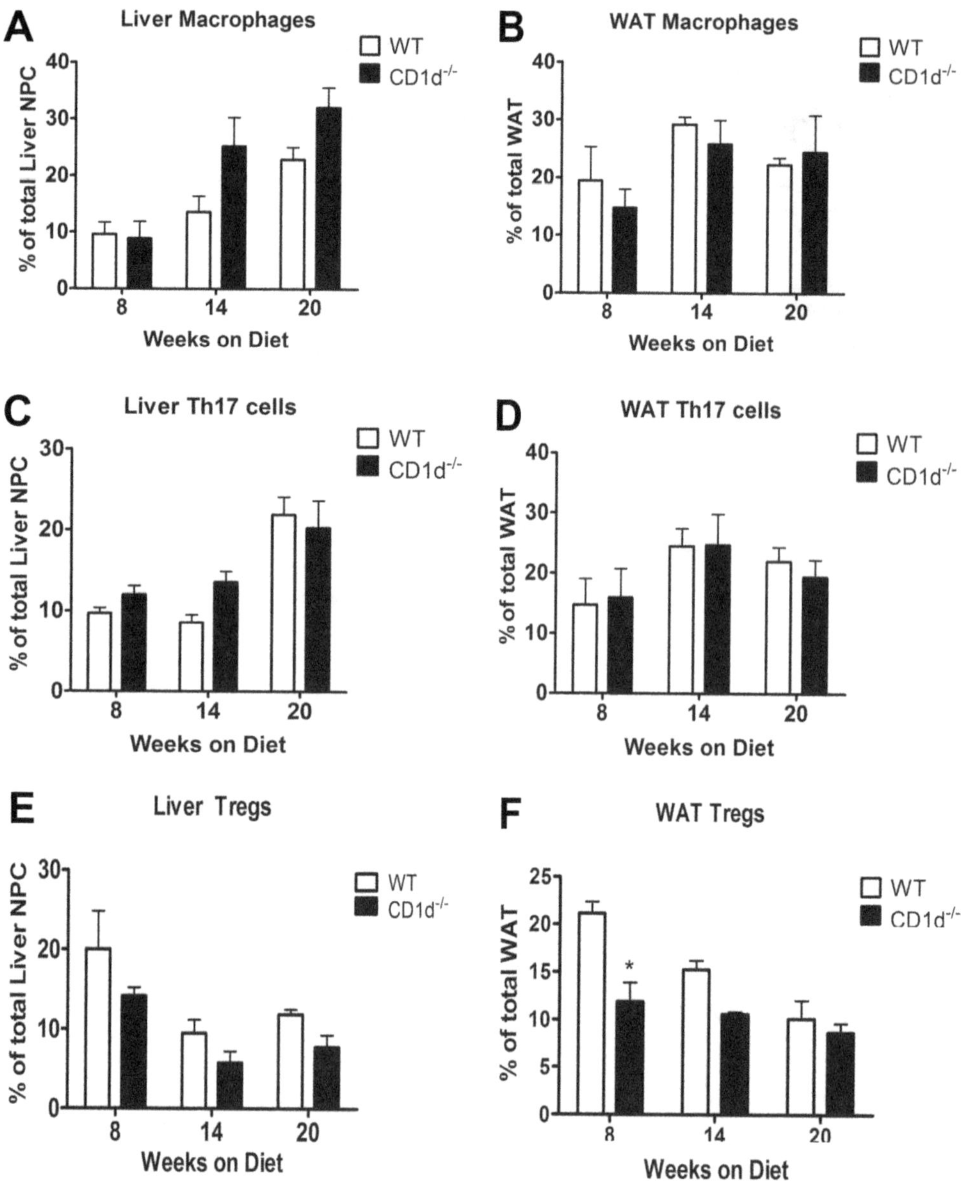

Figure 6. Cellular analysis of the liver and WAT in WT and CD1d$^{-/-}$ mice following HFD feeding. Cells were isolated from the liver and WAT of WT and CD1d$^{-/-}$ mice following 20 weeks HFD feeding. The cells were stained with anti-CD11b PE and anti-F480 antibodies to identify macrophages, anti-CD3 and anti-IL-17 to identify Th17 cells, and anti-CD3 and anti-Foxp3 to identify Treg. Quantification of liver and WAT macrophages (**A and B**), Th17 cells (**C and D**) and Treg (**E and F**) are shown. * $p<0.05$ versus WT mice. Results represent mean ± SEM of 3 mice per group.

and/or the fact that Type I and Type II NKT cells exhibit differing roles as well. A summary of the previous studies examining the role of NKT cells in diet-induced obesity can be found in Table 1 and 2. A few reports that have used both Ja18$^{-/-}$ and CD1d$^{-/-}$ mice on a C57Bl/6 background demonstrated no difference or only marginal differences in lipid accumulation, and mild to moderate changes in glucose tolerance and insulin resistance between NKT cell-deficient and WT mice following HFD [16,35]. Whereas these results suggested that NKT cells have a limited role or no effect in HFD-induced metabolic disorders [16,35], two other recent studies using the same mouse model demonstrated NKT cell-deficient mice to have reduced body weight, smaller adipocytes, milder hepatosteatosis, and improved glucose sensitivity and insulin tolerance compared to WT mice following HFD feeding [22,37]. These studies concluded that NKT cells play a pathogenic role in the development of diet-induced obesity, inflammation, and insulin resistance. In contrast, the most recent publications by [18] demonstrated that compared with WT mice, NKT cell deficient mice gained more body weight, accumulated more lipids in the liver and WAT, and exhibited worsened glucose intolerant and insulin resistant [18]. Consistent with the protective role of NKT cells in metabolic disorders, it has been reported that activation of these cells with α-galactosylceramide causes macrophage polarization to an M2 anti-inflammatory phenotype and improves glucose sensitivity [18,38]. Consistent with the protective function of NKT cells, another study by Miyagi et al. also showed increased liver triglyceride content, increased liver injury and inflammation in Jα18$^{-/-}$ mice compared to WT mice following high fat feeding

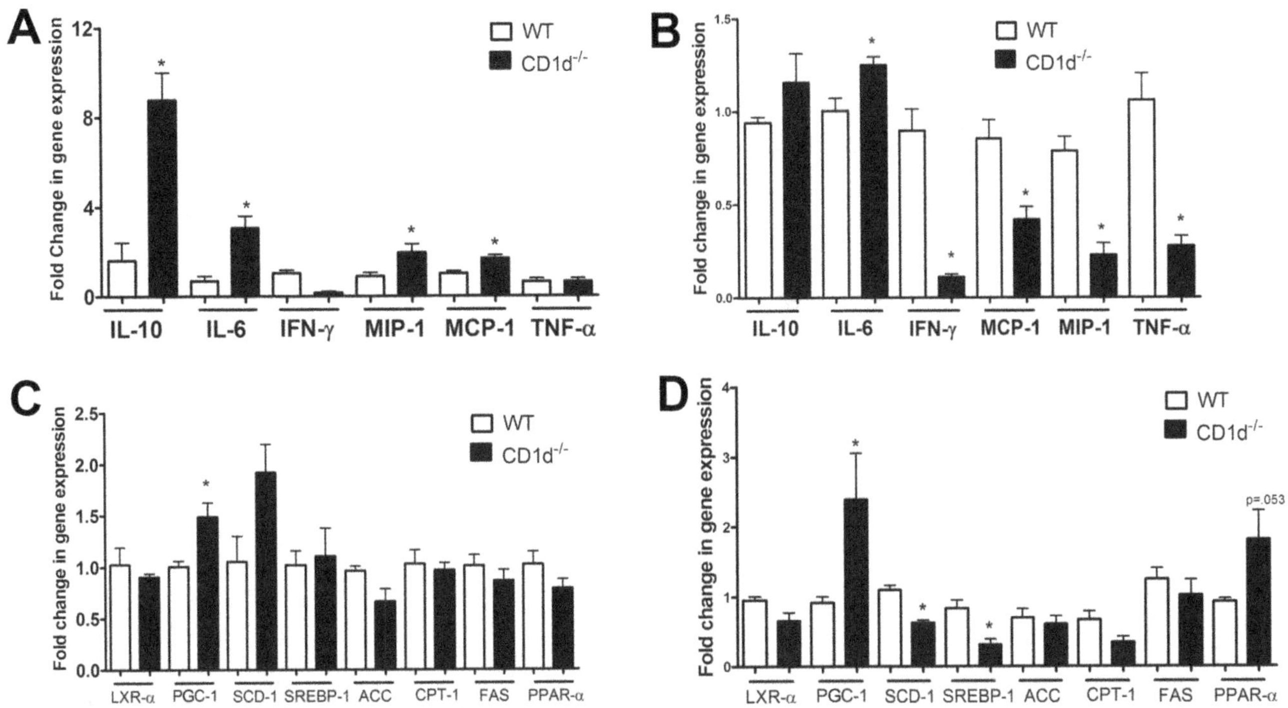

Figure 7. Comparing mRNA expression levels of inflammation- and metabolism-related genes in the liver and WAT of WT and CD1d$^{-/-}$ mice. mRNA levels of various cytokines and chemokines (**A and B**) and metabolic genes (**C and D**) in the liver (**A and C**) and WAT (**B and D**) were measured by qPCR. Fold changes compared with WT mice are shown. * $p<0.05$ versus WT mice. Results represent mean ± SEM of 4 mice per group.

[36]. In contrast to the majority of the published studies using CD1d$^{-/-}$ and Jα18$^{-/-}$ on a C57Bl/6 background, the study by Miyagi et al used Jα18$^{-/-}$ mice on Balb/c background.

It has been reported recently that macrophage numbers and M1 polarization in CD1d$^{-/-}$ mice are increased if compared with their WT counterparts under HFD conditions [39]. However, these changes were not observed in our study. This discrepancy may be due to two main differences between the two studies. First, the CD1d$^{-/-}$ mice used in our study are on Balb/cJ background but the CD1d$^{-/-}$ mice used in the JCI study are on C57B6 background. It has been shown that C57B6 mice are prone to develop obesity and insulin resistance than Balb/c mice [40]. Thus, it is possible that compared with CD1d$^{-/-}$ -Balb/c mice, the CD1d$^{-/-}$ -C57B6mice develop a more severe phenotype with not only worsened insulin resistance but also increased M1-mediated inflammation. Second, the HFD used in the two studies is different. We used Research Diet D12331, and the JCI study used D12451. It has been shown that another type of HFD, D12492, induces greater insulin resistance than D12331 in C57BL/6 mouse due to lard, sodium level and fiber differences [41]. Although D12451 and D12331 have not been compared side-by-side, lard is present in D12451, but not in D12331.

Balb/c and C57Bl/6 mice are two widely used strains throughout biomedical research. These two strains of mice have demonstrated different responses to drug-induced liver injury [42], induction of autoimmune diseases [43], and responses to HFD diet. For example, Balb/c mice have been shown to be resistant to adenovirus type 1 [44] and measles virus [45] whereas C57Bl/6 are more susceptible. Conversely, Balb/c mice are more susceptible to herpes simplex virus [46] and *Leishemonia* [47] and C57Bl/6 are resistant. The difference in susceptibilities to pathogens is hypothesized to be due to the different Th1/Th2 responses in these mice following infection. T cells from C57Bl/6 mice have been shown to preferentially produce Th1 cytokines, such as IFN-γ; whereas, T cells from Balb/c mice produce Th2 cytokines with the favored production of IL-4 [48,49]. Further, isolated splenic DX5^{+} NKT cells from Balb/c and C57Bl/6 mice displayed differential cytokine production following stimulation, with Balb/c producing more Th2 cytokines IL-10 and IL-13 than C57Bl/6J mice [50].

Previous research demonstrates that Balb/c mice express a population of thymic NKT cells that are greater in number and express higher levels of IL-4 compared to C57Bl/6 mice [51]. This may be particularly important in models of obesity, as IL-4 has been linked to protection from metabolic dysregulation. Previous studies have shown IL-4 activation of STAT6 in hepatocytes as important in regulating fatty acid oxidation through the suppression of PPAR-α [52]. Recent work has also shown that IL-4 increases thermogenic gene expression, fatty acid mobilization and energy expenditure, by means of stimulating alternatively activated macrophages [53]. Further, a recent study demonstrated that IL-4 produced by eosinophils, in the visceral adipose tissues is important in protecting mice from HFD-induced obesity, through the maintenance of alternatively activated macrophages [5]. Another report revealed that 4 days of HFD feeding of WT mice was enough to activate NKT cells to produce IL-4, which activated M2 macrophages; however, IL-4 expression was much lower in CD1d$^{-/-}$ mice [54]. These studies suggest that IL-4 produced by NKT cells is an important inhibitor of inflammation, glucose intolerance and insulin resistance. Given the protective role of IL-4 in metabolic regulation we speculate, that in the absence of NKT cells this protection is lost, thus lending NKT cell-deficient mice more susceptible to HFD-induced obesity and metabolic dysfunction. We hypothesize that because the difference

Table 1. Role of NKT cells in diet-induced obesity, summary of previously published work.

Paper	Mouse model	Mouse back-ground	Gender	Diet % Kcal Fat	Change in					
					Body Weight	Total % Fat	Activity	Food Intake	Liver lipids	(WAT) obesity
(Satoh et al., 2012) [37]	$CD1d^{-/-}$	C57	male	32%	$CD1d^{-/-}$ <WT	$CD1d^{-/-}$ <WT	N/A	No	$CD1d^{-/-}$ <WT	$CD1d^{-/-}$ <WT
	$J\alpha18^{-/-}$	C57	male	32%	No difference	No	N/A	No	No	No
(Wu et al., 2012) [22]	$CD1d^{-/-}$	C57	male & female	60%	$CD1d^{-/-}$ <WT	$J\alpha18^{-/-}$ <WT	No	No	$CD1d^{-/-}$ <WT	N/A
	$J\alpha18^{-/-}$	C57	male & female	60%	$J\alpha18^{-/-}$ <WT	$J\alpha18^{-/-}$ <WT	No	No	$J\alpha18^{-/-}$ <WT	$J\alpha18^{-/-}$ <WT
(Miyagi et al., 2010) [36]	$J\alpha18^{-/-}$	Balb/c	male	57%	No difference	N/A	N/A	N/A	$J\alpha18^{-/-}$ >WT	N/A
(Kotas et al., 2011) [16]	$CD1d^{-/-}$	C57	N/A	60%	No difference	No	No	No	$CD1d^{-/-}$ >WT	N/A
	$J\alpha18^{-/-}$	C57	N/A	60%	No difference	N/A	N/A	N/A	No	N/A
(Mantell et al., 2011) [35]	$CD1d^{-/-}$	C57	N/A	44%	No difference	No	No	N/A	No	N/A
(Lynch et al., 2012) [18]	$CD1d^{-/-}$	C57	male	60%	$CD1d^{-/-}$ >WT	$CD1d^{-/-}$ >WT	N/A	No	$CD1d^{-/-}$ >WT	$CD1d^{-/-}$ >WT
	$J\alpha18^{-/-}$	C57	male & female	60%	$J\alpha18^{-/-}$ >WT	$J\alpha18^{-/-}$ >WT	N/A	No	$J\alpha18^{-/-}$ >WT	$J\alpha18^{-/-}$ >WT

of IL-4 levels between WT and NKT cell deficient mice on Balb/c background is greater than the difference between WT and NKT cell deficient mice on C57Bl/6 background, we observed a more severe phenotype in $CD1d^{-/-}$-Balb/c mice following HFD feeding, compared with other studies of $CD1d^{-/-}$-B6 mice. Among published reports thus far, 2 studies [16] comparing WT mice with $CD1d^{-/-}$-B6 showed similar but milder phenotype in $CD1d^{-/-}$-B6 mice than what we observed. Kotas et al showed that $CD1d^{-/-}$-B6 mice to be more glucose intolerant but mildly insulin resistant compared to WT following HFD feeding; however, body weight gain, liver and WAT lipid accumulation were not different between $CD1d^{-/-}$-B6 and WT mice [16]. Lynch et al. showed higher weight gain, higher liver and WAT lipid accumulation, and more severe glucose intolerance in $CD1d^{-/-}$ -B6 than WT mice; however, there was no difference in insulin resistance between WT and $CD1d^{-/-}$-B6 mice [18].

Elevated inflammation has been hypothesized as an important link in the development of insulin resistance. Activated NKT cells are capable of activating other innate and adaptive immune cells and driving both anti-inflammatory and proinflammatory responses, as well as regulating the hepatic recruitment of other types of immunoregulatory cells. We observed trending increase in macrophage accumulation in the liver of $CD1d^{-/-}$ mice over time compared to WT (Figure 6A), and a greater loss of Treg cells in liver and adipose tissue (Figure 6E and 6F). These data suggest that the lack of NKT cells may contribute to activity of other immune cells that contribute to subsequent development of inflammation and fatty liver. We found an elevation of IL-6 mRNA in the liver and adipose tissue of $CD1d^{-/-}$ compared to WT mice (Figures 7A, B). This data is consistent with a diabetic phenotype, as elevated levels of IL-6 in the sera, liver, and WAT correlate with greater BMI, and insulin resistance [55,56]. Further, IL-6 has been shown to enhance circulating triglycerides and glucose levels [57,58]. Contrary to these reports, $IL\text{-}6^{-/-}$ mice develop a mature onset obesity that can in part be reversed by replacing IL-6 [59], suggesting an important therapeutic window for IL-6 levels that may be beneficial compared to levels linked with disease. We further observed a significant increase in MCP-1 and MIP-1 in the liver of $CD1d^{-/-}$ mice (Figure 7A). This data support a previous report by Miyagi et al. which also described elevated MIP-1 levels in the liver of $CD1d^{-/-}$ mice following HFD-feeding [36]. Surprisingly, qPCR analysis of the WAT revealed a significant decrease in IFN-γ, MCP-1 and MIP-1 in $CD1d^{-/-}$ mice compared to WT (Figure 7B), which may reveal an adaptive response of $CD1d^{-/-}$ mice. Overall, the majority of proinflammatory genes were not dramatically higher in the adipose tissues of $CD1d^{-/-}$ mice. This may suggest that inflammation is not the major cause, but rather a result or parallel change, of HFD-induced metabolic disorder in $CD1d^{-/-}$ mice in our model.

In addition, it has been reported that NKT cell deficiency in Nonobese Diabetic (NOD) mice contributes to the susceptibility of NOD mice to autoimmune type 1 diabetes [60] [61]. The absence of NKT cells confers worsened type 1 diabetes, whereas either an increase of NKT cell number or NKT cell activation mitigates the disease [62]. The possible impact of NKT cell deficiency on beta cell function in the model of HFD-induced insulin resistance warrants further investigation in future studies.

In summary, our studies demonstrated that depletion of both Type I and Type II NKT cells resulted in an obese phenotype with insulin resistance, glucose intolerance, body weight gain, and lipid accumulation in the liver and WAT following HFD feeding. Although there have been several studies investigating the role of NKT cells in diet-induced obesity, the findings have been controversial and conflicting. We observed a more dramatic phenotype in NKT cell-deficient mice on Balb/c background, and our findings support a protective role of these cells against development of insulin resistance and metabolic disorders. Although the majority of the published studies focus on the immune modulatory function of NKT cells as an explanation of

Table 2. Role of NKT cells in diet-induced obesity, summary of previously published work.

Paper	Mouse	Insulin Resistance	Glucose Intolerance	Cell infiltration		Cytokine and Chemokine		NKT role in obesity
				Liver	WAT	Liver	WAT	
(Satoh et al., 2012) [37]	CD1d$^{-/-}$	CD1d$^{-/-}$ <WT	CD1d$^{-/-}$ <WT	NKT in WT	NKT in WT	TNF-a and IL6 in WT	N/A	Pathogenic
	Ja18$^{-/-}$	No	No	No	No	No	N/A	No role
(Wu et al., 2012) [22]	CD1d$^{-/-}$	CD1d$^{-/-}$ <WT	N/A	N/A	N/A	N/A	N/A	Pathogenic
	Ja18$^{-/-}$	Ja18$^{-/-}$ <WT	N/A	N/A	Macro in WT	TNF-a, MCP-1, In WT	TNF-a, MCP-1, in WT	
(Miyagi et al., 2010) [36]	Ja18$^{-/-}$	N/A	N/A	CD4^{+} T CD8^{+} T In KO	N/A	TNF-a, IFN-g, IL-10, MIP-2, IP-10, In KO	N/A	Protective
(Kotas et al., 2011) [16]	CD1d$^{-/-}$	No	CD1d$^{-/-}$ >WT	N/A	N/A	N/A	N/A	Minimal protective
	Ja18$^{-/-}$	No	No	N/A	N/A	N/A	N/A	No Role
(Mantell et al., 2011) [35]	CD1d$^{-/-}$	No	No	No	No	No	No	No Role
(Lynch et al., 2012) [18]	CD1d$^{-/-}$	No	CD1d$^{-/-}$ >WT	N/A	Macro in CD1d$^{-/-}$	N/A	Increased CD11c, decreased CD206 in CD1d$^{-/-}$	Protective
	Ja18$^{-/-}$	Ja18$^{-/-}$ >WT	Ja18$^{-/-}$ >WT	N/A	Macro in Ja18$^{-/-}$	N/A	Increased CD11c, decreased CD206 in Ja18$^{-/-}$	Protective

their role either protect or exacerbate diet-induced obesity, our data revealed that CD1d$^{-/-}$ mice are significantly more susceptible to HFD feeding due to excessive energy intake and a trending reduction in physical activity. Further studies are warranted to elucidate the molecular mechanisms involving the role of NKT in the regulation of appetite suppression and overall protection from diet induced obesity.

Author Contributions

Conceived and designed the experiments: BVM QY CJ. Performed the experiments: BVM QY. Analyzed the data: BVM QY HW BD TPR JEF CJ. Contributed reagents/materials/analysis tools: HW BD JEF CJ. Wrote the paper: BVM QY CJ.

References

1. Lumeng CN, Bodzin JL, Saltiel AR (2007) Obesity induces a phenotypic switch in adipose tissue macrophage polarization. J Clin Invest 117: 175–184. PubMed: 17200717.
2. Sell H, Habich C, Eckel J (2012) Adaptive immunity in obesity and insulin resistance. Nat Rev Endocrinol. doi: 10.1038/nrendo.2012.114. PubMed: 22847239.
3. Weisberg SP, McCann D, Desai M, Rosenbaum M, Leibel RL, et al. (2003) Obesity is associated with macrophage accumulation in adipose tissue. J Clin Invest 112: 1796–1808. PubMed: 14679176.
4. Xu H, Barnes GT, Yang Q, Tan G, Yang D, et al. (2003) Chronic inflammation in fat plays a crucial role in the development of obesity-related insulin resistance. J Clin Invest 112: 1821–1830. PubMed: 14679177.
5. Wu D, Molofsky AB, Liang HE, Ricardo-Gonzalez RR, Jouihan HA, et al. (2011) Eosinophils sustain adipose alternatively activated macrophages associated with glucose homeostasis. Science 332: 243–247. doi: 10.1126/science.1201475. PubMed: 21436399.
6. Feuerer M, Herrero L, Cipolletta D, Naaz A, Wong J, et al. (2009) Lean, but not obese, fat is enriched for a unique population of regulatory T cells that affect metabolic parameters. Nat Med 15: 930–939. doi: 10.1038/nm.2002. PubMed: 19633656.
7. Lumeng CN, Liu J, Geletka L, Delaney C, Delproposto J, et al. (2011) Aging is associated with an increase in T cells and inflammatory macrophages in visceral adipose tissue. J Immunol 187: 6208–6216. doi: 10.4049/jimmunol.1102188. PubMed: 22075699.
8. Gao B, Radaeva S, Park O (2009) Liver natural killer and natural killer T cells: immunobiology and emerging roles in liver diseases. J Leukoc Biol 86: 513–528. doi: 10.1189/JLB.0309135. PubMed: 19542050.
9. Exley MA, Koziel MJ (2004) To be or not to be NKT: natural killer T cells in the liver. Hepatology 40: 1033–1040. PubMed: 15486982.
10. Godfrey DI, Hammond KJ, Poulton LD, Smyth MJ, Baxter AG (2000) NKT cells: facts, functions and fallacies. Immunol Today 21: 573–583. PubMed: 11094262.
11. Godfrey DI, MacDonald HR, Kronenberg M, Smyth MJ, Van Kaer L (2004) NKT cells: what's in a name? Nat Rev Immunol 4: 231–237. PubMed: 15039760.
12. Park O, Jeong WI, Wang L, Wang H, Lian ZX, et al. (2009) Diverse roles of invariant natural killer T cells in liver injury and fibrosis induced by carbon tetrachloride. Hepatology 49: 1683–1694. doi: 10.1002/hep.22813. PubMed: 19205035.
13. Durante-Mangoni E, Wang R, Shaulov A, He Q, Nasser I, et al. (2004) Hepatic CD1d expression in hepatitis C virus infection and recognition by resident proinflammatory CD1d-reactive T cells. J Immunol 173: 2159–2166. PubMed: 15265953.
14. Guebre-Xabier M, Yang S, Lin HZ, Schwenk R, Krzych U, et al. (2000) Altered hepatic lymphocyte subpopulations in obesity-related murine fatty livers: potential mechanism for sensitization to liver damage. Hepatology 31: 633–640. PubMed: 10706553.
15. Yang L, Jhaveri R, Huang J, Qi Y, Diehl AM (2007) Endoplasmic reticulum stress, hepatocyte CD1d and NKT cell abnormalities in murine fatty livers. Lab Invest 87: 927–937. PubMed: 17607300.
16. Kotas ME, Lee HY, Gillum MP, Annicelli C, Guigni BA, et al. (2011) Impact of CD1d deficiency on metabolism. PLoS One 6: e25478. doi: 10.1371/journal.pone.0025478. PubMed: 21980475.
17. Elinav E, Pappo O, Sklair-Levy M, Margalit M, Shibolet O, et al. (2006) Adoptive transfer of regulatory NKT lymphocytes ameliorates non-alcoholic steatohepatitis and glucose intolerance in ob/ob mice and is associated with intrahepatic CD8 trapping. J Pathol 209: 121–128. PubMed: 16482497.
18. Lynch L, Nowak M, Varghese B, Clark J, Hogan AE, et al. (2012) Adipose Tissue Invariant NKT Cells Protect against Diet-Induced Obesity and Metabolic Disorder through Regulatory Cytokine Production. Immunity 37: 574–587. doi: 10.1016/j.immuni.2012.06.016. PubMed: 22981538.

19. Margalit M, Shalev Z, Pappo O, Sklair-Levy M, Alper R, et al. (2006) Glucocerebroside ameliorates the metabolic syndrome in OB/OB mice. J Pharmacol Exp Ther 319: 105–110. PubMed: 16815870.
20. Li Z, Oben JA, Yang S, Lin H, Stafford EA, et al. (2004) Norepinephrine regulates hepatic innate immune system in leptin-deficient mice with nonalcoholic steatohepatitis. Hepatology 40: 434–441. PubMed: 15368448.
21. Tajiri K, Shimizu Y, Tsuneyama K, Sugiyama T (2009) Role of liver-infiltrating CD3+CD56+ natural killer T cells in the pathogenesis of nonalcoholic fatty liver disease. Eur J Gastroenterol Hepatol 21: 673–680. doi: 10.1097/MEG.0-b013e32831bc3d6. PubMed: 19318971.
22. Wu L, Parekh VV, Gabriel CL, Bracy DP, Marks-Shulman PA, et al. (2012) Activation of invariant natural killer T cells by lipid excess promotes tissue inflammation, insulin resistance, and hepatic steatosis in obese mice. Proc Natl Acad Sci U S A 109: E1143–E1152. doi: 10.1073/pnas.1200498109. PubMed: 22493234.
23. Fearnside JF, Dumas ME, Rothwell AR, Wilder SP, Cloarec O, et al. (2008) Phylometabonomic patterns of adaptation to high fat diet feeding in inbred mice. PLoS One 3: e1668. doi: 10.1371/journal.pone.0001668. PubMed: 18301746.
24. Folch J, Lees M, Sloane Stanley GH (1957) A simple method for the isolation and purification of total lipides from animal tissues. J Biol Chem 226: 497–509. PubMed: 13428781.
25. Koopman R, Schaart G, Hesselink MK (2001) Optimisation of oil red O staining permits combination with immunofluorescence and automated quantification of lipids. Histochem Cell Biol 116: 63–68. PubMed: 11479724.
26. Jensen DR, Gayles EC, Ammon S, Phillips R, Eckel RH (2001) A self-correcting indirect calorimeter system for the measurement of energy balance in small animals. J Appl Physiol 90: 912–918. PubMed: 11181600.
27. Holt MP, Cheng L, Ju C (2008) Identification and characterization of infiltrating macrophages in acetaminophen-induced liver injury. J Leukoc Biol 84: 1410–1421. doi: 10.1189/jlb.0308173. PubMed: 18713872.
28. Madhur MS, Funt SA, Li L, Vinh A, Chen W, et al. (2011) Role of interleukin 17 in inflammation, atherosclerosis, and vascular function in apolipoprotein e-deficient mice. Arterioscler Thromb Vasc Biol 31: 1565–1572. doi: 10.1161/ATVBAHA.111.227629. PubMed: 21474820.
29. Erbel C, Chen L, Bea F, Wangler S, Celik S, et al. (2009) Inhibition of IL-17A attenuates atherosclerotic lesion development in apoE-deficient mice. J Immunol 183: 8167–8175. doi: 10.4049/jimmunol.0901126. PubMed: 20007582.
30. Cheng X, Yu X, Ding YJ, Fu QQ, Xie JJ, et al. (2008) The Th17/Treg imbalance in patients with acute coronary syndrome. Clin Immunol 127: 89–97. doi: 10.1016/j.clim.2008.01.009. PubMed: 18294918.
31. Bourdi M, Eiras DP, Holt MP, Webster MR, Reilly TP, et al. (2007) Role of IL-6 in an IL-10 and IL-4 double knockout mouse model uniquely susceptible to acetaminophen-induced liver injury. Chem Res Toxicol 20: 208–216. PubMed: 17305405.
32. Koo SH, Satoh H, Herzig S, Lee CH, Hedrick S, et al. (2004) PGC-1 promotes insulin resistance in liver through PPAR-alpha-dependent induction of TRB-3. Nat Med 10: 530–534. PubMed: 15107844.
33. Cai D, Liu T (2011) Hypothalamic inflammation: a double-edged sword to nutritional diseases. Ann N Y Acad Sci 1243: E1–39. doi: 10.1111/j.1749-6632.2011.06388.x. PubMed: 22417140.
34. Umetsu DT (2012) Early exposure to germs and the Hygiene Hypothesis. Cell Res 22: 1210–1211. doi: 10.1038/cr.2012.65. PubMed: 22525335.
35. Mantell BS, Stefanovic-Racic M, Yang X, Dedousis N, Sipula IJ, et al. (2011) Mice lacking NKT cells but with a complete complement of CD8+ T-cells are not protected against the metabolic abnormalities of diet-induced obesity. PLoS One 6: e19831. doi: 10.1371/journal.pone.0019831. PubMed: 21674035.
36. Miyagi T, Takehara T, Uemura A, Nishio K, Shimizu S, et al. (2010) Absence of invariant natural killer T cells deteriorates liver inflammation and fibrosis in mice fed high-fat diet. J Gastroenterol 45: 1247–1254. doi: 10.1007/s00535-010-0272-y. PubMed: 20596733.
37. Satoh M, Andoh Y, Clingan CS, Ogura H, Fujii S, et al. (2012) Type II NKT cells stimulate diet-induced obesity by mediating adipose tissue inflammation, steatohepatitis and insulin resistance. PLoS One 7: e30568. doi: 10.1371/journal.pone.0030568. PubMed: 22383967.
38. Ji Y, Sun S, Xia S, Yang L, Li X, et al. (2012) Short Term High Fat Diet Challenge Promotes Alternative Macrophage Polarization in Adipose Tissue via Natural Killer T Cells and Interleukin-4. J Biol Chem 287: 24378–24386. doi: 10.1074/jbc.M112.371807. PubMed: 22645141.
39. Schipper HS, Rakhshandehroo M, van de Graaf SF, Venken K, Koppen A, et al. (2012) Natural killer T cells in adipose tissue prevent insulin resistance. J Clin Invest 122: 3343–3354. doi: 10.1172/JCI62739. PubMed: 22863618.
40. Alexander J, Chang GQ, Dourmashkin JT, Leibowitz SF (2006) Distinct phenotypes of obesity-prone AKR/J, DBA2J and C57BL/6J mice compared to control strains. Int J Obes (Lond) 30: 50–59. PubMed: 16231032.
41. Omar B, Pacini G, Ahren B (2012) Differential development of glucose intolerance and pancreatic islet adaptation in multiple diet induced obesity models. Nutrients 4: 1367–1381. doi: 10.3390/nu4101367. PubMed: 23201760.
42. You Q, Cheng L, Reilly TP, Wegmann D, Ju C (2006) Role of neutrophils in a mouse model of halothane-induced liver injury. Hepatology 44: 1421–1431. PubMed: 17133481.
43. Gaupp S, Pitt D, Kuziel WA, Cannella B, Raine CS (2003) Experimental autoimmune encephalomyelitis (EAE) in CCR2(-/-) mice: susceptibility in multiple strains. Am J Pathol 162: 139–150. PubMed: 12507897.
44. Guida JD, Fejer G, Pirofski LA, Brosnan CF, Horwitz MS (1995) Mouse adenovirus type 1 causes a fatal hemorrhagic encephalomyelitis in adult C57BL/6 but not BALB/c mice. J Virol 69: 7674–7681. PubMed: 7494276.
45. Niewiesk S, Brinckmann U, Bankamp B, Sirak S, Liebert UG, et al. (1993) Susceptibility to measles virus-induced encephalitis in mice correlates with impaired antigen presentation to cytotoxic T lymphocytes. J Virol 67: 75–81. PubMed: 8093223.
46. Brenner GJ, Cohen N, Moynihan JA (1994) Similar immune response to nonlethal infection with herpes simplex virus-1 in sensitive (BALB/c) and resistant (C57BL/6) strains of mice. Cell Immunol 157: 510–524. PubMed: 8069930.
47. Monroy-Ostria A, Fuentes-Fraga I, Garcia-Flores C, Favila-Castillo L (1994) Infection of BALB/c, C57B1/6 mice and F1 hybrid CB6F1 mice with strains of Leishmania mexicana isolated from Mexican patients with localized or diffuse cutaneous leishmaniasis. Arch Med Res 25: 401–406. PubMed: 7858398.
48. Scott P, Natovitz P, Coffman RL, Pearce E, Sher A (1988) Immunoregulation of cutaneous leishmaniasis. T cell lines that transfer protective immunity or exacerbation belong to different T helper subsets and respond to distinct parasite antigens. J Exp Med 168: 1675–1684. PubMed: 2903212.
49. Heinzel FP, Sadick MD, Holaday BJ, Coffman RL, Locksley RM (1989) Reciprocal expression of interferon gamma or interleukin 4 during the resolution or progression of murine leishmaniasis. Evidence for expansion of distinct helper T cell subsets. J Exp Med 169: 59–72. PubMed: 2521244.
50. Werner JM, Busl E, Farkas SA, Schlitt HJ, Geissler EK, et al. (2011) DX5+NKT cells display phenotypical and functional differences between spleen and liver as well as NK1.1-Balb/c and NK1.1+ C57Bl/6 mice. BMC Immunol 12: 26. doi: 10.1186/1471-2172-12-26. PubMed: 21529347.
51. Lai D, Zhu J, Wang T, Hu-Li J, Terabe M, et al. (2011) KLF13 sustains thymic memory-like CD8(+) T cells in BALB/c mice by regulating IL-4-generating invariant natural killer T cells. J Exp Med 208: 1093–1103. doi: 10.1084/jem.20101527. PubMed: 21482696.
52. Ricardo-Gonzalez RR, Red EA, Odegaard JI, Jouihan H, Morel CR, et al. (2010) IL-4/STAT6 immune axis regulates peripheral nutrient metabolism and insulin sensitivity. Proc Natl Acad Sci U S A 107: 22617–22622. doi: 10.1073/pnas.1009152108. PubMed: 21149710.
53. Nguyen KD, Qiu Y, Cui X, Goh YP, Mwangi J, et al. (2011) Alternatively activated macrophages produce catecholamines to sustain adaptive thermogenesis. Nature 480: 104–108. doi: 10.1038/nature10653. PubMed: 22101429.
54. Ji Y, Sun S, Xia S, Yang L, Li X, et al. (2012) Short Term High Fat Diet Challenge Promotes Alternative Macrophage Polarization in Adipose Tissue via Natural Killer T Cells and Interleukin-4. J Biol Chem 287: 24378–24386. doi: 10.1038/nature10653. PubMed: 22645141.
55. Maachi M, Pieroni L, Bruckert E, Jardel C, Fellahi S, et al. (2004) Systemic low-grade inflammation is related to both circulating and adipose tissue TNFalpha, leptin and IL-6 levels in obese women. Int J Obes Relat Metab Disord 28: 993–997. PubMed: 15211360.
56. Bastard JP, Jardel C, Bruckert E, Blondy P, Capeau J, et al. (2000) Elevated levels of interleukin 6 are reduced in serum and subcutaneous adipose tissue of obese women after weight loss. J Clin Endocrinol Metab 85: 3338–3342. PubMed: 10999830.
57. Nonogaki K, Fuller GM, Fuentes NL, Moser AH, Staprans I, et al. (1995) Interleukin-6 stimulates hepatic triglyceride secretion in rats. Endocrinology 136: 2143–2149. PubMed: 7720663.
58. Tsigos C, Papanicolaou DA, Kyrou I, Defensor R, Mitsiadis CS, et al. (1997) Dose-dependent effects of recombinant human interleukin-6 on glucose regulation. J Clin Endocrinol Metab 82: 4167–4170. PubMed: 9398733.
59. Wallenius V, Wallenius K, Ahren B, Rudling M, Carlsten H, et al. (2002) Interleukin-6-deficient mice develop mature-onset obesity. Nat Med 8: 75–79. PubMed: 11786910.
60. Hammond KJ, Poulton LD, Palmisano LJ, Silveira PA, Godfrey DI, et al. (1998) alpha/beta-T cell receptor (TCR)+CD4-CD8- (NKT) thymocytes prevent insulin-dependent diabetes mellitus in nonobese diabetic (NOD)/Lt mice by the influence of interleukin (IL)-4 and/or IL-10. J Exp Med 187: 1047–1056. PubMed: 9529321.
61. Poulton LD, Smyth MJ, Hawke CG, Silveira P, Shepherd D, et al. (2001) Cytometric and functional analyses of NK and NKT cell deficiencies in NOD mice. Int Immunol 13: 887–896. PubMed: 11431419.
62. Novak J, Griseri T, Beaudoin L, Lehuen A (2007) Regulation of type 1 diabetes by NKT cells. Int Rev Immunol 26: 49–72. PubMed: 17454264.

14

Intake of Farmed Atlantic Salmon Fed Soybean Oil Increases Insulin Resistance and Hepatic Lipid Accumulation in Mice

Lisa Kolden Midtbø[1,2,9], Mohammad Madani Ibrahim[2,3,9], Lene Secher Myrmel[1,2], Ulrike Liisberg Aune[1,2], Anita Røyneberg Alvheim[2], Nina S. Liland[2], Bente E. Torstensen[2], Grethe Rosenlund, Bjørn Liaset[2], Trond Brattelid[2], Karsten Kristiansen[1]*, Lise Madsen[1,2]*

1 Department of Biology, University of Copenhagen, Copenhagen, Denmark, **2** National Institute of Nutrition and Seafood Research, Bergen, Norway, **3** Institute of Biomedicine, University of Bergen, Bergen, NorwayStavanger, Norway

Abstract

Background: To ensure sustainable aquaculture, fish derived raw materials are replaced by vegetable ingredients. Fatty acid composition and contaminant status of farmed Atlantic salmon (*Salmo salar L.*) are affected by the use of plant ingredients and a spillover effect on consumers is thus expected. Here we aimed to compare the effects of intake of Atlantic salmon fed fish oil (FO) with intake of Atlantic salmon fed a high proportion of vegetable oils (VOs) on development of insulin resistance and obesity in mice.

Methodology/principal findings: Atlantic salmon were fed diets where FO was partly (80%) replaced with three different VOs; rapeseed oil (RO), olive oil (OO) or soy bean oil (SO). Fillets from Atlantic salmon were subsequently used to prepare Western diets (WD) for a mouse feeding trial. Partial replacement of FO with VOs reduced the levels of polychlorinated biphenyls (PCB) and dichloro-diphenyl-tricloroethanes (DDT) with more than 50% in salmon fillets, in WDs containing the fillets, and in white adipose tissue from mice consuming the WDs. Replacement with VOs, SO in particular, lowered the n−3 polyunsaturated fatty acid (PUFA) content and increased n−6 PUFA levels in the salmon fillets, in the prepared WDs, and in red blood cells collected from mice consuming the WDs. Replacing FO with VO did not influence obesity development in the mice, but replacement of FO with RO improved glucose tolerance. Compared with WD-FO fed mice, feeding mice WD-SO containing lower PCB and DDT levels but high levels of linoleic acid (LA), exaggerated insulin resistance and increased accumulation of fat in the liver.

Conclusion/Significance: Replacement of FO with VOs in aqua feed for farmed salmon had markedly different spillover effects on metabolism in mice. Our results suggest that the content of LA in VOs may be a matter of concern that warrants further investigation.

Editor: Frances M. Sladek, Univeristy of California Riverside, United States of America

Funding: This study was funded by the Research Council of Norway, project 199626. The funders had no role in study design, data collection, decision to publish or preparation of the manuscript.

Competing Interests: Grete Rosenlund is funded by Skretting Aquaculture Research Centre (ARC). Skretting ARC's role was to produce the salmon for the feeding trial with a fatty acid composition tailored according to the study design.

* E-mail: lise.madsen@nifes.no (LM); kk@bio.ku.dk (KK)

9 These authors contributed equally to this work.

Introduction

The ability of marine n−3 polyunsaturated fatty acids (PUFAs) to protect against the development of cardiovascular disease is well documented [1–3]. Thus, increasing the dietary intake of n−3 PUFAs is currently recommended by several health authorities. During the recent years, there has been increasing focus on the possible ability of n−3 PUFAs to protect against other life-style diseases such as obesity and type 2 diabetes. Although human studies are inconclusive [4], rodent feeding trials demonstrate that marine n−3 PUFAs are able to protect against development of obesity [5–10], and insulin resistance [9,11–15]. Fish and seafood, in particular fatty fish such as Atlantic salmon (*Salmo salar* L.), are rich in n−3 PUFAs. Thus, both health authorities and consumers have accepted farmed Atlantic salmon as part of a healthy diet. Farmed Atlantic salmon have traditionally been fed diets with high levels of fish meal and fish oil (FO), and a single meal of 200 g Atlantic salmon, providing 4 g of n−3 PUFAs, would be sufficient to cover more than the weekly recommended intake of n−3 PUFAs [16]. However, due to the pressure on wild fish stocks, and hence limited access and variable prices of fish meal and FO for the rapidly growing global aquaculture industry [17], efforts are channeled towards development of aqua feed that rely less on fish meal and FO [18,19].

Table 1. Composition of the experimental mice diets (g/kg).

	WD-FO	WD-RO	WD-OO	WD-SO	LF	WD
Components added (g/kg)						
Casein	97	97	97	97	197	197
Protein from salmon	100	100	100	100	-	-
Milk fat, anhydrous	138	131	129	135	-	200
Fat from salmon	62	69	71	65	-	-
Corn oil	10	10	10	10	70	10
Corn Starch	38	46	41	41	-	50
Maltodextrin	100	100	100	100	539	100
Sucrose	340	340	340	340	90	340
Analyzed						
Fat (g/kg)	203	203	195	200	47	194
Crude protein (N*6.25) (g/kg)	171.2	162.9	163.6	163.6	173.1	156.2
Energy kJ/g	21.2	21.1	21.0	21.1	17.1	20.7

All diets were supplemented with 40 mg/kg ethoxyquin, 2g/kg Choline bitartrate, 4g/kg calcium carbonate, 10g/kg Vitamin mix V1001, 35g/kg Mineral mix, 3g/kg L-Methionine and 50g/kg cellulose. Cholesterol levels in WDs were balanced to a final concentration of 1.5 g/kg.
Analyzed values represent the mean of duplicate measurements.

Vegetable oils (VOs) are presently recognized as suitable alternatives in aqua feed [20], and consequently, the nutrient composition in the Atlantic salmon fillets will change [16]. Although the Atlantic salmon have the ability to elongate and desaturate fatty acids [21,22], Atlantic salmon fed vegetable feed have lower content of marine n−3 PUFAs [16,22] and a direct relationship has been reported between marine n−3 PUFA content in aqua feed, Atlantic salmon fillets and plasma in patients with coronary heart disease (CHD) consuming the fillets [23]. Documentation related to the health beneficial effects of fish has almost exclusively been based on trials using FO, and therefore focused on the content of marine n−3 PUFAs in seafood. Thus, an important question is whether the health beneficial effects are preserved when the Atlantic salmon are fed VOs at the expense of FO. A recent study by Alvheim et al. has demonstrated that an increased content of linoleic acid (LA) from soybean oil (SO) in salmon feed increased the endocannabinoid tone, both in the Atlantic salmon and in the mice fed diets containing the salmon fillets [24]. The increased endocannabinoid tone in the mice was accompanied by increased weight gain.

Persistent organic pollutants (POPs) accumulate in lipid-rich food, and thus, Atlantic salmon represent a source of POPs in addition to marine n−3 PUFAs. The levels of POPs in wild fish are determined by factors including fat content, prey and geographic location (Seafood data, www.nifes.no), whereas contamination in farmed fish mainly depends on the composition of the fish feed [25]. Thus, replacing marine ingredients in aqua feed with vegetable sources will change the composition of nutrients and the type and levels of POPs in the fish fillets [25,26]. For instance, Atlantic salmon fed higher amounts of vegetable ingredients have lower fillet levels of dioxins and polychloridinated biphenyl (PCB) congeners compared to salmon fed FO [25]. This may be of importance for the consumers as POP exposure has been associated with development of type 2 diabetes in humans [27–31]. We have recently demonstrated that intake of purified salmon oil attenuated development of insulin resistance and obesity in Wistar rats, whereas intake of crude salmon oil containing POPs exaggerated obesity development [32]. Moreover, we have recently shown that chronic consumption of Atlantic salmon with a high level of POPs caused insulin resistance and obesity in mice [33]. When the levels of POPs in the salmon were reduced, development of insulin resistance and obesity in the mice decreased concomitantly [33].

Since both the nutrient and contaminant status of Atlantic salmon are affected by the use of plant-based feed ingredients, a spillover effect on consumer health might be expected. In the present study we compared the development of insulin resistance and obesity in mice fed a western type diet containing either Atlantic salmon fed FO or Atlantic salmon where the FO in the feed was replaced by a high proportion of VOs. Our results indicate that the altered fatty acid composition, the increased content of linoleic acid (LA) in particular, rather than the altered content of POPs, in fillets from Atlantic salmon, influenced development of insulin resistance and hepatic accumulation of lipids in mice.

Materials and Methods

Ethical Statement

Animal handling and experiments were performed in accordance with the guidelines of the Norwegian State Board of Biological Experiments with Living Animals (Norwegian approval identification nr, FOTS Id: 3196). No adverse events were observed.

Production of Atlantic Salmon

The salmon feeding trial was carried out at Skretting ARC, Fish Trials Station, Stavanger, Norway. A total of 600 Atlantic salmon (*Salmo salar L.*), mean weight 815±28 g, were randomly distributed in 12 tanks. The salmon were divided into four experimental groups and fed different experimental diets for 28 weeks as described earlier [22]. The fat source in the control diet was 100% FO, whereas 80% of the FO was replaced by rapeseed oil (RO), olive oil (OO), or soy bean oil (SO), in the experimental diets. These oils were chosen based on their different n−6 PUFA

Table 2. Fatty acid composition of the experimental mice diets.

	WD-FO	WD-RO	WD-OO	WD-SO	LF	WD
Sum SFA (mg/g)	93.2	78.8	84.2	85.2	7.1	103.5
Sum MUFA (mg/g)	58.2	67.1	73.4	55.4	7.6	50.8
LA, 18:2*n*−6 (mg/g)	9.6	15.6	15.3	25.8	8.0	8.1
AA, 20:4*n*−6 (mg/g)	<0.1	0.3	0.3	<0.1	<0.1	<0.1
Sum *n*−6 (mg/g)	10.5	17.3	17.0	28.5	8.1	8.3
ALA, 18:3*n*−3 (mg/g)	1.8	3.9	2.7	2.7	1.0	1.0
EPA, 20:5*n*−3 (mg/g)	4.1	1.3	1.2	1.2	<0.1	0.1
DHA, 22:6*n*−3 (mg/g)	6.2	2.6	2.5	2.3	<0.1	<0.1
Sum *n*−3 (mg/g)	18.4	10.9	9.2	9.2	1.1	2.5
n−3/n−6 ratio	1.75	0.63	0.54	0.32	0.13	0.29

Data represent mean of duplicate measurements. Sum n−3 and sum n−6 include additional fatty acids not indicated in the table.
Abbreviations: ALA, α-linolenic acid; AA, arachidonic acid; DHA, docosahexaenoic acid; EPA, eicosapentaenoic acid; LA, linoleic acid, MUFA, monounsaturated fatty acids; SFA, saturated fatty acids.

content [22]. In all diets 70% of fish meal was replaced with plant proteins. The complete dietary compositions and analyses of the diets and fillets have been reported earlier [22]. Upon sampling, salmon fillets were freeze dried, homogenized and analyzed for fat and protein content.

Mouse Diets

All diets formulations were based on the standard Western diet (WD), D12079B Research Diets, Inc. NJ, USA prepared by Ssniff Spezialdiäten (Soest, Germany). We replaced 50% of the protein source in the standard Western diet with proteins from salmon fed FO, RO, OO or SO. Since the fat content differed in salmon fed the different diets, milk fat was used to achieve isocaloric diets. The major fatty acid source in the milk fat used was 16:0, 18:1, 14:0 and 18:0, representing, 29, 26, 10 and 11%, respectively. Composition of the mice diets are shown in Table 1. As references, two groups of mice were fed either a casein based standard WD (Ssniff S8672), or a regular low fat diet (LF), D12450B (Ssniff EF R/M Control, Germany). Complete fatty acid composition of the WD and LF diet is available at http://www.ssniff.com/documents/10_catalogue_ef_engl_1.pdf.

Animals

48 male C57BL/6J BomTac mice were obtained from Taconic (Ejby, Denmark) at 8 weeks of age. The mice were maintained in a controlled environment with an artificial 12-h-light/dark cycle at thermoneutrality (30°C). Before the start of the feeding experiment animals were allowed to acclimatize to a regular LF diet for 5 d. After acclimatization, the mice were housed individually and randomly assigned to the experimental diets.

The animals were fed the experimental diets described in Table 1 for 10 weeks *ad libitum*. Throughout the experiment, all mice were weighed once a week and feed intake was assessed every Monday, Wednesday and Friday.

Insulin and Glucose Tolerance Tests (ITT and GTT)

ITT and GTT were performed on conscious mice after 7 and 8 weeks of feeding, respectively. ITT was performed in fed state by intraperitoneal (i.p.) injection of insulin (Actrapid, Novo Nordisk, Bagsværd, Denmark, 0,75 U/kg body weight). GTT was performed in 6 h fasted mice by i.p injection of glucose (2.0 mg/g body weight). Blood was collected from the lateral tail vein and glucose levels were measured at different time-points using a glucometer (Ascensia Contour, Bayer Healthcare, Oslo, Norway). For the GTT, incremental area under the curve (AUC) was calculated as blood glucose concentrations above baseline levels.

Plasma and Tissue Sampling

At the end of the feeding period, overnight fasted mice were sacrificed by cardiac puncture under Isoflurane anesthesia (Isoba-vet, Schering-Plough, Denmark). Liver, muscles, and adipose tissue depots were quickly dissected out, weighed, snap-frozen in liquid nitrogen and stored at −80°C for further analyses. Blood was collected in tubes containing 10 µl heparin (10 mg/ml, Sigma-Aldrich, United Kingdom), and plasma was prepared by centrifugation. Red blood cells (RBCs) and plasma were stored in aliquots at −80°C for further use.

Plasma Analyses

A commercial ELISA kit was used in accordance with the manufacturer's instruction for determination of plasma insulin (Mouse Insulin ultrasensitive ELISA, DRG, Marburg, Germany). Plasma glucose was determined using an automated analyzer (Maxmat PLII, Multi-purpose diagnostic analyzer system, Montpellier, France).

Lipid Analyses

Total fat content in the diets was measured gravimetrically after acidic hydrolysis and petroleum ether extraction. Tissue lipids were extracted from liver and muscle samples with chloroform: methanol, 2:1 (v/v). Lipid classes were analyzed using an automated High Performance Thin Layer Chromatography (HPTLC) system (Camaq, Switzerland) and separated on HPTLC plates coated with silica gel 60 F [34]. Fatty acid composition of total lipids in red blood cells was analyzed on a capillary gas chromatograph with flame ionization detector (Perkin Elmer, USA) [35].

Energy in Feces and Diets

Energy content was determined in a bomb calorimeter following the manufacturer's instruction (Parr Instruments, Moline, IL, USA).

Contaminant Analyses

The levels of 7 polychlorinated biphenyls (7 PCBs) and dichloro-diphenyl-tricloroethanes (DDTs) in salmon fillets, mouse feed, liver and adipose tissue from mice were analyzed as described earlier [33]. The 7 PCBs comprise PCB 28, 52, 101, 118, 138, 153 and 180). DDTs comprise op′-DDT, pp′-DDT, op′-DDD, pp′-DDD, op′-DDE and pp′-DDE.

Statistics

All data are presented as mean ± SEM. Statistical significance was analyzed by using one-way ANOVA, with Dunnett's Multiple Comparisons test as post hoc test. All groups were compared against the group receiving WD containing salmon fed FO. To compare plasma glucose concentrations during the GTT and ITT over time and between dietary treatments, a 2-way repeated-measures ANOVA was applied. Statistical analysis was performed using Graph Pad Prism version 5.04 (GraphPad Software Inc, La Jolla, CA, USA). *, ** and ***represents significant different from WD containing salmon fed FO at $P<0.05$, $P<0.01$ and $P<0.001$ levels, respectively.

Results

Replacing Fish Oil with Vegetable Oils in Fish Feed Reduces the n−3/n−6 Ratio in Atlantic Salmon Fillets and in the Red Blood Cells from Mice Consuming the Salmon Fillets

It is well known that replacing FO with VO in fish feed changes the composition of both nutrients and POPs in Atlantic salmon fillets [22,25], but the spillover effects of such changes for the consumers are not thoroughly examined. To investigate this, Atlantic salmon were fed diets in which 70% of marine proteins were exchanged with vegetable proteins and 80% of the FO were exchanged with VO. The VOs used were rape seed oil (RO), olive oil (OO) and soybean oil (SO), chosen based on their different content of n−6 PUFAs [22]. Compositions of the salmon diets are listed in Liland et al. 2012 [22]. To investigate the potential spillover implications of such changes in the aqua feed for consumers, we prepared standard WDs containing these salmon filets, replacing 50% of the protein source (casein) with protein from salmon (Table 1). The fat content was slightly different in

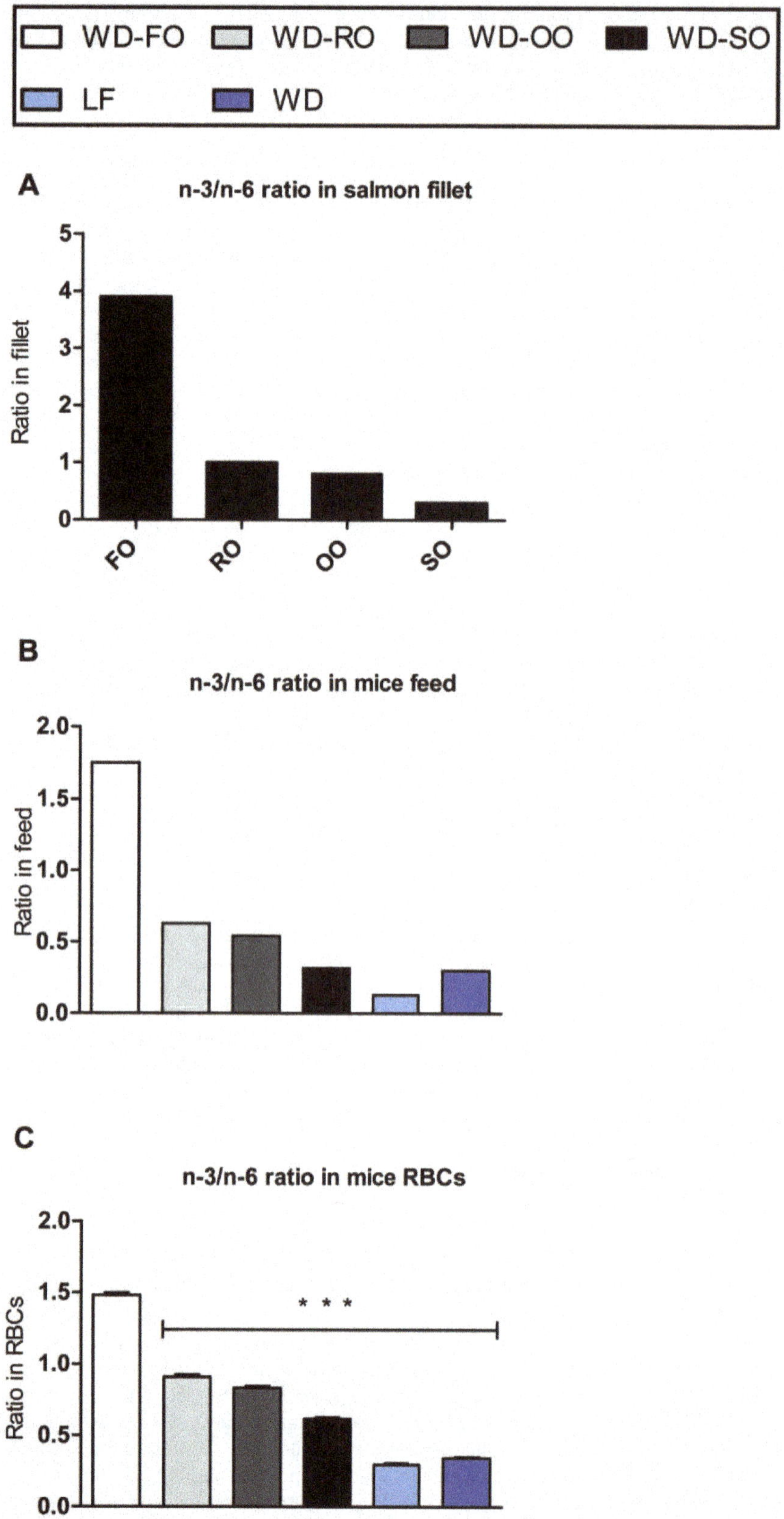

Figure 1. Composition of salmon aqua feed changes n−3/n−6 PUFA ratio in mice consuming the salmon fillets. Fish oil (FO) in aqua feed was partly replaced with rapeseed oil (RO), olive oil (OO) or soy bean oil (SO) and fed Atlantic salmon. The salmon fillets were used in Western diets (WDs) fed male C57BL/6J mice (n = 8/diet) for 10 weeks. Fatty acid composition was measured and the n−3/n−6 PUFA ratio calculated in (A) Atlantic salmon fillets (B) the WDs containing the fillets and (C) red blood cells (RBC) collected from mice consuming the WDs and reference diets. Data represent mean of duplicate measurements in A and B and mean+SEM (n = 5) in C. Asterisk(s) indicates significant different from FO-WD.

Table 3. Fatty acid composition in RBCs from mice after consuming the experimental diets for 10 weeks.

	WD-FO	WD-RO	WD-OO	WD-SO	LF	WD
Sum FA (mg/g)	3.1±0.2	3.1±0.2	3.2±0.1	3.2±0.2	3.1±0.1	3.1±0.1
Sum SFA (mg/g)	1.26±0.06	1.14±0.01*	1.18±0.02	1.19±0.01	1.18±0.01	1.13±0.02*
Sum MUFA (mg/g)	0.58±0.03	0.59±0.01	0.66±0.01*	0.51±0.02	0.61±0.02	0.70±0.02***
LA, 18:2n−6 (mg/g)	0.23±0.02	0.32±0.01***	0.32±0.02**	0.37±0.01***	0.29±0.02*	0.26±0.01
AA, 20:4n−6 (mg/g)	0.22±0.01	0.25±0.01	0.27±0.01**	0.32±0.01***	0.56±0.02***	0.51±0.01***
Sum n−6 (mg/g)	0.49±0.03	0.65±0.02***	0.69±0.01***	0.82±0.02***	0.97±0.01***	0.91±0.02***
EPA, 20:5n−3 (mg/g)	0.21±0.01	0.15±0.01***	0.13±0.01***	0.09±0.01***	0.01±0.00***	0.02±0.00***
DHA, 22:6n−3 (mg/g)	0.40±0.02	0.34±0.00**	0.35±0.00*	0.34±0.01**	0.23±0.01***	0.22±0.01***
Sum n−3 (mg/g)	0.73±0.04	0.59±0.01***	0.58±0.01***	0.51±0.01***	0.28±0.01***	0.31±0.01***
Calculated n−6 HUFA (%)	26.6±0.2	36.1±0.5***	39.4.0±0.6***	47.5±0.5***	71±1***	68.0±0.6***
Calculated n−3 index (%)	19.4±0.1	15.9±0.2***	15.2±0.2***	13.3±0.3***	7.7±0.1***	7.8±0.2***

The n−3 index: EPA+ DHA content of erythrocytes expressed as a percent of total fatty acids in RBCs. Sum n−3 and sum n−6 include additional fatty acids not indicated in the table.
Data are presented as mean ± SEM (n = 5). Asterisk(s) indicates significant different from WD-FO.
*p<0.05,
**p<0.01,
***p<0.005.
Abbreviations: AA, arachidonic acid; DHA, docosahexaenoic acid, EPA, eicosapentaenoic acid, FA, fatty acids; HUFA, highly unsaturated fatty acids (HUFA, ≥20 carbons and ≥3 carbon-carbon double bonds), LA, linoleic acid; MUFA, monounsaturated fatty acids; RBCs, red blood cells; SFA, saturated fatty acids.

salmons fed the different feeds, and milk fat, used as fat source in the standard WD diet, was used to achieve isocaloric diets (Table 1). To verify the expected differences in fatty acid composition in the mouse diets, hereafter referred to as WD-FO, WD-RO, WD-OO, and WD-SO, analyses of the diets were performed (Table 2). The diets containing salmon fed either of the VOs, hereafter collectively referred to as WD-VOs, had significantly lower, but comparable levels of the marine n−3 PUFAs, EPA and DHA, than WD-FO (Table 2). Compared with WD-FO, the levels of n−6 PUFAs were higher in WD-VOs (Table 2). Of note, the levels of LA were comparable in WD-RO and WD-OO, but particularly high in WD-SO (Table 2). Furthermore, the levels of the vegetable n−3 PUFA, α-linolenic acid (ALA) was higher in the WD-RO than the other WD-VOs (Table 2). Thus, the n−3/n−6 ratio varied between the WD-VOs. The n−3/n−6 ratio was lower in WD-OO than in WD-RO, and the lowest n−3/n−6 ratio was measured in the WD-SO (Table 2).

To investigate possible spillover effects for consumers, C57BL/6J mice were fed these diets for 10 weeks and fatty acid composition was measured in the red blood cells (RBC). As references, two groups of mice were fed either a standard casein based WD or a regular low fat (LF) diet. As predicted, the combined levels of n−6 PUFAs were higher and the levels of n−3 PUFAs lower in RBCs in mice fed WD-VOs compared with WD-FO (Table 3). Thus, the n−3/n−6 ratio in RBCs in the mice reflected the ratio in the salmon fillets and mouse diets (Fig. 1). Compared with the WD-FO diet all the WD-VOs significantly reduced the omega-3 index - with over 30% reduction in mice fed the WD-SO diet compared to mice fed the WD-FO diet (Table 3). The omega-3 indices were reduced 18 and 21% in WD-RO and WD-OO fed mice, respectively (Table 3). However, all mice fed diets containing salmon had an omega-3 index higher than 8% [2], indicating that intake of the WD-VO diets still might exert a cardio-protective effect. For comparison, the reference diets resulted in an omega-3 index below the recommended limit of 8%.

Replacing Fish Oil with Vegetable Oils in Fish Feed Reduces the Levels of PCBs and DDTs in Atlantic Salmon Fillets and Accumulation of these in Adipose Tissue from Mice Consuming the Salmon Fillets

When FO was replaced with VO in salmon feed, the levels of PCBs and DDTs were reduced by more than 50% in the salmon fillets (Fig. 2A). PCBs and DDTs are lipid soluble contaminants that accumulate in adipose tissue in rats and mice [32,33]. Thus, the contaminant levels in adipose tissue, but not in liver of the mice mirrored the levels in the salmon fillets and the mouse diets (Fig. 2). Together, changes in the salmon feed were translated into altered fatty acid composition in RBCs and levels of POPs in adipose tissue in mice consuming the salmon fillets.

The Nutrient- and Contaminant Changes in Salmon Fillets do not Influence Obesity Development in Mice

We have previously demonstrated that chronic consumption of commercially available Atlantic salmon with a high level of POPs caused obesity in obesity prone C57BL/6J mice [33]. When the levels of POPs in the salmon were reduced, obesity development in the mice were slightly, but significantly, decreased. Here we demonstrate that although the accumulation of both PCBs and DDTs in adipose tissue was significantly lower in mice fed the various WD-VOs than in mice fed WD-FO, (Fig. 2C) body weight gain (Table 4) and adipose tissue masses (Table 5) were comparable. As expected, mice fed the LF diet, consumed significantly less energy and gained less weight than WD-FO fed mice. However, energy intake and apparent fat digestibility in the WD-VOs fed mice were comparable to those of mice fed the WD-FO (Table 4). Thus, neither reduced levels of PCBs and DDTs nor lower n−3/n−6 ratio in the WD-VOs had any effect on the body weight or obesity development (Table 4 and 5).

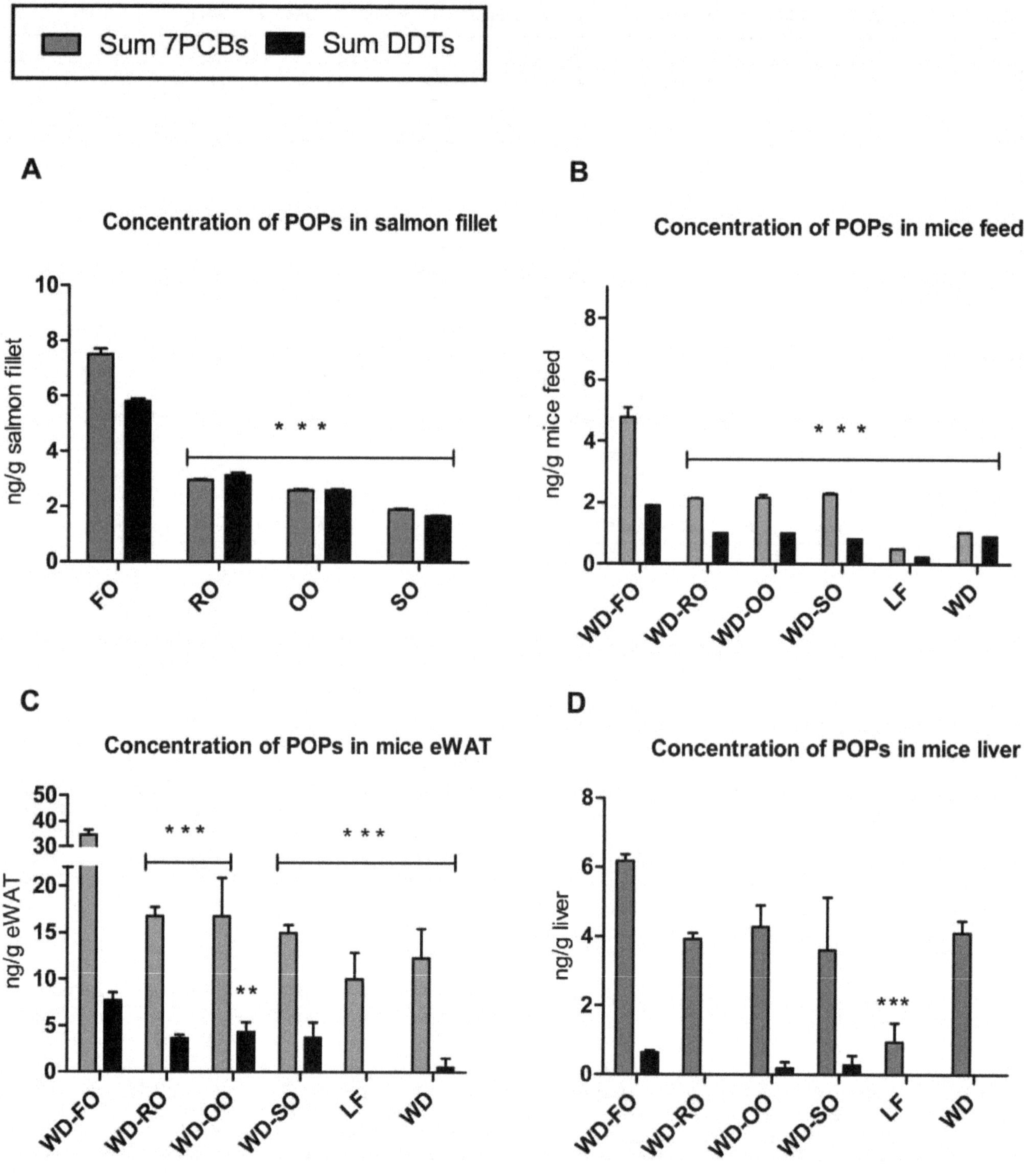

Figure 2. Composition of salmon aqua feed changes accumulation of POPs in mice consuming the salmon fillets. Fish oil (FO) in aqua feed was partly replaced with rapeseed oil (RO), olive oil (OO) or soy bean oil (SO) and fed Atlantic salmon. The salmon fillets were used in Western diets (WDs) fed male C57BL/6J mice (n = 8/diet) for 10 weeks. Concentrations of 7PCBs and DDTs were measured in (A) Atlantic salmon fillets (B) the WDs containing the fillets and (C) epididymal white adipose tissue (eWAT) and (D) liver collected from mice consuming the WDs and a low fat reference diet. Data represent mean of duplicate measurements in A and B. Tissues from two animals were pooled to achieve sufficient material for POP analyzes, and data in C and D thus represent mean+SEM (n = 4). Asterisk(s) indicates significant different from WD-FO.

Table 4. Body weight, energy intake, energy efficiency and apparent fat digestibility in mice fed the different diets for 10 weeks.

	WD-FO	WD-RO	WD-OO	WD-SO	LF	WD
Initial BW (g)	25.4±0.5	25.3±0.4	25.4±0.5	25.5±0.4	25.4±0.6	25.4±0.5
BW gain (g)	18.6±0.6	16.7±0.9	17.0±1.0	18.5±1.1	8.2±0.7***	15.3±0.7*
Total energy intake (kJ)	4125±140	4016±127	4113±231	4032±195	3423±133*	3840±104
Energy efficiency (g/MJ)	4.5±0.2	4.2±0.3	4.2±0.4	4.6±0.2	2.4±0.2***	4.0±0.2
Fat digestibility (%)	97.7±0.3	98.1±0.3	98.5±0.1	98.6±0.1	96.7±0.1	96.2±0.6**

Data are presented as means ± SEM (n = 8). Asterisk(s) indicates significant different from WD-FO.
*p<0.05,
**p<0.01,
***p<0.005.
Abbreviations: BW, body weight.

The Fatty Acid Composition in Salmon Fillets Influences Development of Insulin Resistance and Hepatic Lipid Accumulation in Mice

Given the earlier findings that POPs appear to exacerbate insulin resistance [32,33], whereas n−3 PUFAs have been demonstrated to attenuate development of diet-induced insulin resistance [9,11–15], we measured fasting levels of glucose and insulin, and performed glucose and insulin tolerance tests.

Overnight fasting plasma glucose levels were comparable in all groups (Fig. 3A). Compared with intake of WD-FO, intake of WD-VOs did not affect plasma insulin levels (Fig. 3B). The glucose tolerance in mice fed the WD-FO was comparable to the glucose tolerance in mice fed the standard WD, but lower than in mice fed the LF diet (Fig. 3C and E). WD-RO had a significantly decreased incremental area under the curve (AUC) compared with WD-FO (Fig. 3E) indicating an improved glucose tolerance. During the insulin tolerance test, AUC in WD-RO fed mice was not significantly lower than in mice fed WD-SO, but significantly lower ($p<0.05$) than in WD-FO fed mice (Fig. 3D). Mice receiving WD-SO had significantly higher blood glucose levels at 15 and 45 min after insulin injection than mice fed the WD-FO (Fig. 3D). LF fed mice had lower plasma glucose 30 and 45 min after injection of glucose (Fig. 3D). The difference was confirmed by a repeated-measures ANOVA test during the ITT revealing that the glucose response over time was significantly higher after in WD-SO fed mice as compared to WD-FO fed mice ($p<0.05$), whereas the glucose response over time in LF fed mice was significantly lower ($p<0.01$). Furthermore, mice receiving WD-SO had significantly larger AUC during ITT than mice fed the WD-FO (Fig. 3F). These results suggest that insulin sensitivity in mice fed WD-SO was decreased.

The reduced insulin sensitivity in WD-SO fed mice was not associated with increased adipose tissue mass. However, as not only increased adipose tissue mass, but also ectopic deposition of lipids have been suggested to contribute to the development of insulin resistance [11,36–38] we quantified lipids in liver and the tibialis anterior muscle. We did not observe any significant changes in muscle lipid content (not shown). Hepatic levels of PL and free fatty acids were similar in all groups but mice fed the WD-SO had significantly higher levels of total lipids, free cholesterol, steryl ester (SE) and triacylglycerol (TAG) in the liver than mice fed the WD-FO (Fig. 4). A similar tendency was seen in mice fed the WD-OO, but due to large individual differences this did not reach statistical significance. Given the ability of n−3 PUFAs to protect against diet-induced accumulation of fat in liver [39,40], and the indication of increased accumulation of lipids with increasing amount of n−6 in the diet, our data suggest that fatty acid composition in the salmon fillets appears to play a more important role than the levels of 7 PCBs and DDTs.

Discussion

The acceptance of Atlantic salmon as part of a healthy diet has to a large extent been based on its high content of marine n−3 PUFAs. However, the traditional use of fish-derived raw materials such as fish meal and FO in aquaculture is not sustainable due to the pressure on wild fish stocks. Thus, VOs are presently recognized as suitable alternatives in aqua feed [20]. We recently

Table 5. Organ weights (g) in the mice fed the experimental diets for 10 weeks.

	WD-FO	WD-RO	WD-OO	WD-SO	LF	WD
Liver	1.35±0.06	1.33±0.03	1.54±0.10	1.59±0.14	1.11±0.04	1.47±0.05
eWAT	1.98±0.05	1.97±0.08	1.87±0.16	1.96±0.08	0.70±0.08*	1.79±0.08
iWAT	0.70±0.02	0.68±0.05	0.65±0.09	0.71±0.05	0.25±0.03*	0.63±0.05
iBAT	0.102±0.006	0.085±0.006	0.089±0.008	0.100±0.006	0.080±0.007	0.084±0.005
Muscle (Tibialis)	0.091±0.004	0.081±0.004	0.097±0.006	0.092±0.007	0.089±0.005	0.082±0.003

Data are presented as means ± SEM (n = 8). Asterisk(s) indicates significant different from WD-FO.
*p<0.05,
**p<0.01,
***p<0.005.
Abbreviations; eWAT, epididymal white adipose tissue; iBAT, interscapular brown adipose tissue; iWAT, inguinal white adipose tissue.

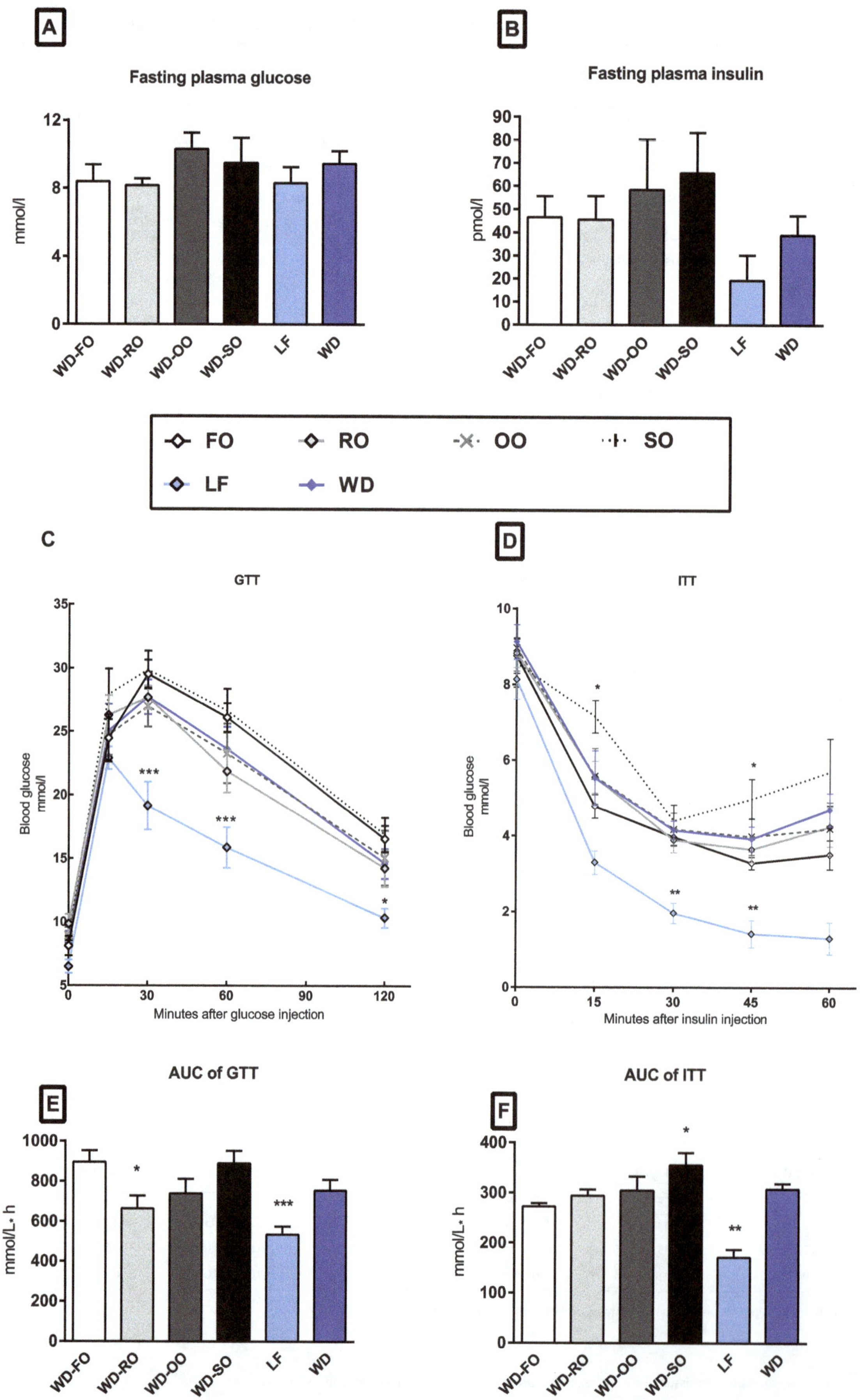
A
Fasting plasma glucose
mmol/l
WD-FO
WD-RO
WD-OO
WD-SO
LF
WD
B
Fasting plasma insulin
pmol/l
FO
RO
OO
SO
LF
WD
C
GTT
Blood glucose mmol/l
Minutes after glucose injection
D
ITT
Blood glucose mmol/l
Minutes after insulin injection
AUC of GTT
E
mmol/L• h
AUC of ITT
F

Figure 3. Fatty acid composition in salmon fillets influences development of insulin resistance in mice. Male C57BL/6J mice (n = 8/diet) were fed WD-FO, WD-RO, WD-OO and WD-SO for 10 weeks. As references, two groups of mice received regular WD or LF diet. Plasma glucose (A) and insulin (B) were measured after overnight fasting. An intraperitoneal glucose tolerance test (GTT) was performed after 7 weeks of feeding (C) and an intraperitoneal insulin tolerance test (ITT) was performed after 8 weeks of feeding (D). Area under the curve (AUC) was calculated from the glucose tolerance (baseline was set to fasted blood glucose levels) (E) and insulin tolerance test (F). Data are presented as means+SEM (n = 8). *represents significant different from WD-FO ($P<0.05$). **represents significant different from WD-FO ($P<0.01$). ***represents significant different from WD-FO ($P<0.005$).

demonstrated that a net production of marine proteins, but not marine n−3 PUFAs, is achievable when 70% of the marine proteins and 80% of the marine oils are replaced by vegetable alternatives [22]. Here we demonstrate that replacing FO with RO, OO or SO, decreased the n−3/n−6 ratio in salmon fillets by 79, 76 and 92%, respectively, with a concomitant reduction in

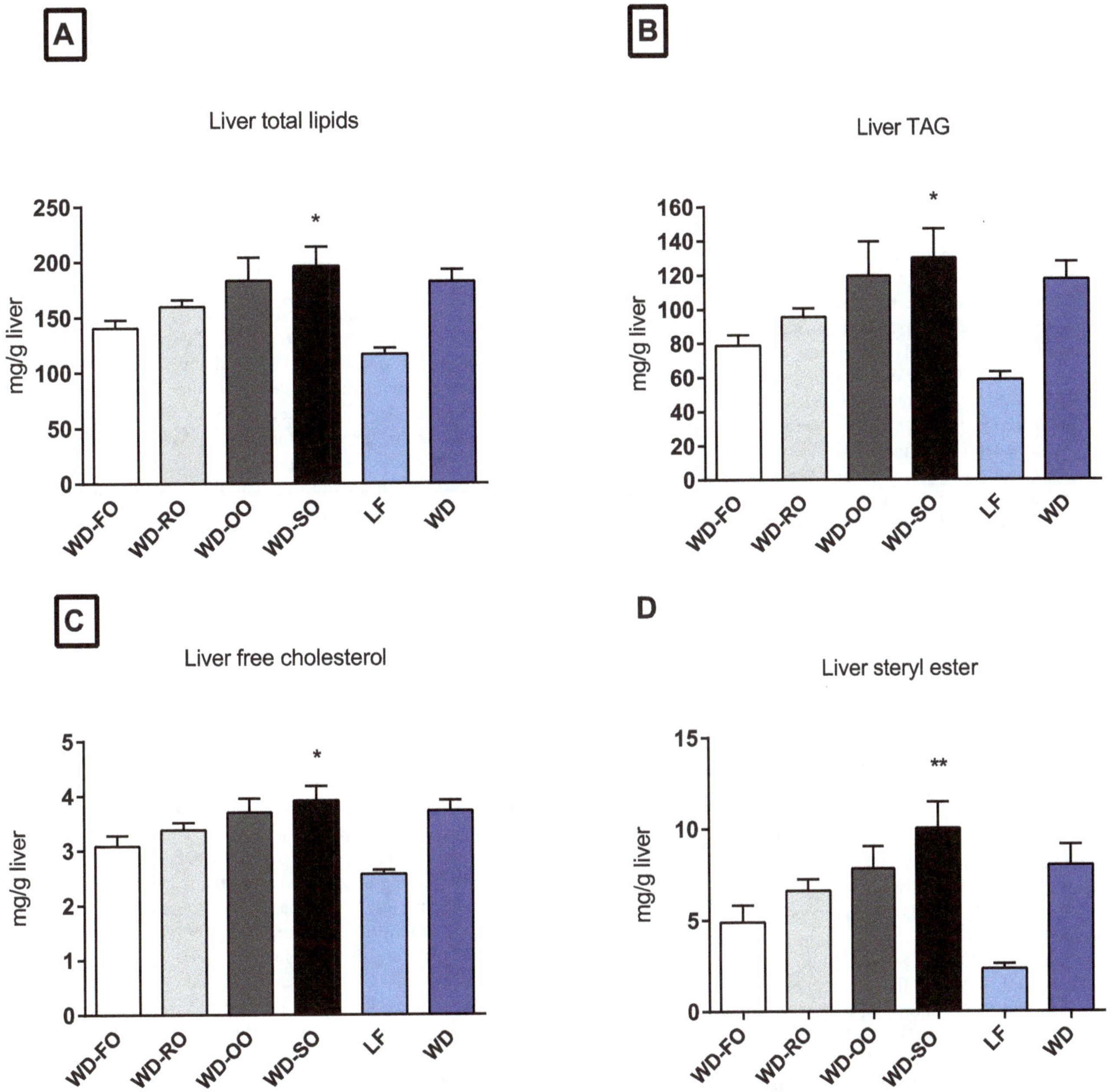

Figure 4. Fatty acid composition in salmon fillets influences development of hepatic lipid accumulation in mice. Male C57BL/6J mice (n = 8/diet) were fed WD-FO, WD-RO, WD-OO and WD-SO for 10 weeks. As references, two groups of mice received standard WD or LF diet. Lipids were extracted from liver and (A) total lipids; (B) triacylglycerol (TAG); (C) free cholesterol, and (D) steryl ester (SE) were quantified. Data are presented as means+SEM (n = 8). Asterisk(s) indicates significant different from WD-FO.

marine n−3 PUFAs in RBCs collected from mice fed WDs containing the salmon fillets. The omega-3 PUFA content in RBC membranes reflects the levels in cardiac membranes, and an omega-3 index below 4% is considered a risk factor for cardiovascular disease [2]. The omega-3 index was lower in mice fed the WD-VOs, WD-SO in particular, than in mice fed the WD-FO, however, the omega-3 index remained above 8% in all mice fed WDs containing salmon. Thus, the cardio-protective effects of salmon ingestion appeared to be maintained in diets based on VO fed salmon.

The ability of marine n−3 PUFAs to protect against development of obesity in rodents is well documented [5–10], whereas n−6 PUFAs, LA in particular, have been associated with increased weight gain [10,41–44]. We recently demonstrated that elevation of dietary LA from 1 to 8en% increased endocannabinoid tone and obesity development in mice, an effect that was prevented by adding 1% EPA and DHA to the 8e% LA diets [10]. Furthermore, excessive dietary LA from SO in salmon feed increased the endocannabinoid tone, both in Atlantic salmon and in mice fed high fat diets containing the salmon fillets. The increased endocannabinoid tone in the mice was accompanied by increased weight gain [24]. Here, the WD-SO contained more n−6 PUFAs, mainly LA, than the WD-FO and the other WD-VOs. Thus, the calculated n−6 HUFA content in WD-SO fed mice was significantly higher than in WD-FO and the other WD-VO fed mice. However, obesity development and weight gain were not influenced by replacing FO with VO in the present study. Compared to WD-FO fed mice, glucose tolerance was comparable in mice fed WD-OO and WD-SO, and actually improved in WD-RO fed mice. Despite similar body weight, adipose tissue mass and glucose tolerance, WD-SO fed mice became more insulin resistant and accumulated more lipids in the liver than WD-FO fed mice. Thus, in this study insulin resistance was accompanied by ectopic fat accumulation rather than obesity. Although a causal relationship is not fully established, hepatic insulin resistance is frequently accompanied by excessive deposition of fat in the liver [37]. The sequence of events leading to insulin resistance is not elucidated, but it was recently demonstrated that development of diet-induced hepatic insulin resistance precedes development of peripheral insulin resistance [45]. The finding that WD-SO fed mice had higher accumulation of hepatic TAG and were more insulin resistant than WD-FO fed mice might thus be related to the fatty acid composition of the diets. A number of studies have demonstrated the ability of marine n−3 PUFAs to prevent diet-induced accumulation of hepatic TAG [2,46,47]. Of note, the levels of the marine omega-3 fatty acids, EPA and DHA, were comparable in all WD-VOs. However, the level of LA was higher in WD-SO than in WD-OO and WD-RO. This might be of great importance for the omega-3 index, as the conversion of LA to arachidonic acid (AA), allows competition between AA and the n−3 PUFAs, EPA and DHA, for incorporation into membrane phospholipids (PL) [10]. In the study by Alvheim et al, 100% replacement of FO with SO in salmon feed led to increased LA and decreased EPA and DHA levels in salmon liver and fillet [24]. The mice fed SO salmon had higher AA and lower EPA and DHA levels in the PLs. Glucose tolerance and insulin resistance were not measured in the study by Alvheim et al., but the lower levels of EPA and DHA were accompanied with a 2.5-fold increased accumulation of hepatic TAG in mice fed SO salmon. Although a cause relationship is not demonstrated, it is possible that the high levels of n−6 PUFAs, LA in particular, in the WD-SO attenuated the ability of marine n−3 PUFA to reduce hepatic TAG, and thereby contributed to the augmented insulin resistance in WD-SO fed mice.

In the study by Alvheim et al., the Atlantic salmon were fed refined and purified FO and SO. However, the oils commonly used in the aquaculture industry contain POPs, and the use of vegetable oils in aqua feed will introduce different POPs in addition to changing the nutrient composition of salmon fillet. This is an important aspect, as the POPs present in commercially available farmed salmon are transferred to mice consuming the salmon, and these POPs may contribute to development of obesity and insulin resistance [32,33]. Chronic long term consumption of commercially available Atlantic salmon with current levels of POPs caused obesity and insulin resistance in mice [33], and the accumulation of POPs in adipose tissue was similar to levels in mice fed the WD-FO. When the levels of POPs in the salmon were reduced, obesity development and insulin resistance were slightly, but significantly decreased [33]. In this study, however, neither obesity nor insulin resistance correlated with accumulation of POPs in adipose tissue. Since obesity in general is often associated with insulin resistance, we cannot exclude the possibility that insulin resistance in the earlier studies [32,33], at least in part, simply reflected the degree of obesity. Laboratory rodents are normally fed a diet where casein is used as the protein source. In a previous salmon study, we replaced 100% of the casein with salmon proteins [33]. Mice receiving salmon as the sole protein source gained significantly more adipose tissue mass than mice receiving casein. The increased adiposity was accompanied with increased digestibility of fat. Thus, in order to limit the difference in fat digestibility, we exchanged only 50% of the casein with proteins from salmon in the present study. The difference in fat digestibility between WD and WD-FO was still significant with higher digestibility in the WD-FO. All the WD-VOs had the same fat digestibility as WD-FO, suggesting that the uptake of fat from the different WDs was comparable.

In the present experiment insulin resistance was more pronounced in mice fed the WD-SO than in mice fed WD-FO although the degree of adiposity was similar in all WD groups. Of note, the levels of PCBs and DDTs reported to accumulate in adipose tissue [33] were comparable to the levels found after 10 weeks feeding with WD-FO in the present study, whereas mice fed the WD-SO diet had lower accumulation of PCBs and DDTs than reported for mice fed Atlantic salmon with reduced POP levels [33]. Obviously, the levels of POPs in adipose tissue are not the sole determining factor of insulin resistance. We cannot exclude the possibility that POPs contributed to the development of insulin resistance, but our results suggest that other factors, such as fatty acid composition in the diets, are of importance.

In view of the limited access to marine fish meal and fish oil for the rapidly growing aquaculture industry, a global contributor to food security, the use of alternative feed ingredients is inevitable. Exchanging FO with VO in aquatic feed reduced the accumulation of POPs in adipose tissue by more than 50% in mice consuming the salmon. Importantly, in relation to replacement of fish oil with vegetable oil in future feed for salmon farming, our data clearly demonstrate that VOs have markedly different spillover effects on metabolism in mice, and that the content of LA may be a matter of concern. This raises the important question as to whether similar effects will be observed in humans consuming Atlantic salmon fed VOs, SO in particular, and in this context our study suggests that RO and/or OO represent a better choice than SO to replace FO.

Acknowledgments

The authors thank Aase Heltveit and Øyvind Reinshol for animal care.

Author Contributions

Conceived and designed the experiments: LM BET KK. Performed the experiments: LKM MMI LSM ULA ARA NSL BET BL TB KK LM GR. Analyzed the data: LKM MMI LSM ULA ARA NSL BET BL TB KK LM. Wrote the paper: LKM MMI KK LM.

References

1. Mozaffarian D, Wu JHY (2012) (n−3) Fatty Acids and Cardiovascular Health: Are Effects of EPA and DHA Shared or Complementary? J Nutr 142: 614S–625S.
2. Harris WS (2010) The omega-3 index: clinical utility for therapeutic intervention. Curr Cardiol Rep 12: 503–508.
3. Abeywardena MY, Patten GS (2011) Role of omega3 long-chain polyunsaturated fatty acids in reducing cardio-metabolic risk factors. Endocr Metab Immune Disord Drug Targets 11: 232–246.
4. Buckley JD, Howe PRC (2010) Long-Chain Omega-3 Polyunsaturated Fatty Acids May Be Beneficial for Reducing Obesity-A Review. Nutrients 2: 1212–1230.
5. Wang H, Storlien LH, Huang XF (2002) Effects of dietary fat types on body fatness, leptin, and ARC leptin receptor, NPY, and AgRP mRNA expression. Am J Physiol Endocrinol Metab 282: E1352–1359.
6. Ukropec J, Reseland JE, Gasperikova D, Demcakova E, Madsen L, et al. (2003) The hypotriglyceridemic effect of dietary n−3 FA is associated with increased beta-oxidation and reduced leptin expression. Lipids 38: 1023–1029.
7. Mori T, Kondo H, Hase T, Tokimitsu I, Murase T (2007) Dietary fish oil upregulates intestinal lipid metabolism and reduces body weight gain in C57BL/6J Mice. J Nutr 137: 2629–2634.
8. Perez-Echarri N, Perez-Matute P, Marcos-Gomez B, Baena MJ, Marti A, et al. (2008) Differential inflammatory status in rats susceptible or resistant to diet-induced obesity: effects of EPA ethyl ester treatment. Eur J Nutr 47: 380–386.
9. Kalupahana NS, Claycombe K, Newman SJ, Stewart T, Siriwardhana N, et al. (2010) Eicosapentaenoic Acid Prevents and Reverses Insulin Resistance in High-Fat Diet-Induced Obese Mice via Modulation of Adipose Tissue Inflammation. J Nutr 140: 1915–1922.
10. Alvheim AR, Malde MK, Osei-Hyiaman D, Hong Lin Y, Pawlosky RJ, et al. (2012) Dietary Linoleic Acid Elevates Endogenous 2-AG and Anandamide and Induces Obesity. Obesity (Silver Spring) 10: 1984–1994.
11. Storlien LH, Kraegen EW, Chisholm DJ, Ford GL, Bruce DG, et al. (1987) Fish oil prevents insulin resistance induced by high-fat feeding in rats. Science 237: 885–888.
12. Jucker BM, Cline GW, Barucci N, Shulman GI (1999) Differential effects of safflower oil versus fish oil feeding on insulin-stimulated glycogen synthesis, glycolysis, and pyruvate dehydrogenase flux in skeletal muscle - A C-13 nuclear magnetic resonance study. Diabetes 48: 134–140.
13. Neschen S, Morino K, Dong JY, Wang-Fischer Y, Cline GW, et al. (2007) N−3 fatty acids preserve insulin sensitivity in vivo in a peroxisome proliferator-activated receptor-alpha-dependent manner. Diabetes 56: 1034–1041.
14. Samane S, Christon R, Dombrowski L, Turcotte S, Charrouf Z, et al. (2009) Fish oil and argan oil intake differently modulate insulin resistance and glucose intolerance in a rat model of dietary-induced obesity. Metabolism 58: 909–919.
15. Oh DY, Talukdar S, Bae EJ, Imamura T, Morinaga H, et al. (2010) GPR120 Is an Omega-3 Fatty Acid Receptor Mediating Potent Anti-inflammatory and Insulin-Sensitizing Effects. Cell 142: 687–698.
16. Torstensen BE, Bell JG, Rosenlund G, Henderson RJ, Graff IE, et al. (2005) Tailoring of Atlantic salmon (Salmo salar L.) flesh lipid composition and sensory quality by replacing fish oil with a vegetable oil blend. J Agric Food Chem 53: 10166–10178.
17. Tacon AGJ (2006) Use of fishery resources as feed inputs to aquaculture development: trends and policy implications; Hasan MR, Subasinghe RP, editors. Rome: Food and Agriculture Organization of the United Nations.
18. Tacon AGJ, Metian M (2008) Global overview on the use of fish meal and fish oil in industrially compounded aquafeeds: Trends and future prospects. Aquaculture 285: 146–158.
19. Torstensen BE, Espe M, Sanden M, Stubhaug I, Waagbo R, et al. (2008) Novel production of Atlantic salmon (Salmo salar) protein based on combined replacement of fish meal and fish oil with plant meal and vegetable oil blends. Aquaculture 285: 193–200.
20. Turchini GM, Torstensen BE, Ng WK (2009) Fish oil replacement in finfish nutrition. Reviews in Aquaculture 1: 10–57.
21. Sargent J, Bell G, McEvoy L, Tocher D, Estevez A (1999) Recent developments in the essential fatty acid nutrition of fish. Aquaculture 177: 191–199.
22. Liland NS, Rosenlund G, Berntssen MHG, Brattelid T, Madsen L, Torstensen BE (2012) Net production of Atlantic salmon (FIFO, Fish in Fish out<1) with dietary plant proteins and vegetable oils. Aquaculture Nutrition, ahead of print, doi: 10.1111/j.1365-2095.2012.00958.x.
23. Seierstad SL, Seljeflot I, Johansen O, Hansen R, Haugen M, et al. (2005) Dietary intake of differently fed salmon; the influence on markers of human atherosclerosis. Eur J Clin Invest 35: 52–59.
24. Alvheim AR, Torstensen BE, Lin YH, Lillefosse HH, Lock EJ, et al. (2012) Dietary linoleic acid elevates endogenous 2-arachidonoylglycerol and anandamide in Atlantic salmon (Salmo salar L.) and mice, and induces weight gain and inflammation in mice. Br J Nutr: 1–10.
25. Berntssen MHG, Lundebye AK, Torstensen BE (2005) Reducing the levels of dioxins and dioxin-like PCBs in farmed Atlantic salmon by substitution of fish oil with vegetable oil in the feed. Aquaculture Nutrition 11: 219–231.
26. Berntssen MHG, Julshamn K, Lundebye AK (2010) Chemical contaminants in aquafeeds and Atlantic salmon (Salmo salar) following the use of traditional-versus alternative feed ingredients. Chemosphere 78: 637–646.
27. Rignell-Hydbom A, Rylander L, Hagmar L (2007) Exposure to persistent organochlorine pollutants and type 2 diabetes mellitus. Hum Exp Toxicol 26: 447–452.
28. Rylander L, Rignell-Hydbom A, Hagmar L (2005) A cross-sectional study of the association between persistent organochlorine pollutants and diabetes. Environ Health 4: 28.
29. Lee DH, Lee IK, Song K, Steffes M, Toscano W, et al. (2006) A strong dose-response relation between serum concentrations of persistent organic pollutants and diabetes: results from the National Health and Examination Survey 1999–2002. Diabetes Care 29: 1638–1644.
30. Airaksinen R, Rantakokko P, Eriksson JG, Blomstedt P, Kajantie E, et al. (2011) Association between type 2 diabetes and exposure to persistent organic pollutants. Diabetes Care 34: 1972–1979.
31. Ukropec J, Radikova Z, Huckova M, Koska J, Kocan A, et al. (2010) High prevalence of prediabetes and diabetes in a population exposed to high levels of an organochlorine cocktail. Diabetologia 53: 899–906.
32. Ruzzin J, Petersen R, Meugnier E, Madsen L, Lock EJ, et al. (2010) Persistent Organic Pollutant Exposure Leads to Insulin Resistance Syndrome. Environ Health Perspect 118: 465–471.
33. Ibrahim MM, Fjaere E, Lock EJ, Naville D, Amlund H, et al. (2011) Chronic Consumption of Farmed Salmon Containing Persistent Organic Pollutants Causes Insulin Resistance and Obesity in Mice. PLoS One 6: e25170.
34. Torstensen BE, Espe M, Stubhaug I, Lie O (2011) Dietary plant proteins and vegetable oil blends increase adiposity and plasma lipids in Atlantic salmon (Salmo salar L.). Br J Nutr 106: 633–647.
35. Arslan G, Brunborg LA, Froyland L, Brun JG, Valen M, et al. (2002) Effects of duodenal seal oil administration in patients with inflammatory bowel disease. Lipids 37: 935–940.
36. Savage DB, Petersen KF, Shulman GI (2007) Disordered lipid metabolism and the pathogenesis of insulin resistance. Physiol Rev 87: 507–520.
37. Farese RV Jr, Zechner R, Newgard CB, Walther TC (2012) The problem of establishing relationships between hepatic steatosis and hepatic insulin resistance. Cell Metab 15: 570–573.
38. Suganami T, Tanaka M, Ogawa Y (2012) Adipose tissue inflammation and ectopic lipid accumulation [Review]. Endocr J 59: 849–857.
39. Perez-Martinez P, Perez-Jimenez F, Lopez-Miranda J (2010) n−3 PUFA and lipotoxicity. Biochim Biophys Acta 1801: 362–366.
40. Ma T, Liaset B, Hao Q, Petersen RK, Fjaere E, et al. (2011) Sucrose counteracts the anti-inflammatory effect of fish oil in adipose tissue and increases obesity development in mice. Plos One 6: e21647.
41. Madsen L, Petersen RK, Kristiansen K (2005) Regulation of adipocyte differentiation and function by polyunsaturated fatty acids. Biochim Biophys Acta 1740: 266–286.
42. Massiera F, Saint-Marc P, Seydoux J, Murata T, Kobayashi T, et al. (2003) Arachidonic acid and prostacyclin signaling promote adipose tissue development: a human health concern? J Lipid Res 44: 271–279.
43. Javadi M, Everts H, Hovenier R, Kocsis S, Lankhorst AE, et al. (2004) The effect of six different C18 fatty acids on body fat and energy metabolism in mice. Br J Nutr 92: 391–399.
44. Ailhaud G, Massiera F, Weill P, Legrand P, Alessandri JM, et al. (2006) Temporal changes in dietary fats: role of n−6 polyunsaturated fatty acids in excessive adipose tissue development and relationship to obesity. Prog Lipid Res 45: 203–236.
45. Kleemann R, van Erk M, Verschuren L, van den Hoek AM, Koek M, et al. (2010) Time-Resolved and Tissue-Specific Systems Analysis of the Pathogenesis of Insulin Resistance. PLoS One 5: e8817.
46. Kajikawa S, Harada T, Kawashima A, Imada K, Mizuguchi K (2009) Highly purified eicosapentaenoic acid prevents the progression of hepatic steatosis by repressing monounsaturated fatty acid synthesis in high-fat/high-sucrose diet-fed mice. Prostaglandins Leukot Essent Fatty Acids 80: 229–238.
47. Tanaka N, Zhang XG, Sugiyama E, Kono H, Horiuchi A, et al. (2010) Eicosapentaenoic acid improves hepatic steatosis independent of PPAR alpha activation through inhibition of SREBP-1 maturation in mice. Biochem Pharmacol 80: 1601–1612.

15

Predicting the Development of Diabetes using the Product of Triglycerides and Glucose: The Chungju Metabolic Disease Cohort (CMC) Study

Seung-Hwan Lee[1,2], Hyuk-Sang Kwon[1,3], Yong-Moon Park[4,5], Hee-Sung Ha[4], Seung Hee Jeong[6], Hae Kyung Yang[1,2], Jin-Hee Lee[7], Hyeon-Woo Yim[4,6], Moo-Il Kang[1,2], Won-Chul Lee[4], Ho-Young Son[1,2], Kun-Ho Yoon[1,2]*

1 Department of Internal Medicine, College of Medicine, The Catholic University of Korea, Seoul, Korea, **2** Division of Endocrinology and Metabolism, Department of Internal Medicine, Seoul St. Mary's Hospital, Seoul, Korea, **3** Division of Endocrinology and Metabolism, Department of Internal Medicine, Yeouido St. Mary's Hospital, Seoul, Korea, **4** Department of Preventive Medicine, College of Medicine, The Catholic University of Korea, Seoul, Korea, **5** Department of Epidemiology and Biostatistics, Arnold School of Public Health, University of South Carolina, Columbia, South Carolina, United States of America, **6** Clinical Research Coordinating Center, College of Medicine, The Catholic University of Korea, Seoul, Korea, **7** Catholic Institute of U-Healthcare, The Catholic University of Korea, Seoul, Korea

Abstract

Background: To determine whether the TyG index, a product of the levels of triglycerides and fasting plasma glucose (FPG) might be a valuable marker for predicting future diabetes.

Methods: A total of 5,354 nondiabetic subjects who had completed their follow-up visit for evaluating diabetes status were selected from a large cohort of middle-aged Koreans in the Chungju Metabolic Disease Cohort study. The risk of diabetes was assessed according to the baseline TyG index, calculated as ln[fasting triglycerides (mg/dL) × FPG (mg/dL)/2]. The median follow-up period was 4.6 years.

Results: During the follow-up period, 420 subjects (7.8%) developed diabetes. The baseline values of the TyG index were significantly higher in these subjects compared with nondiabetic subjects (8.9±0.6 vs. 8.6±0.6; $P<0.0001$) and the incidence of diabetes increased in proportion to TyG index quartiles. After adjusting for age, gender, body mass index, waist circumference, systolic blood pressure, high-density lipoprotein (HDL)-cholesterol level, a family history of diabetes, smoking, alcohol drinking, education level and serum insulin level, the risk of diabetes onset was more than fourfold higher in the highest vs. the lowest quartile of the TyG index (relative risk, 4.095; 95% CI, 2.701–6.207). The predictive power of the TyG index was better than the triglyceride/HDL-cholesterol ratio or the homeostasis model assessment of insulin resistance.

Conclusions: The TyG index, a simple measure reflecting insulin resistance, might be useful in identifying individuals at high risk of developing diabetes.

Editor: Maria Eugenia Saez, CAEBi, Spain

Funding: This study was supported by the National Research Foundation of Korea (NRF) grant funded by the Korea government (MSIP, 2013M3C8A2075675) and the grant from the Catholic Medical Center Research Foundation made in the program year of 2013 (to SHL). The funders had no role in study design, data collection and analysis, decision to publish, or preparation of the manuscript.

Competing Interests: The authors have declared that no competing interests exist.

* E-mail: yoonk@catholic.ac.kr

Introduction

The incidence and prevalence of type 2 diabetes is increasing rapidly worldwide, and is expected to affect 439 million adults by 2030 [1–3]. To overcome the burden of this epidemic, public health strategy should focus on the identification of subjects at high risk of developing diabetes with the aim of prevention and proper intervention. This might lead to favorable outcomes while avoiding unnecessary effort [4]. For this purpose, an easily measurable and widely applicable index with high predictability needs to be developed.

Various risk factors and predictive models have been suggested. In addition to traditional risk factors, inflammatory biomarkers and genetic risk factors are under investigation to improve the prediction of diabetes. However, the additive role of these novel markers is reported to be limited [5–8]. Among traditional risk factors, the levels of fasting plasma glucose (FPG) and triglycerides (TG) are well validated for their role in predicting the development of diabetes. Higher FPG levels have been shown to be an independent risk factor for developing type 2 diabetes even when subjects are within the normoglycemic range [9,10]. Elevations and increases in TG levels over time also enhanced the risk of developing diabetes in various populations [11–14].

The TyG index, the product of FPG and TG, is a novel index that has been suggested as a surrogate of insulin resistance in healthy subjects [15,16]. It was well correlated with the homeostasis model assessment of insulin resistance (HOMA-IR) and total glucose metabolism rates during hyperinsulinemic–euglycemic clamp studies. Given that insulin resistance is the core pathophysiologic mechanism of type 2 diabetes and is already present 1–2 decades before the diagnosis [17,18], surrogate indices of insulin resistance might aid in the prediction of incident diabetes.

In this study, we aimed to determine whether the TyG index could be a valuable marker for predicting diabetes and to compare it with other insulin resistance indices in a large-scale cohort of middle-aged nondiabetic Koreans.

Subjects and Methods

Subjects

The Chungju Metabolic disease Cohort (CMC) study is an ongoing community-based study of metabolic diseases including diabetes, metabolic syndrome and osteoporosis in a population aged 40 years and over living in the rural area of Chungju City, Korea. The first phase (baseline) of the study was performed in 2003–2006. Three hundred thirty-four districts were selected by stratified random cluster sampling and 11,718 subjects participated. These participants were follwed up at 4-year intervals in the second phase of the study (2007–2010) with a follow-up rate of 58%, and the third phase of the study is ongoing (2011–2014). Subjects with known or newly diagnosed diabetes or prediabetes at the baseline study, and those lacking laboratory or anthropometric data were excluded. In this analysis, persons who had completed their follow-up visit at the second phase (n = 3,814) or both second and third phases (n = 1,540) of the study were included (total 5,354 participants). The institutional review board at The Catholic University of Korea approved this study (No. KCMC070T076, KC13OISI0427) and written informed consent was obtained from all participants.

Study Protocol

Investigators were trained in the study protocol prior to carrying out physical examinations and administering the questionnaire. Detailed data on the medical history and lifestyle behavior of the subjects were obtained on the day of the investigation by interview. Data on alcohol drinking (yes/no), average alcohol amount (g/day), cigarette smoking (none, ex-smoker or current smoker), doing exercise at least once a week (yes/no) and education level were collected. Anthropometric measurements were performed with the subjects wearing light clothing, and height, weight, and waist and hip circumferences were measured according to standardized methods. Prior to the measurement of blood pressure (BP), the subjects were asked to rest for 5 min while seated. The BP on the right upper arm was measured twice and the average was recorded. Hypertension was defined on the basis of the Joint National Committee 7 report as ≥140 (systolic BP)/90 (diastolic BP) mmHg or when the subjects reported using antihypertensive medications.

Analytical Methods and Calculations

Blood samples were collected after the subjects had fasted for at least 12 h and analyzed at a central laboratory (Samkwang Medical Laboratories, Seoul, Korea). FPG was measured using the hexokinase method and serum insulin was measured using a radioimmunoassay kit (Dainabot, Tokyo, Japan). Serum creatinine was measured using an enzymatic method. Serum total cholesterol (TC) and TG were measured using enzymatic colorimetric tests; high-density lipoprotein (HDL)-cholesterol was measured using a selective inhibition method and low-density lipoprotein (LDL)-cholesterol was calculated using the Friedewald formula. The intra- and inter-assay coefficient of variances of analytical procedures were less than 4.7% and 4.5%, respectively. In subjects with TG levels greater than 5.6 mmol/L (n = 55), the values of LDL-cholesterol were treated as missing. The homeostasis model assessment estimate of beta-cell function (HOMA-ß) and HOMA-IR were calculated using the following formulae: 20×fasting insulin (mIU/L)/[FPG (mmol/L)–3.5] and FPG (mmol/L)×fasting insulin (mIU/L)/22.5, respectively. [19]. The TyG index was calculated as the ln[fasting triglycerides (mg/dL)×FPG (mg/dL)/2] [15,16].

Definition of Diabetes Mellitus

In the first phase of the study, a 75 g oral glucose tolerance test (OGTT) was performed if the subject's FPG level exceeded 6.1 mmol/L. Diabetes and prediabetes (impaired fasting glucose and/or impaired glucose tolerance) were defined according to the American Diabetes Association criteria published in 1997, which define the normal FPG level as <6.1 mmol/L [20]. In the second phase of the study, an OGTT was performed if the FPG level exceeded 5.6 mmol/L. However, from September 2009, every participant underwent an OGTT, independent of his or her FPG level. The revised report on the diagnosis of diabetes mellitus published in 2003, which set a normal FPG level of <5.6 mmol/L, was used to define the development of diabetes or prediabetes in follow-up studies [21].

Statistical Analysis

All statistical analyses were performed using SAS 9.2 software (SAS Institute Inc., Cary, NC, USA). Data are expressed as the mean ± standard deviation (SD), as medians (25th–75th percentiles) or as proportions. For comparing the characteristics of subgroups according to the development of diabetes or TyG index quartiles, the Wilcoxon rank sum test, Chi squared test or Fisher's exact test were used. Spearman correlation analysis was used to examine the relationships between the TyG index and other parameters. Log-Binomial regression model using Proc GenMod procedure was performed to calculate relative risk (RR), for testing the usefulness of various markers in predicting the development of diabetes. RR and 95% CI values of the upper three quartiles were calculated using the lowest quartile as the reference category. The area under the curve (AUC) of the receiver operating characteristics (ROC) curve and a 95% CI were calculated to compare the predictive power of each index. A P value <0.05 was considered significant.

Results

Baseline Characteristics

The age, body mass index (BMI), and FPG levels of the subjects were 61.6±9.3 years, 24.2±3.2 kg/m^2, and 4.99±0.47 mmol/L, respectively (means ± SDs). Their TyG index value was 8.7±0.6, which was not significantly different between men and women (8.7±0.6 vs. 8.6±0.5; P=0.191). The median (minimum, maximum) duration of follow-up was 4.6 (4.0, 8.8) years. During this period, 420 subjects (7.8%) had developed diabetes. When the baseline characteristics of these subjects were compared with those remaining free of diabetes, the subjects were found to be older, more obese and more hypertensive. FPG levels, fasting insulin levels, HOMA-IR, TC, TG and LDL-cholesterol levels were higher while HOMA-ß and HDL-cholesterol levels were lower in subjects with incident diabetes. They also had higher frequencies of a familiy history of diabetes and of alcohol drinking. The baseline values of the TyG index were significantly higher in

Table 1. Baseline characteristics of subjects according to diabetes status at follow-up.

	Total (n = 5354)	Non-DM (n = 4934)	DM (n = 420)	*P*
Age (years)	61.6±9.3	61.5±9.4	62.9±8.6	0.007
Gender (men, %)	37.7	37.6	39.8	0.375
Height (cm)	155.8±8.6	155.8±8.6	155.7±8.4	0.927
Weight (kg)	58.8±9.7	58.7±9.7	61.0±9.9	<0.0001
BMI (kg/m^2)	24.2±3.2	24.1±3.2	25.1±3.4	<0.0001
Waist circumference (cm)	82.7±8.6	82.4±8.5	86.3±8.6	<0.0001
Hip circumference (cm)	93.8±6.4	93.6±6.3	95.3±7.1	<0.0001
Waist–Hip Ratio	0.881 (0.839–0.924)	0.879 (0.837–0.922)	0.901 (0.861–0.947)	<0.0001
Systolic BP (mmHg)	136.4±19.0	135.9±18.7	143.1±21.1	<0.0001
Diastolic BP (mmHg)	84.5±10.7	84.2±10.6	87.5±11.4	<0.0001
FPG (mmol/L)	4.99±0.47	4.96±0.46	5.31±0.50	<0.0001
Fasting insulin (pmol/L)	35.6±31.2	35.1±30.8	41.5±35.4	<0.0001
HOMA–IR	1.1 (0.7–1.6)	1.0 (0.6–1.6)	1.4 (0.8–2.1)	<0.0001
HOMA–ß	67.3 (41.8–103.8)	67.6 (42.0–104.4)	63.4 (38.7–93.9)	0.035
Total cholesterol (mmol/L)	5.17±0.94	5.15±0.93	5.38±1.01	<0.0001
Triglycerides (mmol/L)	1.40 (0.97–2.03)	1.37 (0.96–1.99)	1.74 (1.15–2.59)	<0.0001
HDL–cholesterol (mmol/L)	1.34±0.32	1.35±0.32	1.30±0.31	0.001
LDL–cholesterol (mmol/L)	3.09±0.85	3.08±0.84	3.20±0.88	0.002
Serum creatinine (umol/L)	79.5±14.7	79.5±14.7	79.3±14.6	0.909
Hypertension (%)	24.5	23.7	34.4	<0.0001
Family history of DM (%)	8.9	8.5	13.4	0.0007
Exercise (%)	13.3	13.2	13.6	0.854
Alcohol drinking (%)	44.6	44.1	50.4	0.013
Average alcohol/day (g)	21.1±30.4	20.9±29.9	24.3±36.4	0.691
Smoking (%)				
None	70.6	70.8	67.9	0.305
Ex-smoker	12.6	12.6	12.7	
Current	16.8	16.6	19.4	
Education (%)				
None	29.4	28.8	36.9	0.008
Elementary school	49.8	50.2	44.6	
Middle school	12.3	12.4	11.3	
High school	7.0	7.1	5.3	
College	1.5	1.5	1.9	
TyG index	8.7±0.6	8.6±0.6	8.9±0.6	<0.0001

Data are expressed as means ± SD, % or median (25th–75th percentiles).
BMI, body mass index; BP, blood pressure; DM, diabetes mellitus; FPG, fasting plasma glucose; HDL, high-density lipoprotein; HOMA-ß, homeostasis model assessment estimate of beta-cell function; HOMA-IR, homeostasis model assessment of insulin resistance; LDL, low-density lipoprotein.

subjects who had developed diabetes compared with nondiabetic subjects (8.9±0.6 vs. 8.6±0.6; $P<0.0001$) (Table 1).

Next, the baseline characteristics of subjects were compared according to the TyG index quartile (Q1–Q4) groups. Subjects in the higher quartile groups were more obese, more hypertensive and had higher frequencies of smoking and alcohol drinking. The values for FPG and fasting insulin, HOMA-IR, HOMA-ß, TC, TG, LDL-cholesterol, and serum creatinine increased and the level of HDL-cholesterol decreased in proportion to the TyG index quartiles (Table 2).

The Association between TyG Index and other Parameters

There were significant correlations between the TyG index and anthropometric indices, BP and lipid profiles. The TyG index was correlated with body weight ($r = 0.185$; $P<0.0001$), BMI ($r = 0.215$; $P<0.0001$), waist circumference ($r = 0.251$; $P<0.0001$), waist-hip ratio ($r = 0.229$; $P<0.0001$), systolic BP ($r = 0.140$; $P<0.0001$), diastolic BP ($r = 0.145$; $P<0.0001$), and with the levels of TC ($r = 0.262$; $P<0.0001$), TG ($r = 0.984$; $P<0.0001$), LDL-cholesterol ($r = 0.029$; $P = 0.039$), and HDL-cholesterol ($r = -0.370$; $P<0.0001$). As expected, the TyG index also showed significant correlations with FPG levels ($r = 0.243$; $P<$

Table 2. Baseline characteristics of subjects according to the TyG index quartiles.

	Q1 (n = 1336)	Q2 (n = 1340)	Q3 (n = 1342)	Q4 (n = 1336)	*P*
Age (years)	61.1±9.8	61.7±9.3	62.0±9.2	61.6±8.8	0.125
Gender (men, %)	37.7	38.0	35.5	39.8	0.142
Height (cm)	155.6±8.6	155.9±8.6	155.3±8.7	156.4±8.6	0.015
Weight (kg)	56.4±9.2	58.3±9.2	59.3±9.8	61.4±10.0	<0.0001
BMI (kg/m^2)	23.3±3.1	24.0±3.2	24.5±3.1	25.0±3.1	<0.0001
Waist circumference (cm)	79.7±8.4	82.1±8.2	83.6±8.4	85.4±8.3	<0.0001
Hip circumference (cm)	92.2±6.2	93.7±6.3	94.2±6.3	94.9±6.5	<0.0001
Waist–Hip Ratio	0.860 (0.818–0.904)	0.876 (0.835–0.916)	0.887 (0.844–0.929)	0.900 (0.861–0.939)	<0.0001
Systolic BP (mmHg)	132.8±18.1	135.5±18.2	137.7±19.2	139.7±19.8	<0.0001
Diastolic BP (mmHg)	82.4±10.4	84.2±10.5	85.1±10.9	86.3±10.6	<0.0001
FPG (mmol/L)	4.82±0.48	4.96±0.45	5.02±0.43	5.14±0.47	<0.0001
Fasting insulin (pmol/L)	29.0±29.7	32.7±26.0	37.1±32.7	43.4±34.1	<0.0001
HOMA–IR	0.814 (0.511–1.243)	0.999 (0.626–1.489)	1.139 (0.713–1.671)	1.378 (0.869–2.088)	<0.0001
HOMA– ß	59.0 (36.0–92.4)	64.6 (39.8–97.7)	70.9 (45.0–106.6)	76.0 (49.3–116.8)	<0.0001
Total cholesterol (mmol/L)	4.83±0.84	5.10±0.89	5.27±0.89	5.48±1.01	<0.0001
Triglycerides (mmol/L)	0.77 (0.65–0.90)	1.17 (1.06–1.29)	1.66 (1.51–1.84)	2.68 (2.31–3.35)	<0.0001
HDL–cholesterol (mmol/L)	1.50±0.35	1.38±0.30	1.31±0.28	1.18±0.26	<0.0001
LDL– cholesterol (mmol/L)	2.97±0.76	3.17±0.82	3.19±0.83	3.02±0.95	<0.0001
Serum creatinine (umol/L)	78.5±14.2	79.4±14.5	79.3±14.5	80.8±15.6	0.001
Hypertension (%)	17.0	23.8	26.9	30.5	<0.0001
Family history of DM (%)	7.6	8.4	9.2	10.2	0.113
Exercise (%)	12.5	13.6	13.4	13.7	0.808
Alcohol drinking (%)	39.3	44.3	45.4	49.3	<0.0001
Average alcohol/day (g)	17.7±29.4	19.5±27.9	19.1±28.4	26.6±34.0	0.0004
Smoking (%)					0.007
None	72.0	71.8	72.4	66.2	
Ex-smoker	12.3	11.4	12.2	14.6	
Current	15.7	16.8	15.4	19.2	
Education (%)					0.148
None	26.7	30.1	30.4	30.4	
Elementary school	49.6	49.7	50.0	49.6	
Middle school	14.1	12.3	11.2	11.7	
High school	8.4	6.0	6.7	6.8	
College	1.2	1.8	1.7	1.4	
TyG index	8.0±0.2	8.4±0.1	8.8±0.1	9.4±0.3	<0.0001

Data are expressed as means ± SD, % or median (25th–75th percentiles).
BMI, body mass index; BP, blood pressure; DM, diabetes mellitus; FPG, fasting plasma glucose; HDL, high-density lipoprotein; HOMA-ß, homeostasis model assessment estimate of beta-cell function; HOMA-IR, homeostasis model assessment of insulin resistance; LDL, low-density lipoprotein.

0.0001), fasting insulin levels (r = 0.249; *P*<0.0001), HOMA-IR (r = 0.273; *P*<0.0001), and HOMA-ß (r = 0.143; *P*<0.0001) indicating that this index could reflect the degree of insulin resistance and compensatory ß-cell function in these study subjects.

The Incidence of Diabetes According to TyG Index Quartiles

Figure 1 shows the incidence of diabetes, which increased in proportion to TyG index quartiles (Q1, 3.3%; Q2, 6.9%; Q3, 7.2%; Q4, 14.1%; *P* for trend <0.0001). Similar results could be observed in both men (Q1, 4.2%; Q2, 7.5%; Q3, 6.3%; Q4, 14.7%; *P* for trend <0.0001) and women (Q1, 2.8%; Q2, 6.5%; Q3, 7.6%; Q4, 13.7%; *P* for trend <0.0001).

Prediction of the Development of Diabetes using the TyG Index

Log-Binomial regression analyses were performed to evaluate the TyG index in predicting the incident diabetes (Table 3). In the initial crude analysis, a statistically significant association was shown between an increased TyG index and an increased risk of incident diabetes in subjects in Q2–Q4 vs. those in Q1. Adjustment for age, gender and BMI (model 1), and further adjustment for waist circumference, systolic BP, HDL-cholesterol,

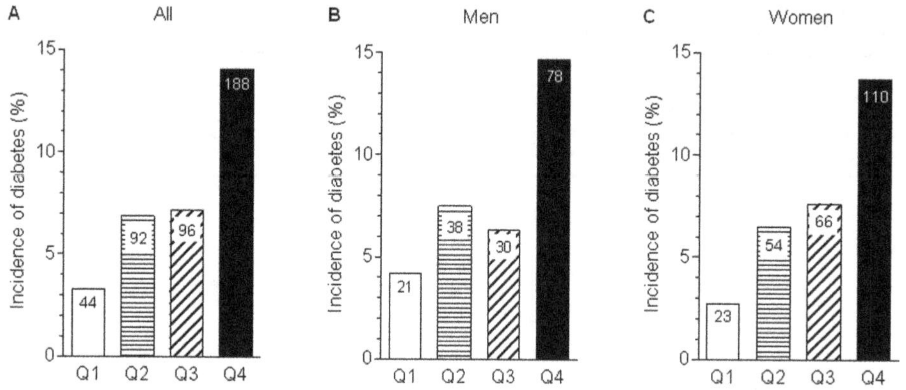

Figure 1. Incidence of diabetes according to the baseline TyG index quartiles in all study subjects (A), men (B), and women (C). The number in the bar indicates the number of participants with incident diabetes.

family history of diabetes, smoking, alcohol drinking and education level (model 2) did not attenuate this association. Even after further adjustment for fasting serum insulin level, which reflects the degree of insulin resistance (model 3), the risk of incident diabetes was more than fourfold higher in the Q4 vs. the Q1 group (RR, 4.095; 95% CI, 2.701–6.207). There were no significant differences in the results of this analysis between men and women or between obese (BMI≥25 kg/m^2) and nonobese (BMI<25 kg/m^2) subjects (Tables S1, S2). To compare the predictive role of TyG index with other indices of insulin resistance, we performed similar analyses with the TG/HDL-cholesterol ratio and HOMA-IR. The TG/HDL-cholesterol ratio also proved to be a useful tool for predicting the development of diabetes, but with a significantly lower RR than the TyG index. After adjusting for age, gender, BMI, waist circumference, systolic BP, family history of diabetes, smoking, alcohol drinking, education level, and insulin, the RR (95% CI) of diabetes risk in the highest quartile vs. the lowest quartile of the TG/HDL-cholesterol ratio was 2.209 (1.566–3.115) (Table 3). Regarding the HOMA-IR values, only subjects in the highest quartile but not in the second or third quartile showed a significantly increased risk of diabetes (RR, 1.621; 95% CI, 1.171–2.243) compared with the lowest quartile group after adjustment for age, gender and BMI. However, this association disappeared after further adjustment for multiple variables (Table 3). The AUC (95% CI) of the ROC curve for the TyG index at 0.645 (0.632–0.659) was significantly higher than that of the TG/HDL-cholesterol ratio at 0.609 (0.595–0.623) or HOMA-IR at 0.592 (0.578–0.606). These results suggest that the TyG index is superior to the TG/HDL-cholesterol ratio or HOMA-IR in predicting the risk of incident diabetes.

Discussion

In this large prospective cohort study, we found that individuals in the highest baseline quartile of TyG index had a fourfold higher risk of developing diabetes than those in the lowest quartile during a median of 4.6 years of follow-up. The predictive value of the TyG index was better than other indices of insulin resistance such as HOMA-IR or TG/HDL-cholesterol ratio. These findings highlight the usefulness of this simple index for identifying individuals with a high risk of developing diabetes.

Prospective studies on the natural history of type 2 diabetes indicate that insulin resistance is a primary defect that can occur many years before the diagnosis [17,18]. Thus, examining the degree of insulin resistance with an accurate measure will be a key factor to improve prediction of incident diabetes. Because the hyperinsulinemic–euglycemic insulin clamp technique, a gold standard method for quantifying the degree of insulin resistance, is difficult to apply in clinical practice, several indices derived from the OGTT have been evaluated. Calculated indices reflecting insulin resistance or both insulin resistance and insulin secretory capacity showed their substantial ability to predict future type 2 diabetes [22–24]. However, simpler indices with a single blood test would be appropriate for a screening tool in large epidemiologic studies.

The TyG index, the product of FPG and TG levels, was proposed by Guerrero-Romero et al. as a surrogate of insulin resistance with a Pearson's correlation coefficient of 0.322 with HOMA-IR, and −0.681 with M rates measured by the hyperinsulinemic–euglycemic clamp test [15,16]. This correlation was similar between men and women, nonobese and obese, and nondiabetic and diabetic individuals. Another study in a Brazilian population supported this correlation [25]. The TyG index was also significantly correlated with insulin-stimulated glucose uptake measured as the steady-state plasma glucose concentration during insulin suppression testing [26], and was better associated with carotid atherosclerosis than HOMA-IR [27]. However, there are no data examining whether this index has a predictive role in identifying individuals with a high risk of developing diabetes. Our data suggest that it has a good performance in this regard. Even after adjusting for several known risk factors of diabetes and insulin level, the association between the baseline TyG index and the risk of incident diabetes was statistically significant, indicating that the TyG index is an independent risk factor. Of note, this association was similar between obese and nonobese subjects, and between men and women suggesting that the TyG index might be applicable to a wide range of subjects. The incidence rate was approximately twofold higher in subjects in the Q2 and Q3 TyG groups and more than fourfold higher in subjects in the Q4 group in this study population.

The TG/HDL-cholesterol ratio is another surrogate measure of insulin resistance demonstrated by several researchers although the relationship might differ by ethnicity [28,29]. This simple index also has been shown to be associated with the risk of future diabetes [30,31]. Our analysis shows that the subjects in the highest quartile of the TG/HDL-cholesterol ratio had a lower RR of diabetes development when compared with those in the Q4 TyG index group. Similarly, the RR of incident diabetes among subjects in the highest quartile of the HOMA-IR was significantly lower than for those in the Q4 TyG index group. This observation

Table 3. Associations of baseline TyG index, TG/HDL-cholesterol ratio and HOMA-IR with the risk of future diabetes.

	Crude	Model 1	Model 2	Model 3
TyG index				
Q1	1 (Ref.)	1 (Ref.)	1 (Ref.)	1 (Ref.)
Q2	2.163 (1.498–3.124)	2.026 (1.400–2.930)	2.099 (1.426–3.090)	2.286 (1.502–3.479)
Q3	2.261 (1.569–3.258)	2.022 (1.399–2.921)	1.960 (1.323–2.903)	2.020 (1.317–3.100)
Q4	4.806 (3.429–6.737)	4.152 (2.947–5.848)	4.098 (2.805–5.987)	4.095 (2.701–6.207)
P for trend	<0.0001	<0.0001	<0.0001	<0.0001
TG/HDL-cholesterol ratio				
Q1	1 (Ref.)	1 (Ref.)	1 (Ref.)	1 (Ref.)
Q2	1.528 (1.100–2.122)	1.409 (1.012–1.960)	1.422 (1.011–1.999)	1.441 (1.001–2.075)
Q3	1.598 (1.154–2.214)	1.418 (1.020–1.971)	1.308 (0.929–1.843)	1.299 (0.898–1.880)
Q4	2.847 (2.107–3.846)	2.446 (1.801–3.322)	2.267 (1.648–3.119)	2.209 (1.566–3.115)
P value	<0.0001	<0.0001	<0.0001	0.0002
HOMA-IR				
Q1	1 (Ref.)	1 (Ref.)	1 (Ref.)	
Q2	0.896 (0.635–1.266)	0.864 (0.610–1.223)	0.845 (0.589–1.212)	
Q3	1.269 (0.921–1.749)	1.152 (0.827–1.604)	1.084 (0.757–1.552)	
Q4	1.986 (1.474–2.676)	1.621 (1.171–2.243)	1.542 (0.997–2.387)	
P value	0.0001	0.015	0.103	

Results are expressed as RRs (95% CI).
Model 1: Adjusted for age, gender, and BMI.
Model 2: Adjusted for model 1+ waist circumference, systolic BP, HDL-cholesterol, family history of diabetes, smoking, alcohol drinking, and education level.
For the TG/HDL-cholesterol ratio, the HDL-cholesterol level was removed as a covariable.
For the HOMA-IR, the TG level was added as a covariable.
Model 3: Adjusted for model 2+ insulin level.
HDL, high-density lipoprotein; HOMA-IR, homeostasis model assessment of insulin resistance; TG, triglycerides.

might be explained by the fact that muscle is the major organ of insulin action and glucose uptake, accounting for 85–90% of the impairment in total body glucose disposal in patients with type 2 diabetes [18,32]. Because elevation of TG levels in blood and skeletal muscle interfere with glucose metabolism in muscle [33], the TyG index seems to mainly reflect muscle insulin resistance while HOMA-IR mainly mirrors hepatic insulin resistance [34]. Therefore, it is possible that the TyG index is superior to previously known indices for diabetes prediction, although our data need to be confirmed in other ethnic populations with different characteristics.

The strength of this study is that the study subjects were from a large scale cohort with long-term follow-up and there were sufficient cases for rigorous analysis. Diagnosis of diabetes by OGTT, although not performed in all participants in the present study, minimizes the number of overlooked cases with isolated post-load hyperglycemia. To our knowledge, this is the first report on the TyG index in an Asian population that has examined its ability as a predictive marker of future diabetes. This study also has limitations. Because the rate of follow-up loss was relatively high, the potential for selection bias needs to be considered. In addition, the findings of our study might not be generalized because it was performed in a semirural area on subjects with similar lifestyles. Although lack of information on the use of lipid-lowering agents might have influenced the result, we think that it would be minimal because only 2.3% of subjects reported that they were diagnosed as having hyperlipidemia. Another limitation is that different criteria for the normal FPG level were used at the baseline and follow-up studies.

It will be interesting to test whether a postprandial TyG index might also have meaningful effects. Because elevated postprandial levels of TG and glucose represent metabolically abnormal responses that reflect insulin resistance [35,36], higher risks of diabetes or cardiovascular events might be associated with a higher postprandial TyG index, which remains to be clarified.

In conclusion, we propose that the TyG index is a valuable marker reflecting the degree of insulin resistance and predicting the risk of future diabetes in both men and women, and in obese and nonobese individuals. Because it can be easily calculated from routine laboratory data, our findings suggest the possibility of applying this index in risk assessment for diabetes in real clinical practice or large epidemiologic studies. Therefore, confirmation of our data in other populations is warranted for further application of this marker.

Acknowledgments

The authors wish to thank all the survey personnel and the officers in Chungju Health Center for continued support.

Author Contributions

Conceived and designed the experiments: SHL HSK YMP KHY. Performed the experiments: SHL HSK YMP HSH JHL HWY WCL HYS KHY. Analyzed the data: SHL HSK YMP SHJ HKY MIK KHY. Wrote the paper: SHL KHY.

References

1. Shaw JE, Sicree RA, Zimmet PZ (2010) Global estimates of the prevalence of diabetes for 2010 and 2030. Diabetes Res Clin Pract 87: 4–14.
2. Yoon KH, Lee JH, Kim JW, Cho JH, Choi YH, et al. (2006) Epidemic obesity and type 2 diabetes in Asia. Lancet 368: 1681–1688.
3. Task Force Team for Basic Statistical Study of Korean Diabetes Mellitus of Korean Diabetes Association, Park IeB, Kim J, Kim DJ, Chung CH, et al. (2013) Diabetes epidemics in Korea: reappraise nationwide survey of diabetes "diabetes in Korea 2007". Diabetes Metab J 37: 233–239.
4. Knowler WC, Barrett-Connor E, Fowler SE, Hamman RF, Lachin JM, et al. (2002) Reduction in the incidence of type 2 diabetes with lifestyle intervention or metformin. N Engl J Med 346: 393–403.
5. Dallmeier D, Larson MG, Wang N, Fontes JD, Benjamin EJ, et al. (2012) Addition of inflammatory biomarkers did not improve diabetes prediction in the community: the framingham heart study. J Am Heart Assoc 1: e000869.
6. Kashima S, Inoue K, Matsumoto M, Akimoto K (2013) Do non-glycaemic markers add value to plasma glucose and hemoglobin a1c in predicting diabetes? Yuport health checkup center study. PLos One 8: e66899.
7. Echouffo-Tcheugui JB, Dieffenbach SD, Kengne AP (2013) Added value of novel circulating and genetic biomarkers in type 2 diabetes prediction: A systematic review. Diabetes Res Clin Pract 101: 255–269.
8. Schulze MB, Weikert C, Pischon T, Bergmann MM, Al-Hasani H, et al. (2009) Use of multiple metabolic and genetic markers to improve the prediction of type 2 diabetes: the EPIC-Potsdam Study. Diabetes Care 32: 2116–2119.
9. Tirosh A, Shai I, Tekes-Manova D, Israeli E, Pereg D, et al. (2005) Normal fasting plasma glucose levels and type 2 diabetes in young men. N Engl J Med 353: 1454–1462.
10. Rhee SY, Woo JT (2011) The prediabetic period: review of clinical aspects. Diabetes Metab J 35: 107–116.
11. Dotevall A, Johansson S, Wilhelmsen L, Rosengren A (2004) Increased levels of triglycerides, BMI and blood pressure and low physical activity increase the risk of diabetes in Swedish women. A prospective 18-year follow-up of the BEDA study. Diabet Med 21: 615–622.
12. Hjellvik V, Sakshaug S, Strøm H (2012) Body mass index, triglycerides, glucose, and blood pressure as predictors of type 2 diabetes in a middle-aged Norwegian cohort of men and women. Clin Epidemiol 4: 213–224.
13. Wilson PW, Meigs JB, Sullivan L, Fox CS, Nathan DM, et al. (2007) Prediction of incident diabetes mellitus in middle-aged adults: the Framingham Offspring Study. Arch Intern Med 167: 1068–1074.
14. Tirosh A, Shai I, Bitzur R, Kochba I, Tekes-Manova D, et al. (2008) Changes in triglyceride levels over time and risk of type 2 diabetes in young men. Diabetes Care 31: 2032–2037.
15. Simental-Mendía LE, Rodríguez-Morán M, Guerrero-Romero F (2008) The product of fasting glucose and triglycerides as surrogate for identifying insulin resistance in apparently healthy subjects. Metab Syndr Relat Disord 6: 299–304.
16. Guerrero-Romero F, Simental-Mendía LE, González-Ortiz M, Martínez-Abundis E, Ramos-Zavala MG, et al. (2010) The product of triglycerides and glucose, a simple measure of insulin sensitivity. Comparison with the euglycemic-hyperinsulinemic clamp. J Clin Endocrinol Metab 95: 3347–3351.
17. Warram JH, Martin BC, Krolewski AS, Soeldner JS, Kahn CR (1990) Slow glucose removal rate and hyperinsulinemia precede the development of type II diabetes in the offspring of diabetic parents. Ann Intern Med 113: 909–915.
18. DeFronzo RA (2009) From the triumvirate to the ominous octet: a new paradigm for the treatment of type 2 diabetes mellitus. Diabetes 58: 773–795.
19. Matthews DR, Hosker JP, Rudenski AS, Naylor BA, Treacher DF, et al. (1985) Homeostasis model assessment: insulin resistance and beta-cell function from fasting plasma glucose and insulin concentrations in man. Diabetologia 28: 412–419.
20. The expert committee on the diagnosis and classification of diabetes mellitus (1997) Report of the expert committee on the diagnosis and classification of diabetes mellitus. Diabetes Care 20: 1183–1197.
21. The expert committee on the diagnosis and classification of diabetes mellitus (2003) Follow-up report on the diagnosis of diabetes mellitus. Diabetes Care 26: 3160–3167.
22. Abdul-Ghani MA, Williams K, DeFronzo RA, Stern M (2007) What is the best predictor of future type 2 diabetes? Diabetes Care 30: 1544–1548.
23. Hanley AJ, Williams K, Gonzalez C, D'Agostino RB Jr, Wagenknecht LE, et al. (2003) Prediction of type 2 diabetes using sample measures of insulin resistance: combined results from the San Antonio Heart Study, the Mexico City Diabetes Study, and the Insulin Resistance Atherosclerosis Study. Diabetes 52: 463–469.
24. Lorenzo C, Hazuda HP, Haffner SM (2012) Insulin resistance and excess risk of diabetes in Mexican-Americans: the San Antonio Heart Study. J Clin Endocrinol Metab 97: 793–799.
25. Vasques AC, Novaes FS, de Oliveira Mda S, Souza JR, Yamanaka A, et al. (2011) TyG index performs better than HOMA in a Brazilian population: a hyperglycemic clamp validated study. Diabetes Res Clin Pract 93: e98–e100.
26. Abbasi F, Reaven GM (2011) Comparison of two methods using plasma triglyceride concentration as a surrogate estimate of insulin action in nondiabetic subjects: triglycerides × glucose versus triglyceride/high-density lipoprotein cholesterol. Metabolism 60: 1673–1676.
27. Irace C, Carallo C, Scavelli FB, De Franceschi MS, Esposito T, et al. (2013) Markers of insulin resistance and carotid atherosclerosis. A comparison of the homeostasis model assessment and triglyceride glucose index. Int J Clin Pract 67: 665–672.
28. McLaughlin T, Abbasi F, Cheal K, Chu J, Lamendola C, et al. (2003) Use of metabolic markers to identify overweight individuals who are insulin resistant. Ann Intern Med 139: 802–809.
29. Kim-Dorner SJ, Deuster PA, Zeno SA, Remaley AT, Poth M (2010) Should triglycerides and the triglycerides to high-density lipoprotein cholesterol ratio be used as surrogates for insulin resistance? Metabolism 59: 299–304.
30. He S, Wang S, Chen X, Jiang L, Peng Y, et al. (2012) Higher ratio of triglyceride to high-density lipoprotein cholesterol may predispose to diabetes mellitus: 15-year prospective study in general population. Metabolism 61: 30–36.
31. Hadaegh F, Hatami M, Tohidi M, Sarbakhsh P, Saadat N, et al. (2010) Lipid ratios and appropriate cut off values for prediction of diabetes: a cohort of Iranian men and women. Lipids Health Dis 9: 85.
32. DeFronzo RA, Gunnarsson R, Björkman O, Olsson M, Wahren J (1985) Effects of insulin on peripheral and splanchnic glucose metabolism in noninsulin-dependent (type II) diabetes mellitus. J Clin Invest 76: 149–155.
33. Kelley DE, Goodpaster BH, Storlien L (2002) Muscle triglyceride and insulin resistance. Annu Rev Nutr 22: 325–346.
34. Tripathy D, Almgren P, Tuomi T, Groop L (2004) Contribution of insulin-stimulated glucose uptake and basal hepatic insulin sensitivity to surrogate measures of insulin sensitivity. Diabetes Care 27: 2204–2210.
35. Bansal S, Buring JE, Rifai N, Mora S, Sacks FM, et al. (2007) Fasting compared with nonfasting triglycerides and risk of cardiovascular events in women. JAMA 298: 309–316.
36. Kolovou GD, Mikhailidis DP, Kovar J, Lairon D, Nordestgaard BG, et al. (2011) Assessment and clinical relevance of non-fasting and postprandial triglycerides: an expert panel statement. Curr Vasc Pharmacol 9: 258–270.

IGFBP-3 Inhibits Cytokine-Induced Insulin Resistance and Early Manifestations of Atherosclerosis

Lathika Mohanraj[1], Ho-Seong Kim[2], Wei Li[3], Qing Cai[1], Ki Eun Kim[4], Hye-Jung Shin[5], Yong-Jae Lee[6], Woo Jung Lee[2], Jung Hyun Kim[2], Youngman Oh[1,3]*

1 Department of Pathology, Virginia Commonwealth University, Richmond, Virginia, United States of America, **2** Department of Pediatrics, Institute of Endocrinology, Yonsei University College of Medicine, Seoul, Korea, **3** Biocure Pharma LLC, Richmond, Virginia, United States of America, **4** Department of Pediatrics, CHA University College of Medicine, Seoul, Korea, **5** Department of Pediatrics, National Medical Center, Seoul, Korea, **6** Department of Family Medicine, Yonsei University College of Medicine, Seoul, Korea

Abstract

Metabolic syndrome is associated with visceral obesity, insulin resistance and an increased risk of cardiovascular diseases. Visceral fat tissue primarily consists of adipocytes that secrete cytokines leading to a state of systemic inflammation in obese conditions. One of the IGF-independent functions of IGFBP-3 is its role as an anti-inflammatory molecule. Our study in obese adolescents show a decrease in total IGFBP-3 levels and increase in proteolyzed IGFBP-3 in circulation when compared to their normal counterparts and establishes a positive correlation between IGFBP-3 proteolysis and adiposity parameters as well as insulin resistance. In human adipocytes, we show that IGFBP-3 inhibits TNF-α-induced NF-κB activity in an IGF-independent manner, thereby restoring the deregulated insulin signaling and negating TNF-α-induced inhibition of glucose uptake. IGFBP-3 further inhibits TNF-α, CRP and high glucose-induced NF-κB activity in human aortic endothelial cells (HAECs) and subsequently suppresses monocyte adhesion to HAEC through the IGFBP-3 receptor. In conclusion, these findings suggest that reduced levels of IGFBP-3 in circulation and reduced expression of IGFBP-3 in macrophages in obesity may result in suppression of its anti-inflammatory functions and therefore IGFBP-3 may present itself as a therapeutic for obesity-induced insulin resistance and for events occurring in the early stages of atherosclerosis.

Editor: Josep Bassaganya-Riera, Virginia Tech, United States of America

Funding: This work was supported by United States Department of Defense (DOD) grant (PC061151) to YO and the Yonsei University College of Medicine-MSD Grant (6-2006-0151) to HK. The funders had no role in study design, data collection and analysis, decision to publish, or preparation of the manuscript.

Competing Interests: YO is the founder of BioCure Pharma LLC and WL is an employee of BioCure Pharma LLC.

* E-mail: yoh@mcvh-vcu.edu

These authors contributed equally to this work.

Introduction

Over the past two decades obesity has dramatically increased resulting in one-third of the adults in the United States being obese [1]. Obesity is a complex disorder and is a major risk factor associated with the incidence of diabetes, insulin resistance, cardiovascular diseases (CVD), hypertension, diabetic retinopathy and other metabolic disorders [2]. The endocrine paradigm suggests that visceral fat in obesity, consisting primarily of adipocytes, secretes various pro-inflammatory and pro-atherogenic adipokines such as TNF-α, C-reactive protein (CRP) [3], IL-6 and others [4] creating a state of local inflammation further resulting in chronic systemic inflammation and accelerating the events leading to metabolic disorders.

The IGF system plays a major role in growth, development and maintenance of homeostasis in normal cells. Insulin-like growth factor binding protein-3 (IGFBP-3), the major binding protein in circulation [5] has been shown to be associated with CVD, coronary events [6] and thickness of the intima-media [7]. A study comparing the concentrations of IGFs and IGFBP-3 with respect to BMI and body fat revealed that these levels are decreased in obese women [8]. IGFBP-3 overexpression in the retinal endothelium has also been shown to restore vascular integrity, suggesting that IGFBP-3 may represent treatment of diabetic retinopathy [9]. These observations clearly indicate involvement of IGFBP-3 in CVD, obesity and insulin resistance; however the mechanisms responsible for the role of IGFBP-3 in metabolic syndrome remains poorly understood.

In addition to IGF-dependent functions, IGF-independent functions of IGFBP-3 have also been studied [10]. Some of the disease states that show IGF-independent actions of IGFBP-3 include cancer [11] and asthma [12]. IGFBP-3 exerts antitumor and anti-inflammatory effects via a specific receptor (IGFBP-3R) that involves activation of caspase pathway and cross-talk with NF-κB signaling [11,13]. Another interesting attribute that may regulate the functions of IGFBP-3 is proteolytic cleavage of IGFBP-3 that has been reported in several physiological and pathological conditions, including cancer, type 1 and 2 diabetes, burn injuries, and surgery, suggesting that catabolic states increase degradation of circulating IGFBP-3 [14–18]. In line with the potential anti-inflammatory role of IGFBP-3 in cancers and other diseases [11–13,15,16] and its crosstalk with the NF-κB pathway, our study investigates the relationship between proteolyzed IGFBP-3 in circulation and the parameters of adiposity and the potential role of IGFBP-3 in obesity-induced insulin resistance and its involvement in the progression of atherosclerosis and CVD.

Results

IGFBP-3 Profile in Normal and Obese Adolescents

A total of 197 adolescents aged 12 to 13 years were classified into control, overweight and obese groups according to BMI for age and gender. Comparisons of clinical features in all groups (Table 1) show that the obese group had significantly higher height, weight, BMI, waist circumference, systolic BP and diastolic BP than controls. HDL-cholesterol levels were markedly decreased in the obesity group. The obesity group had much higher levels of triglycerides, LDL-cholesterol and ALT than the controls (Table 2). Fasting insulin levels differed significantly in the obesity compared with other groups. The levels of fasting glucose were increased in the overweight and obesity compared to the control but was not significantly different between each other. HOMA-IR increased similarly (Table 3). Serum IGF-1 was increased in overweight and obese individuals compared with the normal group whereas total IGFBP-3 showed a slight increase in overweight individuals. However both IGF-1 and total IGFBP-3 levels showed a significant decrease in obese individuals compared to overweight individuals. Total IGFBP-3 levels in particular were less even when compared to the normal group (Table 1). The data further shows an increase in the IGF-1/IGFBP-3 in both overweight and obese groups when compared to the control group. In order to further analyze the IGFBP-3 levels, we determined the presence and distribution of proteolyzed IGFBP-3 in the overweight and obese subjects by Western immunoblot assay as well as protease activity assay. The western blot analysis of the serum samples shows a robust presence of IGFBP-3 proteolytic fragments (29-kDa and 18-kDa) in the obese and overweight groups, but low or no detection of these fragments were seen in controls. Densitometric analysis of the proteolytic IGFBP-3 fragments showed a 183 percent and a 184 percent increase in the overweight and obese groups respectively when compared to the control group (Figure 1A).

To investigate this further protease activity assay was performed on the samples, in which recombinant human glycosylated IGFBP-3 was biotinylated and IGFBP-3 protease activity was measured as the ability of serum samples from control, overweight and obese individuals to proteolyze biotinylated IGFBP-3. Results show that IGFBP-3 protease activity increased in overweight and obese individuals compared to the control group, but did not differ between the overweight and obese groups (Figure 1B).

Further statistical analyses revealed that proteolyzed IGFBP-3 positively correlates with adiposity parameters such as waist circumference ($r = 0.608$, $P<0.001$), BMI ($r = 0.4651$, $P<0.001$), fasting insulin ($r = 0.307$, $P = 0.001$), and insulin resistance index (HOMA-IR) ($r = 0.313$, $P<0.001$) in overweight and obese population (Figure 1C), suggesting that predisposition to insulin resistance and other consequences of increased visceral fat can occur even in overweight individuals and not necessarily only in obese population.

Taken together, based on our data and previous studies demonstrating IGFBP-3 proteolysis in patients with type 2 diabetes [17], we speculate that increased proteolytic IGFBP-3 fragments in overweight and obese individuals probably result in reduced levels of intact IGFBP-3 thereby inhibiting its IGF-independent anti-inflammatory functions. Based on these findings, we further investigated the effect of IGFBP-3 and its underlying mechanism in cytokine-induced insulin resistance in adipocytes and early manifestations of atherosclerosis in HAECs.

TNF-α Activates the NF-κB Pathway in Adipocytes in an *in vitro* System

Visceral adipocytes are highly responsive to TNF-α mediated activation of NF-κB pathway [18]. In order to confirm that the NF-κB pathway was intact in fully differentiated human primary adipocytes (ASCs), cells were treated with TNF-α and the pattern of NF-κB activation was analyzed. Figure 2A clearly indicates the cyclic phosphorylation pattern of IκBα and a time dependent increase in the levels of phospho-NF-κBp65. These results indicate that TNF-α activates the NF-κB pathway in ASCs.

Activation of the NF-κB Pathway Affects Insulin Signaling in Adipocytes

Cytokines such as TNF-α, interferes with insulin signaling by decreasing the levels of Insulin receptor substrate-1 (IRS-1) and Glucose transporter-4 (GLUT4) [19,20]. Deficient levels of adiponectin, an insulin sensitizing and anti-inflammatory adipokine are observed in individuals with visceral fat [21]. Our experiment was to determine the effect of TNF-α on IRS-1, GLUT4 and adiponectin levels in *in vitro* ASCs. Figure 2B demonstrates that TNF-α treatment decreases the transcriptional levels of IRS-1, GLUT4 and adiponectin in a dose dependent manner and treatment with IKK inhibitor shows that the reduced mRNA levels of our genes of interest were restored, confirming that TNF-α exerts its effect through the NF-κB pathway in adipocytes. This was confirmed by the decrease in the protein levels of IRS-1 with dose dependent TNF-α treatment (Figure 2C).

IGFBP-3 Inhibits the NF-κB Activity in Primary Human Adipocytes

To investigate the anti-inflammatory function of IGFBP-3 on TNF-α-induced NF-κB pathway and insulin signaling in ASCs, TNF-α treated cells were infected with adenoviral constructs containing IGFBP-3 sequence (Ad:IGFBP-3). ASCs produce no detectable basal level of IGFBP-3 and TNF-α-treatment shows no change in IGFBP-3 at the mRNA and protein levels (Figure 3). TNF-α inhibits IRS-1, GLUT4 and adiponectin in TNF-α-treated control cells, however, infection with Ad:IGFBP-3 restored IRS-1, GLUT4 and adiponectin mRNA (Figure 3A) and protein levels (Figure 3B). Overexpressed IGFBP-3 inhibits TNF-α-mediated induction of MCP-1 at both mRNA (Figure 3A) and protein levels (Figure 3B). Cells treated with IKK inhibitor confirmed involvement of the NF-κB pathway. These data show that IGFBP-3 inhibits the TNF-α-induced NF-κB activity, thereby restoring insulin signaling in ASCs.

IGFBP-3 Inhibits NF-κB Pathway in Human Adipocytes in an IGF-independent Manner

In order to decipher if IGFBP-3 inhibits the NF-κB pathway in adipocytes in an IGF- independent manner, we used IGFBP-3 ^{GGG} mutant, which has no binding affinity to IGF and therefore any effect of this mutant would be an IGF independent effect [22]. On infection with Ad:EV, Ad:IGFBP-3 and Ad:IGFBP-3^{GGG} mutant, semi-quantitative PCR shows that the effect of Ad:IGFBP-3^{GGG} on the mRNA levels of GLUT4, IRS-1, adiponectin and MCP-1 was similar to Ad:IGFBP-3 suggesting that IGFBP-3 effect on the NF-κB pathway in adipocytes was IGF-independent (Figure 3C). Protein expression of IRS-1, GLUT4, adiponectin and MCP-1 confirmed that IGFBP-3 inhibits the NF-κB pathway and successfully restores the repressed levels of IRS-1, GLUT4 and adiponectin in ASCs in an IGF-independent manner (Figure 3D).

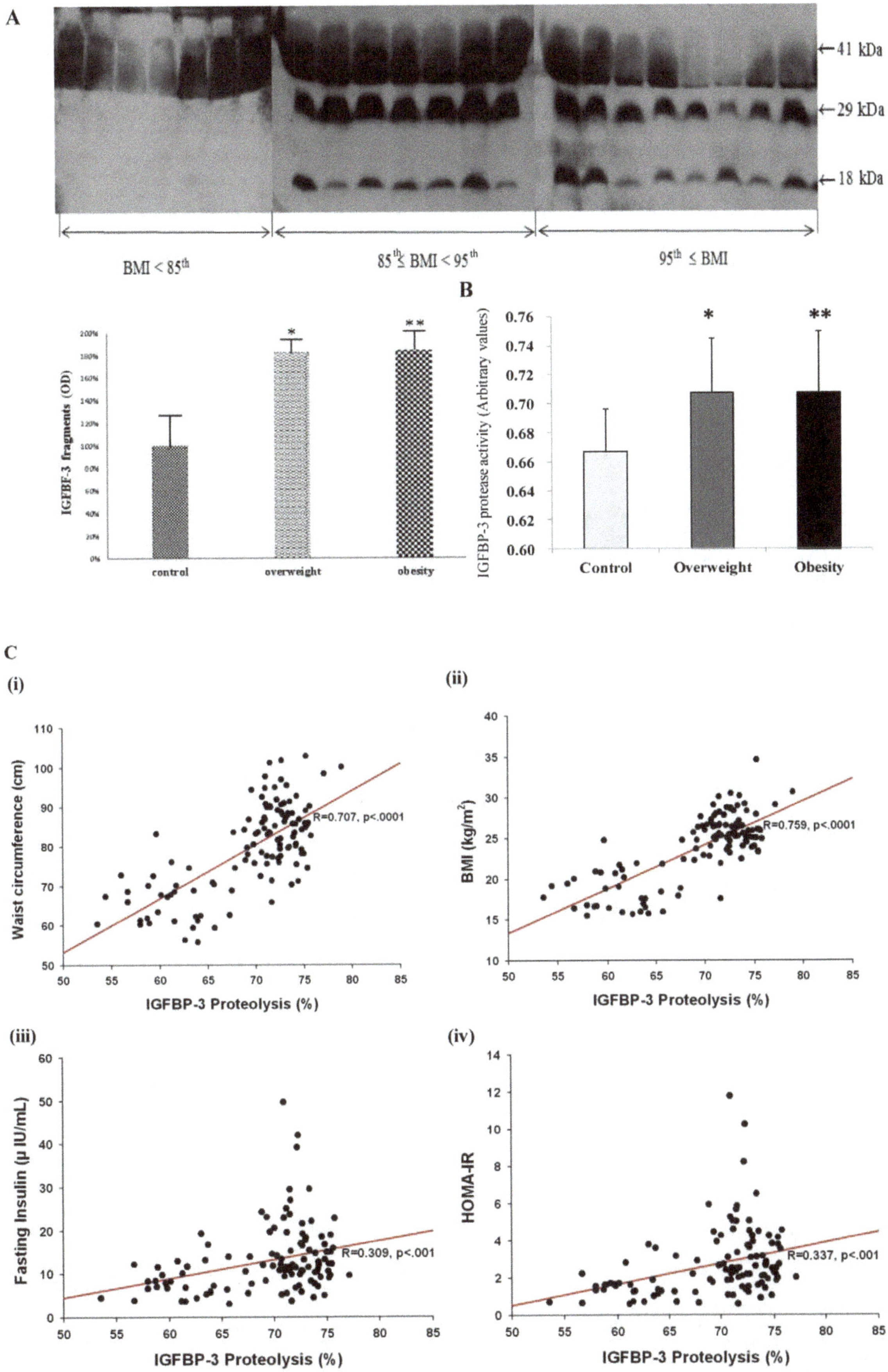
A
41 kDa
29 kDa
18 kDa
BMI < 85th
85th ≤ BMI < 95th
95th ≤ BMI
IGFBP-3 fragments (OD)
control
overweight
obesity
B
IGFBP-3 protease activity (Arbitrary values)
Control
Overweight
Obesity
C
(i)
Waist circumference (cm)
R=0.707, p<.0001
IGFBP-3 Proteolysis (%)
(ii)
BMI (kg/m2)
R=0.759, p<.0001
IGFBP-3 Proteolysis (%)
(iii)
Fasting Insulin (μ IU/mL)
R=0.309, p<.001
IGFBP-3 Proteolysis (%)
(iv)
HOMA-IR
R=0.337, p<.001
IGFBP-3 Proteolysis (%)

Figure 1. Increased IGFBP-3 proteolysis in obese adolescents. (A) The IGFBP-3 proteolytic fragments were detected by Western blot assay. Optical density was significantly increased in the overweight and obesity. *, control vs. overweight, 2.09±1.32 (100%) vs. 3.83±0.37 (183%), P<0.001; **, control vs. obesity, 2.09±1.32 (100%) vs. 3.85±0.63 (184%), P<0.001). (B) Protease activity assay was performed to determine IGFBP-3 proteolysis. The activity was measured as optical density and it was significantly higher in the overweight and obese group. *, control vs. overweight, 0.667±0.030 vs. 0.707±0.038, P=0.001; **, control vs. obesity, 0.667±0.030 vs. 0.708±0.043, P=0.002). (C) Relationship between IGFBP-3 proteolysis and (i) waist circumference (r=0.707, P<0.0001), (ii) BMI (r=0.759, P<0.0001), (iii) fasting insulin (r=0.309, P<0.001), and (iv) HOMA-IR (r=0.337, P<0.001) were calculated by Pearson's correlation coefficient.

TNF-α Induces Insulin Resistance in Human Adipocytes

The dose dependent effect of insulin on increasing glucose uptake in ASCs has been demonstrated in Figure 3E. However, visceral obesity is accompanied by release of various adipokines that leads to an inflammatory state resulting in insulin resistance wherein cells cease to respond to insulin presence. Figure 3F shows that increase in glucose uptake in the adipocytes on addition of insulin is inhibited in the presence of TNF-α, showing its role in insulin resistance. The IKK inhibitor treatment restores glucose uptake by the cells indicating that the decrease in glucose uptake by TNF-α was mediated via the NF-κB pathway.

IGFBP-3 Negates TNF-α Induced Inhibition of Glucose Uptake in Human Adipocytes

In order to determine the effect of IGFBP-3 on TNF-α-induced insulin resistance, adipocytes were infected with IGFBP-3 alone and in the presence of TNF-α and insulin. Figure 3G shows that insulin alone increased the glucose uptake to almost 400 percent, however no change in glucose uptake was observed in the presence of IGFBP-3 alone, suggesting that IGFBP-3 under normal conditions does not regulate glucose metabolism. On the contrary, cells treated with TNF-α and insulin together showed more than a 50 percent decrease in glucose uptake but infection with IGFBP-3 abolished the TNF-α effect and restored levels of glucose uptake. Therefore, IGFBP-3 abrogates TNF-α-mediated inhibition of glucose uptake in human adipocytes and does not affect normal glucose metabolism.

TNF-α Activates the NF-κB Pathway in HAECs

In obesity, cytokines like TNF-α are elevated in circulation and result in cardiovascular endothelial dysfunction, plaque formation and CVD [23]. We studied the effect of TNF-α on cardiovascular endothelial cells by treating HAECs with TNF-α and observed a cyclic pattern in the levels of phospho-IκBα and total IκBα and an increase in phospho-p65 levels (Figure 4A). Figure 4B, shows that the downstream targets of the NF-κB pathway, ICAM-1, VCAM-1 and MCP-1 mRNA levels increased in a dose dependent manner ranging 0–100 ng/ml of TNF-α treatment and Figure 4C shows a dose dependent increase in the protein expression of ICAM-1 and VCAM-1 with TNF-α treatment.

Expression Pattern of IGFBPs in HAECs

Figure 4D shows detectable endogenous levels of IGFBP-3 mRNA; however levels of other IGFBPs were not detected. Furthermore, Figure 5E shows no detectable levels of IGFBP-3 at the protein level and TNF-α treatment alone does not alter the levels of IGFBP-3 protein secreted in the conditioned media.

IGFBP-3 Inhibits TNF-α Induced Activation of NF-κB Activity in HAECs

To determine if IGFBP-3 also plays an anti-inflammatory role in HAECs, TNF-α treated HAECs were infected with Ad:IGFBP-3 and the mRNA and expression levels of NF-κB-regulated target genes were analyzed. Figure 5A shows that IGFBP-3 alone has no effect on the mRNA levels however, infection with Ad:IGFBP-3, in the presence of TNF-α (50 ng/ml) significantly downregulates the mRNA levels of TNF-α-induced ICAM-1, VCAM-1 and MCP-1. IKK inhibitor treatment confirms that TNF-α and IGFBP-3 mediate their effects by regulating the NF-κB pathway. Figure 5B shows the protein profile for ICAM-1, confirming that

Table 1. Clinical and anthropometric characteristics of subjects.

	Controls	Overweight	Obese	P value
n (M:F)	100 (49:51)	41 (19:22)	56 (25:31)	NS
Age (years)	12.2±0.4	12.2±0.4	12.2±0.3	NS
Weight (kg)	47.2±6.9	61.0±6.9	69.7±7.7	a
Height (cm)	156.9±7.1	157.9±7.2	160±5.7	b
BMI (kg/m ^{2})	19.1±1.9	24.4±1.0	27.2±1.8	a
Waist Circumference (cm)	68.5±6.2	80.8±5.6	87.9±7.0	a
Systolic BP (mmHg)	101.2±10.8	107.9±10.6	114.8±10.7	a
Diastolic BP (mmHg)	63.6±6.4	65.6±7.5	69.9±7.8	c
IGF-1 (ng/ml)	120.3±63.4	153.6±88.1	145.5±73.8	d
IGFBP-3 (ug/mL)	7.11±1.16	7.47±1.02	6.82±1.28	e
IGF-1/IGFBP-3 molar ratio	0.129±0.051	0.162±0.068	0.161±0.08	f

NS, not significant; BMI, body mass index. Values are expressed as mean ± SD. Each group was classified by the BMI percentile according to 2007 Korea Growth Charts.

[a]control *vs.* overweight; overweight *vs.* obesity; control *vs.* obesity; respectively, *P*<0.01.

[b]control *vs.* overweight (*P*<0.01), and overweight *vs.* obesity (*P*<0.01).

[c]control *vs.* overweight (*P*<0.01), and control *vs.* obesity (*P*<0.01).

[d]control *vs.* overweight (*P*<0.05), and control *vs.* obesity (*P*<0.05).

[e]overweight *vs.* obese (*P*<0.05).

[f]control *vs.* overweight (*P*<0.004), and control *vs.* obesity (*P*<0.01).

Table 2. Biochemical characteristics of subjects.

	Controls	Overweight	Obese	*P* value
Total cholesterol (mg/dL)	145.4±32.3	158.6±29.0	150.3±34.0	NS
HDL-cholesterol (mg/dL)	53.1±13.3	53.6±11.4	46.5±10.6	a
Triglycerides (mg/dL)	82.9±37.6	110.9±47.7	103.2±36.8	b
LDL-cholesterol (mg/dL)	75.9±24.2	82.9±23.3	84.7±26.5	c
AST (IU/L)	21.8±12.6	22.9±10.3	26.0±17.6	NS
ALT (IU/L)	11.4±21.4	17.2±2.7	20.9±20.8	a
hs-CRP (mg/dL)	0.07±0.13	0.07±0.13	0.11±0.11	NS

Values are expressed as mean ± SD.

[a]control *vs.* obesity (*P*<0.01), and overweight *vs.* obesity (*P*<0.01).

[b]control *vs.* overweight (*P*<0.01), and control *vs.* obesity (*P*<0.01).

[c]control *vs.* overweight (*P*<0.05), and control *vs.* obesity (*P*<0.05).

P values were calculated by one-way ANOVA.

Table 3. Insulin resistance of subjects.

	Controls	Overweight	Obese	*P* value
Fasting glucose (mg/dL)	75.8±11.3	86.3±12.5	85.3±7.2	a
Fasting insulin (μIU/Ml)	8.0±4.0	12.9±8.7	16.9±9.5	b
HOMA-IR	1.5±0.8	2.9±3.2	3.6±2.2	a

[a]control *vs.* overweight ($P<0.001$), and control *vs.* obesity ($P<0.001$).
[b]control *vs.* overweight, overweight *vs.* obesity, and control *vs.* obesity, respectively; $P<0.001$.
P values were calculated by one-way ANOVA.

IGFBP-3 inhibits TNF-α induced NF-κB activity in HAECs.

IGFBP-3 Suppresses MCP-1 Levels and Inhibits Monocyte Adhesion to HAEC Monolayer

One of the consequences of chronic inflammatory state induced by the adipokines secreted by the visceral adipose tissue is increase in the recruitment of monocytes to cardiovascular endothelial cells, eventually leading to plaque formation. *In vitro* data shows that TNF-α-treated HAECs show increase in MCP-1 levels, whereas IGFBP-3 abolishes TNF-α effects (Figure 5C). Since MCP-1 levels are indicative of monocyte adhesion in cells, we performed a monocyte adhesion experiment that showed that HAECs treated with TNF-α lead to a two-fold increase in monocyte adhesion to a monolayer of heart cells and infection with Ad:IGFBP-3 inhibited monocyte adhesion to HAEC cells (Figure 5D). This confirms that IGFBP-3 inhibits a biological effect of TNF-α-induced pro-inflammatory activity in HAECs.

IGFBP-3 Inhibits the Action of CVD Risk Factors, CRP and High Glucose

Other factors in circulation that adversely contribute towards CVD include insulin resistance-induced high glucose and CRP. Increase in the mRNA levels of ICAM-1, VCAM-1 and MCP-1 was observed on addition of CRP (Figure 5E) or high glucose (Figure 5G) and infection with IGFBP-3 significantly decreased these levels. We also confirm that both CRP (Figure 5F) and high glucose (Figure 5H) have a similar effect even on the protein levels of the NF-κB downstream targets and HAEC cells infected with Ad:IGFBP-3 reduce these levels.

IGFBP-3 Inhibits the NF-κB Pathway in an IGF-independent Manner

In order to elucidate the underlying mechanism in the inhibition of NF-κB pathway by IGFBP-3, and to determine if this effect was an IGF-independent, HAECs were infected with Ad:IGFBP-3^{GGG} and then treated with TNF-α. Figure 6A shows that infection with Ad: IGFBP-3^{GGG} followed by TNF-α treatment inhibits the mRNA levels of ICAM-1 and VCAM-1 similar to Ad:IGFBP-3 compared to the control. This pattern was also seen in protein expression (Figure 6B). An MCP-1 ELISA assay determined that both Ad:IGFBP-3^{GGG} and Ad:IGFBP-3 inhibited TNF-α- induced MCP-1 levels (Figure 6C). Ad:IGFBP-3^{GGG} also inhibited monocyte adhesion to the HAECs comparable to the effect of Ad:IGFBP-3 (Figure 6D). Furthermore, to determine if IGFBP-3 inhibits the NF-κB pathway and its downstream targets, through IGFBP-3R, HAECs were transfected with siRNA to knockdown endogenous levels of IGFBP-3R (Figure 6E). Figure 6F shows that Ad:IGFBP-3 inhibited expression of ICAM-1 by 40 percent and knockdown of IGFBP-3R negates the inhibitory effect of IGFBP-3 on TNF-α-induced levels of downstream target of the NF-κB pathway and restores the levels of ICAM-1.

Differential Expression of IGFBP-3 in Classically and Alternately Activated Macrophages

In addition to adipocytes, tissue macrophages have also been shown to be responsible for maintaining an inflammatory response in adipose tissue [24]. Based on specific environmental stimuli, macrophage activation can be categorized into two responses: classical (M1) or alternative (M2) macrophages [25]. It has been shown that obesity induces a phenotypic switch from an anti-inflammatory M2 state to a pro-inflammatory M1 state [26]. To determine if M1 and M2 activation affects the levels of IGFBP-3, we used human monocytes (THP-1 cells) and differentiated them to M1 and M2 macrophages using phorbol-12-myristate-13-acetate (PMA)+IFN-γ+LPS and PMA+IL4 respectively. We used CCR-7 and fibronectin as markers for M1 and M2 to confirm that our treatments did differentiate the monocytes to M1 and M2 macrophages respectively [27]. Monocytes treated with PMA+IFN-γ+LPS show higher levels of CCR7 (M1 marker) and those treated with PMA+IL4 show increased levels of fibronectin (M2 marker) (Figure 7A). On confirming macrophage differentiation, we analyzed the mRNA and protein levels of IGFBP-3. Figure 7B shows that M2 macrophages express approximately 5.5 fold higher levels of IGFBP-3 mRNA when compared to M1 macrophages. Further protein analysis of IGFBP-3 in the

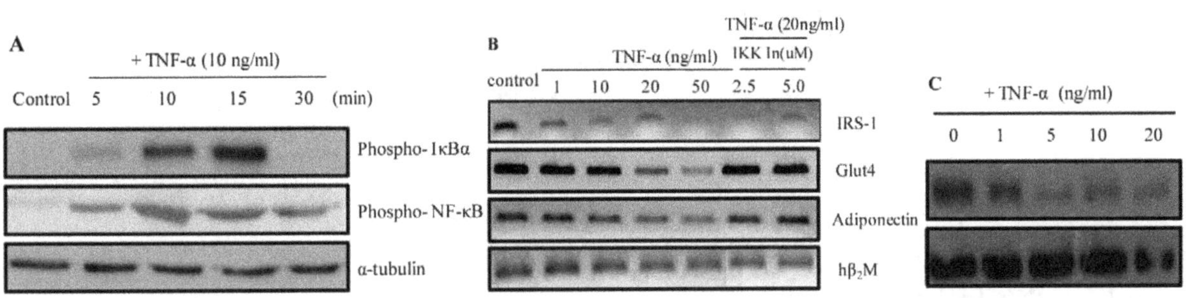

Figure 2. Effect of TNF-α on NF-κB signaling in adipocytes. (A) Differentiated adipocytes were treated with 10 ng/ml TNF-α for 0, 5, 10, 15 and 30 minutes respectively and its effect on the levels of phospho-IκBα and phospho-NF-κB was detected by western blotting. α-tubulin served as the loading control. (B) Differentiated adipocytes were treated with different concentration (1, 10, 20 and 50 ng/ml) of TNF-α for 18 hours followed by analysis of the mRNA levels of IRS-1, GLUT4 and adiponectin by RT-PCR. Cells were treated with 2.5 and 5.0 μM of IKK-IV inhibitor followed by treatment with 20 ng/ml TNF-α. hβ2M was used as the internal control for normalizing mRNA levels. (C) Cells were treated with 1, 5, 10 and 20 ng/ml TNF-α for 24 hour and immunoblotted for IRS-1 and α-tubulin.

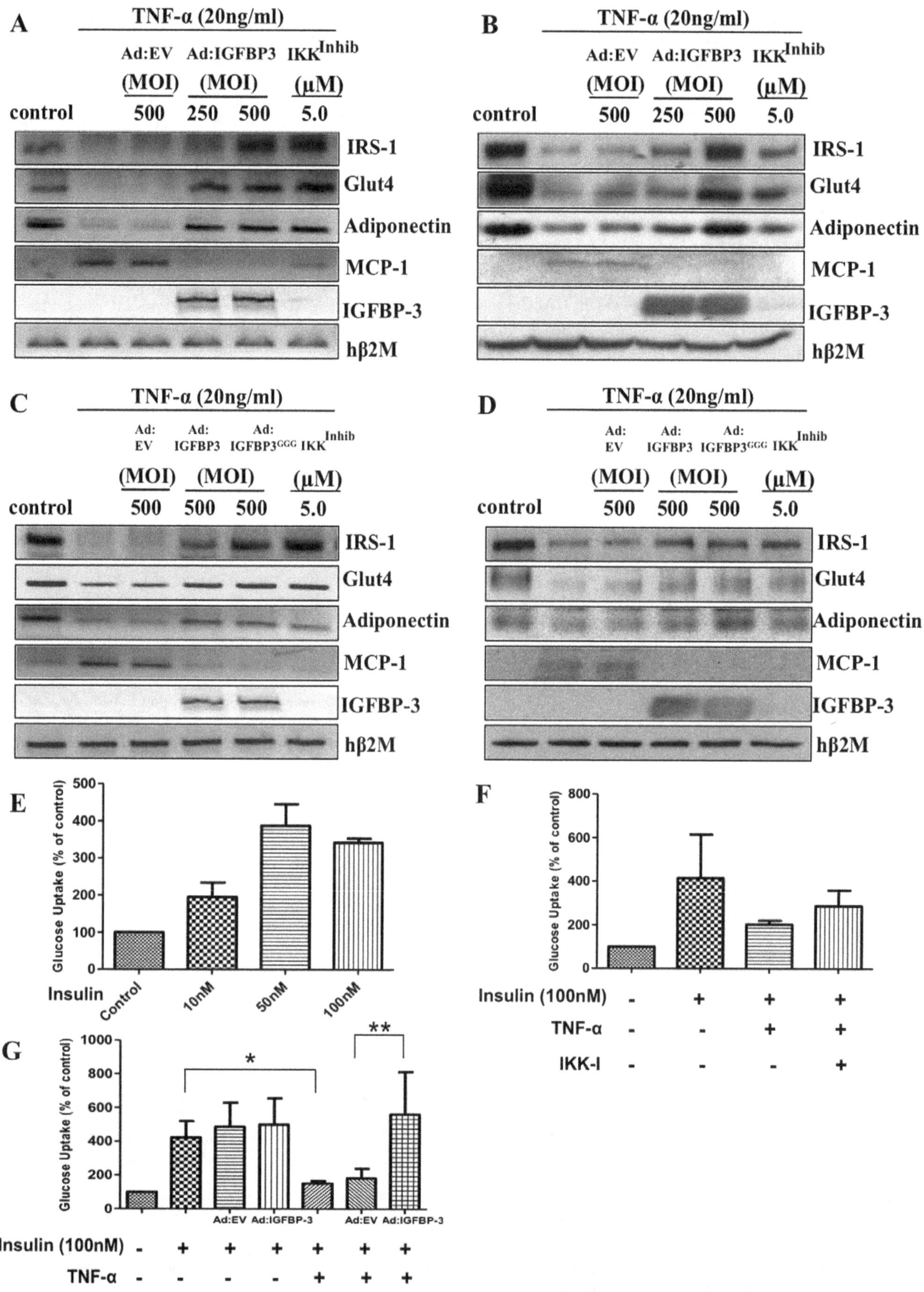
A
TNF-α (20ng/ml)
Ad:EV Ad:IGFBP3 IKKInhib
(MOI) (MOI) (μM)
control 500 250 500 5.0
IRS-1
Glut4
Adiponectin
MCP-1
IGFBP-3
hβ2M
B
TNF-α (20ng/ml)
Ad:EV Ad:IGFBP3 IKKInhib
(MOI) (MOI) (μM)
control 500 250 500 5.0
IRS-1
Glut4
Adiponectin
MCP-1
IGFBP-3
hβ2M
C
TNF-α (20ng/ml)
Ad: EV Ad: IGFBP3 Ad: IGFBP3GGG IKKInhib
(MOI) (MOI) (μM)
control 500 500 500 5.0
IRS-1
Glut4
Adiponectin
MCP-1
IGFBP-3
hβ2M
D
TNF-α (20ng/ml)
Ad: EV Ad: IGFBP3 Ad: IGFBP3GGG IKKInhib
(MOI) (MOI) (μM)
control 500 500 500 5.0
IRS-1
Glut4
Adiponectin
MCP-1
IGFBP-3
hβ2M
E
Glucose Uptake (% of control)
500
400
300
200
100
0
Insulin
Control
10nM
50nM
100nM
F
Glucose Uptake (% of control)
800
600
400
200
0
Insulin (100nM) - + + +
TNF-α - - + +
IKK-I - - - +
G
Glucose Uptake (% of control)
1000
800
600
400
200
0
*
**
Ad:EV
Ad:IGFBP-3
Ad:EV
Ad:IGFBP-3
Insulin (100nM) - + + + + + +
TNF-α - - - - + + +

Figure 3. IGFBP-3 inhibits the NF-κB pathway in primary human adipocytes in an IGF-independent manner. Effect of IGFBP-3 on IRS-1, GLUT4, adiponectin and MCP-1 levels induced upon treatments with TNF-α (20 ng/ml) was analyzed by (A) RT-PCR (18 hours) and (B) immunoblot analysis (36 hours). Similar experiments were performed by infecting adipocytes with mutant-Ad:IGFBP3GGG followed by treatment with TNF-α and analyzing IRS-1, GLUT4, adiponectin and MCP-1 levels by (C) RT-PCR and (D) immunoblotting. Overexpressed IGFBP-3 levels were confirmed in these experiments. Cells were infected with either Ad:EV (m.o.i. 500), Ad:IGFBP-3 (m.o.i. 250, 500), Ad:IGFBP-3GGG (m.o.i. 500) or IKK IV inhibitor at a concentration of 5.0 μM. (E) Differentiated adipocytes were treated with 10, 50 and 100 nM of insulin and a glucose uptake assay was performed on these cells. (F) The inhibitory effect of TNF-α (20 ng/ml) alone and in the presence of IKK IV inhibitor on the biological functions of insulin was analyzed by the glucose uptake assay. (G) Human adipocytes were treated with TNF-α in the presence of insulin (100 nM) and the insulin sensitizing effect of IGFBP-3 was analyzed by glucose uptake assay. Cells were infected with either Ad:EV or Ad:IGFBP-3 (m.o.i. 250), n = 3, in duplicate; *, $p<0.001$;**, $p<0.05$.

conditioned media reiterates that M2 macrophages express higher levels of IGFBP-3 than M1 macrophages without any detectable proteolyzed fragments (Figure 7C). This result suggests that in addition to reduced levels of biologically active, intact IGFBP-3 in circulation in obese state due to increased proteolysis, another possible mechanism for reduced anti-inflammatory function of IGFBP-3 in the adipose tissue could be due to reduction in the presence of anti-inflammatory M2 macrophages resulting in reduced expression of IGFBP-3.

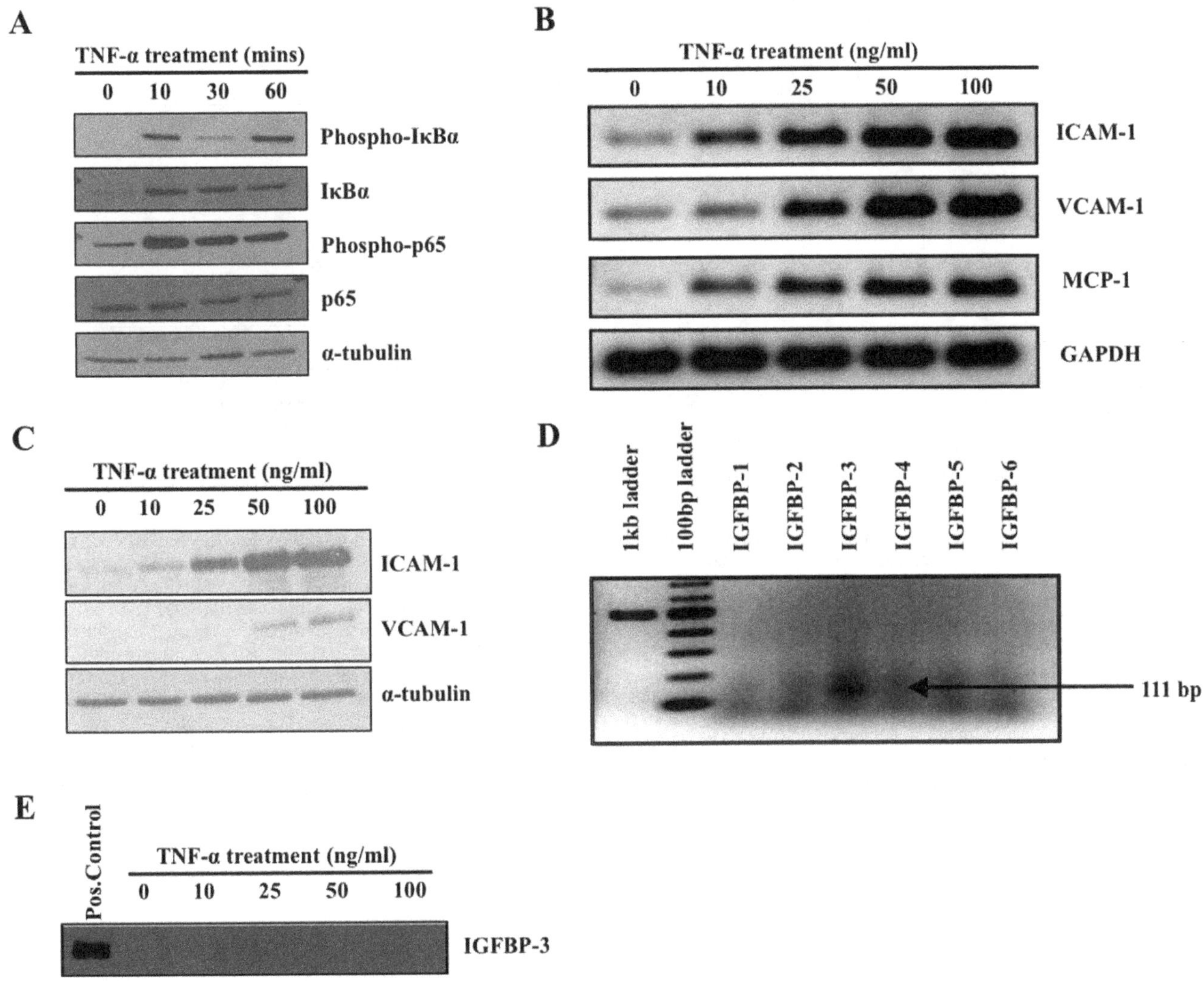

Figure 4. TNF-α activates NF-κB pathway in HAEC cells. (A) HAECs were treated with 50 ng/ml TNF-α and lysates were collected at 0, 10, 30 and 60 minutes. The cell lysates were analyzed by western blotting to observe the activation of NF-κB pathway. The figure shows phospho-IκBα and phospho-p65 confirming activation of NF-κB pathway by TNF-α in HAEC. (B) Dose dependent increase in the mRNA levels of ICAM-1, VCAM-1 and MCP-1 upon TNF-α treatment was analyzed by RT-PCR and GAPDH was the internal control for normalizing mRNA levels. (C) Dose dependent increase in protein levels of ICAM-1 and VCAM-1 by immunoblotting. α-tubulin was used as the loading control. (D) The expression profile of IGFBPs in HAECs was analyzed by RT-PCR using primers IGFBP-1 through IGFBP-6. PCR products were run on a 2% agarose gel. (E) HAEC cells were treated with TNF-α for 48 hours and subsequently analyzed for IGFBP-3 expression in conditioned media (CM). HAECs infected with Ad:IGFBP-3 was used a positive control.

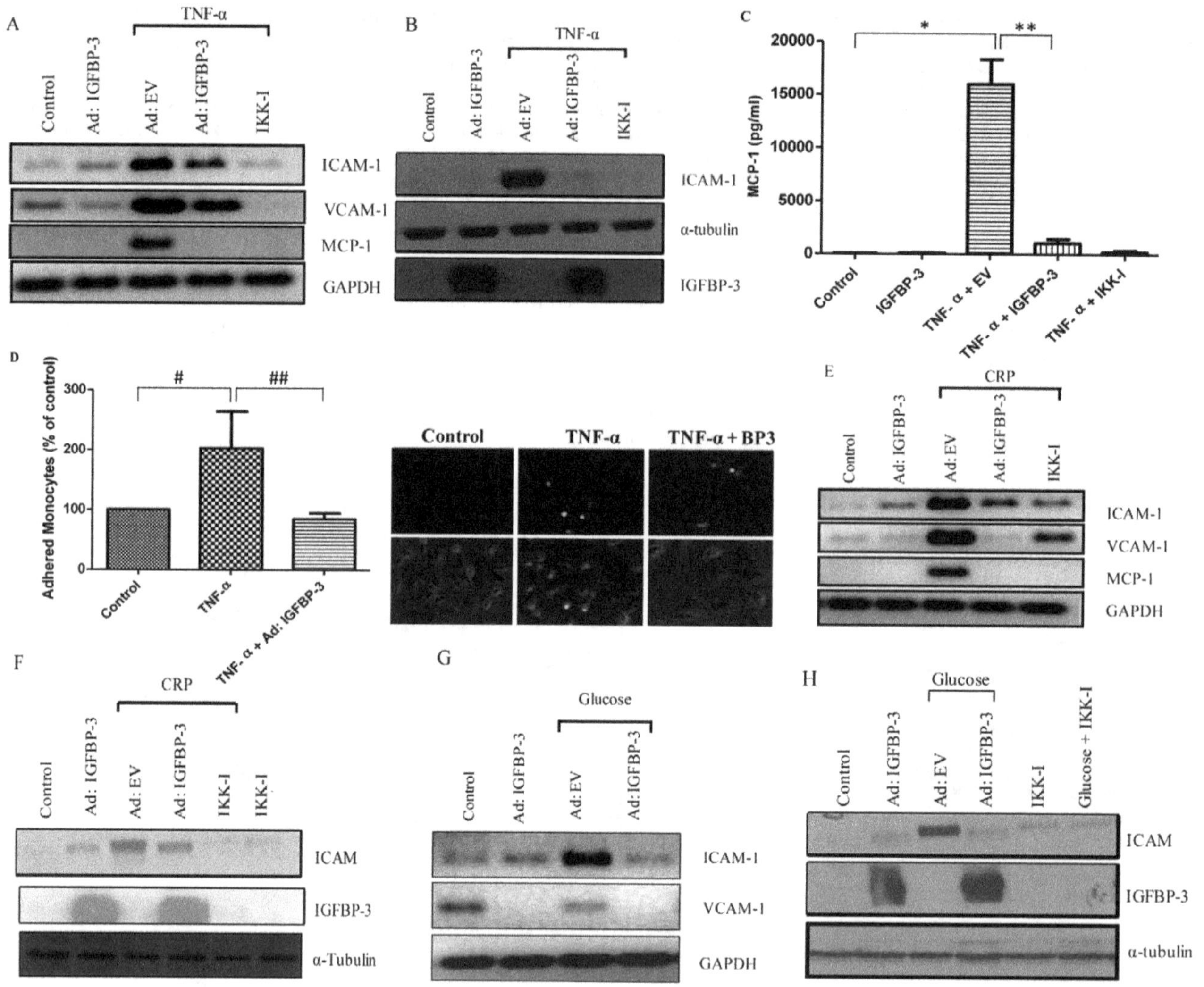

Figure 5. Effect of IGFBP-3 on NF-κB pathway in HAECs: Effect of IGFBP-3 on TNF-α induced NF-κB activation in HAEC cells. HAEC cells were infected with Ad:EV (m.o.i.100) or Ad:IGFBP-3 (m.o.i.100) for 24 hours followed by TNF-α treatment (50 ng/ml) for 24 hours and were analyzed for mRNA and protein expression by RT-PCR and western blotting respectively. Cells were also treated with 2.5 μM IKK-IV inhibitor. Figure (A) shows the mRNA levels for ICAM-1, VCAM-1 and MCP-1 for the treated samples and (B) shows protein expression for ICAM-1, IGFBP-3 and α-tubulin after IGFBP-3 infection by western blotting. IGFBP-3 blot confirms expression after adenovirus infection. HAECs were treated with IKK Inhibitor to confirm the involvement of the NF-κB pathway. The data demonstrates that IGFBP-3 inhibits TNF-α-induced NF-κB activity consequently inhibiting the mRNA and protein levels of ICAM-1, VCAM-1 and MCP-1. (C) A similar experiment was performed with IGFBP-3 infection and TNF-α treatment and MCP-1 levels were quantified in the CM using ELISA. n = 3, in duplicates; *, $p<0.001$;**, $p<0.001$. (D) HAEC cells were infected with Ad:IGFBP-3 and treated with 50 ng/ml of TNF-α. At the end of the incubation, monocyte cell adhesion assay was performed. 1*105 monocytes were stained with Calcein AM fluorescent dye and the stained cell suspension was layered over the HAEC cells. After 30 minutes of incubation non-adherent cells were removed and only the adhered cells were analyzed by fluorescent microscopy. The figure shows a representative field of each well. The number of adhered monocytes on the HAEC monolayer is depicted as a bar graph. n = 2, in triplicates; #, $p<0.05$;##, $p<0.01$. Effect of IGFBP-3 on CRP- and glucose-induced NF-κB activation in HAEC cells: HAEC cells were infected with adenovirus constructs for control and IGFBP-3. Simultaneously, cells were treated with 50 ng/ml CRP for 6 hrs or 30 mM of glucose for five days respectively. Cells were analyzed for effect on the mRNA levels (E, G) and protein expression (F, H) respectively after CRP or glucose treatment.

Discussion

Visceral fat obesity and not subcutaneous fat obesity, correlates significantly with insulin resistance [28], hypertension [29] and cardiac dysfunction [30]. In obesity, fat depots increase the levels of cytokines that act in a paracrine manner further entering circulation and resulting in a state of systemic inflammation [31].

In addition to its ability to modulate IGF availability, IGFBP-3 has also been shown to have IGF-independent effects [10]. IGFBP-3 has been shown to be associated with CVD [7], obesity [8] and insulin resistance [32]. We and others have shown that IGFBP-3 acts as an anti-inflammatory factor, capable of inhibiting the NF-κB pathway [21,22,33]. Reports suggest that IGFBP-3 may act as an insulin antagonist. IGFBP-3 has been shown to inhibit insulin-stimulated glucose uptake in adipocytes, human omental adipose tissue, and in Sprague-Dawley rats [34,35]. It is of note that these studies characterize IGFBP-3 function in a normal physiological setting. However, we, in our study show that IGFBP-3 may have a distinct function in pathologic, disease states. Nevertheless, our data demonstrate that IGFBP-3 does not affect insulin-induced glucose uptake under normal conditions (Figure 3G) A recent study shows that diet-induced obese rats

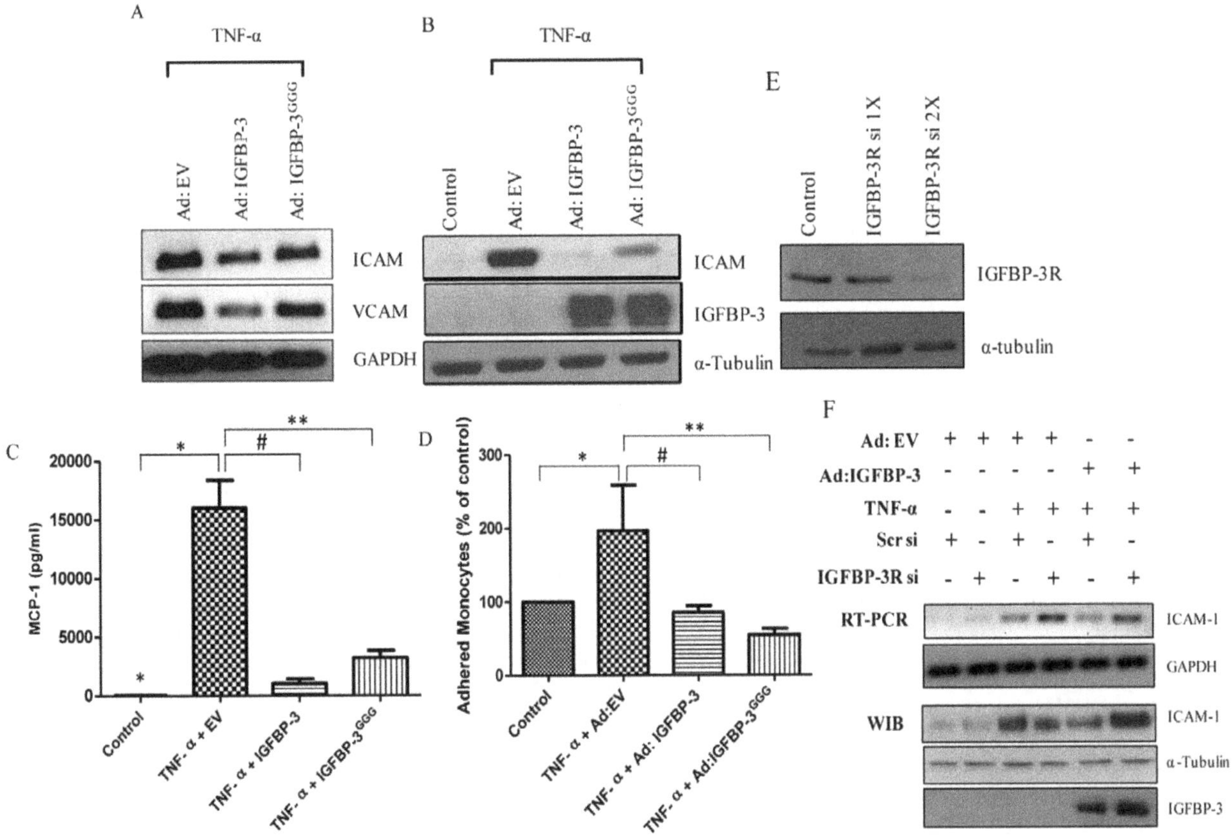

Figure 6. IGFBP-3 inhibits NF-κB activity in an IGF-independent manner in HAECs. HAEC cells were infected with Ad:EV (m.o.i.100) or Ad:IGFBP-3 (m.o.i.100) and Ad:IGFBP-3GGG (m.o.i. 100) followed by TNF-α treatment for 24 hours and were analyzed for mRNA (A) and protein expression (B) by RT-PCR and western blotting respectively. (C) A similar experiment was performed with infection with Ad:EV, Ad:IGFBP-3 or Ad:IGFBP-3GGG and TNF-α treatment and MCP-1 levels were quantified in the CM using ELISA. n = 2, in triplicates; *,#,**, $p<0.001$ (D) HAEC cells were infected with Ad:IGFBP-3 or Ad:IGFB3GGG and treated with 50 ng/ml of TNF-α. At the end of the incubation period, monocyte cell adhesion assay was performed. The numbers of adhered monocytes on the HAEC monolayer are depicted as a bar graph. n = 2 in triplicates; *, p = 0.05; #, **, $p<0.05$. (E) HAEC cells were transfected with siRNA against IGFBP-3R once or two consecutive times and cells were harvested to determine the knockdown of IGFBP-3R by western blotting. HAEC cells were transfected with either scrambled siRNA or siRNA against IGFBP-3R. (F) The cells were then infected with Ad:EV (m.o.i.100) or Ad:IGFBP-3 (m.o.i.100) followed by TNF-α treatment for 24 hours and were analyzed for mRNA and protein expression.

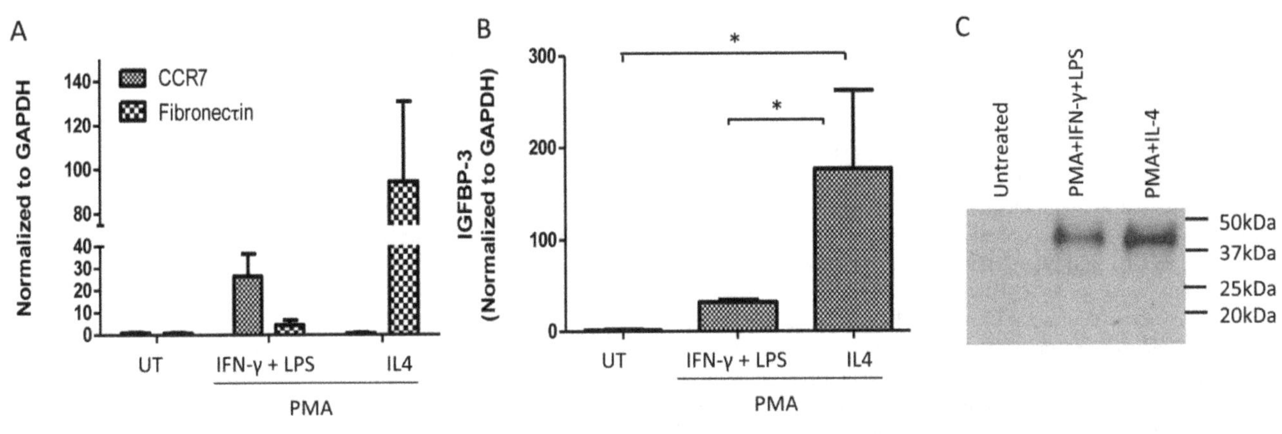

Figure 7. Differential expression of IGFBP-3 in classically and alternately activated macrophages. PMA treated macrophages were differentiated into M1 and M2 macrophages by treating them with IFN-γ+LPS and IL-4 respectively. Figure (A) shows that M1 shows increased levels of CCR7 (M1 marker) mRNA and Fibronectin (M2 marker) levels are higher in M2 when compared to Untreated (B) The bar graph below shows that mRNA levels of IGFBP-3 are higher in M2 when compare to both untreated and M1 differentiated macrophages, * $p<0.05$. For protein analysis, equal numbers of THP-1 cells were plated and differentiated to M1 and M2 as mentioned above and IGFBP-3 protein levels were analyzed on a western blot by loading equal volumes of conditioned media (C).

show a downregulation of IGFBP-3 expression in mesenteric fat when compared to their lean counterparts, suggesting that IGFBP-3 may have a protective effect against obesity [36].

IGF-1 has been shown to increase insulin sensitivity and improve glycemic control in patients with type 2 diabetes [37]. In our data, we see that insulin resistance exists in both overweight and obese adolescents, in spite of the levels of IGF-1 increasing in the overweight and obese individuals. In some instances, it has been shown that at low concentrations, IGF-1 stimulates proliferation of arterial smooth muscle cells and at high concentrations it inhibits smooth muscle cell proliferation. This suggests that IGF-1 could be both a pro-atherogenic and an anti-atherogenic factor [38] indicating that IGFBP-3 levels and its regulation on IGF-1 may be a better indicator and marker of insulin resistance.

Proteolytic degradation of IGFBP-3 has been reported in several catabolic conditions and proteases found in a variety of biological fluids can degrade IGFBP-1-6 into fragments that greatly reduce affinity for IGF-I and IGF-II, thereby increasing the concentration of free IGF [39]. Therefore, IGFBP proteolysis directly regulates IGF receptor signaling [40]. However, it is not known if the proteolyzed IGFBP-3 fragments still possess intrinsic biological functions of intact IGFBP-3 such as IGF-independent anti-inflammatory function of IGFBP-3. It is of note that the mid region of IGFBP-3 molecule possesses an IGFBP-3R binding domain [13] whereas IGFBP-3 proteases appear to cleave the IGFBP-3 mid region [41,42]. Taken together, these findings strongly suggest that IGFBP-3 proteolysis may result in loss of IGFBP-3R binding ability and subsequent its anti-inflammatory function. In this study we show that IGFBP-3 proteolysis was significantly increased in overweight as well as obesity groups compared to normal controls by both western blotting and protease activity assay. Its correlation with HOMA-insulin resistance suggests that proteolysis of IGFBP-3 may be involved in the pathogenesis of obesity-induced insulin resistance. Though there are conflicting reports about the effect of obesity on IGFBP-3 proteolysis [43] it is evident that IGFBP-3 proteolysis is increased in patients with non insulin-dependent diabetes mellitus [17]. This further raises an interesting concept that IGFBP-3 proteolysis may result in decrease of intact IGFBP-3 in circulation and the local environment, thereby suppressing the intrinsic anti-inflammatory function of IGFBP-3. Also, studies show that adipose tissue of a lean mice have a macrophage content of less than 10% of the total cell nuclei count, whereas obese mice present more than 50% of macrophage content [24,44]. It has been shown that obesity induces a phenotypic switch from an anti-inflammatory M2 state to a pro-inflammatory M1 state [26]. On the other hand, Lumeng *et al* in his study suggests that during obesity, adipose tissue macrophages are newly recruited from monocyte precursors and these macrophages display M1 characteristics [45]. M2 macrophages are known to maintain glucose tolerance, insulin sensitivity and general adipocyte function that can prevent development of obesity due to diet and type-2 diabetes [25,45]. In both humans and mice, lipidystrophy has been associated with overexpression of the M1 phenotype of macrophages [46,47]. In accordance with the role of macrophages and the anti-inflammatory properties of IGFBP-3, in our study we show that M2 macrophages express higher levels of IGFBP-3 than M1, suggesting that decreased expression of IGFBP-3 by macrophages in addition to occurrence of IGFBP-3 proteolysis in circulation may contribute towards obesity and insulin resistance.

Visceral adipocytes are highly responsive to TNF-α mediated activation of NF-κB pathway [18]. Our study shows that IGFBP-3 inhibits TNF-α-induced NF-κB activity in differentiated human adipocytes, inhibiting TNF-α-mediated deregulation of insulin signaling in ASCs. IGFBP-3 restores the levels of IRS-1, GLUT4 and adiponectin and inhibits MCP-1 levels. NF-κB pathway has been shown to be active in human atherosclerotic plaques and in contrast, healthy vessels are devoid of such increased activity. Presence of activated NF-κB pathway is observed in smooth muscle cells, endothelial cells of atherosclerotic lesions [48] and in the intimal cells of the coronary arteries of pigs that are fed a hypercholesterolemic diet [49]. Many genes regulated by the NF-κB pathway such as ICAM-1, VCAM-1, IL-8 and MCP-1 help in the recruitment of monocytes to the arterial intima. This further leads to the migration and proliferation of smooth muscle cells resulting in plaque formation and atherosclerosis. Since pharmacological inhibition or genetic knockdown of adhesion molecules, MCP-1 and TNF-α is known to retard the progression of CVD in atherosclerotic models [50,51], in our study we investigated and determined that in HAECs, IGFBP-3 inhibits TNF-α-induced adhesion molecules; ICAM-1, VCAM-1 and MCP-1, downstream of the NF-κB pathway. In addition to inhibiting TNF-α-induced MCP-1 levels in the cells, IGFBP-3 also prevents adhesion of monocytes to HAECs. High glucose and CRP, that are pro-atherogenic and pro-inflammatory factors also activate the NF-κB pathway, upregulating adhesion proteins and recruiting monocytes to the vascular endothelium [52] and our data shows that IGFBP-3 also inhibits CRP- and high glucose-induced NF-κB pathway in HAECs.

Taken together, these *in vitro* data provide convincing evidence that IGFBP-3 negates obesity-induced NF-κB activity in adipocytes and HAECs. Our data with IGFBP-3^{GGG} mutant further confirms that this inhibition of the NF-κB activity occurs in an IGF-independent manner. IGFBP-3R [13], is involved in the inhibition of TNF-α induced NF-κB signaling cascade via the activation of caspases and eventual apoptosis in cancer cells [11]. IGFBP-3 also inhibits NF-κB signaling in normal lung epithelial cells via activation of the IGFBP-3R that involves activation of caspase pathway and degradation of IκBα and p65-NF-κB proteins, thereby inhibiting TNF-α-induced activation of NF-κB signaling cascades and blocking the physiological manifestations of asthma and bronchial inflammation [12]. Not surprisingly, knockdown of endogenous IGFBP-3R in our *in vitro* heart cell system negates the biological effect of IGFBP-3 and restores the levels of ICAM-1, thereby suggesting that IGFBP-3 inhibits the NF-κB pathway via an IGFBP-3/IGFBP-3R axis.

In conclusion, these new discoveries for the inhibitory role of IGFBP-3 in obesity-induced insulin resistance and in the events occurring in the early stages of atherosclerosis, set the stage for a potential therapeutic role of IGFBP-3 in various aspects of metabolic syndrome.

Materials and Methods

Subjects

The study consisted of 197 subjects aged 12 to 13 years old among adolescents who visited the National Medical Center, Korea for medical examinations. The BMI percentiles for age and gender according to 2007 Korea Growth Charts for assessment of obesity were utilized. At the time of study enrollment no subject had either a chronic disease or acute illness, was taking medications for any condition, or had a history of smoking. The Hospital Ethnics Committee of the Severance Children's hospital reviewed and approved the study, and written informed consent was obtained from guardians and study subjects.

Anthropometric Measurements

Weight, height, BP and waist circumference were measured as previously described [24,29].

Blood Samples Analyses

All subjects were fasted for more than 12 hours. Whole blood samples were obtained by venipuncture. Sera were used for biochemical and hormonal assay within 8 hours and immunoblot assay was performed.

Biochemical and Hormonal Analyses

Level of fasting serum glucose, insulin, total cholesterol, triglycerides, AST, ALT and HDL cholesterol were measured. Levels of LDL cholesterol were calculated as follows: LDL-cholesterol = total cholesterol − HDL-cholesterol–(triglyceride/5). CRP concentrations were measured by IMMAGE assay (Beckman Coulter, CA, USA), and fasting insulin levels were measured by electroluminescence immunoassay. HOMA-IR was calculated as follows: HOMA-IR = [fasting insulin (μIU/mL) x fasting glucose (mg/dL)/18]/22.5 [25].

IGFBP-3 Protease Activity Assay

Recombinant human glycosylated IGFBP-3 was biotinylated by Biotin-XX microscale protein labeling kit (Invitrogen). Two ul sera and 5 ul biotinylated IGFBP-3 were incubated at 37°c for 15 minutes and subjected to WIB. IGFBP-3 protease activity was calculated from WIB as the sum of density of the fragment bands at 29 and 18 kDa divided by the sum of all fragments and intact IGFBP-3 at approximately 43, 29, and 18 kDa.

ELISA Assays for IGF-I, IGFBP-3 and MCP-1 ELISA Assays

Human IGF-I ELISA (ALPCO,NH, USA), total IGFBP-3 (MEDIAGNOST, Reutlingen, Germany) and MCP-1 ELISA kits (BD Biosciences) were purchased and assays were performed according to manufacturer's protocol.

Reagents

Isobutyl-methylxanthine, dexamethasone, indomethacin, insulin glucose, TNF-α were purchased from Sigma, IKK inhibitor and CRP were obtained from Calbiochem, whereas Calcein AM from Molecular probes.

Semi Quantitative and Quantitative PCR Analysis

Total RNA was extracted and reverse transcripted, and RTQ-PCR was performed with designed primers (Table 4) [18].

Adenoviral Constructs

Ad:IGFBP-3 and Ad:IGFBP-3^{GGG} were generated and characterized as previously described [13].

Growth, Differentiation and Maintenance of ASCs

Cells were grown to 100% confluence in the growth medium supplemented with 10% FBS. Confluent cells were incubated in DM for 6 days (change medium every 3 days), 1 day in MM and then switched to DM again. This cycle was repeated for a period of 21 days until cells were differentiated.

Macrophage Differentiation

Cells were treated with 20 ng/ml PMA for 8 hours followed by treatment with 20 ng/ml of IFN-γ and 20 ng/ml LPS for differentiating them into M1 macrophages and 20 ng/ml IL-4 for M2 macrophages. The cells were then harvested for mRNA analysis after 20 hours and cell lysates and conditioned media were collected at 72 hours.

Table 4. Primer Sequences.

Genes	Primer sequence
IRS-1 fwd	5′-CCTGGATTTGGTCAAGGACT-3′
IRS-1 rev	5′-TCATTCTGCTGTGATGTCCA-3′
Glut4 fwd	5′- TTATTCGACCAGCATCTTCG-3′
Glut4 rev	5′-AGCAGAGCCACAGTCATCAG-3′
Adiponectin fwd	5′-TGCTGGGAGCTGTTCTACTG-3′
Adiponectin rev	5′-GTTTCACCGATGTCTCCCTT-3′
MCP-1 fwd	5′ - ATCAATGCCCCAGTCACC - 3′
MCP-1 rev	5′-AGTCTTCGGAGTTTGGG-3′
hβ2M fwd	5′- GTGCTCGCGCTACTCTCTCT-3′
hβ2M rev	5′- TCAATGTCGGATGGATGAAA-3′
IGFBP-3R fwd	5′- AGACAGGAACAAGACCCGGACATT -3′
IGFBP-3R rev	5′- ATAGGCAGGTTCCTGCAGTCCTTT-3′
ICAM-1 fwd	5′-CTGCAGACAGTGACCATC-3′
ICAM-1 rev	5′- GTCCAGTTTCCCGGACAA-3′
VCAM-1 fwd	5′- AGATGGCGCCTATACCATCCGAAA -3′
VCAM-1 rev	5′- AGAGCACGAGAAGCTCAGGAGAAA -3′
IGFBP-1 fwd	5′- AGGCTCTCCATGTCACCAACATCA -3′
IGFBP-1 rev	5′- TGTCTCCTGTGCCTTGGCTAAACT –3′
IGFBP-2 fwd	5′- GCATGGCCTGTACAACCTCAAACA-3′
IGFBP-2 rev	5′- AGCCTCCTGCTGCTCATTGTAGA -3′
IGFBP-3 fwd	5′- CAGAGCACAGATACCCAGAACTTC-3′
IGFBP-3 rev	5′-CACATTGAGGAACTTCAGGTGATT-3′
IGFBP-4 fwd	5′- TGCAGAAGCACTTCGCCAAA-3′
IGFBP-4, rev	5′- ATGATGTAGAGGTCCTCGTGGGTG-3′
IGFBP-5 fwd	5′- AAAGAGCTACCGCGAGCAAGTCAA -3′
IGFBP-5 rev	5′- ACAAACTTGGACTGGGTCAGCTTC-3′
IGFBP-6 fwd	5′- AACCGCAGAGACCAACAGAGGAAT-3′
IGFBP-6 rev	5′- TGGTCACAATTGGGCACGTAGAGT -3′
GAPDH fwd	5′- CCAATAGGCGCTCACTGTTCT -3′
GAPDH rev	5′- GCGAACTCACCCGTTGACT -3′

Monocyte Adhesion Assay

Equal numbers of HAEC cells were plated, followed by adenovirus infection with Ad: EV, Ad: IGFBP-3 or Ad: IGFBP-3^{GGG} as required followed by TNF-α treatment with in respective wells. A fixed number of monocytes (THP-1) were stained with 2 μM Calcein AM and the adhered monocytes were counted using a fluorescence microscope for three representative fields.

Glucose Uptake Assay

Differentiated adipocytes were cultured in serum free low glucose medium for 2 hours. In experiments involving adenovirus infection, two hours after infection cells were treated with 20 ng/ml of TNF-α. After 24 hours of incubation, cells were incubated with or without insulin in KRPH buffer for 20 min and subjected to glucose uptake assay.

siRNA Transfection

Cells were transfected with siRNAs against IGFBP-3R (siGENOME SMARTpool, Dharmacon) as described previously [23].

Statistical Analyses

To determine the statistical differences in clinical characteristics among the three groups, we used one-way analysis of variance (ANOVA). Pearson's correlation coefficients were calculated to evaluate the relationship between the degree of IGFBP-3 proteolysis and clinical features. Results were considered significant when $P<0.05$. All statistical analyses were performed with SAS 9.13 service pack3 (SAS Institute, Cary, NC, USA). Statistical analyses for *in vitro* experiments in differentiated adipocytes and HAECs were performed by t-test.

Author Contributions

Conceived and designed the experiments: YO LM HK. Performed the experiments: LM HK QC WL KK HS YL WL JK. Analyzed the data: YO LM HK. Contributed reagents/materials/analysis tools: YO HK. Wrote the paper: YO LM HK.

References

1. Ogden CL, Carroll MD, Curtin LR, Lamb MM, Flegal KM (2010) Prevalence of high body mass index in US children and adolescents, 2007–2008. JAMA 303: 242–249.
2. Dubuc PU (1976) The development of obesity, hyperinsulinemia, and hyperglycemia in ob/ob mice. Metabolism 25: 1567–1574.
3. Ouchi N, Kihara S, Funahashi T, Nakamura T, Nishida M, et al. (2003) Reciprocal association of C-reactive protein with adiponectin in blood stream and adipose tissue. Circulation 107: 671–674.
4. Neels JG, Olefsky JM (2006) Inflamed fat: what starts the fire? J Clin Invest 116: 33–35.
5. Hwa V, Oh Y, Rosenfeld RG (1999) The insulin-like growth factor-binding protein (IGFBP) superfamily. Endocr Rev 20: 761–787.
6. Kaplan RC, McGinn AP, Pollak MN, Kuller LH, Strickler HD, et al. (2007) Association of total insulin-like growth factor-I, insulin-like growth factor binding protein-1 (IGFBP-1), and IGFBP-3 levels with incident coronary events and ischemic stroke. J Clin Endocrinol Metab 92: 1319–1325.
7. Spilcke-Liss E, Friedrich N, Dorr M, Schminke U, Volzke H, et al. (2011) Serum Insulin-like Growth Factor-I and its Binding Protein 3 in their Relation to Intima Media Thickness: Results of the Study of Health in Pomerania (SHIP). Clin Endocrinol (Oxf).
8. Gomez JM, Maravall FJ, Gomez N, Navarro MA, Casamitjana R, et al. (2004) The IGF-I system component concentrations that decrease with ageing are lower in obesity in relationship to body mass index and body fat. Growth Horm IGF Res 14: 91–96.
9. Kielczewski JL, Hu P, Shaw LC, Li Calzi S, Mames RN, et al. (2011) Novel protective properties of IGFBP-3 result in enhanced pericyte ensheathment, reduced microglial activation, increased microglial apoptosis, and neuronal protection after ischemic retinal injury. Am J Pathol 178: 1517–1528.
10. Oh Y, Muller HL, Lamson G, Rosenfeld RG (1993) Insulin-like growth factor (IGF)-independent action of IGF-binding protein-3 in Hs578T human breast cancer cells. Cell surface binding and growth inhibition. J Biol Chem 268: 14964–14971.
11. Han J, Jogie-Brahim S, Harada A, Oh Y (2011) Insulin-like growth factor-binding protein-3 suppresses tumor growth via activation of caspase-dependent apoptosis and cross-talk with NF-kappaB signaling. Cancer Lett 307: 200–210.
12. Lee YC, Jogie-Brahim S, Lee DY, Han J, Harada A, et al. (2011) Insulin-like growth factor-binding protein-3 (IGFBP-3) blocks the effects of asthma by negatively regulating NF-kappaB signaling through IGFBP-3R-mediated activation of caspases. J Biol Chem 286: 17898–17909.
13. Ingermann AR, Yang YF, Han J, Mikami A, Garza AE, et al. (2010) Identification of a novel cell death receptor mediating IGFBP-3-induced anti-tumor effects in breast and prostate cancer. J Biol Chem 285: 30233–30246.
14. Hossenlopp P, Segovia B, Lassarre C, Roghani M, Bredon M, et al. (1990) Evidence of enzymatic degradation of insulin-like growth factor-binding proteins in the 150K complex during pregnancy. J Clin Endocrinol Metab 71: 797–805.
15. AM HZ, Collard TJ, Malik K, Hicks DJ, Paraskeva C, et al. (2006) Induction of apoptosis by the 16-kDa amino-terminal fragment of the insulin-like growth factor binding protein 3 in human colonic carcinoma cells. Int J Oncol 29: 1279–1286.
16. Jogie-Brahim S, Feldman D, Oh Y (2009) Unraveling insulin-like growth factor binding protein-3 actions in human disease. Endocr Rev 30: 417–437.
17. Bang P, Brismar K, Rosenfeld RG (1994) Increased proteolysis of insulin-like growth factor-binding protein-3 (IGFBP-3) in noninsulin-dependent diabetes mellitus serum, with elevation of a 29-kilodalton (kDa) glycosylated IGFBP-3 fragment contained in the approximately 130- to 150-kDa ternary complex. J Clin Endocrinol Metab 78: 1119–1127.
18. Maury E, Noel L, Detry R, Brichard SM (2009) In vitro hyperresponsiveness to tumor necrosis factor-alpha contributes to adipokine dysregulation in omental adipocytes of obese subjects. J Clin Endocrinol Metab 94: 1393–1400.
19. Skolnik EY, Marcusohn J (1996) Inhibition of insulin receptor signaling by TNF: potential role in obesity and non-insulin-dependent diabetes mellitus. Cytokine Growth Factor Rev 7: 161–173.
20. Olson AL, Pessin JE (1996) Structure, function, and regulation of the mammalian facilitative glucose transporter gene family. Annu Rev Nutr 16: 235–256.
21. Matsuzawa Y (2010) Adiponectin: a key player in obesity related disorders. Curr Pharm Des 16: 1896–1901.
22. Buckway CK, Wilson EM, Ahlsen M, Bang P, Oh Y, et al. (2001) Mutation of three critical amino acids of the N-terminal domain of IGF-binding protein-3 essential for high affinity IGF binding. J Clin Endocrinol Metab 86: 4943–4950.
23. Ouwens DM, Sell H, Greulich S, Eckel J (2010) The role of epicardial and perivascular adipose tissue in the pathophysiology of cardiovascular disease. J Cell Mol Med 14: 2223–2234.
24. Weisberg SP, McCann D, Desai M, Rosenbaum M, Leibel RL, et al. (2003) Obesity is associated with macrophage accumulation in adipose tissue. J Clin Invest 112: 1796–1808.
25. Odegaard JI, Chawla A (2011) Alternative macrophage activation and metabolism. Annu Rev Pathol 6: 275–297.
26. Dalmas E, Clement K, Guerre-Millo M (2011) Defining macrophage phenotype and function in adipose tissue. Trends Immunol 32: 307–314.
27. Martinez FO, Gordon S, Locati M, Mantovani A (2006) Transcriptional profiling of the human monocyte-to-macrophage differentiation and polarization: new molecules and patterns of gene expression. J Immunol 177: 7303–7311.
28. Yamashita S, Nakamura T, Shimomura I, Nishida M, Yoshida S, et al. (1996) Insulin resistance and body fat distribution. Diabetes Care 19: 287–291.
29. Kanai H, Matsuzawa Y, Kotani K, Keno Y, Kobatake T, et al. (1990) Close correlation of intra-abdominal fat accumulation to hypertension in obese women. Hypertension 16: 484–490.
30. Nakamura T, Tokunaga K, Shimomura I, Nishida M, Yoshida S, et al. (1994) Contribution of visceral fat accumulation to the development of coronary artery disease in non-obese men. Atherosclerosis 107: 239–246.
31. Guzik TJ, Mangalat D, Korbut R (2006) Adipocytokines - novel link between inflammation and vascular function? J Physiol Pharmacol 57: 505–528.
32. Kim HS, Ali O, Shim M, Lee KW, Vuguin P, et al. (2007) Insulin-like growth factor binding protein-3 induces insulin resistance in adipocytes in vitro and in rats in vivo. Pediatr Res 61: 159–164.
33. Williams AC, Smartt H, AM HZ, Macfarlane M, Paraskeva C, et al. (2007) Insulin-like growth factor binding protein 3 (IGFBP-3) potentiates TRAIL-induced apoptosis of human colorectal carcinoma cells through inhibition of NF-kappaB. Cell Death Differ 14: 137–145.
34. Silha JV, Gui Y, Murphy LJ (2002) Impaired glucose homeostasis in insulin-like growth factor-binding protein-3-transgenic mice. Am J Physiol Endocrinol Metab 283: E937–945.
35. Moses AC, Young SC, Morrow LA, O'Brien M, Clemmons DR (1996) Recombinant human insulin-like growth factor I increases insulin sensitivity and improves glycemic control in type II diabetes. Diabetes 45: 91–100.
36. Palau N, Rebuffat SA, Altirriba J, Piquer S, Hanzu FA, et al. (2012) Role of IGFBP-3 in the regulation of beta-cell mass during obesity: adipose tissue/beta-cell cross talk. Endocrinology 153: 177–187.
37. Gatenby VK, Kearney MT (2010) The role of IGF-1 resistance in obesity and type 2 diabetes-mellitus-related insulin resistance and vascular disease. Expert Opin Ther Targets 14: 1333–1342.
38. Schuler-Luttmann S, Monnig G, Enbergs A, Schulte H, Breithardt G, et al. (2000) Insulin-like growth factor-binding protein-3 is associated with the presence and extent of coronary arteriosclerosis. Arterioscler Thromb Vasc Biol 20: E10–15.
39. Maile LA, Holly JM (1999) Insulin-like growth factor binding protein (IGFBP) proteolysis: occurrence, identification, role and regulation. Growth Horm IGF Res 9: 85–95.
40. Bunn RC, Fowlkes JL (2003) Insulin-like growth factor binding protein proteolysis. Trends Endocrinol Metab 14: 176–181.
41. Bang P, Fielder PJ (1997) Human pregnancy serum contains at least two distinct proteolytic activities with the ability to degrade insulin-like growth factor binding protein-3. Endocrinology 138: 3912–3917.
42. Firth SM, Baxter RC (1995) The role of glycosylation in the action of IGFBP-3. Prog Growth Factor Res 6: 223–229.
43. Ballerini MG, Ropelato MG, Domene HM, Pennisi P, Heinrich JJ, et al. (2004) Differential impact of simple childhood obesity on the components of the growth hormone-insulin-like growth factor (IGF)-IGF binding proteins axis. J Pediatr Endocrinol Metab 17: 749–757.
44. Xu H, Barnes GT, Yang Q, Tan G, Yang D, et al. (2003) Chronic inflammation in fat plays a crucial role in the development of obesity-related insulin resistance. J Clin Invest 112: 1821–1830.

45. Lumeng CN, Deyoung SM, Bodzin JL, Saltiel AR (2007) Increased inflammatory properties of adipose tissue macrophages recruited during diet-induced obesity. Diabetes 56: 16–23.
46. Odegaard JI, Ricardo-Gonzalez RR, Red Eagle A, Vats D, Morel CR, et al. (2008) Alternative M2 activation of Kupffer cells by PPARdelta ameliorates obesity-induced insulin resistance. Cell Metab 7: 496–507.
47. Kang K, Reilly SM, Karabacak V, Gangl MR, Fitzgerald K, et al. (2008) Adipocyte-derived Th2 cytokines and myeloid PPARdelta regulate macrophage polarization and insulin sensitivity. Cell Metab 7: 485–495.
48. Brand K, Page S, Rogler G, Bartsch A, Brandl R, et al. (1996) Activated transcription factor nuclear factor-kappa B is present in the atherosclerotic lesion. J Clin Invest 97: 1715–1722.
49. Wilson SH, Caplice NM, Simari RD, Holmes DR Jr, Carlson PJ, et al. (2000) Activated nuclear factor-kappaB is present in the coronary vasculature in experimental hypercholesterolemia. Atherosclerosis 148: 23–30.
50. Van der Heiden K, Cuhlmann S, Luong le A, Zakkar M, Evans PC (2010) Role of nuclear factor kappaB in cardiovascular health and disease. Clin Sci (Lond) 118: 593–605.
51. Tikellis C, Jandeleit-Dahm KA, Sheehy K, Murphy A, Chin-Dusting J, et al. (2008) Reduced plaque formation induced by rosiglitazone in an STZ-diabetes mouse model of atherosclerosis is associated with downregulation of adhesion molecules. Atherosclerosis 199: 55–64.
52. Jialal I, Devaraj S (2001) Inflammation and atherosclerosis: the value of the high-sensitivity C-reactive protein assay as a risk marker. Am J Clin Pathol 116 Suppl: S108–115.

17

The Role of the Niemann-Pick Disease, Type C1 Protein in Adipocyte Insulin Action

Rachael Fletcher[1¶], Christopher Gribben[1¶], Xiuquan Ma[1], James G. Burchfield[1], Kristen C. Thomas[1], James R. Krycer[1,2], David E. James[1,3], Daniel J. Fazakerley[1]*

1 Diabetes and Obesity Program, Garvan Institute of Medical Research, Sydney, New South Wales, Australia, **2** School of Biotechnology and Biomolecular Sciences, The University of New South Wales, Sydney, New South Wales, Australia, **3** Charles Perkins Centre, School of Molecular Bioscience, The University of Sydney, Sydney, Australia

Abstract

The Niemann-Pick disease, type C1 (*NPC1)* gene encodes a transmembrane protein involved in cholesterol efflux from the lysosome. SNPs within *NPC1* have been associated with obesity and type 2 diabetes, and mice heterozygous or null for *NPC1* are insulin resistant. However, the molecular mechanism underpinning this association is currently undefined. This study aimed to investigate the effects of inhibiting NPC1 function on insulin action in adipocytes. Both pharmacological and genetic inhibition of NPC1 impaired insulin action. This impairment was evident at the level of insulin signalling and insulin-mediated glucose transport in the short term and decreased *GLUT4* expression due to reduced liver X receptor (LXR) transcriptional activity in the long-term. These data show that cholesterol homeostasis through NPC1 plays a crucial role in maintaining insulin action at multiple levels in adipocytes.

Editor: Mikel Garcia-Marcos, Boston University School of Medicine, United States of America

Funding: This work was supported by an NHMRC program grant (D.E.J.). D.E.J. is an NHMRC Senior Principal Research Fellow. D.J.F. is a Sir Henry Wellcome Postdoctoral Fellow. The funders had no role in study design, data collection and analysis, decision to publish, or preparation of the manuscript.

Competing Interests: The authors have declared that no competing interests exist.

* E-mail: d.fazakerley@garvan.org.au

¶ These authors contributed equally to this work.

Introduction

Metabolic diseases such as insulin resistance and type 2 diabetes (T2D) are major and escalating health concerns. Despite extensive research we have a rudimentary understanding of the molecular mechanisms that underpin insulin resistance in insulin target tissues. Recent advances in large-scale analysis platforms have offered the opportunity to reveal novel links between genes and disease phenotypes. For example, genome wide association studies (GWAS) have identified more than 70 genetic loci that associate with T2D [1–6], but for many of these the molecular basis for the association remains unknown. Studies to interrogate how genes associated with these loci impact whole body glucose metabolism are required.

One example of an associated gene is Niemann-Pick disease, type C1 (*NPC1)* which encodes a transmembrane protein that has been primarily studied in the context of Niemann-Pick type C (NPC) disease. NPC disease is a rare lysosomal storage disease characterized at the cellular level by the accumulation of cholesterol and sphingolipids within the late endosomal/lysosomal compartment [7]. NPC1 cooperates with NPC2 in the egress of cholesterol from the late endosomal/lysosomal system [8,9], though the vast majority of NPC disease cases arise from mutations in *NPC1* [10]. Single nucleotide polymorphisms (SNPs) within the *NPC1* gene have been associated with early onset and morbid obesity and, independently of obesity, insulin resistance in humans [11–13]. Further, mice heterozygous for NPC1 have increased susceptibility to weight gain and display abnormal metabolic characteristics such as hyperinsulinemia and glucose intolerance [14], and this impairment in glucose tolerance is independent of body weight [15]. Taken together, these data suggest a role for NPC1 function in maintaining metabolic homeostasis and in predisposition to metabolic diseases.

NPC1 has been reported to influence insulin signalling in the spontaneous murine (nih) model of NPC disease [16]. Insulin acts largely via activating the serine/threonine Kinase Akt (PKB) through its phosphorylation at S473 and T308. NPC1 (nih) mice exhibited reduced phosphorylation of Akt and its substrate GSK3β in the brain, which was attributed to a marked decrease in insulin receptor substrate 1 (IRS1) expression. Also, pharmacological and genetic inhibition of NPC1 function reduced phosphorylation of Akt in endothelial cells due to inhibition of mTORC2 activity, which is responsible for phosphorylating Akt at S473 [17]. In light of the GWAS association, the metabolic profile of NPC1 null mice and these molecular data, we speculated that disruption of NPC1 function may impact metabolic homeostasis through reduced insulin-stimulated Akt activation and that the association between *NPC1* and insulin resistance may be due to effects on insulin action in its target tissues. We report that inhibition of NPC1 activity in an adipocyte cell model reduced insulin-stimulated glucose uptake through disruption of multiple sites: Akt activation, exocytosis of the insulin-responsive glucose transporter GLUT4, and total levels of GLUT4.

Materials and Methods

Cell Culture

3T3-L1 fibroblasts were cultured in Dulbecco's modified Eagle's medium (DMEM) (Life Technologies) supplemented with 10% focal calf serum (Thermo Scientific) and 1% Glutamax (Life Technologies) at 37°C in 10% CO_2. Fibroblasts were grown to confluence before differentiation into adipocytes in DMEM containing 100 ng/ml dexamethosone, 100 ng/ml biotin, 2 μg/ml insulin and 50 μM 3-isobutyl-1-methyl-xanthine (IBMX) for 3 days. Following this cells were post differentiated for a further 3 days in DMEM containing 2 μg/ml insulin. 3T3-L1 adipocytes were used for experiments 10–14 days after initiation of differentiation. HA-GLUT4 expressing 3T3-L1 adipocytes were generated as previously described [18]. Cells were treated for specified periods of time with 0.1% DMSO as a vehicle control or 10 μg/ml U18666a (Sigma-Aldrich). U18666a was not present during the basal period (DMEM, Glutamax, 0.2% BSA). Incubations with the LXR agonist GW3965 at 10 μM (Sigma-Aldrich) were performed during the final 16 h of 72 h U18666a treatment. Control (K1) and NPC1 knockout (2–2) CHO cells were a kind gift from Dr. Andrew Brown (UNSW, Sydney, Australia). CHO cells were cultured in DMEM F-12 nutrient medium supplemented with 10% foetal calf serum and 1% Glutamax at 37°C in 10% CO_2.

Transient Transfection and siRNA Mediated Knock Down

NPC1-YFP was kindly provided by Dr. Hongyuan Robert Yang (UNSW, Sydney, Australia). NPC1-YFP was transfected into CHO cells using Lipofectamine LTX (Life Technologies) following the manufacturer's guidelines. For siRNA experiments approximately 2 million cells were used for each nucleofection with scrambled siRNA as a control (sense 5′-CAGTCGCGTTTGCGACTGGTT-3′) or siRNA to NPC1 (sense 5′-GGGAAAGAAUUCAUGAAAUUU-3′) (Thermo Scientific) using the Amaxa Kit and reagents following the manufacturers guidelines (Lonza). Cells were reseeded onto matrigel (BD Biosciences) coated plates and experiments were performed 4 d later.

Preparation of Whole Cell Lysates and Western Blotting

Cells were serum starved in serum-free media for 2 h before incubation with 100 nM insulin for 20 min. Cells were lysed in lysis buffer (2% w/v SDS in phosphate buffered saline (PBS), pH 7.4, protease inhibitors (Roche), 1 mm sodium pyrophosphate, 2 mm sodium vanadate, 10 mm sodium fluoride) sonicated for 12s and centrifuged at 13,000×*g*. The protein concentration of the supernatant was determined by BCA assay (Thermo Scientific). 10 μg samples of protein were resolved by SDS-PAGE and transferred to PVDF membranes. Membranes were blocked in 5% skim milk powder in TBS-T (0.1% v/v Tween-20 in tris-buffered saline) for 1 h followed by an overnight incubation at 4°C with specific 1° antibody solutions. Membranes were incubated with an appropriate secondary antibody for 1 h before signals were detected using ECL (Thermo Scientific) or on the Odyssey infrared imaging system (LI-COR). Anti-Akt, anti-pT473 Akt and anti-pT308 Akt antibodies were obtained from Cell Signaling Technology. Anti-IRS1 antibody, anti-insulin receptor β antibody and anti-14-3-3 antibodies were from Santa Cruz Biotechnology. Anti-AS160 was from Upstate, anti-pT642 AS160 was from Symansis, anti-NPC1 antibody was from Abcam and anti-TfR antibody was from Zymed. IRAP, GLUT1 and GLUT4 antibodies were generated in-house.

Filipin Staining

For imaging of U18666a-treated 3T3-L1 adipocytes cells were seeded into individual collagen type IV coated wells of μ-Slide 8 well chambered slides (Ibidi) prior to U18666a treatment as described above. Cells were at room temperature with 3% paraformaldehyde (PFA) in PBS for 30 minutes. PFA was quenched with 20 mM glycine and cells were blocked with 2% BSA in PBS. Filipin (Sigma-Aldrich) was added to cells at 125 μg/ml at room temperature for 30 min. Cells were imaged in PBS with 5% glycerol (Sigma) and 2.5% 1,4-diazabicyclo[2.2.2]octane (Sigma) on a Leica DMI 6000 SP8 MP microscope (Leica) using a 63×/1.20 water corrected objective. Z-stacks were acquired for the entire sample thickness up to 50 μm with a voxel size of 0.12×0.12×0.43 μm. The Filipin signal was imaged using multiphoton excitation at 725 nm and emission was detected at 450–550 nm.

For imaging of siRNA-treated cells, 3T3-L1 adipocytes were electroporated with scrambled siRNA or siRNA directed to NPC1 as described above. Cells were and seeded onto matrigel coated 42 mm coverslips (#1.5). Cells were fixed and stained as above. Cells were washed, mounted and imaged on a Leica DMI 6000 SP8 confocal microscope (Leica) using a 63×/1.20 water corrected objective. The Filipin signal was imaged using 405 nm excitation and emission was detected at 450–550 nm, voxel size 0.07×0.07×0.34 μm.

Cholesterol Assay

3T3-L1 adipocytes were homogenised in HES buffer (10 mM Hepes, pH 7.4, 1 mM EDTA, 250 mM sucrose, protease inhibitors (Roche)) by 12 strokes of a dounce homogeniser. Cell debris was pelleted at 700×*g* for 10 min and a total membrane preparation acquired by centrifugation at 235,000×*g* for 75 min. Lipid was extracted by chloroform:methanol extraction. Briefly, membrane preparation was added to chloroform:methanol (2:1) mix, vortexed and shaken for 10 minutes. ddH_2O was added and samples were centrifuged for 10 minutes to generate a clear interface. The lower phase was removed and evaporated to dryness. Lipid residue was reconstituted in 100 μl 10% (v/v) Triton X-100 in Isopropanol and cholesterol levels determined using an Amplex Red based cholesterol detection assay following the manufacturer's instructions (Life Technologies).

2-[3H]deoxyglucose Uptake Assay

3T3-L1 adipocytes were serum starved in serum-free DMEM for 2 hours before being washed in PBS (x3) and incubated in Krebs Ringer buffer (KRP) (0.6 mM Na_2HPO_4, 0.4 mM NaH_2PO_4, 120 mM NaCl, 6 mM KCl, 1 mM $CaCl_2$, 1.2 mM $MgSO_4$ and 12.5 mM Hepes (pH 7.4)) with 0.2% BSA. Cells were stimulated with 100 nM insulin for 20 min. To determine non-specific glucose uptake, 25 μM cytochalasin B was added into the wells before addition of 2-[3H]deoxyglucose. During the final 5 min, 2-deoxyglucose transport was initiated by addition of 2-[3H]deoxyglucose (PerkinElmer). Following three rapid washes in ice-cold PBS, cells were solubilized in 1% (v/v) Triton X-100 in PBS. Scintillation counts were normalized for protein content.

Subcellular Fractionation

3T3-L1 adipocytes cultured in 15cm plates were harvested in HES buffer and dounce homogenised. Subcellular fractionation was carried out as previously described [19].

HA-GLUT4 Assay

The determination of plasma membrane HA-GLUT4 levels was carried out as previously described [20].

qPCR

3T3-L1 adipocytes cultured in 6 well plates were lysed in 1 mL TRIzol (Life Technologies). 0.2 mL of chloroform was added samples were mixed well. Samples were centrifuged at 12,000×*g* for 15 min at 4°C and the aqueous phase collected. Following addition of 0.5 mL 100% isopropanol, samples were incubated for 10 min at RT and centrifuged at 12,000×*g* for 10 min at 4°C. The pellet was washed with 1 mL 75% ethanol and centrifuged as 7,500×*g* for 5 min at 4°C. The RNA pellet was resuspended in RNase-free water and incubated at 60°C for 10–15 min. A master mix was prepared for the reverse-transcription reaction comprised of 10 x Buffer RT, 5 mM dNTP, 10 µM Oligo dT primer, 10 U/µl RNase inhibitor, Omniscript Reverse Transcriptase (Qiagen) and RNase-free water. 2 µg Template RNA was added to the master mix which was then briefly vortexed, centrifuged and incubated for 60 min at 37°C. qPCR was performed using the LightCycler 480 (Roche) using the LightCycler480 Master reagent (Roche), according to the manufacturer's instructions. Primers for target genes were 5′-gcagatcaagcatcccaact-3′ and 5′- ccagagaatgtttcattgtcca-3′ for *ABCA1*, 5′- tgctctgggtaccatgacatc-3′ and 5′- cccacaaatgtcgcaacc -3′ for *ABCG1*, 5′-agaccctggaggctaaggac-3′ and 5′-agagccttcatcttcgcaat-3′ for *APOE*, 5′-catgagggaaatcaatgatcg-3′ and 5′-ctaaagctgagagagtgtgagagc-3′ for *TfR*, 5′-agtgttcatatctacgaaccgtacc-3′ and 5′-tcaatggcgatctgtaagtcc-3′ for *NPC1*, 5′-gacctgtcctcaagattggtg-3′ and 5′-gatggtgtgccttcatctgtc-3′ for *IRAP*, 5′- cagccggcacagctagag -3′ and 5′- agcactgctcctcccaca -3′ for *GLUT1*, 5′- gacggacactccatctgttg -3′ and 5′- gccacgatggagacatagc -3′ for *GLUT4* and 5′-ttcttcataaccacagtcaagacc-3′ and 5′-accttccgtaccacatccat-3′ for *CYPB*.

Results

Genetic Ablation of NPC1 Inhibited Insulin Signalling

To initially assess the role of NPC1 activity on insulin signalling we utilised CHO 2–2 cells, an NPC1 knockout cell line [21]. These cells do not express NPC1 due to a frame-shift in the gene transcript (Figure 1A). We did not observe any changes in the total levels of the insulin signalling molecules Akt or Akt substrate AS160 (TBC1D4) between this cell line and wild type CHO (K1) cells (Figure 1B). However, differences were apparent upon insulin stimulation. In wild type CHO (K1) cells, insulin stimulated phosphorylation of Akt at S473 and T308 and AS160 at T642. This effect was reduced in 2–2 cells (Figure 1C).

We validated the specificity of this approach by rescuing NPC1 expression. NPC1-YFP was transfected into both K1 and in 2–2 cells (Figure 1A). NPC1 overexpression enhanced phosphorylation of Akt and AS160 in K1 cells suggesting that increasing NPC1 activity in wild type cells can augment insulin responses. Rescue of NPC1 expression in 2–2 cells restored insulin-stimulated phosphorylation of Akt at S473 and T308 and AS160 at T642 towards the levels observed in K1 cells, although the degree of phosphorylation at these sites did not fully revert to levels in control cells (Figure 1C). Overall, introduction of exogenous NPC1 improved signalling in both wild type and NPC1 KO cells.

Inhibition of NPC1 Impaired Insulin Signalling in 3T3-L1 Adipocytes

Having shown that NPC1 regulates insulin signalling in CHO cells, we investigated whether this link also exists in 3T3-L1 adipocytes, a more physiologically relevant cell model for insulin signalling. We first took a pharmacological approach to reduce NPC1 activity. U18666a is an agent used to induce an NPC disease phenotype and is reported to interact directly with NPC1 [22]. Incubation of adipocytes with U18666a for 24, 48, and 72 h resulted in redistribution of cholesterol from the plasma membrane to intracellular structures most likely due to the accumulation of cholesterol in lysosomes (Figure 2A). Treatment with U18666a also led to increased concentrations of cholesterol within the crude membrane fraction (Figure 2B). Both these readouts indicated effective NPC1 inhibition [7].

We used this model to interrogate the effect of NPC1 inhibition on insulin signalling in 3T3-L1 adipocytes. We treated 3T3-L1 adipocytes with U18666a for 24, 48, and 72 h prior to examining insulin signalling. Insulin-stimulated phosphorylation of Akt (T308 and S473), and AS160 (T642) was substantially reduced in U18666a treated cells (Figure 2C). To investigate why we observed this defect in insulin signalling, we measured the expression levels of proteins comprising key nodes within the insulin signalling pathway (Figure 2D). Total Akt levels were unchanged with U18666a treatment. However, expression of both the insulin receptor (IR) and insulin receptor substrate 1 (IRS1) were reduced in adipocytes incubated with U18666a for prolonged periods (48–72 h). However, these changes in total expression levels are unlikely to fully account for the reduced Akt phosphorylation since the change in IR and IRS1 occurred much later than the defect in Akt phosphorylation. In fact changes in IR and IRS1 corresponded better with redistribution of cholesterol from the PM to intracellular sites (Figure 2A).

NPC1 Activity was Required for Full Akt Activation

To confirm our observations using a pharmacologic inhibitor of NPC1 we next used siRNA knock down to determine if this achieved the same outcome. Introduction of an NPC1-targetted siRNA into adipocytes was sufficient to achieve an approximately 50% reduction in cellular NPC1 levels and inhibit NPC1 function as indicated by the accumulation of cholesterol at intracellular sites (Figures 2E, F). Consistent with our studies with U18666a, phosphorylation of Akt at both 308 and 473 was reduced by approximately 50% (Figures 2G). In addition, AS160 phosphorylation at T642 was decreased in NPC1 knock down cells (Figures 2G). Intriguingly we did not observe any significant change in the levels of either IR or IRS1 with NPC1 siRNA (Figure 2F) in contrast to that seen with U18666a. This is consistent with our observation in drug treated cells the impairment in Akt signalling precedes the reduction in IR and IRS1 levels. To further confirm that defects at Akt were not due to reduced IRS levels we next examined the regulation of Akt by PDGF in 3T3-L1 adipocytes overexpressing the PDGF receptor. Unlike insulin, PGDF activates Akt through a direct interaction between the PDGF receptor and PI3K [23] and so initiation of Akt signalling in response to PDGF is independent of IRS1. We observed a reduction in PDGF-stimulated Akt activation in U18666a treated cells (Figure 2I). Based on these findings we conclude that that inhibition of NPC1 influences Akt function independently of its effects on IRS1 protein abundance.

Inhibition of NPC1 Reduced Insulin-stimulated Glucose Uptake in 3T3-L1 Adipocytes

Since we observed considerable impairment of insulin signalling in response to NPC1 inhibition, we next measured whether this had downstream consequences; specifically on insulin-stimulated glucose transport. Insulin stimulates glucose transport in adipocytes through promoting trafficking of GLUT4 to the cell surface [24]. U18666a treatment substantially reduced insulin-stimulated

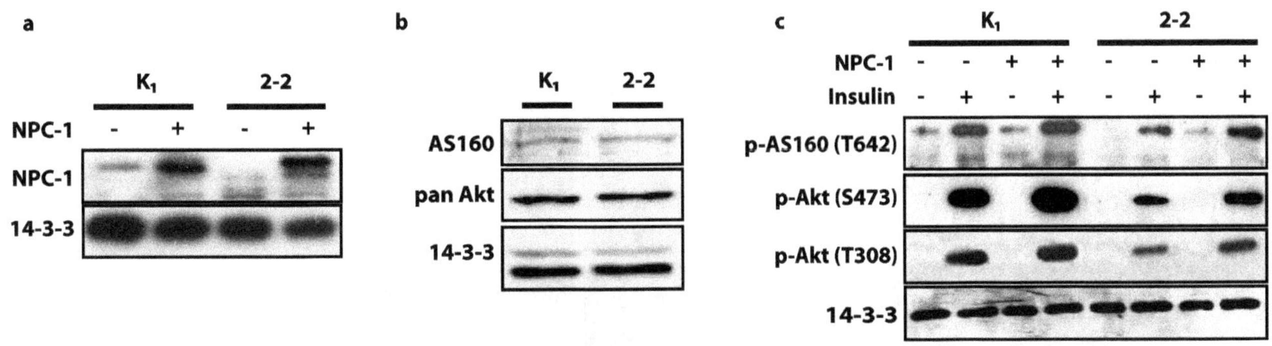

Figure 1. NPC1 knockout inhibited insulin signalling in CHO cells. (**a**) Total cell lysates of K1 CHO cells and 2–2 CHO cells were immunoblotted with anti-NPC1 antibody to determine expression levels of endogenous NPC1 and overexpressed NPC1-YFP. (**b**) Total cells lysates of K1 CHO cells and 2–2 CHO cells were immunoblotted with anti-Akt and AS160 antibodies to compare expression levels between K1 and 2–2 CHO cells. (**c**) Total cell lysates from unstimulated and insulin-stimulated cells (100 nM, 20 min) were immunoblotted with phospho-T308 Akt, phospho-S473 Akt, phospho-T642 AS160 and 14-3-3 antibodies to assess insulin signalling.

2-deoxyglucose uptake, and this phenotype worsened over the time course of NPC1 inhibition (Figure 3A). However, the extent of this defect was blunted compared to the level of Akt phosphorylation (Figure 2C). In addition, 2-deoxyglucose uptake in the absence of insulin was increased with U18666a treatment over time (Figure 3A). Although no defect in 2-deoxyglucose transport in NPC1-knockdown cells was observed at 100 nM insulin, there was a blunted effect at 0.1 nM (Figure 3B), indicating reduced sensitivity to insulin.

Inhibition of NPC1 Altered GLUT4 Trafficking

Considering that basal and insulin-stimulated glucose uptake was affected by U18666a treatment, we hypothesised that GLUT4 trafficking to the PM in response to insulin would be altered in U18666a treated cells. We isolated PM fractions from unstimulated and insulin-stimulated adipocytes treated with or without U18666a and determined the levels of GLUT4 and IRAP, a protein that co-traffics with GLUT4 [25](Figure 3C). A striking observation was the reduction in PM GLUT4 and IRAP under basal conditions. PM caveolin levels were also reduced in U18666a treated cells. Although the major effect of U18666a treatment appeared to be in reducing GLUT4 levels in PM fractions from both basal and insulin-stimulated adipocytes, there also appeared to be a reduction in the fold-stimulation of GLUT4 translocation to the PM in U18666a-treated cells. To confirm this defect in GLUT4 translocation, we performed a complementary assay in 3T3-L1 adipocytes overexpressing GLUT4 with a HA-epitope in the primary exofacial loop (HA-GLUT4) to measure PM levels of GLUT4 [20]. The advantage of this assay is that PM HA-GLUT4 levels can be readily expressed relative to total HA-GLUT4 expression levels allowing determination of the level of HA-GLUT4 translocation to the PM independent of any effects on GLUT4 expression which may confound interpretation when assaying endogenous GLUT4 levels. PM GLUT4 was increased in the basal state and decreased in the insulin-stimulated state in response to U18666a. The extent of increased PM HA-GLUT4 under unstimulated conditions and inhibition of insulin-stimulated HA-GLUT4 translocation was more pronounced with increasing U18666a treatment length (Figure 3D). Overall, U18666a treatment resulted in modest but significant changes in GLUT4 trafficking under both unstimulated and insulin stimulated conditions.

Total GLUT4 Levels were Reduced by U18666a Treatment

Despite observing changes in GLUT4 trafficking, the major observation from our subfractionation studies was reduced GLUT4 in the PM fraction. We next determined whether this was due to mislocalisation of GLUT4 or to a reduction in total levels of GLUT4. GLUT4 protein levels were considerably decreased, after 72h of U18666a treatment (Figure 4A). We compared this to effects on the levels of other trafficking proteins. Intriguingly the levels of IRAP and the transferrin receptor (TfR) were also reduced in cells exposed to U18666a for 72 h, but to a lesser extent than GLUT4. In contrast to effects on GLUT4, levels of another GLUT isoform, GLUT1, was increased in the U18666a treated cells (Figure 4A), indicating that U18666a treatment did not lead to a global reduction in trafficking protein expression.

Inhibition of NPC1 Reduced LXR-mediated GLUT4 Transcription

To assess whether the change in GLUT isoform, IRAP and TfR protein expression was mediated transcriptionally, we measured transcript levels in control and U18666a treated cells by qPCR. U18666a resulted in down-regulation of *GLUT4* mRNA to 32% of that of control cells and of *TFR* to 36% of that in control cells (Figure 4B). In contrast, *GLUT1* transcription was up-regulated approximately 2-fold while *IRAP* transcript levels were unchanged implying that changes in IRAP protein were not mediated transcriptionally. We next measured mRNA levels of these genes in cells treated with NPC siRNA. This analysis confirmed NPC1 knockdown and also revealed a significant decrease in *GLUT4* expression which did not translate to a change in GLUT4 protein levels in these cells (89.9% ±7.1% S.E.M, $n = 4$, $p = 0.25$ by two sample t-test) (Figures 4C, D). The extent of *GLUT4* down-regulation at the mRNA and protein level was substantially less than observed in U18666a-treated cells. *GLUT1*, *TFR* and *IRAP* transcripts were not altered in NPC1 knockdown cells (Figure 4C).

It has previously been reported that the activity of the liver X receptor (LXR), a nuclear receptor that recognises oxysterol ligands, is reduced under NPC1 inhibition [26]. Further, LXR has been implicated in regulating *GLUT4* expression [27]. Therefore we tested whether LXR activity was reduced in adipocytes treated with U18666a through measuring the expression of classical LXR target genes *ABCA1*, *ABCG1*, and *APOE*. These genes were down-regulated by 44%, 64%, and 53% respectively, indicative of reduced LXR activity (Figure 4E). To test whether *GLUT4*

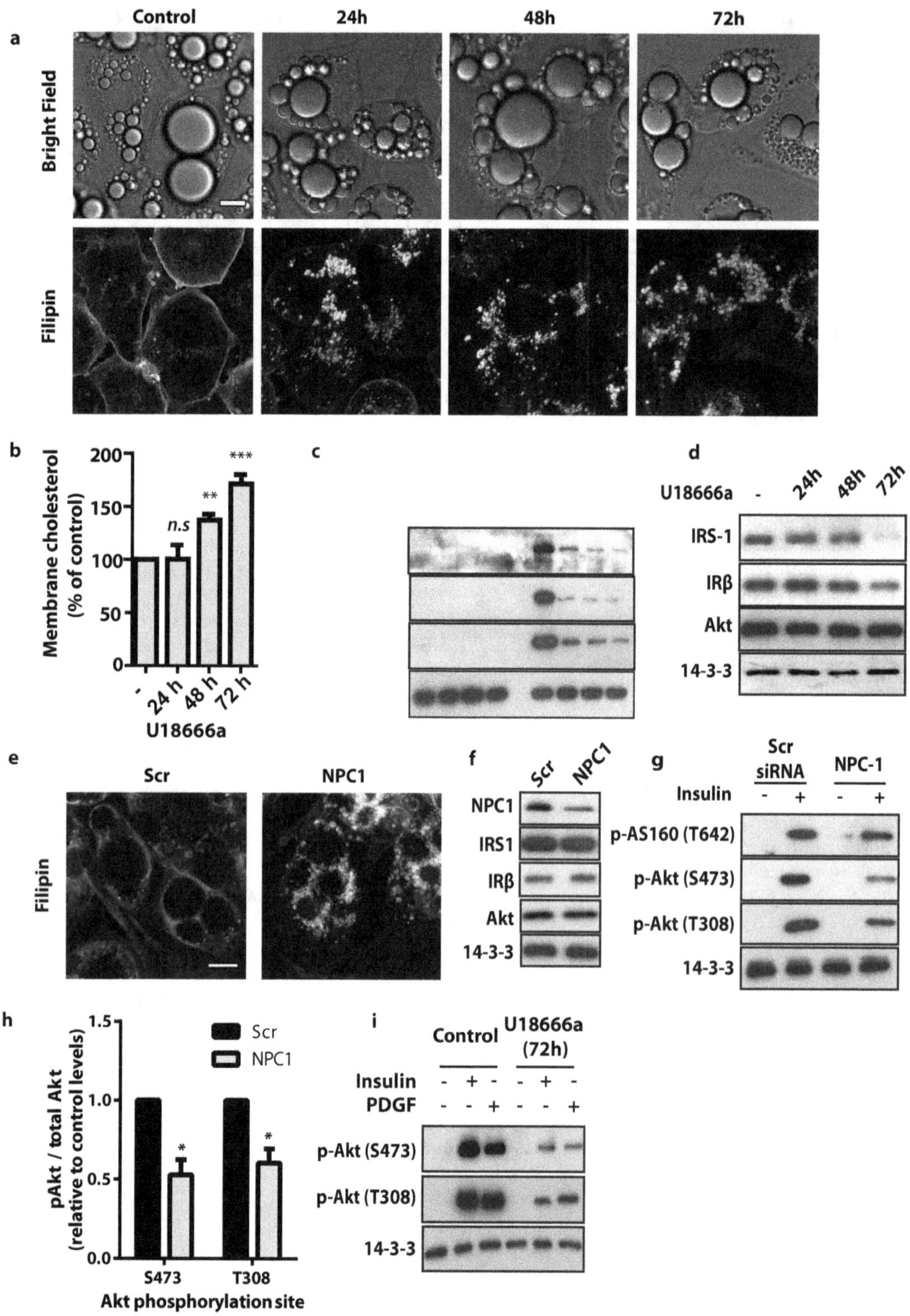

Figure 2. Pharmacological and genetic inhibition of NPC1 reduced insulin signalling in 3T3-L1 adipocytes. NPC1 was inhibited in 3T3-L1 adipocytes through treatment with U18666a or through siRNA-mediated knockdown of NPC1. (**a**) Subcellular localisation of cholesterol in 3T3-L1 adipocytes after treatment with U18666a for indicated times was visualised by Filipin staining (scale bar = 10 μm), bottom panel. Corresponding bright field images are provided (top panel). Images are representative of n ≥300 cells viewed per condition over 3 experiments. (**b**) Total membrane cholesterol levels within the total membrane fraction. Data are mean ± S.E.M, n = 3 independent experiments, one-way ANOVA. (**c**) Insulin signalling was assessed by immunoblotting total cell lysates of unstimulated and insulin-stimulated (100 nM, 20 min) 3T3-L1 adipocytes for phospho-T308 Akt, phospho-S473 Akt, phospho-T642 AS160 and 14-3-3. (**d**) Total protein expression of key proteins in the insulin pathway determined by immunoblotting for IRS-1, IRβ and Akt. (**e**) Subcellular localisation of cholesterol after treatment with scrambled or NPC1 siRNA was visualised by Filipin staining (scale bar = 10 μm). Images are representative of n≥300 cells viewed per condition over 3 experiments. (**f**) The extent of siRNA mediated knockdown of NPC1 and the effect of knockdown on expression of proximal insulin signalling components was measured by probing for NPC1, IRS-1, IRβ and Akt. (**g**) The effect of NPC1 knock-down on insulin signalling was assessed by immunoblotting with phospho-T308 Akt, phospho-

S473 Akt, phospho-T642 AS160 and 14-3-3 antibodies. (**h**) The levels of insulin-stimulated pS473 and pT308 of Akt in cells NPC1 knockdown cells was quantified relative to control cells. Data are mean ± S.E.M, n = 3 independent experiments, two-sample t-test. (**i**) 3T3-L1 adipocytes overexpressing PDGF receptor were treated with U18666a for 72 hr prior to assessment of insulin and PDGF-mediated (20 ng/mL, 20 min) signalling. Signalling was assessed by immunoblotting with phospho-T308 Akt, phospho-S473 Akt and 14-3-3 antibodies. All data are representative of at least n = 3 independent experiments, significance calculated compared to control cells, n.s = non-significant, *, = p<0.05 ** = p<0.01 *** = p<0.001, statistical tests as indicated.

expression was decreased as a function of reduced LXR activity we utilised GW3965, which activates LXR independently of cellular sterol status. GW3965 increased the expression of the classic LXR target genes as well as GLUT4 in control cells (Figure 4E). Applying GW3965 to cells pre-treated with U18666a for 72 h rescued the expression of *ABCA1* and *ABCG1* above the levels observed in untreated control cells, towards levels observed in control cells treated with GW3965. *APO-E* and *GLUT4* expression was increased towards levels observed in untreated control cells. For *GLUT4*, the increase in expression in response to GW3965 was significantly greater in cells pretreated with U18666a than in control cells (Figure 4E, F). This rescue of *GLUT4* mRNA levels also resulted in increased protein expression (Figure 4G). To ensure that reduced LXR activity was a result of NPC1 inhibition by U18666a and not an off target effect we also assessed LXR target gene expression in NPC1 knockdown cells. NPC1 knockdown altered LXR activity cells as *ABCA1* and *ABCG1* transcript levels were significantly reduced (Figure 4H). However, *APOE* levels were not changed. Nevertheless, these data indicate that decreased LXR activity partially accounts for reduced *GLUT4* gene expression upon NPC1 inhbition.

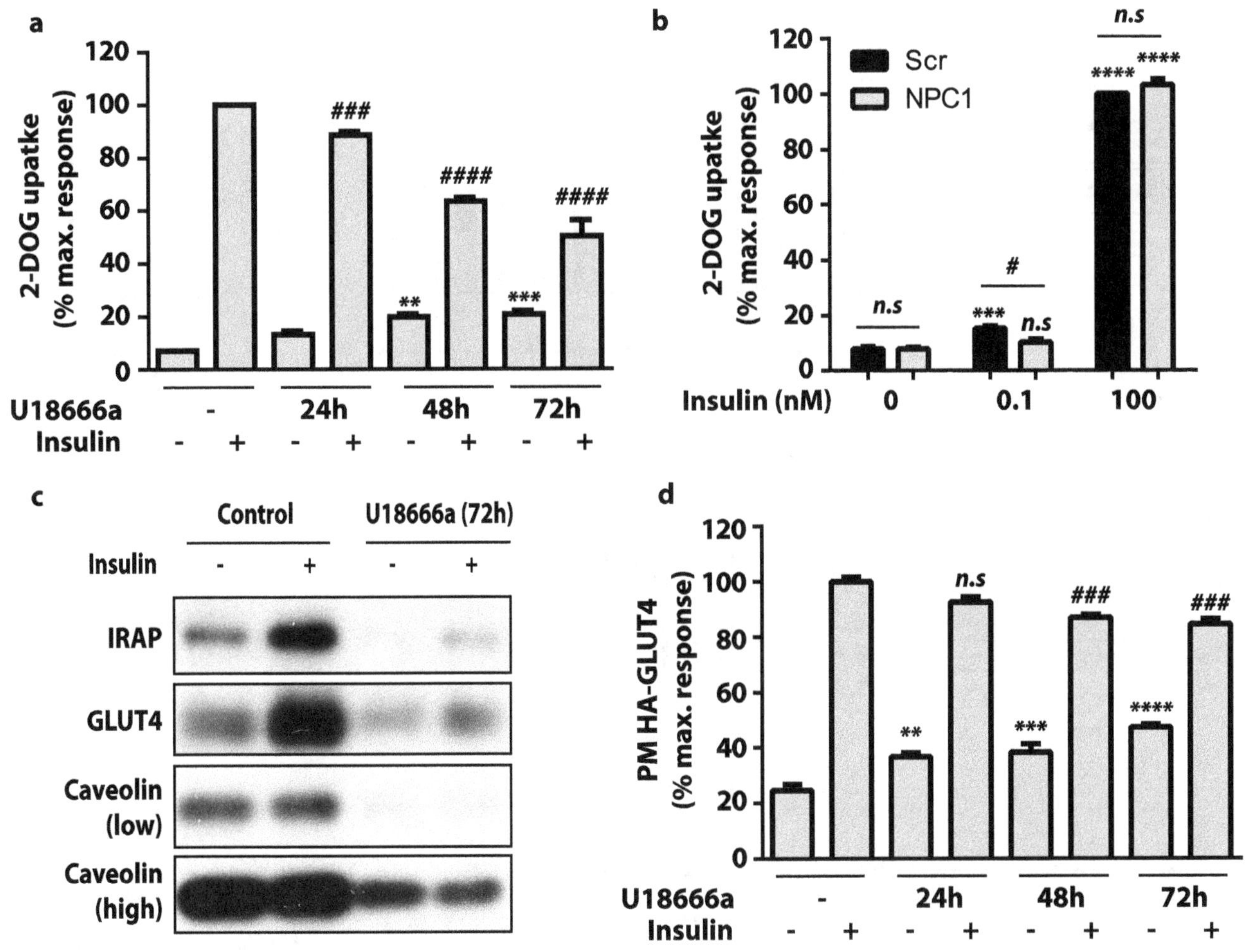

Figure 3. Inhibition of NPC1 repressed insulin-stimulated glucose uptake. (**a**) 3T3-L1 adipocytes were treated with U18666a for indicated periods of time before radiolabelled 2-deoxy-D-glucose uptake assays were performed on basal and insulin-stimulated cells. Data are mean ±S.E.M, n = 4 independent experiments. (**b**) 3T3-L1 adipocytes electroporated with scrambled (Scr) or siRNA directed to NPC1 (NPC1) were subjected to radiolabelled 2-deoxy-D-glucose uptake assays under basal and insulin-stimulated conditions. Insulin doses as indicated. Data are mean ±S.E.M, n = 3 independent experiments. (**c**) Plasma membrane (PM) levels of IRAP, GLUT4 and Caveolin 1 in unstimulated and insulin-stimulated (100 nM, 20 min) adipocytes were determined by immunoblotting. (**d**) PM levels of HA-GLUT4 was measured using a fluorescence based assay in 3T3-L1 adipocytes overexpressing HA-GLUT4 treated with U18666a for indicated periods of time. Data are mean ±S.E.M, n = 3 independent experiments. Significance calculated by two-way ANOVA. Comparisons to unstimulated cells (a, b, d) indicated by n.s = non-significant, * = p<0.05 ** = p<0.01 *** = p<0.001 **** = p<0.0001. Comparisons to insulin-stimulated cells (a, b, d) indicated by n.s = non-significant, # = p<0.05 ## = p<0.01 ### = p<0.001 #### = p<0.0001.

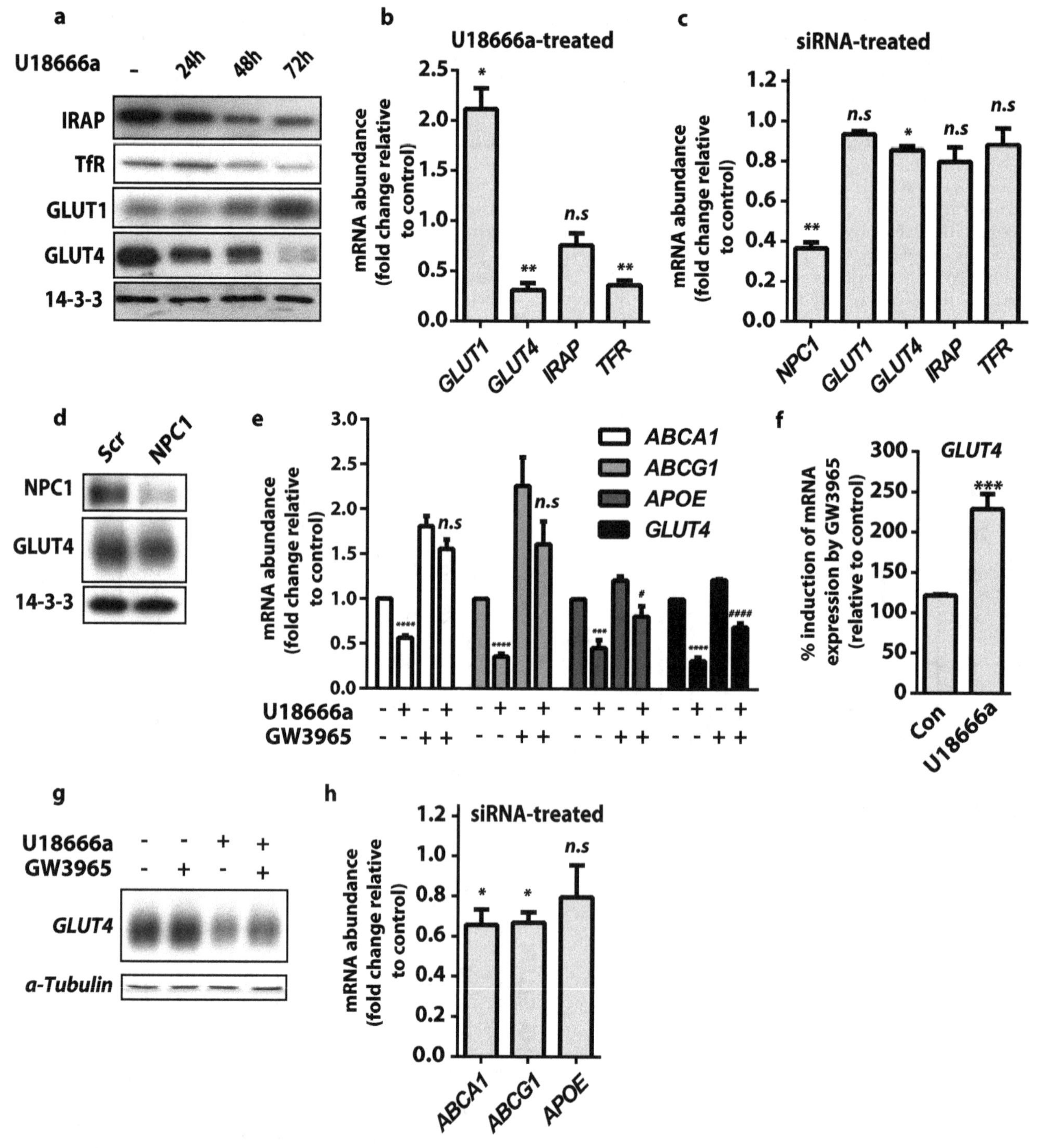

Figure 4. Inhibition of NPC1 reduced *GLUT4* expression via lower LXR activity. (**a**) Total protein levels of IRAP, Transferrin, GLUT1 and GLUT4 were determined by immunoblotting of whole cell lysates from cells with U18666a for indicated times. (**b**) *GLUT1, GLUT4, IRAP,* and *TFR* mRNA levels in 3T3-L1 adipocytes treated with U18666a for 72 h were determined by qPCR and presented relative to expression in control cells. Data are mean ±S.E.M, n = 3–5 independent experiments. (**c**) *NPC1, GLUT1, GLUT4, IRAP* and *TFR* mRNA levels in 3T3-L1 adipocytes treated with NPC1 siRNA were determined by qPCR and presented relative to expression in control cells. Data are mean ±S.E.M, n = 3 independent experiments. (**d**) Total protein levels of NPC1 and GLUT4 were determined by immunoblotting of whole cell lysates from control and NPC1 knockdown cells. (**e**) mRNA levels of *ABCA1, ABCG1* and *APO-E* and *GLUT4* were determined by qPCR. Control and U18666a (72 h) pre-treated adipocytes were treated with the LXR agonist GW3965 (10 μM) for 16 h. Data are mean ±S.E.M and expressed relative to mRNA levels for each gene in control cells. All data are n = 3–5 independent experiments. (**f**) Percentage change in *GLUT4* mRNA levels following GW3095 addition was calculated from (f). (**g**) Total GLUT4 protein levels were determined by immunoblotting of whole cell lysates from control cells and cells treated with U18666a and/or GW3095 as indicated. (**h**) *ABCA1, ABCG1 and APOE* mRNA levels in 3T3-L1 adipocytes treated with NPC1 siRNA were determined by qPCR and presented relative to expression in control cells. Data are mean ±S.E.M, n = 3 independent experiments. Significance calculated by two sample t-test (b,c,f,h) or two-way ANOVA (e) and indicated p values are compared to control cells n.s = non-significant, * = p<0.05 ** = p<0.01 *** = p<0.001 **** = p<0.0001 or cells treated with U18666a (f) n.s = non-significant, # = p<0.05 #### = p<0.0001 (e).

Discussion

The molecular mechanisms of insulin resistance remain unresolved. Recent genome-wide studies have begun to reveal associations of genetic loci with insulin resistance. Indeed, GWAS data and genetic studies in mice have uncovered a link between insulin resistance and NPC1 [4]. Although this gene has been previously implicated in insulin resistance and glucose intolerance [14], the mechanism underpinning this association is undefined. Here we report that pharmacological or genetic inhibition of NPC1 function causes considerable defects at four major nodes of insulin signalling to glucose transport; at the level of IRS1 expression, Akt activation, GLUT4 trafficking and GLUT4 transcription. Additionally, these nodes appear to be differentially sensitive to NPC1 inhibition. These data strongly implicate NPC1 function and cholesterol homeostasis in the maintenance of insulin sensitivity in adipocytes.

One of the major phenotypes associated with reduced NPC1 levels or activity was reduced insulin signalling. Insulin-stimulated Akt and AS160 phosphorylation were reduced in an NPC1 KO CHO cell line (2–2) and in 3T3-L1 adipocytes in which NPC1 levels were depleted using siRNA (Figure 1C and 2G, H). The fact that this was observed in two cell lines supports the concept that NPC1 function is required in multiple cell types to maintain insulin responsiveness. U18666a treatments further disrupted insulin signalling to Akt and AS160 (Figure 2C), but also led to decreased levels of the insulin receptor and IRS1 (Figure 2D). This matches observations from NPC1−/− mice [16]. However, we did not observe the same reduction in these proximal signalling molecules in siRNA treated cells (Figure 2F). We speculate that this discrepancy may be due to the severity of NPC1 inhibition, with prolonged U18666a treatment possibly more potently inhibiting NPC1 function than the partial knockdown with siRNA. We observed a reduction in PM cholesterol and an increase in intracellular membrane cholesterol levels following U18666a treatment and siRNA-mediated NPC knock down (Figures 2A, B, E). However, only under conditions where PM cholesterol is undetectable relative to internal staining do we begin to observe reductions in IR and IRS1 levels (Figure 2A, D –48 h, 72 h). However, we cannot rule out that U18666a is having effects other than on NPC1, which may account for this difference. For example, U18666a is known to inhibit sterol synthesis [28], which could exacerbate the cholesterol trafficking defects observed in U18666a treated cells (Figure 2A). However, considering that cholesterol trafficking defects and IRS1 levels appear to correlate it may be that cholesterol-rich caveolae, within which IR resides [29], were disrupted by U18666a treatment. We observed a large reduction in caveolin at the PM in U18666a treated cells (Figure 3B) but no change in total cellular caveolin (data not shown), indicative of increased internal caveolin which has been reported to occur in response to PM cholesterol depletion [30]. Since there is evidence for a role for caveolin in stabilising IRS1 [31–33] and for caveolin as a promoter of insulin signalling [34], we favour the possibility that reduced IR and IRS1 levels are caused by a loss of PM cholesterol and subsequent loss of lipid rafts.

In addition to these IR and IRS1 effects, we also detected specific inhibition of Akt phosphorylation which was IRS1-independent. We provide several avenues of evidence for this conclusion. Firstly, we observed reduced Akt phosphorylation prior to impaired IRS1 expression in U18666a-treated cells, although we cannot rule out that IRS1 is mislocalised at earlier time points (Figure 2C and 2D). Secondly, a reduction in phospho-Akt was detected in siRNA-treated cells without changes in IR and IRS1 levels (Figures 2F, G). Thirdly, PDGF-dependent Akt signalling was also reduced (Figure 2I). These data indicate that NPC1 activity is required for complete activation of Akt and that this requirement is independent of the alterations in IRS1 protein levels. These findings shed new light on insulin signalling defects in the NPC1−/− mice, which had been previously attributed to solely reduced IRS1 expression [16]. Since we observed IRS1-independent inhibition of Akt phosphorylation in response to NPC1 inhibition, a defect is likely to lie at the level of phosphatidylinositol-3-kinase (PI3K) or at the upstream kinases of Akt, PDK1 and/or mTORC2. A number of components of this signalling nexus have been localised to cholesterol-rich lipid raft domains including phosphatidylinostol-2-phosphate (PIP2) [35–37] the substrate for PI3K and both PDK1 [38] and mTORC2 [39]. Further, PTEN, a negative regulator of Akt phosphorylation has been reported to be excluded from these domains [38]. Taken together, one possibility for the pronounced defect in insulin signalling downstream to Akt in the context of NPC1 inhibition is the loss of the localisation of these signalling molecules upon disruption of cholesterol trafficking.

Downstream of Akt signalling we also observed a defect in insulin-stimulated glucose transport following U18666a treatment (Figure 3A) and at low dose insulin in NPC1 knockdown cells (Figure 3B) indicative of NPC1 inhibition reducing insulin sensitivity. The time lag between reduced signalling and the defects in GLUT4 translocation and glucose uptake observed in U18666a-treated cells is of interest (Figures 2C, 3A,3D); U18666a treatment for 24 h caused a relatively small decrease in glucose transport and GLUT4 translocation, while Akt phosphorylation was considerably reduced at this time point. Furthermore, the level of insulin signalling is similar between 48 h and 72 h of U18666a treatment, whereas it is between these time points that major effects upon glucose uptake and GLUT4 translocation are observed. One explanation for this is the redundancy within the Akt signalling network. Only 5% of maximal Akt activation is required to elicit full glucose transport effects [40]. Additionally, disruption to other components comprising the insulin responsive system may also account for this. We observed increasingly aberrant GLUT4 trafficking over the 72 h U18666a treatment (Figures 2A, B). This manifested itself as increased PM GLUT4 (as a percentage of total levels) under unstimulated conditions and reduced insulin stimulated GLUT4 PM levels (Figure 3D). Decreased PM cholesterol has previously been reported to inhibit GLUT4 internalisation, which may explain increased proportion of total GLUT at the PM under basal conditions [41]. Further, disruption of cholesterol trafficking has been found to reduce SNARE machinery, specifically SNAP23 and syntaxin-4, at the PM [42]. These SNAREs mediate GLUT4 fusion with the PM [24] and thus impaired SNARE assembly at the PM or at other cellular organelles [43] may contribute to the reduced GLUT4 translocation in U18666a treated cells (Figure 3C and D).

Although we observed modest effects on glucose transport at times when signalling was reduced by U18666a (24 h) or siRNA-mediated NPC1 knockdown, the major disruption of regulated glucose transport only occurred in unison with large reductions in GLUT4 protein levels (table 1). Considering these data, we speculate that the metabolic complications associated with reduced NPC1 expression [14,15] may be due, in part, to decreased GLUT4 expression in adipose since adipose-specific KO of GLUT4 confers insulin resistance and glucose intolerance [44]. Concomitant with decreases in *GLUT4* gene expression, we measured reduced in *TFR* but increased *GLUT1* expression (Figure 3B, C). Increased GLUT1 protein expression likely explains raised basal 2-deoxyglucose uptake rates observed in

Table 1. Summary of phenotypes with different modes of NPC1 inhibition.

	24 h U18666a	48 h U18666a	72 h U18666a	NPC1 siRNA
Akt signalling	↓↓	↓↓	↓↓	↓
GLUT4 translocation	=	↓↓	↓↓	NM
GLUT4 protein	↓	↓	↓↓	=
GLUT4 mRNA	NM	NM	↓↓	↓
Glucose (2DOG) uptake	↓↓	↓↓↓	↓↓↓	↓ (at low dose insulin)

Number of arrows indicates severity of phenotype. NM = not measured.

U18666a treated cells (Figure 3A). Although we detected a defect in GLUT4 trafficking in unstimulated cells under U18666a treatment (Figure 3D) this probably does not contribute to increased basal 2-deoxyglucose uptake as absolute levels of GLUT4 at the PM were severely reduced (Figure 3C).

The effects of NPC1 inhibition described here are similar to those described in cholesterol depleted adipocytes [45]. This includes the change in expression of GLUT isoforms and induction of insulin resistance. Reduced cholesterol availability reduces LXR activity [46], which is a master transcriptional regulator of cholesterol homeostasis. LXR has been reported to regulate GLUT4 expression in adipocytes [27], and the LXR target gene *ABCA1* was reported to be down-regulated in cholesterol depleted adipocytes that also displayed reduced GLUT4 expression [45]. LXR activity was reduced in response to U18666a, as measured by target gene expression levels. The use of the LXR agonist GW3965 partially rescued the reduction in *GLUT4* gene expression (Figure 4F, G). In addition to *GLUT4*, *GLUT1* may also be LXR responsive. It has been shown previously to respond to an LXR agonist [47]; we found that GW3965 treatment similarly stimulated GLUT1 expression (data not shown). However, it responds differently to canonical LXR target genes in response to U18666a, suggesting that other transcriptional regulators are at play. Nevertheless, it is clear that changes in cholesterol homeostasis and LXR activity influence adipocyte GLUT isoform expression.

The data presented here indicate that it is the change in GLUT4 levels that has the biggest impact on insulin-regulated glucose transport and that it is possible to achieve marked reduction in Akt and AS160 phosphorylation without any major impact on insulin-regulated glucose transport at high doses of insulin. This is consistent with our previous work that highlights the spareness in signalling components comprising the PI3K/Akt signalling network [15,48]. However, such spareness does not exist for GLUT4 and so models of GLUT4 repression are invariably associated with defective insulin action at the level of insulin-stimulated glucose transport. These include models of insulin resistance in 3T3-L1 adipocytes [49–51], transgenic models in mice [52], adipose tissue from insulin resistance mice [53] and adipose tissue from insulin resistant humans [54].

Inhibiting NPC1 and so disrupting cholesterol trafficking in 3T3-L1 adipocytes resulted in a complex phenotype culminating in a reduced response to insulin. Inhibiting NPC1 function resulted in both reductions in IR and IRS1 proteins levels possibly via instability created by disrupting cell surface lipid rafts and reduced activation of Akt by upstream kinases again possibly due to disruption of PM micro-domains. Further, it reduced GLUT4 levels partly through inhibition of LXR activity. Taken together, our data reveal the importance of NPC1 activity in the maintenance of adipocyte insulin sensitivity and implicates cholesterol homeostasis in regulating several nodes of the insulin response.

Author Contributions

Conceived and designed the experiments: RF CG JRK DEJ DJF. Performed the experiments: RF CG XM JGB KCT JRK DJF. Analyzed the data: RF CG XM JGB DJF. Wrote the paper: RF CG JRK DJF.

References

1. Morris AP, Voight BF, Teslovich TM, Ferreira T, Segre AV, et al. (2012) Large-scale association analysis provides insights into the genetic architecture and pathophysiology of type 2 diabetes. Nat Genet 44: 981–990.
2. Zeggini E, Scott LJ, Saxena R, Voight BF, Marchini JL, et al. (2008) Meta-analysis of genome-wide association data and large-scale replication identifies additional susceptibility loci for type 2 diabetes. Nat Genet 40: 638–645.
3. Voight BF, Scott LJ, Steinthorsdottir V, Morris AP, Dina C, et al. (2010) Twelve type 2 diabetes susceptibility loci identified through large-scale association analysis. Nat Genet 42: 579–589.
4. Dupuis J, Langenberg C, Prokopenko I, Saxena R, Soranzo N, et al. (2010) New genetic loci implicated in fasting glucose homeostasis and their impact on type 2 diabetes risk. Nat Genet 42: 105–116.
5. Shu XO, Long J, Cai Q, Qi L, Xiang YB, et al. (2010) Identification of new genetic risk variants for type 2 diabetes. PLoS Genet 6: e1001127.
6. Yamauchi T, Hara K, Maeda S, Yasuda K, Takahashi A, et al. (2010) A genome-wide association study in the Japanese population identifies susceptibility loci for type 2 diabetes at UBE2E2 and C2CD4A-C2CD4B. Nat Genet 42: 864–868.
7. Vanier MT (2010) Niemann-Pick disease type C. Orphanet J Rare Dis 5: 16.
8. Infante RE, Radhakrishnan A, Abi-Mosleh L, Kinch LN, Wang ML, et al. (2008) Purified NPC1 protein: II. Localization of sterol binding to a 240-amino acid soluble luminal loop. J Biol Chem 283: 1064–1075.
9. Kwon HJ, Abi-Mosleh L, Wang ML, Deisenhofer J, Goldstein JL, et al. (2009) Structure of N-terminal domain of NPC1 reveals distinct subdomains for binding and transfer of cholesterol. Cell 137: 1213–1224.
10. Lloyd-Evans E, Platt FM (2010) Lipids on trial: the search for the offending metabolite in Niemann-Pick type C disease. Traffic 11: 419–428.
11. Robiou-du-Pont S, Bonnefond A, Yengo L, Vaillant E, Lobbens S, et al. (2013) Contribution of 24 obesity-associated genetic variants to insulin resistance, pancreatic beta-cell function and type 2 diabetes risk in the French population. Int J Obes (Lond) 37: 980–985.
12. Meyre D, Delplanque J, Chevre JC, Lecoeur C, Lobbens S, et al. (2009) Genome-wide association study for early-onset and morbid adult obesity identifies three new risk loci in European populations. Nat Genet 41: 157–159.
13. Al-Daghri NM, Cagliani R, Forni D, Alokail MS, Pozzoli U, et al. (2012) Mammalian NPC1 genes may undergo positive selection and human polymorphisms associate with type 2 diabetes. BMC Med 10: 140.
14. Jelinek D, Millward V, Birdi A, Trouard TP, Heidenreich RA, et al. (2011) Npc1 haploinsufficiency promotes weight gain and metabolic features associated with insulin resistance. Hum Mol Genet 20: 312–321.
15. Jelinek D, Castillo JJ, Garver WS (2013) The C57BL/6J Niemann-Pick C1 mouse model with decreased gene dosage has impaired glucose tolerance independent of body weight. Gene 527: 65–70.
16. Ong QR, Lim ML, Chua CC, Cheung NS, Wong BS (2012) Impaired insulin signaling in an animal model of Niemann-Pick Type C disease. Biochem Biophys Res Commun 424: 482–487.

17. Xu J, Dang Y, Ren YR, Liu JO (2010) Cholesterol trafficking is required for mTOR activation in endothelial cells. Proc Natl Acad Sci U S A 107: 4764–4769.
18. Shewan AM, van Dam EM, Martin S, Luen TB, Hong W, et al. (2003) GLUT4 recycles via a trans-Golgi network (TGN) subdomain enriched in Syntaxins 6 and 16 but not TGN38: involvement of an acidic targeting motif. Mol Biol Cell 14: 973–986.
19. Piper RC, Hess LJ, James DE (1991) Differential sorting of two glucose transporters expressed in insulin-sensitive cells. Am J Physiol 260: C570–580.
20. Govers R, Coster AC, James DE (2004) Insulin increases cell surface GLUT4 levels by dose dependently discharging GLUT4 into a cell surface recycling pathway. Mol Cell Biol 24: 6456–6466.
21. Dahl NK, Reed KL, Daunais MA, Faust JR, Liscum L (1992) Isolation and characterization of Chinese hamster ovary cells defective in the intracellular metabolism of low density lipoprotein-derived cholesterol. J Biol Chem 267: 4889–4896.
22. Sugimoto Y, Ninomiya H, Ohsaki Y, Higaki K, Davies JP, et al. (2001) Accumulation of cholera toxin and GM1 ganglioside in the early endosome of Niemann-Pick C1-deficient cells. Proc Natl Acad Sci U S A 98: 12391–12396.
23. Coughlin SR, Escobedo JA, Williams LT (1989) Role of phosphatidylinositol kinase in PDGF receptor signal transduction. Science 243: 1191–1194.
24. Bryant NJ, Govers R, James DE (2002) Regulated transport of the glucose transporter GLUT4. Nat Rev Mol Cell Biol 3: 267–277.
25. Keller SR (2003) The insulin-regulated aminopeptidase: a companion and regulator of GLUT4. Front Biosci 8: s410–420.
26. Rigamonti E, Helin L, Lestavel S, Mutka AL, Lepore M, et al. (2005) Liver X receptor activation controls intracellular cholesterol trafficking and esterification in human macrophages. Circ Res 97: 682–689.
27. Laffitte BA, Chao LC, Li J, Walczak R, Hummasti S, et al. (2003) Activation of liver X receptor improves glucose tolerance through coordinate regulation of glucose metabolism in liver and adipose tissue. Proc Natl Acad Sci U S A 100: 5419–5424.
28. Cenedella RJ (2009) Cholesterol synthesis inhibitor U18666A and the role of sterol metabolism and trafficking in numerous pathophysiological processes. Lipids 44: 477–487.
29. Gustavsson J, Parpal S, Karlsson M, Ramsing C, Thorn H, et al. (1999) Localization of the insulin receptor in caveolae of adipocyte plasma membrane. FASEB J 13: 1961–1971.
30. Thorn H, Stenkula KG, Karlsson M, Ortegren U, Nystrom FH, et al. (2003) Cell surface orifices of caveolae and localization of caveolin to the necks of caveolae in adipocytes. Mol Biol Cell 14: 3967–3976.
31. Gonzalez-Munoz E, Lopez-Iglesias C, Calvo M, Palacin M, Zorzano A, et al. (2009) Caveolin-1 loss of function accelerates glucose transporter 4 and insulin receptor degradation in 3T3-L1 adipocytes. Endocrinology 150: 3493–3502.
32. Chen J, Capozza F, Wu A, Deangelis T, Sun H, et al. (2008) Regulation of insulin receptor substrate-1 expression levels by caveolin-1. J Cell Physiol 217: 281–289.
33. Pederson TM, Kramer DL, Rondinone CM (2001) Serine/threonine phosphorylation of IRS-1 triggers its degradation: possible regulation by tyrosine phosphorylation. Diabetes 50: 24–31.
34. Couet J, Sargiacomo M, Lisanti MP (1997) Interaction of a receptor tyrosine kinase, EGF-R, with caveolins. Caveolin binding negatively regulates tyrosine and serine/threonine kinase activities. J Biol Chem 272: 30429–30438.
35. Pike LJ, Casey L (1996) Localization and turnover of phosphatidylinositol 4,5-bisphosphate in caveolin-enriched membrane domains. J Biol Chem 271: 26453–26456.
36. Pike LJ, Miller JM (1998) Cholesterol depletion delocalizes phosphatidylinositol bisphosphate and inhibits hormone-stimulated phosphatidylinositol turnover. J Biol Chem 273: 22298–22304.
37. Laux T, Fukami K, Thelen M, Golub T, Frey D, et al. (2000) GAP43, MARCKS, and CAP23 modulate PI(4,5)P(2) at plasmalemmal rafts, and regulate cell cortex actin dynamics through a common mechanism. J Cell Biol 149: 1455–1472.
38. Gao X, Lowry PR, Zhou X, Depry C, Wei Z, et al. (2011) PI3K/Akt signaling requires spatial compartmentalization in plasma membrane microdomains. Proc Natl Acad Sci U S A 108: 14509–14514.
39. Partovian C, Ju R, Zhuang ZW, Martin KA, Simons M (2008) Syndecan-4 regulates subcellular localization of mTOR Complex2 and Akt activation in a PKCalpha-dependent manner in endothelial cells. Mol Cell 32: 140–149.
40. Hoehn KL, Hohnen-Behrens C, Cederberg A, Wu LE, Turner N, et al. (2008) IRS1-independent defects define major nodes of insulin resistance. Cell Metab 7: 421–433.
41. Blot V, McGraw TE (2006) GLUT4 is internalized by a cholesterol-dependent nystatin-sensitive mechanism inhibited by insulin. EMBO J 25: 5648–5658.
42. Reverter M, Rentero C, de Muga SV, Alvarez-Guaita A, Mulay V, et al. (2011) Cholesterol transport from late endosomes to the Golgi regulates t-SNARE trafficking, assembly, and function. Mol Biol Cell 22: 4108–4123.
43. Nishimura T, Uchida Y, Yachi R, Kudlyk T, Lupashin V, et al. (2013) Oxysterol-binding protein (OSBP) is required for the perinuclear localization of intra-Golgi v-SNAREs. Mol Biol Cell.
44. Abel ED, Peroni O, Kim JK, Kim YB, Boss O, et al. (2001) Adipose-selective targeting of the GLUT4 gene impairs insulin action in muscle and liver. Nature 409: 729–733.
45. Le Lay S, Krief S, Farnier C, Lefrere I, Le Liepvre X, et al. (2001) Cholesterol, a cell size-dependent signal that regulates glucose metabolism and gene expression in adipocytes. J Biol Chem 276: 16904–16910.
46. Wong J, Quinn CM, Brown AJ (2006) SREBP-2 positively regulates transcription of the cholesterol efflux gene, ABCA1, by generating oxysterol ligands for LXR. Biochem J 400: 485–491.
47. Ross SE, Erickson RL, Gerin I, DeRose PM, Bajnok L, et al. (2002) Microarray analyses during adipogenesis: understanding the effects of Wnt signaling on adipogenesis and the roles of liver X receptor alpha in adipocyte metabolism. Mol Cell Biol 22: 5989–5999.
48. Tan SX, Ng Y, Meoli CC, Kumar A, Khoo PS, et al. (2012) Amplification and demultiplexing in insulin-regulated Akt protein kinase pathway in adipocytes. J Biol Chem 287: 6128–6138.
49. Stephens JM, Pekala PH (1991) Transcriptional repression of the GLUT4 and C/EBP genes in 3T3-L1 adipocytes by tumor necrosis factor-alpha. J Biol Chem 266: 21839–21845.
50. Kozka IJ, Clark AE, Holman GD (1991) Chronic treatment with insulin selectively down-regulates cell-surface GLUT4 glucose transporters in 3T3-L1 adipocytes. J Biol Chem 266: 11726–11731.
51. Flores-Riveros JR, McLenithan JC, Ezaki O, Lane MD (1993) Insulin down-regulates expression of the insulin-responsive glucose transporter (GLUT4) gene: effects on transcription and mRNA turnover. Proc Natl Acad Sci U S A 90: 512–516.
52. Rossetti L, Stenbit AE, Chen W, Hu M, Barzilai N, et al. (1997) Peripheral but not hepatic insulin resistance in mice with one disrupted allele of the glucose transporter type 4 (GLUT4) gene. J Clin Invest 100: 1831–1839.
53. Pedersen O, Kahn CR, Flier JS, Kahn BB (1991) High fat feeding causes insulin resistance and a marked decrease in the expression of glucose transporters (Glut 4) in fat cells of rats. Endocrinology 129: 771–777.
54. Garvey WT, Maianu L, Huecksteadt TP, Birnbaum MJ, Molina JM, et al. (1991) Pretranslational suppression of a glucose transporter protein causes insulin resistance in adipocytes from patients with non-insulin-dependent diabetes mellitus and obesity. J Clin Invest 87: 1072–1081.

Obesity has an Interactive Effect with Genetic Variation in the Activating Transcription Factor 6 Gene on the Risk of Pre-Diabetes in Individuals of Chinese Han Descent

Nan Gu, Xiaowei Ma*, Junqing Zhang, Aimei Dong, Mengmeng Jin, Nan Feng, Hong Zhang, Xiaohui Guo

Endocrinology Department, First Hospital, Peking University, Beijing, China

Abstract

Endoplasmic reticulum (ER) stress is one of the contributing factors to the development of β-cell failure in type 2 diabetes. ER stress response through ATF6 has been shown to play an important role in insulin resistance and pancreatic β-cell function. We investigated whether genetic polymorphisms in ATF6 were associated with the risk of pre-diabetes in a Chinese Han population, and whether they had a synergistic effect with obesity. Our samples included 828 individuals who were diagnosed as pre-diabetic, and 620 controls. The minor allele A at rs2340721 was associated with increased risk for pre-diabetes($p = 0.013$), and this association was still significant after adjusting for gender, age, body mass index (BMI), and waist-hip ratio($p' = 0.011$). BMI, treated as a continuous variable, and rs2340721 had an interactive effect on pre-diabetic risk(p for interaction $= 0.003$, $\beta = 0.106$). Carriers of GG at rs7522210 were also at a higher risk compared to non-carriers (OR = 1.390, 95%CI:1.206–1.818, $p = 0.013$, adjusted OR′ = 1.516, 95%CI:1.101–2.006, $p' = 0.006$). GG homozygotes had increased fasting blood glucose (FBG) levels(GG vs CX: 5.6±0.52 vs 5.5±0.57 mmol/L, $p = 0.016$), lower insulin levels (0,30,120 minutes after glucose load) ($p < 0.05$), and reduced areas under the insulin curve than non-carriers(GG vs CX:67.3(44.2–102.3) vs 73.1(49.4–111.4), $p = 0.014$). rs10918270 was associated with FBG, and rs4657103 with 2 hour glucose levels after a 75 g glucose load. We also identified a haplotype of TTAG composed of rs4657103, rs2134697, rs2340721, and rs12079579, which was associated with pre-diabetes. The genetic variation in ATF6 is associated with pre-diabetes and has interactive effects with BMI on pre-diabetes in the Chinese Han population.

Editor: Victor Sanchez-Margalet, Virgen Macarena University Hospital, School of Medicine, University of Seville, Spain

Funding: This work was supported by National Natural Science Foundation of China (NSFC 30771033) and by Specialized Research Fund for the Doctoral Program of Higher Education of China (Grant No. 20110001120047). The funders had no role in study design, data collection and analysis, decision to publish, or preparation of the manuscript.

Competing Interests: The authors have declared that no competing interests exist.

* Email: mxiaowei@yahoo.com

Introduction

Prevalence of type 2 diabetes has been rising rapidly, and it has been a major public health challenge worldwide, especially in China. Pancreatic β-cell dysfunction is a key causal factor in the development and progression of type 2 diabetes. In the early stage of the disease, pre-diabetes, characterized by impaired fasting glucose (IFG) and/or impaired glucose tolerance (IGT) [1], pancreatic β-cell dysfunction and insulin resistance have already presented. Several genetic and environmental factors are likely to contribute to the progressive abnormality or even failure of pancreatic β-cell function, but the precise mechanism is still unknown. Endoplasmic reticulum (ER) stress is thought to be a contributing factor. The unfolded protein response (UPR), induced by the accumulation of unfolded or misfolded proteins in the ER, plays an important role in chronic metabolic diseases, such as insulin resistance and type 2 diabetes. ATF6 is an ER stress-regulated transmembrane transcription factor in the UPR signaling pathway that activates the transcription of ER molecular chaperons to alleviate ER stress. We inferred that the genetic variability in ATF6 may contribute to the changes in pancreatic β-cell function or insulin sensitivity. To test this hypothesis, we studied the genetic variations in ATF6 in a sample of pre-diabetic Chinese individuals.

Materials and Methods

Ethics statement

The study protocol and informed written consent forms were approved by the research ethics committee of Peking University First Hospital, and the study was carried out in compliance with the Helsinki Declaration. All patients signed an informed written consent form to participate in the study.

Study population

Subjects were recruited from the database for the Epidemiological Survey on Diabetes that was conducted in three large communities in Beijing from 2007 to 2009. A total of 1,448 non-consanguineous subjects with complete medical records were enrolled in the study. Based on the oral glucose tolerance test (75 g OGTT), and according to the 1999 WHO diagnostic criteria for diabetes and pre-diabetes, 828 subjects were confirmed pre-diabetic (defined as fasting glucose [FBG] between 6.1 mmol/L [100 mg/dL] and 7.0 mmol/L [126 mg/dL], or 2 hours post-OGTT glucose [PBG] between 7.8 mmol/L [140 mg/dL] and

11.1 mmol/L [200 mg/dL], or both). Another 620 healthy individuals who had no family history of diabetes and were ≥55 years of age served as controls.

Methods

All subjects underwent a standardized clinical and laboratory evaluation. A standard questionnaire for epidemiological survey was used, and the items included general information, family history, medical history, and medication. During the evaluation, body height, body weight, waist circumference, hip circumference, and blood pressure were measured. In the morning, fasting blood was collected for the measurement of glucose and lipid levels (Table 1). The remaining 2–4 ml of venous blood was used for DNA extraction using the salting-out method [20]. Homeostasis model assessments of insulin resistance (HOMA-IR) and β-cell function (HOMA-β) were calculated using the formula described by Matthews et al. [2]. Fasting and 2 hours PBG were measured enzymatically. The coefficient of variation was <2.5% and inter-assay coefficient of variation was <3.5%. Total cholesterol (TC), triglycerides (TG), and high-density lipoprotein cholesterol (HDL-C) were measured using the Hitachi 7600 automatic biochemical analyzer with the coefficient of variation of <1.5% and inter-assay coefficient of variation of <3.0%. Fasting insulin levels (INS0), post-OGTT30′ insulin levels (INS30) and 2 hour post-OGTT insulin levels (INS120) were measured by chemiluminescence using Roche Cobas e 601 Analyzer, while the coefficient of variation was 1.8%–2.0%, and the inter-assay coefficient of variation was 4.7%–7.9%. Homeostasis model assessments of insulin resistance (HOMA-IR), β-cell function (HOMA-β), and areas under the curve for insulin (AUCi) were calculated using the formula [HOMA-IR = fasting insulin × fasting plasma glucose/ 22.5, and HOMA-β = 20× fasting insulin/(fasting plasma glucose - 3.5)] described by Matthews et al. [15].

Genotyping

Genomic DNA was extracted from 2–4 ml of peripheral blood using the salting-out method [20]. Six haplotype-tagging SNPs (r^2<0.8, MAF≥0.05) in the ATF6 gene (16 exons spanning 193 kb on chromosome 1q21–23) were selected from CHB data (Han Chinese in Beijing) in HapMap Phase II (R#23, http://www.hapmap.org). They were rs10918270 (G>A), rs12079579 (G>A), rs2134697 (G>A), rs2340721 (A>C), rs4657103 (G>T), and rs7522210 (G>C). The genotypes of all the 6 SNPs were determined by the MassArray system (Sequenom iPLEXassay, San Diego, United States) [21].

Statistical analysis

All statistical analyses were performed using the SPSS statistical package (version 13.0; SPSS, Chicago, IL). Genotype distributions were tested at each polymorphic locus for departure from Hardy-Weinberg equilibrium. The clinical and laboratory values were expressed as means ± standard deviation (SD) or as medians (lower–upper quartiles). Comparisons of the clinical and laboratory parameters between the pre-diabetes and control groups, as well as between the genotypic groups, were performed with unpaired Student's *t*-tests or χ^2 analysis, as appropriate. As a descriptive measure of the association between genotypes and pre-diabetes, odds ratios (ORs) were calculated along with 95% confidence intervals (CIs). Multifactor model analysis was used to assess hybrid effect. Pairwise LD was estimated using the combined data (cases and controls) by calculating $|D'|$ and r^2 using Haploview (version 4.1) (http://www.broadinstitute.org/haploview/haploview) [13]. Haplotype block structure was determined using a CI algorithm [14] and haplotype frequencies were estimated with an expectation-maximization algorithm [15] using Haploview (v4.1). Bonferroni correction was used to correct for multiple comparisons.

Results

Genotype distributions were in Hardy-Weinberg equilibrium at all six loci (p>0.01). Pre-diabetics were younger, and had higher BMI and waist-hip ratio (WHR), higher TG levels and lower HDL-C levels than control individuals (Table 1).

Carriers of genotype AA at rs2340721 had a higher risk for pre-diabetes than non-carriers (OR = 1.309, p = 0.013, β = 0.263). Using a multifactor model analysis to adjust for gender, age, BMI and WHR, the association of rs2340721 with pre-diabetes was significant (OR′ = 1.341, p' = 0.011, β = 0.308). At rs7522210, GG homozygotes had a higher risk for pre-diabetes compared to non-carriers (OR = 1.390, p = 0.013, β = 0.316, adjusted OR′ = 1.516, p' = 0.006, β = 0.366) (Table 2).

Table 1. Clinical characteristics of pre-diabetic cases and controls in China.

	Controls (n = 621)	p-DM (n = 845)	*P*-value
Gender (M/F)	240/381	291/554	0.099
Age (y)	65.91±7.07	61.75±11.3	0.000
BMI (kg/m²)	25.11±3.43	26.53±3.77	0.000
WHR	0.87±0.06	0.89±0.31	0.041
FPG (mmol/L)	5.26±0.42	5.72±0.57	0.000
2hPPG (mmol/L)	6.01±1.07	8.57±1.33	0.000
TC (mmol/L)	5.24±1.00	5.28±1.11	0.523
TG (mmol/L)	1.54±0.99	1.86±1.28	0.000
HDL-C (mmol/L)	1.35±0.33	1.29±0.35	0.005
LDL-C (mmol/L)	3.23±0.94	3.25±1.50	0.732

p-DM, pre-diabetes;BMI, body mass index; WHR, waist-to-hip ratio; FBG, fasting blood glucose; 2hPPG, post OGTT 2 hours blood glucose; TC, total cholesterol; TG, triglycerides; HDL-C, high-density lipoprotein; LDL-C, low-density lipoprotein.

Table 2. Association between pre-diabetes and SNPs at the ATF6 locus.

SNPs /Genotypes	controls (n = 621)	p-DM (n = 845)	OR	95% CI	*p-value*	OR′	95% CI′	p′
rs10918270								
GG	343	447	0.955	0.775–1.177	0.666	1.006	0.807–1.254	0.956
AX	277	378	1					
rs12079579								
GG	396	515	0.940	0.757–1.166	0.573	0.951	0.762–1.186	0.653
AX	224	310	1					
rs2134697								
GG	396	515	1.039	0.734–1.470	0.380	1.000	0.693–1.443	0.999
AX	224	310	1					
rs2340721								
AA	222	347	1.309	1.050–1.613	0.013	1.341	1.063–1.669	0.011
CX	398	478	1					
rs4657103								
TT	491	677	1.202	0.924–1.564	0.171	1.177	0.891–1.554	0.251
GX	129	148	1					
rs7522210								
GG	88	152	1.390	1.206–1.818	0.013	1.516	1.101–2.006	0.006
CX	532	673	1					

SNPs,single nucleotide polymorphisms; p-DM, pre-diabetes.
OR′: adjusted for gender, age, BMI, and WHR.
p′: adjusted for gender, age, BMI, and WHR.

We also analyzed the interaction between environmental factors and SNPs on the risk of pre-diabetes. When BMI is treated as a continuous variable, there is a significant interaction with rs2340721 on pre-diabetic risk (p for the interaction = 0.003, β = 0.106).

The SNPs were distributed in two Linkage disequilibrium (LD) blocks. We also compared the haplotype distributions between pre-diabetes and controls. In block 1, haplotype TTAG (composed of rs4657103, rs2134697, rs2340721, and rs12079579) was found associated with pre-diabetes (p = 0.009) (Table 3).In block 2,haplotype (composed of rs10918270 and rs7522210) distributions between pre-diabetes and controls showed no statistical significant difference.

Of the 1,448 individuals, 748 had plasma insulin measured following 75 g OGTT. GG homozygotes at rs7522210 had higher FBG (GG vs. CX: 5.6±0.52 vs. 5.5±0.57 mmol/L, p = 0.016), lower HOMA-β (GG vs. CX: 77.0 vs. 79.6%, p = 0.004) and HOMA-IR levels (GG vs. CX: 1.79 vs. 1.84, p = 0.011), lower insulin levels (0, 30, and 120 minutes after glucose load, $p<0.05$), reduced AUCi (GG vs. CX: 67.3 [44.2–102.3] vs. 73.1 [49.4–111.4], p = 0.014) than non-carriers mainly in individuals with pre-diabetes (Table 4).

We also found that the carriers of the GG genotype at rs10918270 had higher FBG (GG vs. AX: 5.568±0.548 vs. 5.501±0.580 mmol/L, p = 0.023), and rs4657103 was associated with PBG after 75 g glucose load (TT vs. GX: 7.590±1.726 vs. 7.316±1.785 mmol/L, p = 0.023).

Discussion

The ER is a complicated membranous network in eukaryotic cells, and is the site for synthesis, folding, assembly, and posttranslational modification of proteins. It includes a highly conserved system of proteins that facilitates protein folding and processing, and protects cells from the toxic effects of accumulating unfolded proteins (i.e., ER stress). When these measures fail, it initiates apoptosis. This system, known as the UPR, is activated by the accumulation of unfolded proteins [3–5]. The UPR pathway is particularly important in secretory cells, including pancreatic β-cells, hepatocytes and adipocytes [3]. Many studies have demonstrated that UPR (including ATF6) is related to pancreatic β-cell function [16], and ATF6α may be important for maintaining β-cell survival [17,18].

ATF6 is a key proximal sensor in the UPR pathway and is transported to the Golgi complex, where it is cleaved by proteases to yield an active cytoplasmic domain that upregulates chaperone proteins. It activates the UPR by regulating a group of genes encoding molecular chaperones and folding enzymes [6]. Its encoding gene includes 16 exons and spans 193 kb on chromosome 1q21–23, a region that is linked to type 2 diabetes in eight different populations [7,8].

In this study, subjects with pre-diabetes were observed to determine the genetic factors that contribute to the very early stage of pancreatic β-cell dysfunction and thus play a role in the progression of type 2 diabetes.

Previous studies identified several SNPs in ATF6 associated with type 2 diabetes in different populations. In Pima Indians, rs2070150 (P145A) and rs1135983 (S157P) are associated with type 2 diabetes and reduced insulin response to oral glucose [12]; in Caucasians and African Americans, rs4579731, rs3820449 and rs10918215 are also associated with these traits [6,9–12].

Two of the six haplotype-tagging SNPs selected for this study, rs2340721 and rs7522210, were respectively in high LD with two previously reported SNPs rs2070150 and rs1135983, in Caucasians (r^2 = 1) and CHB (r^2 = 1.0) in HapMap database. Also, the selected SNP rs4657103 was in high LD with the reported SNP rs4579731 in CHB (r^2 = 1.0). The SNPs linked to those found in other populations may be associated with Chinese pre-diabetes.

We found that rs2340721 was, indeed, associated with pre-diabetes. The carriers of genotype AA had a higher risk than non-carriers, even after adjusting for gender, age, BMI, and WHR. Furthermore, when BMI was treated as a continuous variable, it had an interaction effect with the locus on pre-diabetic risk.

The haplotype TTAG, composed of 4 SNPs including rs2340721 and rs4657103, was associated with pre-diabetes. rs7522210 was associated with FBG, insulin levels (0, 30, and 120 minutes after glucose load), AUCi, and HOMA-IR; rs10918270 was associated with FBG and rs4657103 with post-75 g glucose load (2 hour) glucose levels. These data suggest that genetic variation in ATF6 is associated with pre-diabetes and regulates pancreatic β-cell function in the population. BMI had a synergistic effect with genetic variation on the risk of pre-diabetes, which can be interpreted thatin clinical practice, individuals at a

Table 3. Association analyses of haplotypes at the ATF6 locus with pre-diabetes.

	Haplotype frequencies		
Haplotype	**p-DM**	**Controls**	***p*-value**
Block 1 (rs4657103-rs2134697-rs2340721-rs12079579)			
TTCG	0.556	0.643	0.066
TTAG	0.493	0.399	0.009
TCAA	0.260	0.253	0.765
GCAG	0.100	0.120	0.123
TCAG	0.012	0.013	0.877
Block2 (rs10918270-rs7522210)			
GG	0.752	0.673	0.143
GC	0.446	0.515	0.074
AC	0.356	0.348	0.800

p-DM, pre-diabetes.
P-value: comparison between pre-diabetes and control.

Table 4. β-cell function and insulin resistance for genotype groups at rs7522210 in pre-diabetes individuals.

	GG	CX	
	(n = 121)	(n = 627)	*P*
FBG (mmol/L)*	5.78±0.54	5.74±0.58	0.365
PBG30′ (mmol/L)*	10.08±1.95	10.06±1.73	0.928
PBG-2h (mmol/L)*	8.53±1.31	8.68±1.25	0.187
INS 0′#	8.1 (5.06–8.69)	9.8 (6.4–11.9)	0.001
INS 30′#	44.7 (25.7–52.6)	55.6 (27.3–70.8)	0.037
INS 120′#	59.8 (32.6–73.1)	79.3 (38.8–90.2)	0.031
HOMA-β#	72.7 (46.1–85.9)	90.3 (56.5–105.9)	0.107
HOMA-IR#	2.1 (1.26–2.36)	2.53 (1.61–3.13)	0.002
AUCi#	78.6 (50.5–101.5)	100.1 (54.3–117.7)	0.013
INS 30′/PBG30	21.90 (4.48–12.64)	13.10 (4.69–14.80)	0.336
INS 120′/PBG-2h	33.59 (10.66–33.20)	39.67 (10.97–38.56)	0.528

*data shown as mean ± SD.
#data shown as medians (lower-upper quartiles).
P′: adjusted for age, sex, and BMI.
BMI, body mass index; FBG, fasting blood glucose; PBG, post-OGTT glucose; INS0′#, fasting insulin levels; INS30′#, post-OGTT30′ insulin levels; INS120′#, 2 hours post-OGTT insulin levels;HOMA-β#, β-cell function; HOMA-IR#, homeostasis model assessments of insulin resistance; AUCi#, area under the curve for insulin;INS30′/PBG30, the ratio of INS30′ and PBG30; INS120′/PBG-2h, the ratio of INS120′ and PBG-2h.

high risk of pre-diabetes will benefit from losing body weight; with the risk reduced by 10% per kg/m^2 reduction in BMI. To date, no studies on the ATF6 gene specifically consider individuals with pre-diabetes.

In 2011, Hu et al. [19] reported no association between genetic variations in ATF6 and type 2 diabetes and its traits in a Chinese population. However, our data suggests that the genetic variants in ATF6 are associated with pre-diabetes, the early stage of type 2 diabetes,and its related traits. Firstly, the control subjects in our study were strictly screened, especially by age at 55 years or over. The high quality of control samples seem to be optimal for the studies on genetic factors. Secondly, some of the SNPs selected in the study were different from Hu's study, with SNPs rs2340721 and rs7522210 in common and none shared in the haplotype patterns. Thirdly, the individuals in our study were northern Chinese Han descent, living in Beijing, while eastern Chinese Hans in Hu's. Finally, we studied the subjects with pre-diabetes, rather than type 2 diabetes. This difference may indicate that the genetic variations in ATF6 play a more important role in the pre-diabetic stage than in the diabetic stage in the Chinese population, or likely there exists genetic heterogeneity within Chinese Han race. Additional studies are needed to confirm the hypothesis in different populations.

However, our study has some limitations. The small sample size might bias the results. Also, further functional studies are necessary. Our findings should be confirmed in prospective studies before ATF6 polymorphisms can be used to predict the risk of pre-diabetes in the Chinese population.

Conclusion

The genetic variation in the ATF6 gene is associated with pre-diabetes and has interactive effects with BMI on pre-diabetes in the Chinese Han population.

Acknowledgments

We thank our colleagues from the Department of Statistics in Peking University First Hospital for their help in data collection.

Author Contributions

Conceived and designed the experiments: NG XWM JQZ XHG. Performed the experiments: NG AMD MMJ NF HZ. Analyzed the data: NG XWM MMJ. Contributed reagents/materials/analysis tools: NF HZ XHG. Wrote the paper: NG XWM.

References

1. American Diabetes Association (2004) Diagnosis and classification of diabetes mellitus. Diabetes Care 27 Suppl 1: S5–S10.
2. Matthews DR, Hosker JP, Rudenski AS, Naylor BA, Treacher DF, et al. (1985) Homeostasis model assessment: insulin resistance and beta-cell function from fasting plasma glucose and insulin concentrations in man. Diabetologia 28(7): 412–419.
3. Rutkowski DT, Kaufman RJ (2004) A trip to the ER: coping with stress. Trends Cell Biol 14(1): 20–28.
4. Kaufman RJ (2002) Orchestrating the unfolded protein response in health and disease. J Clin Invest 110(10): 1389–1398.
5. Sartor MA, Kaufman RJ (2005) The mammalian unfolded protein response. Annu Rev Biochem 74: 739–789.
6. Zhang K, Kaufman RJ (2004) Signaling the unfolded protein response from the endoplasmic reticulum. J Biol Chem 279(25): 25935–25938.
7. McCarthy MI (2003) Growing evidence for diabetes susceptibility genes from genome scan data. Curr Diab Rep 3(2): 159–167.
8. Elbein SC, Hoffman MD, Teng K, Leppert MF, Hasstedt SJ (1999) A genome-wide search for type 2 diabetes susceptibility genes in Utah Caucasians. Diabetes 48(5): 1175–1182.
9. Chu WS, Das SK, Wang H, Chan JC, Deloukas P, et al. (2007) Activating transcription factor 6 (ATF6) sequence polymorphisms in type 2 diabetes and pre-diabetic traits. Diabetes 56(3): 856–862.
10. Das SK, Chu WS, Hale TC, Wang X, Craig RL, et al. (2006) Polymorphisms in the glucokinase-associated, dual-specificity phosphatase 12 (DUSP12) gene under chromosome 1q21 linkage peak are associated with type 2 diabetes. Diabetes 55(9): 2631–2639.
11. Meex SJ, van Greevenbroek MM, Ayoubi TA, Vlietinck R, van Vliet-Ostaptchouk JV, et al. (2007) Activating transcription factor 6 polymorphisms

and haplotypes are associated with impaired glucose homeostasis and type 2 diabetes in Dutch Caucasians. J Clin Endocrinol Metab 92(7): 2720–2725.

12. Thameem F, Farook VS, Bogardus C, Prochazka M (2006) Association of amino acid variants in the activating transcription factor 6 gene (ATF6) on 1q21-q23 with type 2 diabetes in Pima Indians. Diabetes 55(3): 839–842.
13. Barrett JC, Fry B, Maller J, Daly MJ (2005) Haploview: analysis and visualization of LD and haplotype maps. Bioinformatics 21(2): 263–265.
14. Gabriel SB, Schaffner SF, Nguyen H, Moore JM, Roy J, et al. (2002) The structure of haplotype blocks in the human genome. Science 296(5576): 2225–2229.
15. Qin ZS, Niu T, Liu JS (2002) Partition-ligation-expectation-maximization algorithm for haplotype inference with single-nucleotide polymorphisms. Am J Hum Genet 71(5): 1242–1247.
16. Back SH, Kang SW, Han J, Chung HT (2012) Endoplasmic reticulum stress in the β-cell pathogenesis of type 2 diabetes. Experimental Diabetes Research. Available: http://www.hindawi.com/journals/jdr/2012/618396/. Accepted 6 July 2011.
17. Teodoro T, Odisho T, Sidorova E, Volchuk A (2012) Pancreatic β-cells depend on basal expression of active ATF6α-p50 for cell survival even under non-stress conditions.Am J Physiol Cell Physiol 302: 992–1003.
18. Usui M, Yamaguchi S, Tanji Y, Tominaga R, Ishigaki Y, et al. (2012) ATF6α-null mice are glucose intolerant due to pancreatic β-cell failure on a high-fat diet but partially resistant to diet-induced insulin resistance. 61(8): 1118–1128.
19. Hu C, Zhang R, Wang C, Ma X, Wang J, et al. (2011) Lack of association between genetic polymorphisms within DUSP12-ATF6 locus and glucose metabolism related traits in a Chinese population. BMC Medical Genetics 12: 3.
20. Miller SA, Dykes DD, Polesky HF (1988) A simple salting-out procedure for extracting DNA from human nucleated cells. Nucleic Acids Res 16(3): 1215–1218.
21. Gabriel S, Ziaugra L, Tabbaa D (2009) SNP genotyping using the Sequenom Mass ARRAY iPLEX platform.Curr Protoc Hmu Genet 60: 2.12:2.12.1–2.12.16.

Chemokine-Like Receptor 1 Deficiency does not Affect the Development of Insulin Resistance and Nonalcoholic Fatty Liver Disease in Mice

Nanda Gruben[1], Marcela Aparicio Vergara[1], Niels J. Kloosterhuis[1], Henk van der Molen[1], Stefan Stoelwinder[1], Sameh Youssef[2], Alain de Bruin[2], Dianne J. Delsing[3], Jan Albert Kuivenhoven[1], Bart van de Sluis[1], Marten H. Hofker[1]❡, Debby P. Y. Koonen[1]*❡

1 University of Groningen, University Medical Center Groningen, Department of Pediatrics, Molecular Genetics Section, Groningen, the Netherlands, **2** Utrecht University, Faculty of Veterinary Medicine, Dutch Molecular Pathology Center, Utrecht, the Netherlands, **3** Merck Research Laboratories, MSD, Department of Immune Therapeutics, Oss, the Netherlands

Abstract

The adipokine chemerin and its receptor, chemokine-like receptor 1 (*Cmklr1*), are associated with insulin resistance and nonalcoholic fatty liver disease (NAFLD), which covers a broad spectrum of liver diseases, ranging from simple steatosis to nonalcoholic steatohepatitis (NASH). It is possible that chemerin and/or *Cmklr1* exert their effects on these disorders through inflammation, but so far the data have been controversial. To gain further insight into this matter, we studied the effect of whole-body *Cmklr1* deficiency on insulin resistance and NAFLD. In view of the primary role of macrophages in hepatic inflammation, we also transplanted bone marrow from *Cmklr1* knock-out (*Cmklr1*$^{-/-}$) mice and wild type (WT) mice into low-density lipoprotein receptor knock-out (*Ldlr*$^{-/-}$) mice, a mouse model for NASH. All mice were fed a high fat, high cholesterol diet containing 21% fat from milk butter and 0.2% cholesterol for 12 weeks. Insulin resistance was assessed by an oral glucose tolerance test, an insulin tolerance test, and by measurement of plasma glucose and insulin levels. Liver pathology was determined by measuring hepatic inflammation, fibrosis, lipid accumulation and the NAFLD activity score (NAS). Whole-body *Cmklr1* deficiency did not affect body weight gain or food intake. In addition, we observed no differences between WT and *Cmklr1*$^{-/-}$ mice for hepatic inflammatory and fibrotic gene expression, immune cell infiltration, lipid accumulation or NAS. In line with this, we detected no differences in insulin resistance. In concordance with whole-body *Cmklr1* deficiency, the absence of *Cmklr1* in bone marrow-derived cells in *Ldlr*$^{-/-}$ mice did not affect their insulin resistance or liver pathology. Our results indicate that *Cmklr1* is not involved in the pathogenesis of insulin resistance or NAFLD. Thus, we recommend that the associations reported between *Cmklr1* and insulin resistance or NAFLD should be interpreted with caution.

Editor: Silvia C. Sookoian, Institute of Medical Research A Lanari-IDIM, University of Buenos Aires-National Council of Scientific and Technological Research (CONICET), Argentina

Funding: This study was performed within the framework of CTMM, the Center for Translational Molecular Medicine (www.ctmm.nl), project PREDICCt (grant 01C-104), and supported by the Dutch Heart Foundation, the Dutch Diabetes Research Foundation (grant 2009.80.016; 2004.00.018) and the Dutch Kidney Foundation. The funders had no role in study design, data collection and analysis, decision to publish, or preparation of the manuscript.

Competing Interests: Dianne J. Delsing is employed by Merck Research Laboratories.

* E-mail: d.p.y.koonen@umcg.nl

❡ These authors contributed equally to this work.

Introduction

Obesity is accompanied by the development of the metabolic syndrome, a cluster of metabolic abnormalities, which includes low-grade inflammation, dyslipidemia and insulin resistance. Since nonalcoholic fatty liver disease (NAFLD) is the hepatic manifestation of the metabolic syndrome, its increasing prevalence follows the increasing rates of obesity seen worldwide. As a result, NAFLD has become one of the main causes of chronic liver disease in Western societies [1]. NAFLD describes a broad spectrum of liver diseases, ranging from simple steatosis (intrahepatic fat accumulation) to nonalcoholic steatohepatitis (NASH), fibrosis, and cirrhosis [2]. NASH can be distinguished from simple steatosis by the presence of inflammation. It is unknown how NAFLD develops or which factors provoke its progression into NASH.

Recently, an adipokine named chemerin has been implicated in the metabolic syndrome and the progression of NAFLD. Chemerin was first identified as a chemo-attractant protein, attracting immune cells expressing the chemerin receptor chemokine-like receptor 1 (*Cmklr1*, also known as *ChemR23*) [3]. This suggests that chemerin has a pro-inflammatory role. However, studies investigating the role of *Cmklr1* in inflammation are controversial. *Cmklr1* knock-out (*Cmklr1*$^{-/-}$) mice have been reported to be protected against central nervous system inflammation [4], but they were more susceptible to lipopolysaccharide-induced lung inflammation [5] and viral pneumonia [6]. As inflammation is thought to play a key role in the progression of insulin resistance and NAFLD, chemerin and *Cmklr1* may be involved in these disorders. Indeed, in several human populations, elevated plasma chemerin levels correlate positively with characteristics of the metabolic syndrome, including inflammation, insulin resistance, plasma lipids and body mass index [7–9]. In addition, elevations in serum chemerin levels were found in patients with NAFLD and NASH compared to healthy controls [10] and have been shown to positively correlate with markers of liver pathology, including fibrosis, portal inflammation and NAFLD activity score (NAS) [11]. In contrast, expression of chemerin in visceral adipose tissue in morbidly obese individuals correlated negatively with hepatic inflammation (unpublished data). Moreover, data on hepatic expression of *chemerin* and *Cmklr1* in human and mouse NAFLD are inconsistent, since both reduced and increased levels of these genes have been found [12–14]. Although these studies indicate that chemerin and its receptor may be involved in the pathogenesis of insulin resistance and NAFLD, a causative role remains to be established.

Thus far, only a few studies have investigated the effect of *Cmklr1* deficiency in metabolic disease and, similar to the studies investigating inflammation, the results have been controversial. In one study it was shown that *Cmklr1* deficiency induced glucose intolerance in mice [15], whereas another study showed no effect of *Cmklr1* deficiency on glucose intolerance [16]. In addition, *Cmklr1*$^{-/-}$ mice were found to have reduced hepatic steatosis on a low fat diet, but not on a high fat diet, whereas hepatic inflammation was reduced in *Cmklr1*$^{-/-}$ mice on both diets [15]. However, differences in inflammation were not confirmed by histological analyses and differences in body weight gain could not be excluded as a confounding factor in this study [15]. Moreover, despite the controversial role of *Cmklr1* deficiency in inflammation, the role of *Cmklr1* in NASH has not been investigated. In the current study, we investigated the effect of whole-body *Cmklr1* deficiency on insulin resistance and NAFLD. In view of the primary role of macrophages in NASH, we also transplanted bone marrow from *Cmklr1*$^{-/-}$ mice and wild type (WT) mice into low-density lipoprotein receptor knock-out (*Ldlr*$^{-/-}$) mice. These mice develop hepatic inflammation when fed a high fat, high cholesterol (HFC) diet and can be regarded as a mouse model for NASH.

Materials and Methods

Ethics Statement

The University of Groningen ethics committee approved all the animal experiments described in this paper (permit numbers 5964A and 5964E) and the animals' discomfort was kept to a minimum.

Mice and Bone Marrow Transplantation

Male mice deficient for *Cmklr1* on a C57BL/6J background and wild type (WT) littermates were kindly provided by MSD (Oss, the Netherlands) and kept on a 12-hour light/12-hour dark cycle, with *ad libitum* access to food and water. Starting at 3–4 months of age, they were fed a high fat, high cholesterol (HFC) diet, containing 21% fat from milk butter and 0.2% cholesterol (Scientific Animal Food and Engineering, Villemoisson-sur-Orge, France), for 12 weeks to induce NAFLD. To investigate the loss of *Cmklr1* in bone marrow-derived cells, female low-density lipoprotein receptor knock-out (*Ldlr*$^{-/-}$) mice on a C57BL/6J background (bred in-house) were irradiated with 9.5 Gy [17] using X-Rad 320 (Precision X-ray, CT, USA) at 2–5 months of age. The next day, these mice were transplanted with bone marrow from WT or *Cmklr1*$^{-/-}$ mice by intravenous injection. To allow hematopoietic cells to replenish, the mice were allowed to recover on a regular chow diet after the transplantation procedure. After 10 weeks recovery, chimerism was confirmed with DNA isolated from whole blood (data not shown) and the *Ldlr*$^{-/-}$ mice were then fed a HFC diet for 12 weeks to induce NASH.

Oral Glucose Tolerance Test and Insulin Tolerance Test

After 6 hours of fasting, the mice were subjected to an oral glucose tolerance test (OGTT) or an insulin tolerance test (ITT). For the OGTT, mice received a bolus of glucose (2 g/kg) and glucose was measured with a glucose meter in blood samples taken beforehand and at 15, 30, 60 and 120 minutes after gavage. For the ITT, mice were injected intraperitoneally with 0.7 U/kg insulin (WT and *Cmklr1*$^{-/-}$ mice) or 0.5 U/kg insulin (bone marrow-transplanted *Ldlr*$^{-/-}$ mice) (Actrapid, Novo Nordisk Canada Inc., Ontario, Canada) and blood glucose levels were measured at the same time points.

Blood and Tissue Collection

Mice were euthanized by a heart puncture under general anesthesia for the collection of blood and tissues. Blood was spun at 3000 g for 10 minutes at 4°C and plasma was stored at −20°C. Tissues were snap-frozen in liquid nitrogen or fixed in 4% paraformaldehyde.

Hepatic Lipid Extraction and Analysis

Lipids were extracted from crushed liver samples according to Bligh and Dyer's method [18]. Hepatic cholesterol and triglyceride levels were determined using commercially available kits (Roche, Mannheim, Germany).

Plasma Measurements

Plasma cholesterol, triglycerides and free fatty acid levels were measured with commercially available kits (cholesterol and triglycerides: Roche; free fatty acids: DiaSys, Holzheim, Germany). Chemerin and insulin were determined in plasma from mice that had fasted for 6 hours, using commercially available ELISA kits (chemerin: R&D systems, Abingdon, UK; insulin: Alpco Diagnostics, Salem, NH).

Real-time PCR

RNA from homogenized liver, visceral and subcutaneous adipose tissue (VAT and SAT) samples was isolated according to the manufacturer's instructions using Qiazol reagent (Qiagen, Venlo, the Netherlands). For real-time (RT)-PCR, cDNA was synthesized with a commercially available kit (Quantitect Reverse Transcription, Qiagen). RT-PCR was performed using Sybr Green Supermix (Bio-Rad, Veenendaal, the Netherlands) according to the manufacturer's instructions. The primer sequences are listed in Table S1.

Histological Analysis

For histological analysis, paraffin-embedded liver, VAT and SAT sections (4 μm) were stained with Hematoxylin-Eosin (HE). HE-stained liver sections were scored for steatosis, lobular inflammation and hepatocyte ballooning by a board certified veterinary pathologist based on the Kleiner Scoring System [19]. The sum of these findings was used to determine the NAFLD activity score (NAS). HE-stained VAT and SAT sections were scanned using the NanoZoomer 2.0-HT slide scanner (Hamamatsu, Herrsching am Ammersee, Germany). To estimate adipocyte size, the number of adipocytes per mm^2 were determined on scanned sections by manually counting all the

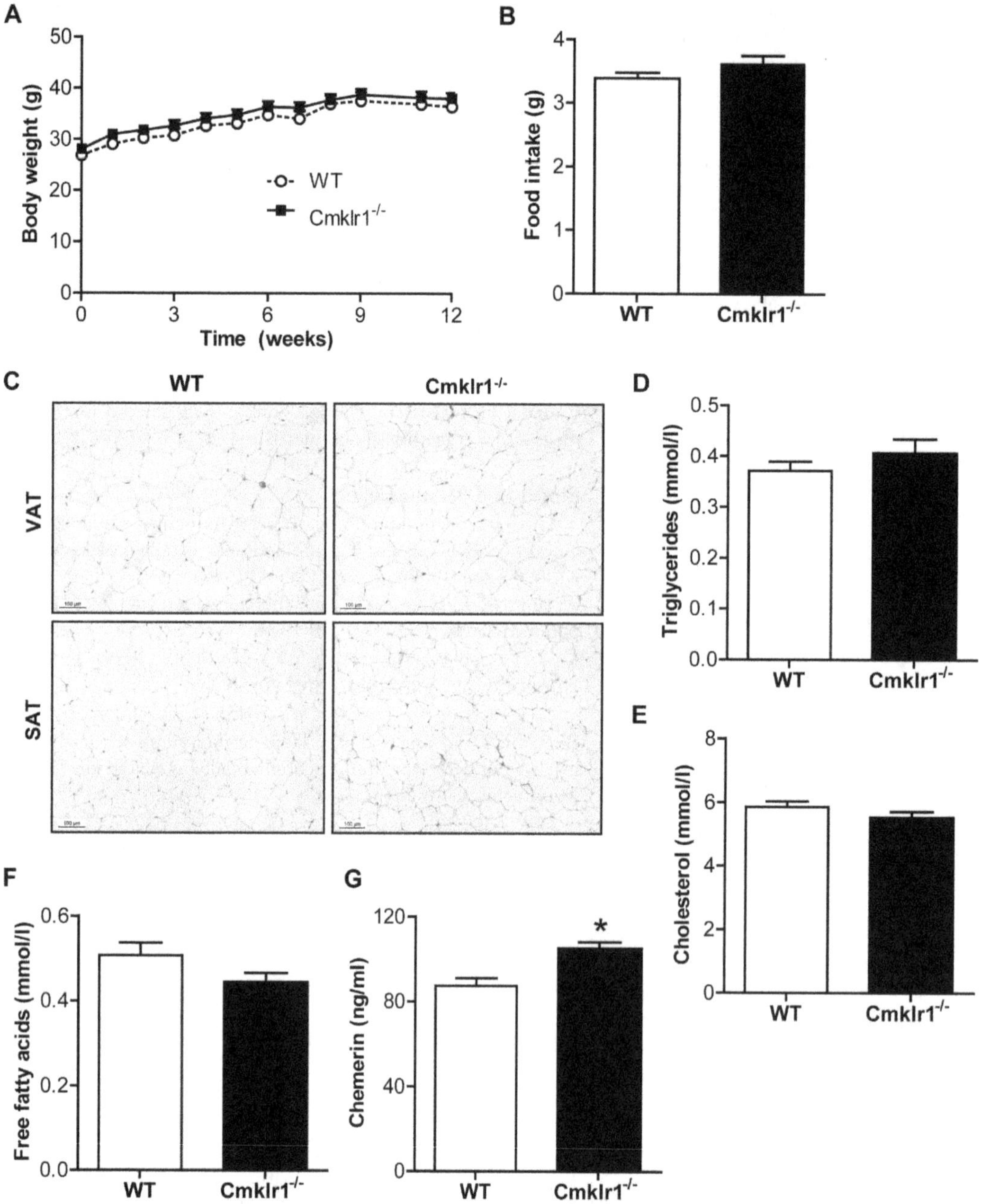

Figure 1. *Cmklr1* deficiency does not affect body weight, food intake or plasma lipid levels. Body weight (A) and food intake (B) were measured throughout the 12-week high fat, high cholesterol diet period. Food intake was expressed as average food intake per day. (C) Representative pictures were taken of Hematoxylin-Eosin (HE) stained visceral and subcutaneous adipose tissue (VAT and SAT) sections. Blood obtained by a heart puncture at the time of euthanasia was used to determine plasma triglycerides (D), plasma cholesterol (E) and plasma free fatty acids (F). (G) Chemerin levels were determined in blood obtained from the tail vein of mice that had fasted for 6 hours at the end of the diet period. Abbreviations: WT, wild type; *Cmklr1*$^{-/-}$, chemokine-like receptor 1 knock-out. N = 7–8 for all experiments. Data are expressed as mean ± SEM. * $p < 0.05$ vs WT.

adipocytes in an area of 4–5 mm^2 using Aperio ImageScope (Leica Biosystems Imaging Inc., CA, USA). Frozen-cut liver sections (5 µm) were fixed in 4% paraformaldehyde and stained with antibodies against the macrophage markers CD68 and CD11b.

Statistical Analysis

For statistical analysis, non-parametric t-tests were performed using GraphPad Prism 5.0 (San Diego, USA). Data were expressed as mean ± SEM and the threshold for significance was set at $p<0.05$.

Results

Cmklr1 Deficiency Does not Affect Body Weight or Food Intake

As *Cmklr1* is known to be necessary for adipocyte differentiation [20] and *Cmklr1*$^{-/-}$ mice were shown to have reduced body weight and fat mass compared to WT mice [15], we evaluated body weight gain and food intake in mice fed a HFC diet for 12 weeks. No differences in body weight or food intake were observed between WT and *Cmklr1*$^{-/-}$ mice (Figs. 1A and 1B, respectively).

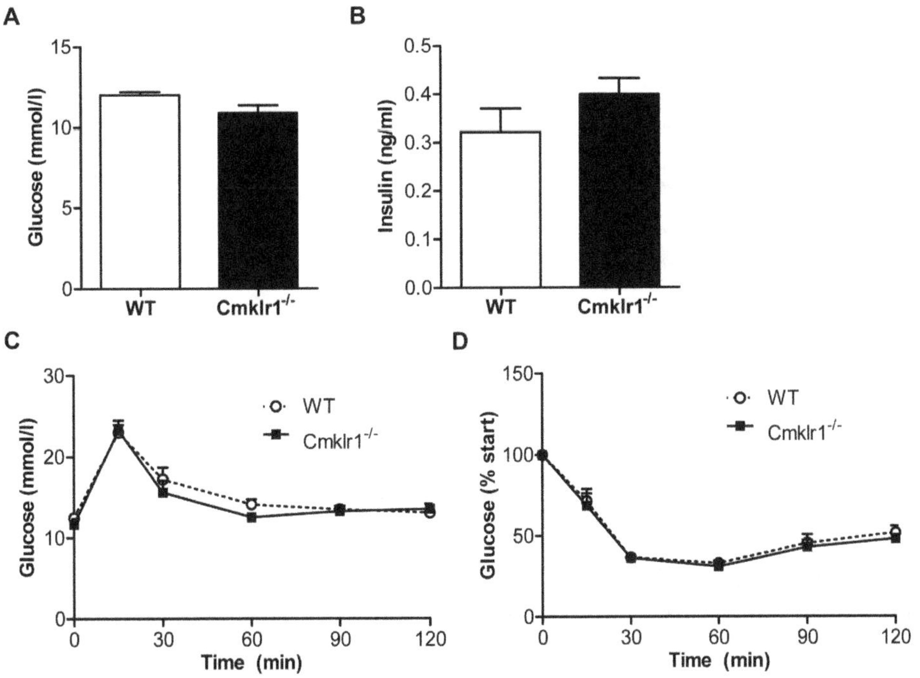

Figure 2. ***Cmklr1*** **deficiency does not affect insulin resistance.** To determine insulin resistance, glucose (A) and insulin levels (B) were measured in mice that had fasted for 6 hours at the end of the 12-week high fat, high cholesterol diet period. In addition, an oral glucose tolerance test (C) and an insulin tolerance test (D) were performed. Abbreviations: WT, wild type; *Cmklr1*$^{-/-}$, chemokine-like receptor 1 knock-out. N = 7–8 for all experiments. Data are expressed as mean ± SEM. * $p<0.05$ vs WT.

Moreover, we observed no differences in the number of adipocytes per mm^2 in visceral and subcutaneous adipose tissue (VAT and SAT) (VAT: WT, 143 cells/mm^2±10; *Cmklr1*$^{-/-}$, 155 cells/mm^2±4, SAT: WT, 301 cells/mm^2±10; *Cmklr1*$^{-/-}$, 345 cells/mm^2±31), indicating that adipose tissue morphology was similar in WT and *Cmklr1*$^{-/-}$ mice (Fig. 1C). In addition, plasma triglycerides (Fig. 1D), cholesterol (Fig. 1E) and free fatty acid levels (Fig. 1F) were the same in both genotypes. However, plasma chemerin levels were significantly increased in *Cmklr1*$^{-/-}$ mice fed a HFC diet compared to WT mice (Fig. 1G), suggesting a compensatory upregulation of the receptor ligand. To identify the origin of these increased plasma chemerin levels, we measured *chemerin* expression in liver, visceral and subcutaneous adipose tissue (VAT and SAT). *Chemerin* expression was significantly higher in VAT and SAT, but not in the liver (Fig. S1A). As chemerin has two other receptors, G protein coupled receptor 1 (*Gpr1*) and (C-C motif) receptor-like 2 (*Ccrl2*) [21,22] we also measured whether the expression of these receptors was altered. No differences were found in the expression of these receptors in either liver tissue, VAT or SAT (Figs. S1B and S1C).

Cmklr1 Deficiency Does not Affect the Development of Systemic Insulin Resistance

As the chemerin-*Cmklr1* system has previously been implicated in the development of insulin resistance [15,23,24], we next assessed the glucose tolerance and insulin sensitivity in WT and *Cmklr1*$^{-/-}$ mice fed a HFC diet for 12 weeks. However, plasma glucose (Fig. 2A) and insulin levels (Fig. 2B) did not differ between the genotypes, and the mice responded similarly to an oral bolus of glucose (Fig. 2C) and an intraperitoneal insulin injection (Fig. 2D). This indicates that *Cmklr1* deficiency does not affect the glucose tolerance and insulin sensitivity of mice fed a HFC diet.

Cmklr1 Deficiency Does not Affect the Development of NAFLD

To investigate whether *Cmklr1* plays a role in the development of diet-induced NAFLD, we analyzed lipid levels and gene expression in the livers of *Cmklr1*$^{-/-}$ mice fed a HFC diet for 12 weeks. Although liver weight, expressed as a percentage of body weight, was lower in *Cmklr1*$^{-/-}$ mice (WT, 5.70%±0.21; *Cmklr1*$^{-/-}$, 5.16%±0.041, $p<0.05$), hepatic triglyceride content did not differ between WT and *Cmklr1*$^{-/-}$ mice (Fig. 3A). In line with this, no difference in hepatic cholesterol was observed between the genotypes (Fig. 3B). The expression of genes encoding for proteins involved in macrophage activation and infiltration (*Cd68* and *Cd11b*), inflammation (*Mcp-1* and *Tnfα*) and fibrosis (*αSma*, *Col1a1*, *Timp1* and *Mmp9*) was similar in *Cmklr1*$^{-/-}$ mice and WT mice (Fig. 3C). However, *Il-1β* gene expression was slightly, but significantly, reduced in *Cmklr1*$^{-/-}$ mice (Fig. 3C). Furthermore, immunostaining for CD68 and CD11b demonstrated that *Cmklr1* deficiency did not affect the activation or infiltration of macrophages in the livers of mice fed a HFC diet (Fig. 3D). Pathological examination of HE-stained liver sections (Fig. 3D) confirmed these findings (Figs. S2A-C) and revealed no difference in NAS (Fig. 3E).

Hematopoietic Deletion of *Cmklr1* Does not Affect the Development of Insulin Resistance or NASH

To further investigate if *Cmklr1* deficiency affects the progression of insulin resistance and NAFLD, we transplanted bone marrow from *Cmklr1*$^{-/-}$ mice or WT mice into *Ldlr*$^{-/-}$ mice. *Ldlr*$^{-/-}$ mice fed a HFC diet can be regarded as a model for NASH that is specifically driven by Kupffer cell activation and the recruitment of macrophages [25,26]. *Ldlr*$^{-/-}$ mice transplanted with *Cmklr1*$^{-/-}$ bone marrow cells (*Ldlr*-BMT$^{Cmklr1-/-}$) had a greater gain in body weight than *Ldlr*$^{-/-}$ mice transplanted with WT bone marrow cells

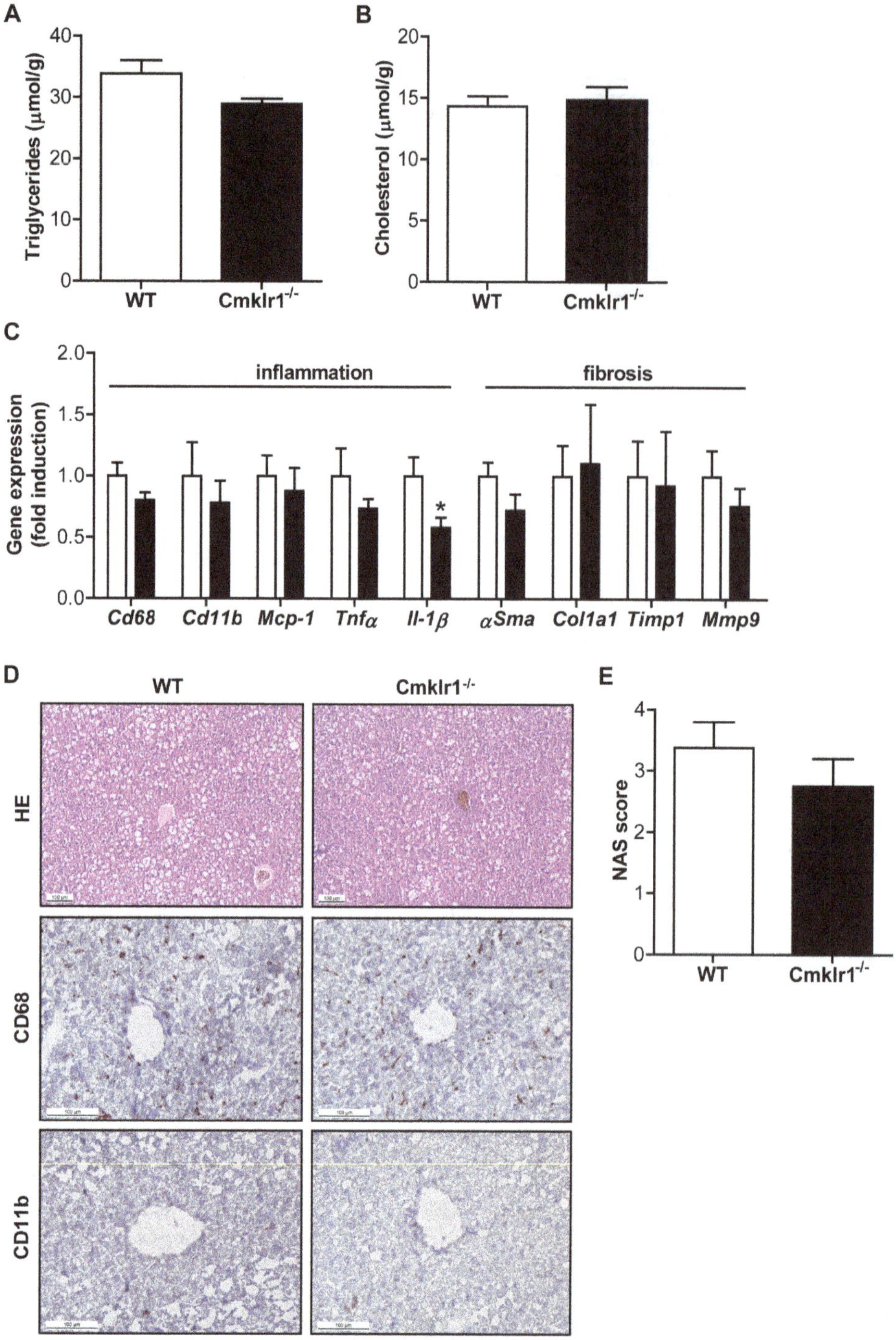

Figure 3. NAFLD progression is not affected by ablation of *Cmklr1*. To investigate the progression of NAFLD, hepatic triglyceride (A) and cholesterol (B) accumulation were measured in mice fed a high fat, high cholesterol diet for 12 weeks. (C) To determine the amount of inflammation and fibrosis in the liver, the inflammatory and pro-fibrotic gene expression were measured in WT mice (white bars) and *Cmklr1*$^{-/-}$ mice (black bars). (D) In addition, a staining for the macrophage markers CD68 and CD11b was performed on frozen-cut liver sections. (E) NAFLD Activity Score (NAS) was determined by pathological examination of Hematoxylin-Eosin (HE) stained liver sections. Abbreviations: WT, wild type; *Cmklr1*$^{-/-}$, chemokine-like receptor 1 knock-out; *Cd68*, cluster of differentiation 68; *Cd11b*, alpha M integrin (*Mac1*); *Mcp-1*, monocyte chemo-attractant protein 1; *Tnfα*, tumor necrosis factor α; *Il1-β*, interleukin 1β; *αSma*, α-smooth muscle actin; *Col1a1*, collagen type 1 alpha 1; *Timp1*, tissue inhibitor of metalloproteinase 1; *Mmp9*, matrix metallopeptidase 9. N = 7–8 for all experiments. Data are expressed as mean ± SEM. * $p<0.05$ vs WT.

(*Ldlr*-BMT^{WT}) (Fig. 4A), and this could not be explained by differences in food intake (Fig. S3A). In concordance, the number of adipocytes per mm^2 was lower in *Ldlr*-BMT$^{Cmklr1-/-}$ mice compared to *Ldlr*-BMT^{WT} mice in both VAT (*Ldlr*-BMT^{WT}, 245 cells/mm^2±26; *Ldlr*-BMT$^{Cmklr1-/-}$, 178 cells/mm^2±15; p = 0.07) and SAT (*Ldlr*-BMT^{WT}, 474 cells/mm^2±51; *Ldlr*-BMT$^{Cmklr1-/-}$, 302 cells/mm^2±30; $p<0.05$), indicating that *Ldlr*-BMT$^{Cmklr1-/-}$ mice have larger adipocytes (Fig. S3B). In contrast,

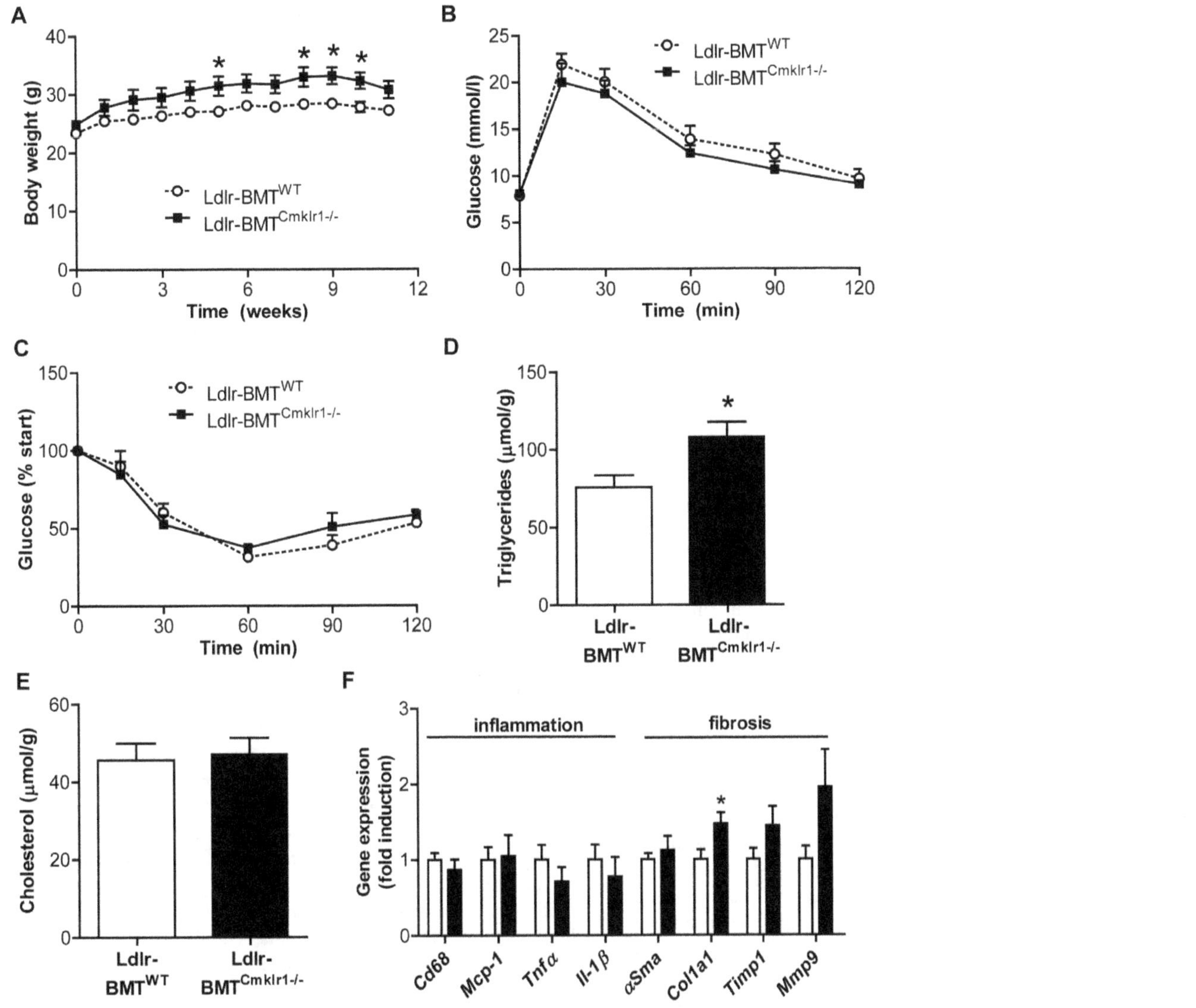

Figure 4. Hematopoietic deletion of *Cmklr1* does not affect NASH development in *Ldlr*$^{-/-}$ mice. (A) Body weight of *Ldlr*-BMT^{WT} and *Ldlr*-BMT$^{Cmklr1-/-}$ mice was measured during the high fat, high cholesterol diet period of 12 weeks. Insulin resistance was assessed by an oral glucose tolerance test (B) and an insulin tolerance test (C). NASH progression was investigated by measuring hepatic triglyceride (D) and cholesterol (E) accumulation and by determining hepatic inflammatory and pro-fibrotic gene expression (F) in *Ldlr*-BMT^{WT} mice (white bars) and *Ldlr*-BMT$^{Cmklr1-/-}$ mice (black bars). Abbreviations: *Ldlr*-BMT^{WT}, low-density lipoprotein receptor knock-out mice transplanted with wild type bone marrow cells; *Ldlr*-BMT$^{Cmklr1-/-}$, low-density lipoprotein receptor knock-out mice transplanted with chemokine-like receptor 1 knock-out bone marrow cells; *Cd68*, cluster of differentiation 68; *Mcp-1*, monocyte chemo-attractant protein 1; *Tnfα*, tumor necrosis factor α; *Il1-β*, interleukin 1β; *αSma*, α-smooth muscle actin; *Col1a1*, collagen type 1 alpha 1; *Timp1*, tissue inhibitor of metalloproteinase 1; *Mmp9*, matrix metallopeptidase 9. N = 5–7 for all experiments. Data are expressed as mean ± SEM. * $p<0.05$ vs WT.

we found no significant differences in plasma triglyceride, cholesterol, glucose and insulin levels between the two groups of mice (Figs. S3C-F). Moreover, hematopoietic deletion of *Cmklr1* did not affect glucose tolerance (Fig. 4B) or insulin tolerance (Fig. 4C). Whereas liver weight, expressed as a percentage of body weight, was slightly lower in *Ldlr*-BMT$^{Cmklr1-/-}$ mice compared to *Ldlr*-BMT^{WT} mice (*Ldlr*-BMT^{WT}, 5.49%±0.086; *Ldlr*-BMT$^{Cmklr1-/-}$, 5.08%±0.10, $p<0.05$), the *Ldlr*-BMT$^{Cmklr1-/-}$ mice showed a small increase in their hepatic triglyceride content and hepatic steatosis (Fig. 4D and Fig. S3G). No differences were observed in hepatic cholesterol accumulation (Fig. 4E). As in the whole-body knock-out model, no differences in inflammatory gene expression (*Cd68*, *Mcp-1*, *Tnfα* and *Il-1β*) were observed (Fig. 4F). Examination of pro-fibrotic genes revealed a trend towards an increase of fibrosis in *Ldlr*-BMT$^{Cmklr1-/-}$ mice. However, the differences were only significant for *Col1a1* (Fig. 4F). Overall, these data indicate that whole-body or hematopoietic ablation of *Cmklr1* does not impact on the development of systemic insulin resistance and NAFLD in mice.

Discussion

The role of *Cmklr1* in the development of insulin resistance and NAFLD is controversial. Our data show that whole-body as well as hematopoietic deletion of *Cmklr1* in *Ldlr*$^{-/-}$ mice did not affect the development of insulin resistance or NAFLD when the mice were fed a HFC-diet for 12 weeks. These results raise the question whether the alterations in serum chemerin levels and hepatic chemerin and *Cmklr1* expression found in rodent models of NAFLD [7,12,14] are causally involved in the development and/or progression of this disease.

In contrast to our findings, others previously reported that *Cmklr1*$^{-/-}$ mice have reduced hepatic inflammation compared to WT mice [15], which may be related to the reduced body weight and fat mass found in these *Cmklr1*$^{-/-}$ mice. In line with this, the same investigators showed that *Cmklr1*$^{-/-}$ mice have reduced steatosis on a low fat diet. However, these differences were not present on a high fat diet [15]. Our results confirm their latter findings. Consistent with our results, another paper observed no differences in body weight, fat mass and glucose tolerance between WT and *Cmklr1*$^{-/-}$ mice at a young age. In that study, *Cmklr1*$^{-/-}$ mice started to gain more fat mass than WT mice only from age 8 months onwards [16]. The increased body weight gain (Fig. 4A) and adipocyte size (Fig. S3B) found in *Ldlr*$^{-/-}$ mice with a hematopoietic deletion of *Cmklr1* might therefore be an age-induced effect. These mice were euthanized at 7–10 months of age, whereas the whole-body knock-outs were euthanized at 6–7 months of age. These results suggest that hematopoietic cells might be responsible for the age-induced weight gain of *Cmklr1*$^{-/-}$ mice. In contrast to *Cmklr1*$^{-/-}$ mice, the *Ldlr*-BMT$^{Cmklr1-/-}$ mice had increased hepatic triglyceride levels (Fig. 4D), increased hepatic steatosis (Fig. S3G) and a tendency towards an increased expression of pro-fibrotic genes (Fig 4F). However, these differences were small and may well be explained by the increased body weight gain seen in these mice.

As neither whole-body *Cmklr1* deficiency and hematopoietic deletion of *Cmklr1* in *Ldlr*$^{-/-}$ mice affected the development of NAFLD, the alterations in chemerin and *Cmklr1* levels found in humans and mouse models of NAFLD may be a secondary effect of the metabolic syndrome and NAFLD [10–12,14]. In these disorders, many of the factors that can regulate chemerin and *Cmklr1* expression become dysregulated. First, chemerin is an adipokine and its secretion rises with increasing adiposity. Second, plasma TNFα levels and *Tnfα* expression in adipose tissue and the liver are higher in NASH [27,28]. This cytokine has been shown to increase chemerin expression from adipose tissue [29,30] and to modulate chemerin activity [31]. Finally, FXR, a nuclear receptor that regulates glucose and lipid homeostasis, induces chemerin expression [12]. The alterations in chemerin levels found in rodent models of NAFLD may thus be caused by increased adiposity, increased *Tnfα* levels [30] or altered FXR activity in NAFLD. Expression of *Cmklr1* in hepatocytes is upregulated by adiponectin [14]. This adipokine protects against steatosis and inflammation and is reduced in human patients with NAFLD [32]. Thus, the reduced expression of *Cmklr1* in patients with NAFLD may be explained by reduced adiponectin levels and it may not be causally involved in the development of NAFLD.

A few limitations to our study must be taken into account. In our model we studied the effects of the absence of *Cmklr1*, but the other receptors that can bind chemerin, *Gpr1* and *Ccrl2*, were still present [21,22]. It is possible that the increased plasma chemerin levels found in our *Cmklr1*$^{-/-}$ mice (Fig. 1G), which most likely originate from the adipose tissue and not from the liver (Fig. S1A), act on these receptors to compensate for the loss-of-function of *Cmklr1*. So far, however, no signaling function has been described for these receptors [33]. Moreover, we did not find any differences in the expression of *Gpr1* and *Ccrl2* in liver, VAT or SAT between WT and *Cmklr1*$^{-/-}$ mice, indicating that there is no compensatory upregulation of these receptors due to *Cmklr1* deficiency (Figs. S1B and S1C). In addition to the other chemerin receptors, *Cmklr1* has another ligand, named resolvin E1 (RvE1). RvE1 is derived from omega-3 polyunsaturated fatty acids and has been described to inhibit NF-κB activity via *Cmklr1* [34]. RvE1 has also been shown to reduce fat accumulation and macrophage infiltration in the liver and to protect against hepatocyte death [35]. This makes it even more remarkable that *Cmklr1* deficiency does not appear to affect NAFLD development. To fully elucidate the role of *Cmklr1* in NAFLD, experiments in mice deficient for chemerin, RvE1, or both, need to be performed.

In summary, our results show that whole-body and hematopoietic deletion of *Cmklr1* in *Ldlr*$^{-/-}$ mice do not affect the development of systemic insulin resistance and NAFLD in mice. This makes it less likely that the alterations in chemerin and *Cmklr1* levels found in mouse models of NAFLD [12,14] are causally related to the development and/or progression of this disease. We feel the associations between chemerin or *Cmklr1* levels and NAFLD should therefore be interpreted with caution.

Supporting Information

Figure S1 The expression of chemerin is increased in adipose tissue, but not in the liver. The expression of *chemerin* (A) and its receptors, *Gpr1* (B) and *Ccrl2* (C), was measured in liver, visceral and subcutaneous adipose tissue of WT mice (white bars) and *Cmklr1*$^{-/-}$ mice (black bars) fed a high fat, high cholesterol diet for 12 weeks. Abbreviations: WT, wild type; *Cmklr1*$^{-/-}$, chemokine-like receptor 1 knock-out; VAT, visceral adipose tissue; SAT, subcutaneous adipose tissue; *Gpr1*, G protein-coupled receptor 1; *Ccrl2*, (C-C) motif receptor-like 2. N = 6-8 for all experiments. Data are expressed as mean ± SEM.

Figure S2 Steatosis, lobular inflammation and ballooning scores were not affected by *Cmklr1* deficiency. Hematoxylin-Eosin (HE) stained liver sections of mice fed a high fat, high cholesterol diet for 12 weeks were scored for steatosis (A), lobular inflammation (B) and ballooning (C) by a certified veterinary pathologist. Abbreviations: WT, wild type; *Cmklr1*$^{-/-}$, chemokine-like receptor 1 knock-out. N = 8 for all experiments. Data are expressed as mean ± SEM.

Figure S3 Characteristics of bone marrow transplanted *Ldlr*$^{-/-}$ mice. (A) Food intake was measured throughout the 12-week high fat, high cholesterol (HFC) diet period and calculated in grams per day. (B) Representative pictures were taken of Hematoxylin-Eosin (HE) stained visceral and subcutaneous adipose tissue (VAT and SAT) sections. Plasma triglycerides (C), cholesterol (D), glucose (E) and insulin (F) levels were determined after 12 weeks of HFC feeding. (G) Paraffin-embedded liver sections were stained with HE for histological analysis. Abbreviations: *Ldlr*-BMT^{WT}, low-density lipoprotein receptor knock-out mice transplanted with wild type bone marrow cells; *Ldlr*-BMT$^{Cmklr1-/-}$, low-density lipoprotein receptor knock-out mice transplanted with chemokine-like receptor 1 knock-out bone marrow cells. N = 5–7 for all experiments. Data are expressed as mean ± SEM.

Table S1 Primer sequences.

Acknowledgments

We thank Paulina Bartuzi, Fareeba Sheedfar, Daphne Dekker, Dr. Anouk Funke and Dr. Pascal Hommelberg for their excellent technical assistance and Dr. Hans Jonker for helpful discussions. We thank Jackie Senior for editing the manuscript.

Author Contributions

Conceived and designed the experiments: NG MAV DPYK. Performed the experiments: NG MAV NJK HVDM SS SY. Analyzed the data: NG MAV NJK SS SY AB DJD JAK BVDS MHH DPYK. Contributed reagents/materials/analysis tools: DJD. Wrote the paper: NG MAV NJK HVDM SS SY AB DJD JAK BVDS MHH DPYK.

References

1. Blachier M, Leleu H, Peck-Radosavljevic M, Valla DC, Roudot-Thoraval F (2013) The burden of liver disease in europe: A review of available epidemiological data. J Hepatol 58: 593–608.
2. Cohen JC, Horton JD, Hobbs HH (2011) Human fatty liver disease: Old questions and new insights. Science 332: 1519–1523.
3. Wittamer V, Franssen JD, Vulcano M, Mirjolet JF, Le Poul E, et al. (2003) Specific recruitment of antigen-presenting cells by chemerin, a novel processed ligand from human inflammatory fluids. J Exp Med 198: 977–985.
4. Graham KL, Zabel BA, Loghavi S, Zuniga LA, Ho PP, et al. (2009) Chemokine-like receptor-1 expression by central nervous system-infiltrating leukocytes and involvement in a model of autoimmune demyelinating disease. J Immunol 183: 6717–6723.
5. Luangsay S, Wittamer V, Bondue B, De Henau O, Rouger L, et al. (2009) Mouse ChemR23 is expressed in dendritic cell subsets and macrophages, and mediates an anti-inflammatory activity of chemerin in a lung disease model. J Immunol 183: 6489–6499.
6. Bondue B, Vosters O, de Nadai P, Glineur S, De Henau O, et al. (2011) ChemR23 dampens lung inflammation and enhances anti-viral immunity in a mouse model of acute viral pneumonia. PLoS Pathog 7: e1002358.
7. Bozaoglu K, Bolton K, McMillan J, Zimmet P, Jowett J, et al. (2007) Chemerin is a novel adipokine associated with obesity and metabolic syndrome. Endocrinology 148: 4687–4694.
8. Bozaoglu K, Segal D, Shields KA, Cummings N, Curran JE, et al. (2009) Chemerin is associated with metabolic syndrome phenotypes in a mexican-american population. J Clin Endocrinol Metab 94: 3085–3088.
9. Fatima SS, Bozaoglu K, Rehman R, Alam F, Memon AS (2013) Elevated chemerin levels in Pakistani men: An interrelation with metabolic syndrome phenotypes. PLoS One 8: e57113.
10. Kukla M, Zwirska-Korczala K, Hartleb M, Waluga M, Chwist A, et al. (2010) Serum chemerin and vaspin in non-alcoholic fatty liver disease. Scand J Gastroenterol 45: 235–242.
11. Sell H, Divoux A, Poitou C, Basdevant A, Bouillot JL, et al. (2010) Chemerin correlates with markers for fatty liver in morbidly obese patients and strongly decreases after weight loss induced by bariatric surgery. J Clin Endocrinol Metab 95: 2892–2896.
12. Deng Y, Wang H, Lu Y, Liu S, Zhang Q, et al. (2013) Identification of chemerin as a novel FXR target gene down-regulated in the progression of nonalcoholic steatohepatitis. Endocrinology 154: 1794–1801.
13. Docke S, Lock JF, Birkenfeld AL, Hoppe S, Lieske S, et al. (2013) Elevated hepatic chemerin mRNA expression in human non-alcoholic fatty liver disease. Eur J Endocrinol 169: 547–557.
14. Wanninger J, Bauer S, Eisinger K, Weiss TS, Walter R, et al. (2012) Adiponectin upregulates hepatocyte CMKLR1 which is reduced in human fatty liver. Mol Cell Endocrinol 349: 248–254.
15. Ernst MC, Haidl ID, Zuniga LA, Dranse HJ, Rourke JL, et al. (2012) Disruption of the chemokine-like receptor-1 (CMKLR1) gene is associated with reduced adiposity and glucose intolerance. Endocrinology 153: 672–682.
16. Rouger L, Denis GR, Luangsay S, Parmentier M (2013) ChemR23 knockout mice display mild obesity but no deficit in adipocyte differentiation. J Endocrinol 219: 279–289.
17. Zoetelief J, Broerse JJ, Davies RW, Octave-Prignot M, Rezvani M, et al. (2001) Protocol for X-ray dosimetry in radiobiology. Int J Radiat Biol 77: 817–835.
18. Bligh EG, Dyer WJ (1959) A rapid method of total lipid extraction and purification. Can J Biochem Physiol 37: 911–917.
19. Kleiner DE, Brunt EM, Van Natta M, Behling C, Contos MJ, et al. (2005) Design and validation of a histological scoring system for nonalcoholic fatty liver disease. Hepatology 41: 1313–1321.
20. Goralski KB, McCarthy TC, Hanniman EA, Zabel BA, Butcher EC, et al. (2007) Chemerin, a novel adipokine that regulates adipogenesis and adipocyte metabolism. J Biol Chem 282: 28175–28188.
21. Barnea G, Strapps W, Herrada G, Berman Y, Ong J, et al. (2008) The genetic design of signaling cascades to record receptor activation. Proc Natl Acad Sci U S A 105: 64–69.
22. Zabel BA, Nakae S, Zuniga L, Kim JY, Ohyama T, et al. (2008) Mast cell-expressed orphan receptor CCRL2 binds chemerin and is required for optimal induction of IgE-mediated passive cutaneous anaphylaxis. J Exp Med 205: 2207–2220.
23. Ernst MC, Issa M, Goralski KB, Sinal CJ (2010) Chemerin exacerbates glucose intolerance in mouse models of obesity and diabetes. Endocrinology 151: 1998–2007.
24. Becker M, Rabe K, Lebherz C, Zugwurst J, Goke B, et al. (2010) Expression of human chemerin induces insulin resistance in the skeletal muscle but does not affect weight, lipid levels, and atherosclerosis in LDL receptor knockout mice on high-fat diet. Diabetes 59: 2898–2903.
25. Wouters K, van Gorp PJ, Bieghs V, Gijbels MJ, Duimel H, et al. (2008) Dietary cholesterol, rather than liver steatosis, leads to hepatic inflammation in hyperlipidemic mouse models of nonalcoholic steatohepatitis. Hepatology 48: 474–486.
26. Bieghs V, Van Gorp PJ, Wouters K, Hendrikx T, Gijbels MJ, et al. (2012) LDL receptor knock-out mice are a physiological model particularly vulnerable to study the onset of inflammation in non-alcoholic fatty liver disease. PLoS One 7: e30668.
27. Crespo J, Cayon A, Fernandez-Gil P, Hernandez-Guerra M, Mayorga M, et al. (2001) Gene expression of tumor necrosis factor alpha and TNF-receptors, p55 and p75, in nonalcoholic steatohepatitis patients. Hepatology 34: 1158–1163.
28. Abiru S, Migita K, Maeda Y, Daikoku M, Ito M, et al. (2006) Serum cytokine and soluble cytokine receptor levels in patients with non-alcoholic steatohepatitis. Liver Int 26: 39–45.
29. Catalan V, Gomez-Ambrosi J, Rodriguez A, Ramirez B, Rotellar F, et al. (2013) Increased levels of chemerin and its receptor, chemokine-like receptor-1, in obesity are related to inflammation: Tumor necrosis factor-alpha stimulates mRNA levels of chemerin in visceral adipocytes from obese patients. Surg Obes Relat Dis 9: 306–314.
30. Parlee SD, Ernst MC, Muruganandan S, Sinal CJ, Goralski KB (2010) Serum chemerin levels vary with time of day and are modified by obesity and tumor necrosis factor-{alpha}. Endocrinology 151: 2590–2602.
31. Parlee SD, McNeil JO, Muruganandan S, Sinal CJ, Goralski KB (2012) Elastase and tryptase govern TNFalpha-mediated production of active chemerin by adipocytes. PLoS One 7: e51072.
32. Buechler C, Wanninger J, Neumeier M (2011) Adiponectin, a key adipokine in obesity related liver diseases. World J Gastroenterol 17: 2801–2811.
33. Bondue B, Wittamer V, Parmentier M (2011) Chemerin and its receptors in leukocyte trafficking, inflammation and metabolism. Cytokine Growth Factor Rev 22: 331–338.
34. Arita M, Bianchini F, Aliberti J, Sher A, Chiang N, et al. (2005) Stereochemical assignment, antiinflammatory properties, and receptor for the omega-3 lipid mediator resolvin E1. J Exp Med 201: 713–722.
35. Gonzalez-Periz A, Horrillo R, Ferre N, Gronert K, Dong B, et al. (2009) Obesity-induced insulin resistance and hepatic steatosis are alleviated by omega-3 fatty acids: A role for resolvins and protectins. FASEB J 23: 1946–1957.

20

Vitamin A and Feeding Statuses Modulate the Insulin-Regulated Gene Expression in Zucker Lean and Fatty Primary Rat Hepatocytes

Wei Chen, Meredith L. Howell, Yang Li, Rui Li, Guoxun Chen*

Department of Nutrition, University of Tennessee at Knoxville, Knoxville, Tennessee, United States of America

Abstract

Unattended hepatic insulin resistance predisposes individuals to dyslipidemia, type 2 diabetes and many other metabolic complications. The mechanism of hepatic insulin resistance at the gene expression level remains unrevealed. To examine the effects of vitamin A (VA), total energy intake and feeding conditions on the insulin-regulated gene expression in primary hepatocytes of Zucker lean (ZL) and fatty (ZF) rats, we analyze the expression levels of hepatic model genes in response to the treatments of insulin and retinoic acid (RA). We report that the insulin- and RA-regulated glucokinase, sterol regulatory element-binding protein-1c and cytosolic form of phosphoenolpyruvate carboxykinase expressions are impaired in hepatocytes of ZF rats fed chow or a VA sufficient (VAS) diet ad libitum. The impairments are partially corrected when ZF rats are fed a VA deficient (VAD) diet ad libitum or pair-fed a VAS diet to the intake of their VAD counterparts in non-fasting conditions. Interestingly in the pair-fed ZL and ZF rats, transient overeating on the last day of pair-feeding regimen changes the expression levels of some VA catabolic genes, and impairs the insulin- and RA-regulated gene expression in hepatocytes. These results demonstrate that VA and feeding statuses modulate the hepatic insulin sensitivity at the gene expression level.

Editor: Mengwei Zang, Boston University School of Medicine, United States of America

Funding: This work was financially supported by research grant from Allen Foundation Inc (to G.C.), start-up fund from the University of Tennessee at Knoxville (to G.C.), and Scientist Development Grant from American Heart Association (09SDG2140003, to G.C.). W.C., Y.L. and R.L. received financial support from the China Scholarship Council. The funders had no role in study design, data collection and analysis, decision to publish, or preparation of the manuscript.

Competing Interests: The authors have declared that no competing interests exist.

* Email: gchen6@utk.edu

Introduction

The liver is critical for glucose and lipid homeostasis, which is achieved partially through the regulation of hepatic gene expression in response to hormonal and nutritional stimuli [1,2]. The disturbance of these responses may lead to the development of metabolic diseases, including obesity and type 2 diabetes [1]. Even though the pathogenesis of these diseases has not been fully elucidated, insulin resistance is a common feature [3]. Current theory postulates that overnutrition triggers system inflammation, dysregulates lipid metabolism, and alters gastrointestinal microbiota, all of which may interplay and lead to impaired insulin action in the body [4].

The insulin-regulated hepatic metabolism is partially attributed to the regulation of hepatic genes expression. For instance, in primary rat hepatocytes, insulin induces the glucokinase (GCK, gene *Gck*) expression to promote glycolysis and suppresses the phosphoenolpyruvate carboxykinase (PEPCK-C, gene *Pck1*) expression to reduce gluconeogenesis [5,6]. Insulin also induces hepatic lipogenesis via inducing sterol regulatory element-binding protein 1c (SREBP-1c, gene *Srebp-1c*) expression. SREBP-1c stimulates the expression of hepatic lipogenic genes, such as acetyl-coenzyme A carboxylase and fatty acid synthase [7]. In the insulin-resistant liver, insulin is unable to suppress the expression of gluconeogenic genes. But it is able to concurrently induce the expression of lipogenic genes [2]. This phenomenon demonstrates the coexistence of hyperglycemia and hyperlipidemia in type 2 diabetes.

As an essential and lipophilic micronutrient, vitamin A (VA, retinol) is implicated in the regulation of glucose and lipid metabolism [1]. Two stepwise cytosolic enzymatic reactions convert retinol to retinal and then into retinoic acid (RA, all-*trans* RA or 9-*cis* RA), which then enters the nucleus and modules gene expression through the activation of retinoid acid receptors and retinoid X receptors [8]. We have reported that the insulin-regulated gene expression is impaired in primary hepatocytes from Zucker fatty (ZF) rats fed ad libitum [9]. Recent reports by our group also show that RA synergizes with insulin to induce the *Gck* and *Srebp-1c* expressions in primary rat hepatocytes [10,11]. RA attenuates the insulin-suppressed *Pck1* expression in the same cells [12]. These data suggest that micronutrient status can affect hepatic insulin sensitivity at the gene expression level. However, the roles of caloric intake and micronutrient composition in the hepatic insulin resistance at the gene expression level have not been investigated.

Here, we chose Zucker lean (ZL) and ZF rats as insulin sensitive and resistant models, respectively, to investigate the effects of energy intake and VA status on the hepatic insulin sensitivity at the gene expression level. We demonstrate that VA deficiency partially corrects the impaired insulin-regulated gene expression in ZF primary hepatocytes. More importantly, transient overeating in ZL and ZF rats causes the impairment of insulin-regulated gene expression in their primary hepatocytes.

Materials and Methods

Reagents

The reagents for primary hepatocyte isolation and culture including Medium 199, Dulbecco's Modification of Eagle Medium (DMEM), liver perfusion buffer and liver digest buffer were obtained from Invitrogen (Carlsbad, CA). For RNA extraction, RNA STAT-60 was purchased from TEL-TEST (Friendswood, TX). The reagents for cDNA synthesis and real-time PCR were obtained from Applied Biosystems (Foster city, CA). All real-time PCR primer sets used in this study were synthesized by Sigma-Aldrich (St. Louis, MO). All other reagents and materials were purchased from Fisher Scientific (Pittsburgh, PA) unless described otherwise.

Animals and rodent diets

Zucker rats (Harlan Laboratories) were bred and housed on a 12 hour light-dark cycle under constant temperature and humidity in the animal facility at University of Tennessee at Knoxville. Breeding pairs were kept on Teklad rodent chow (#8640, Harlan Laboratories, Indianapolis, IN). Weaned male ZL (fa/+ or +/+) and ZF (fa/fa) rats (21 days old) were fed experimental diets for 8 weeks before primary hepatocyte isolation. Synthetic VA sufficient (VAS, #5755, 22.1 IU/g VA) and VA deficient (VAD, #5822, 0 IU/g VA) diets were isocaloric diets from TestDiet (Richmond, VA). All procedures (Protocol #1256, #1863) were approved by the Institutional Animal Care and Use Committee at the University of Tennessee at Knoxville.

Pair-feeding study

Male ZL or ZF rats (VAD-AD group, and VAD ad libitum, 5 rats per group) had free access to the VAD diet and water for 56 days. The body mass and food intake were recorded every 2 days. Primary hepatocytes were isolated on Day 56. Two pair-feeding groups were set up to circumvent a potential caveat on the last day of pair-feeding. Since VAD animals consume significantly less diet than their VAS counterparts in ad libitum feeding condition [13–15], the VAS pair-fed rats would conceivably consume the last day's ration rapidly. This caveat would result in a fasting status in these rats and affect the analysis of insulin-regulated hepatic gene expression. Therefore, 10 rats with matching genotypes were paired up with rats in VAD-AD group according to weaning body mass. They were pair-fed the VAS diet for 55 days to the intakes of their VAD-AD counterparts. During the course of pair-feeding, unfinished food pellets were rolled over to ensure that equal total calories were provided. The body mass and food intake of these rats were recorded daily. On Day 56, one group, VAS-PF-AD (VAS pair-feeding last day ad libitum), was allowed to have free access to the VAS diet to prevent fasting energy status. The other group, VAS-PF-4M (VAS pair-feeding last day 4 meals), was fed the VAS diet to the amount consumed by the VAD-AD group. One fourth of the ration was provided to VAS-PF-4M rats every 6 hours, so that they remained non-fasted energy status till the end of the study. Before primary hepatocyte isolation, the tail tip whole blood glucose was measured using a LifeScan OneTouch Ultramini glucometer (Milpitas, CA).

Primary hepatocyte isolation

The primary hepatocytes were isolated according to previously described protocol [9]. The rat was euthanized by primary carbon dioxide asphyxiation, and then secondary cervical dislocation according to the protocol. A peristaltic pump with the flow rate of 10 ml/min was set up to infuse about 120 ml liver perfusion buffer and 120 ml liver digestion buffer. A catheter connected to the pump was inserted into the portal vein. The inferior vena cava was punctured to allow the outflow of blood and buffers. The liver was then excised and put into a cell culture dish containing liver digestion buffer to remove connective tissues. The released hepatocytes were filtered through a 100 μm cell strainer and collected by 50× g centrifugation for 3 minutes. The hepatocytes were washed twice with high glucose DMEM containing 8% fetal bovine serum, 1% penicillin/streptomycin. Isolated hepatocytes were seeded on 60-mm collagen type I coated dishes at 2×10^6 cells per dish and incubated in high glucose DMEM containing 8% fetal bovine serum, 1% penicillin/streptomycin at 37°C and 5% CO_2 for 3 hours. The attached hepatocytes were washed once with PBS and pretreated in medium A (Medium 199 with 100 nM dexamethasone, 100 nM 3,3′,5-triiodo-L-thyronine (T3), and 1% penicillin/streptomycin) containing 1 nM insulin at 37°C and 5% CO2 for 14–16 hours.

Insulin and RA treatments, RNA extraction and real-time PCR

The pretreated hepatocytes were washed once with PBS, and then treated for 6 hours at 37°C and 5% CO2 with medium A containing indicated concentrations of insulin (0 nM to 100 nM) with or without 5 μM RA. The methods for total RNA extraction and cDNA synthesis were described elsewhere [16]. In essence, total RNA was extraction from the treated hepatocytes with RNA STAT-60 according to the manufacture's protocol. The contaminated DNA in RNA samples was removed using the DNA-free kit. First strand cDNA was synthesized with 2 μg total RNA by cDNA synthesis kit. The gene expression level was determined by real-time PCR with respective primer sets, and normalized to the mRNA level of ribosomal gene 36B4. The data were presented as either minus Δ cycle threshold (Ct) or the induction fold (ΔΔCt) for which the control treatment group was arbitrarily set as 1.

Statistical analysis

Statistical analyses were performed using SPSS 19.0 software. Student t-test was used to compare the means between two treatments. One-way ANOVA with LSD post-hoc test was used to compare the means of three or more treatments. Two-way ANOVA with Bonferroni's post-hoc test was used to determine the effects of diets and genotypes on hepatic gene expression. Data were presented as means ± S.E.M. The number of experiments indicates hepatocyte isolations from different animals. A p value less than 0.05 is considered statistically significant.

Results

The insulin- and RA-regulated *Gck*, *Pck1*, and *Srebp-1c* expressions were impaired in primary hepatocytes from ZF rats fed chow ad libitum

We compared the insulin-regulated gene expression in primary hepatocytes from ZL and ZF rats fed chow ad libitum. Insulin dose-dependently induced the *Gck* and *Srebp-1c* expressions (Figure 1A and 1C), and suppressed the *Pck1* expression (Figure 1B) in ZL hepatocytes. RA (5 μM) synergized with insulin to induce the *Gck* and *Srebp-1c* expressions (Figure 1A and 1C).

The elevated *Pck1* level in the presence of RA was still lowered by insulin at 1 nM or higher (Figure 1B). Comparably in ZF hepatocytes, the fold inductions of *Gck* expression by insulin (marked by *) and RA + insulin (marked by #) at the corresponding concentrations were significantly lower than that in ZL hepatocytes (Figure 1A). The inductions of *Srebp-1c* by insulin (0.1 to 100 nM) and RA + insulin (0.1 to 100 nM) were abolished in ZF hepatocytes (Figure 1C). Additionally, the insulin-mediated suppression of *Pck1* was less profound in ZF hepatocytes compared with that in ZL hepatocytes (Figure 1B, marked by * and #, and Figure S1 in File S1). Furthermore, the expressions of liver type pyruvate kinase gene (*Pklr*) in primary hepatocytes from either ZL or ZF rats were not affected by insulin and RA treatments (Figure 1D). These data confirmed our previous observations [9] and demonstrated the hepatic insulin resistance at the gene expression level in ZF rats fed chow ad libitum.

The insulin- and RA-regulated *Gck*, *Pck1* and *Srebp-1c* expressions were partially recovered in the primary hepatocytes from ZF rats fed a VAD diet ad libitum

VA deficiency reduced food intake, body mass, plasma insulin and triglyceride levels in Zucker rats [9]. Hence, it may attenuate the impairment of the insulin-regulated gene expression in ZF rat hepatocytes. Figure 2A (left panel) showed that, in both VAD and VAS ZL primary hepatocytes, insulin dose-dependently induced the *Gck* expression (first and second column clusters), and RA synergized with insulin to induce its expression (third and fourth column clusters). The fold inductions of *Gck* expression by insulin (marked by *) or by RA + insulin (marked by #) in the VAS ZL hepatocytes were significantly higher than that in VAD ZL hepatocytes at the corresponding insulin concentrations. In comparison, the insulin-induced *Gck* expression was impaired in both VAD and VAS ZF hepatocytes regardless of RA (Figure 2A, right panel).

Insulin dose-dependently suppressed the *Pck1* expression in both VAD and VAS ZL hepatocytes (Figure 2B, left panel, first and second column clusters). RA induced the *Pck1* expression. Insulin at 1 to 100 nM suppressed the *Pck1* expression by over 90% in both VAD and VAS ZL hepatocytes (third and fourth column clusters, Figure S2B in File S1). The net *Pck1* mRNA levels in the presence of RA were higher than that in the absence of RA. On the other hand, the insulin-suppressed *Pck1* expression was impaired in VAS ZF hepatocytes. Insulin at 0.1 nM or 1 nM only suppressed 10% or 40% of the *Pck1* expression level, respectively. However, in VAD ZF hepatocytes, the suppression of *Pck1* expression by 0.1 nM or 1 nM insulin was 40% or 60%, respectively, suggesting improved regulation by insulin (Figure 2B, right panel, first and second column clusters, Figure S2A in File S1). RA induced the *Pck1* expression in VAD and VAS ZF hepatocytes (right panel, third and fourth column clusters). Insulin at 0.1 nM or 1 nM respectively suppressed the *Pck1* expression by 50% or 70% in VAD ZF hepatocytes, which was greater than 20% or 50% in VAS ZF hepatocytes (Figure S2B in File S1).

Insulin dose-dependently induced the *Srebp-1c* expression, and RA synergized with insulin to induce its expression in both VAD and VAS ZL hepatocytes (Figure 2C, left panel). The fold inductions of *Srebp-1c* expression by insulin (marked by *) or by insulin and RA (marked by #) in VAS ZL hepatocytes were significantly lower than that in VAD ZL hepatocytes. In VAS ZF hepatocytes, the insulin-induced *Srebp-1c* expression in the absence or presence of RA was abolished (Figure 2C, right panel). Interestingly in VAD ZF hepatocytes, insulin (1 to 100 nM) partially regained the ability to induce the *Srebp-1c* expression, showing improved regulation (first and third cluster).

ZL or ZF rats pair-fed the VAS diet tended to overeat when sufficient amount of diet was provided

Rats fed a VAD diet after weaning reduced food intakes at around 5 weeks [13]. To determine how total and acute food intakes affect the insulin-regulated hepatic gene expression, an 8-week pair-feeding experiment was designed. Rats were divided into three groups, VAD-AD, VAS-PF-AD and VAS-PF-4M (Figure 3A, see Materials and Methods for detail). Figure 3B shows that VAS-PF-AD ZL and ZF rats ingested 54% and 112% more food on the last day than VAD-AD ZL and ZF rats did, respectively, demonstrating the overeating of VAS-PF-AD rats. The overeating of VAS-PF-AD rats did not significantly increase the total caloric intake over the entire pair-feeding period compared to VAD-AD and VAS-PF-4M counterparts (Figure 3C). Correspondingly, VAS-PF-AD ZL and ZF rats gained 4% and 6% of body mass on the last day, respectively (Figure 3D). Before sacrifice, the tail tip whole blood glucose levels of VAS-PF-AD ZF rats were significantly higher than those of VAD-AD and VAS-PF-4M rats (Figure 3E).

ZL and ZF rats pair-fed the VAS diet had higher body mass and feed efficiency than their VAD fed counterparts after the reduction of food intake

During the 56-day pair-feeding regimen, the two-day food intake of VAD-AD ZL rats gradually increased from ~10 g initially to ~40 g on days 33–34, and kept relatively stable until days 41–42 (Figure 4A, left panel). As anticipated [13–15], the food intake then started to decline until the end of the dietary manipulation. The two-day food intake of VAD-AD ZF rats quickly rose from ~10 g initially to ~60 g on days 17–18, leveled off between days 20 to 34, started to decline on days 35–36, reached ~30 g on days 47–48, and leveled off again until the end of the dietary manipulation (right panel). During the same period, all VAS pair-fed ZL and ZF rats received the same amount of the isocaloric VAS diet to match the energy intake of VAD-AD rats. The body mass of VAD-AD ZL and ZF rats ceased to increase after 36 days of dietary manipulation (Figure 4B). From day 34, the body mass of VAD-AD ZL or ZF rats was significantly lower than that of VAS-PF ZL or ZF rats, respectively (marked by *). Furthermore, the cumulative feed efficiency of all three groups decreased over time. However, VAS-PF ZL or ZF rats had significantly higher feed efficiency than VAD-AD ZL or ZF rats after 36 or 22 days, respectively (Figure 4C).

Transient overeating impaired the insulin-induced *Gck* expression in primary hepatocytes of VAS-PF-AD ZL and ZF rats

In ZL hepatocytes, insulin dose-dependently induced the *Gck* expression (Figure 5A). Without or with RA, the fold inductions by insulin in VAS-PF-AD ZL hepatocytes were significantly lower than that in VAD-AD hepatocytes (marked by *) and VAS-PF-4M ZL hepatocytes (marked by $), suggesting an impaired insulin regulation. Additionally, the fold inductions by insulin in VAD-AD ZL hepatocytes were lower than that of VAS-PF-4M ZL hepatocytes without or with RA (marked by #). These results match the data shown in Figure 2A and indicate that VA status of ZL rats affects the insulin-stimulated *Gck* expression in their hepatocytes.

In ZF hepatocytes, insulin dose-dependently induced the *Gck* expression regardless of RA (Figure 5B). Without RA, the fold inductions by insulin (1 and 10 nM) in VAS-PF-AD ZF hepatocytes were significantly lower than that in VAS-PF-4M ZF hepatocytes (Figure 5B, left panel, marked by $). With RA

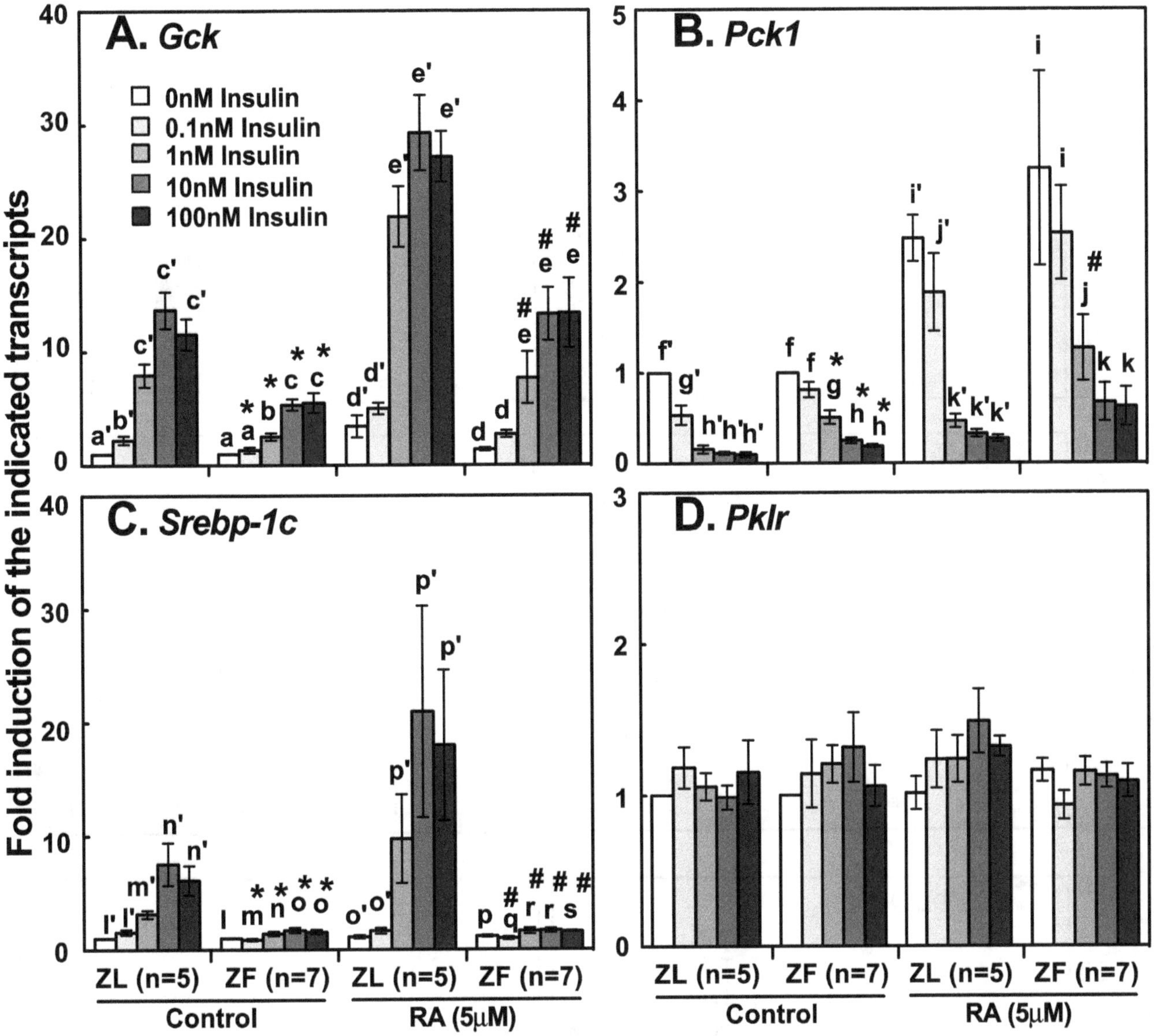

Figure 1. Impaired insulin-regulated gene expression in primary hepatocytes of ZF rats fed chow ad libitum. ZL and ZF rats were fed standard chow for eight weeks before primary hepatocytes were harvested. The primary hepatocytes were incubated in medium A with increasing concentrations of insulin (0 nM to 100 nM) in the absence or presence of RA (5 μM) for 6 hours. Total RNA was extracted, synthesized into cDNA, and then subjected to real-time PCR analysis for the expression levels of *Gck* (A), *Pck1* (B), *Srebp-1c* (C), and *Pklr* (D). The expression level of each gene transcript in ZL or ZF hepatocytes treated with vehicle control was arbitrarily set to 1. The data were expressed as fold induction. The numbers of hepatocyte isolation are presented in parenthesis. All $p<0.05$; for (A), $a'<b'<c'$, $a<b<c$, $d'<e'$, $d<e$; for (B), $f'>g'>h'$, $f>g>h$, $i'>j'$, $i>k$; for (C), $l'<m'<n'$, $m<o$, $p'<q'$, $r<s$ using one-way ANOVA; * or # for comparing ZL or ZF at corresponding treatments using Student's t-test, respectively.

(Figure 5B, right panel), the fold inductions by insulin in VAS-PF-AD ZF hepatocytes were significantly lower than that in VAD-AD (0.1 to 100 nM, marked by *) and VAS-PF-4M (1 to 100 nM, marked by $) ZF hepatocytes. These data demonstrate the impairment of the insulin-induced *Gck* expression in VAS-PF-AD ZF hepatocytes.

The insulin-suppressed *Pck1* expression was partially impaired in primary hepatocytes of VAS-PF-AD ZL rats

In VAD-AD and VAS-PF-4M ZL hepatocytes, insulin at 0.1 nM suppressed *Pck1* expression of by 60% and 70%, respectively (Figure 6A). The insulin-mediated suppression reached over 90% at 1 to 100 nM (left panel). In VAS-PF-AD ZL hepatocytes, the *Pck1* expression levels in the presence of 1 to 100 nM insulin were significantly higher than that in VAD-AD and VAS-PF-4M ZL hepatocytes (marked by * and $, respectively). In the presence of RA, insulin at 0.1 to 100 nM reduced the elevated *Pck1* mRNA levels in all three groups of ZL hepatocytes (Figure 6A, right panel).

For ZF hepatocytes, insulin at 0.1 to 100 nM significantly suppressed the *Pck1* expression in VAD-AD, VAS-PF-AD and VAS-PF-4M groups (Figure 6B, left panel). With RA, insulin reduced the elevated *Pck1* mRNA levels in VAS-PF-AD (0.1 to 100 nM), VAD-AD (1 to 100 nM) and VAS-PF-4M (1 to 100 nM) ZF hepatocytes (right panel). Interestingly, the *Pck1* expression levels in VAS-PF-AD ZF hepatocytes were significantly lower than

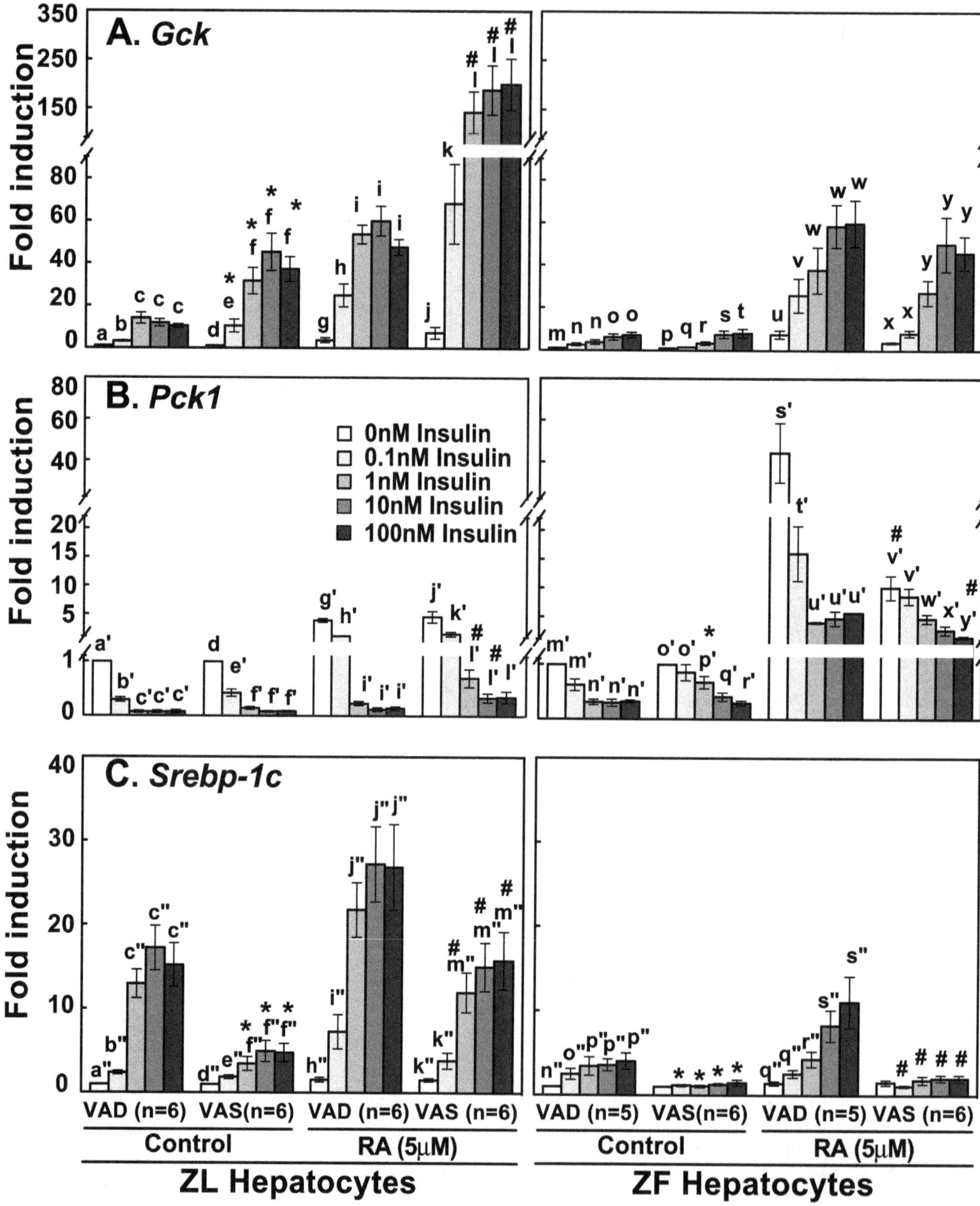

Figure 2. VAD diet partially recovered the impaired insulin-regulated gene expression in ZF primary rat hepatocytes. ZL and ZF rats were fed either a VAS or VAD diet for 8 weeks. Primary hepatocytes were isolated from rats in ad libitum. Cells were incubated in medium A with increasing concentrations of insulin (0 nM to 100 nM) in the absence or presence of RA (5 μM) for 6 hours. Total RNA was extracted, synthesized into cDNA, and then subjected to real-time PCR analysis for the expression levels of *Gck* (A), *Pck1* (B), and *Srebp-1c* (C). The data were expressed as fold induction. The gene transcript levels from the no treatment group (0 nM insulin, no RA) for both ZL and ZF were arbitrarily set to 1. The numbers of hepatocyte isolation are presented in parenthesis. All $p<0.05$; for (A), $a<b<c$, $d<e<f$, $g<h<i$, $j<k<l$, $m<o$, $p<r/s/t$, $q<s/t$, $r<t$, $x<y$; for (B), $a'>b'>c'$, $d'>e'>f'$, $g'>h'>i$, $j'>k'>l'$, $m'>n'$, $o'>q'/r'$, $p'>r'$, $s'>t'>u'$, $v'>x'/y'$, $w'>y'$; for (C), $a''<b''<c''$, $d''<e''<f''$, $h''<i''<j''$, $k''<m''$, $n''<p''$, $q''<s''$, using one-way ANOVA. * or # for comparing ZL and ZF at corresponding treatments using Student's t-test, respectively.

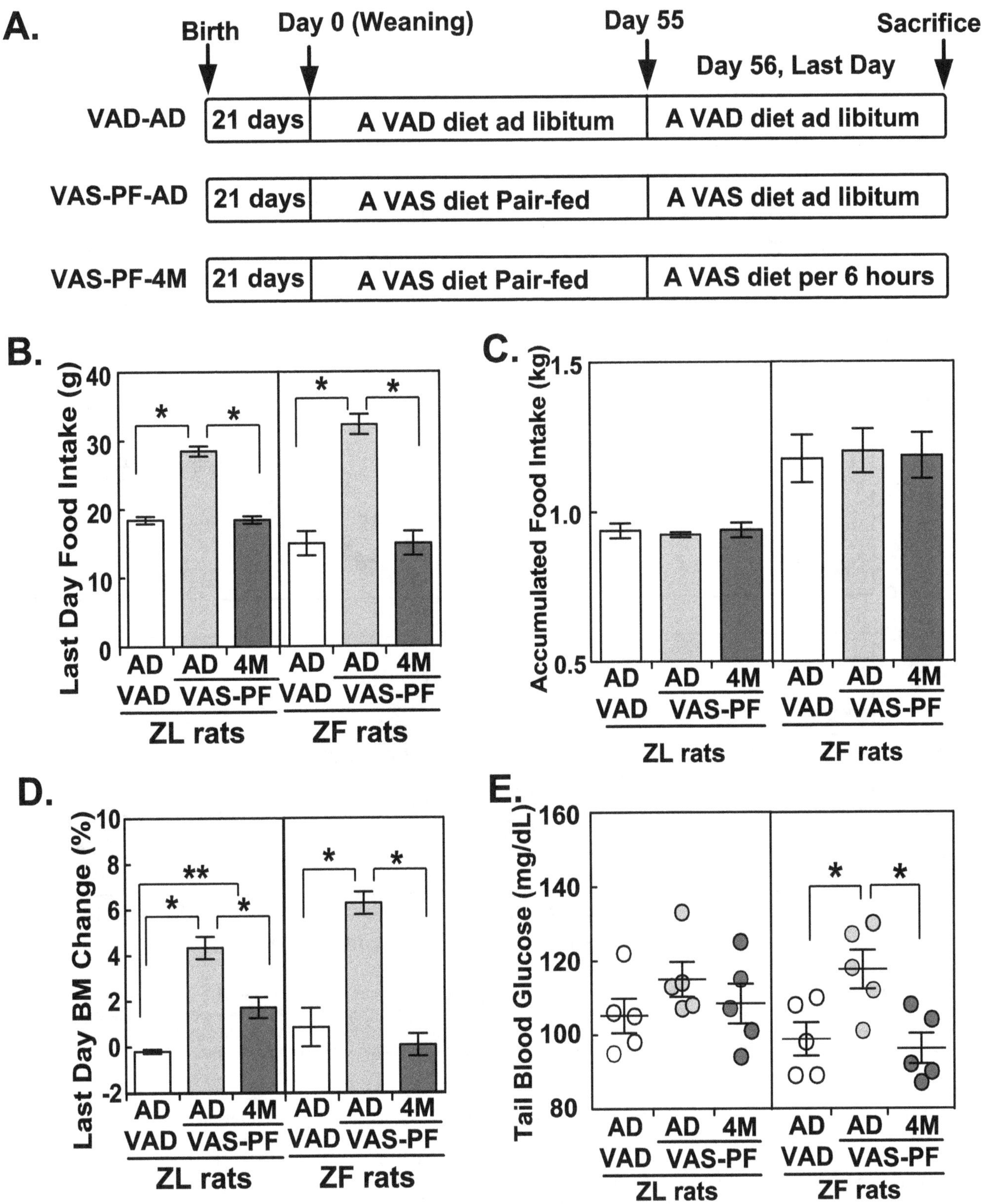

Figure 3. VAS-PF-AD ZL and ZF overate on the last day when sufficient VAS diet was provided. (A) The schematic graph of the setup for the pair-feeding regimen. VAD ad libitum (VAD-AD, n = 5), VAS pair-feeding last day ad libitum (VAS-PF-AD, n = 5), VAS pair-feeding last day 4 meals (VAS-PF-4M, n = 5) (B) Tail tip whole blood glucose from ZL and ZF rats before sacrifice. Each circle represents a value from an individual animal. The bars represent mean ± S.E.M. * Indicates $p<0.05$ using one-way ANOVA with LSD post-hoc test. (C) The accumulative food intake for ZL and ZF rats over 56 days of pair-feeding regimen. (D) The food intake and (E) body mass change for ZL and ZF rats on day 56 of the pair-feeding regimen. * Indicates $p<0.05$ using one-way ANOVA with LSD post-hoc test.

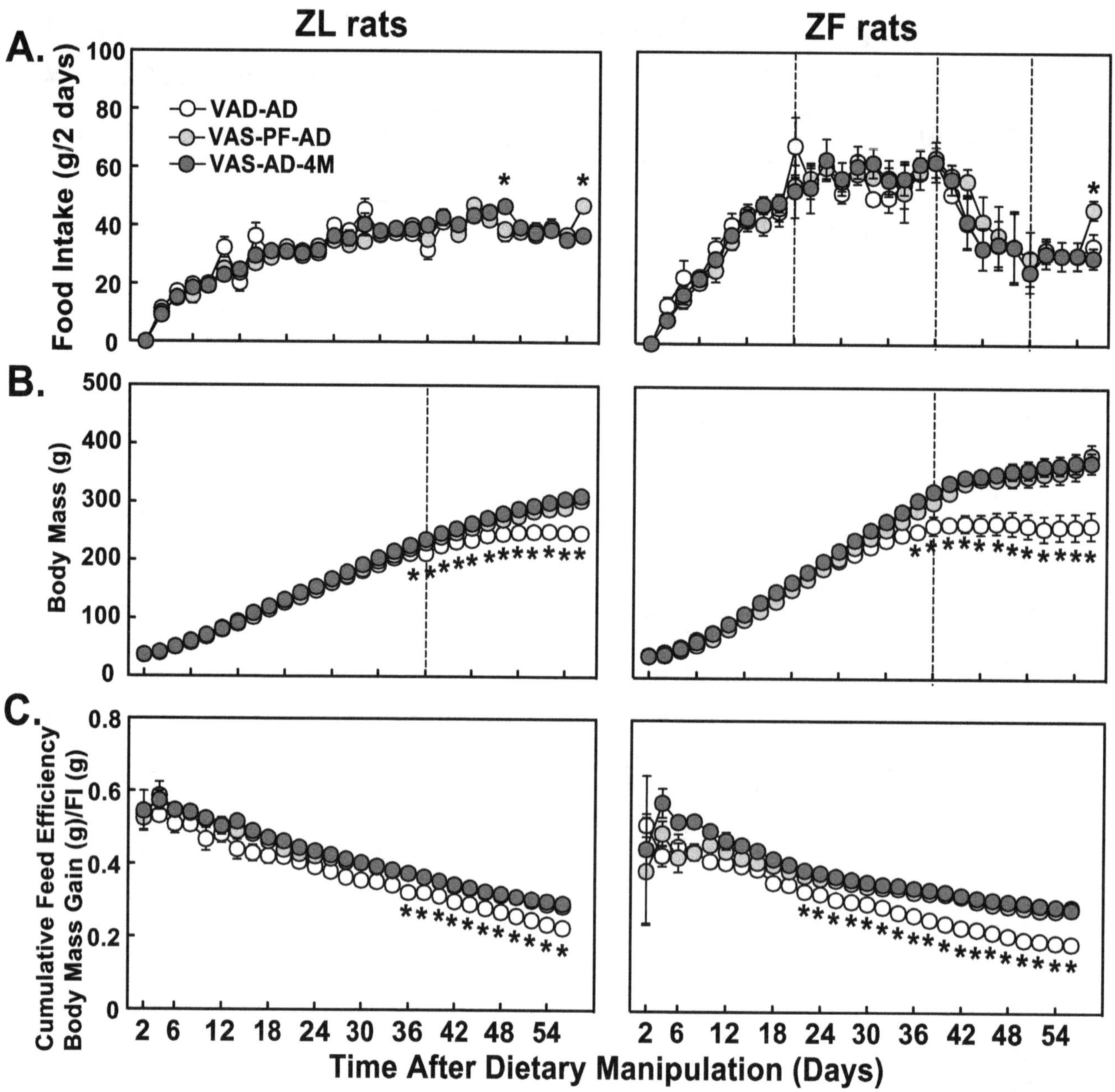

Figure 4. The food intake, body mass and cumulative feed efficiency over 56 days of dietary manipulation. (A) Two-day food intake of ZL and ZF on VAD ad libitum (VAD-AD, n = 5), VAS-Pair-feeding Last Day ad libitum (VAS-PF-AD, n = 5), VAS-Pair-feeding Last Day 4 meals (VAS-PF-4M, n = 5) (B) Body mass of ZL and ZF on VAD AD, VAS-PF AD and VAS-PF 4M. (C) Cumulative feed efficiency (unit weight gain per unit diet consumed) of ZL and ZF on VAD-AD, VAS-PF-AD and VAS-PF-4M. * Indicates $p<0.05$ using one-way ANOVA with LSD post-hoc test.

those in VAD-AD ZF hepatocytes at every concentration (marked by *).

The insulin-induced *Srebp-1c* expression was impaired by transient overeating in hepatocytes of VAS-PF-AD ZL and ZF rats

In VAD-AD and VAS-PF-4M ZL hepatocytes, insulin at 0.1 to 100 nM induced the *Srebp-1c* expression with or without RA (Figure 7A). The fold inductions of *Srebp-1c* by insulin (1 to 100 nM) and insulin + RA (10 to 100 nM) in VAS-PF-AD ZL hepatocytes were significantly lower than that in VAD-AD (marked by *) and VAS-PF-4M (marked by $) ZL hepatocytes at the corresponding treatments.

In VAD-AD and VAS-PF-4M ZF hepatocytes, insulin at 1 to 100 nM induced the *Srebp-1c* expression with or without RA (Figure 7B). In contrast, the insulin-mediated inductions of *Srebp-1c* expression were abolished in VAS-PF-AD ZF hepatocytes regardless of RA. As a result, the fold inductions in VAS-PF-AD ZF hepatocytes were significantly lower than that in VAD-AD (marked by *) and VAS-PF-4M ZF (marked by $) hepatocytes. These data demonstrate that the transient overeating of VAS-PF-AD rats impairs the insulin-induced *Srebp-1c* expression in their hepatocytes.

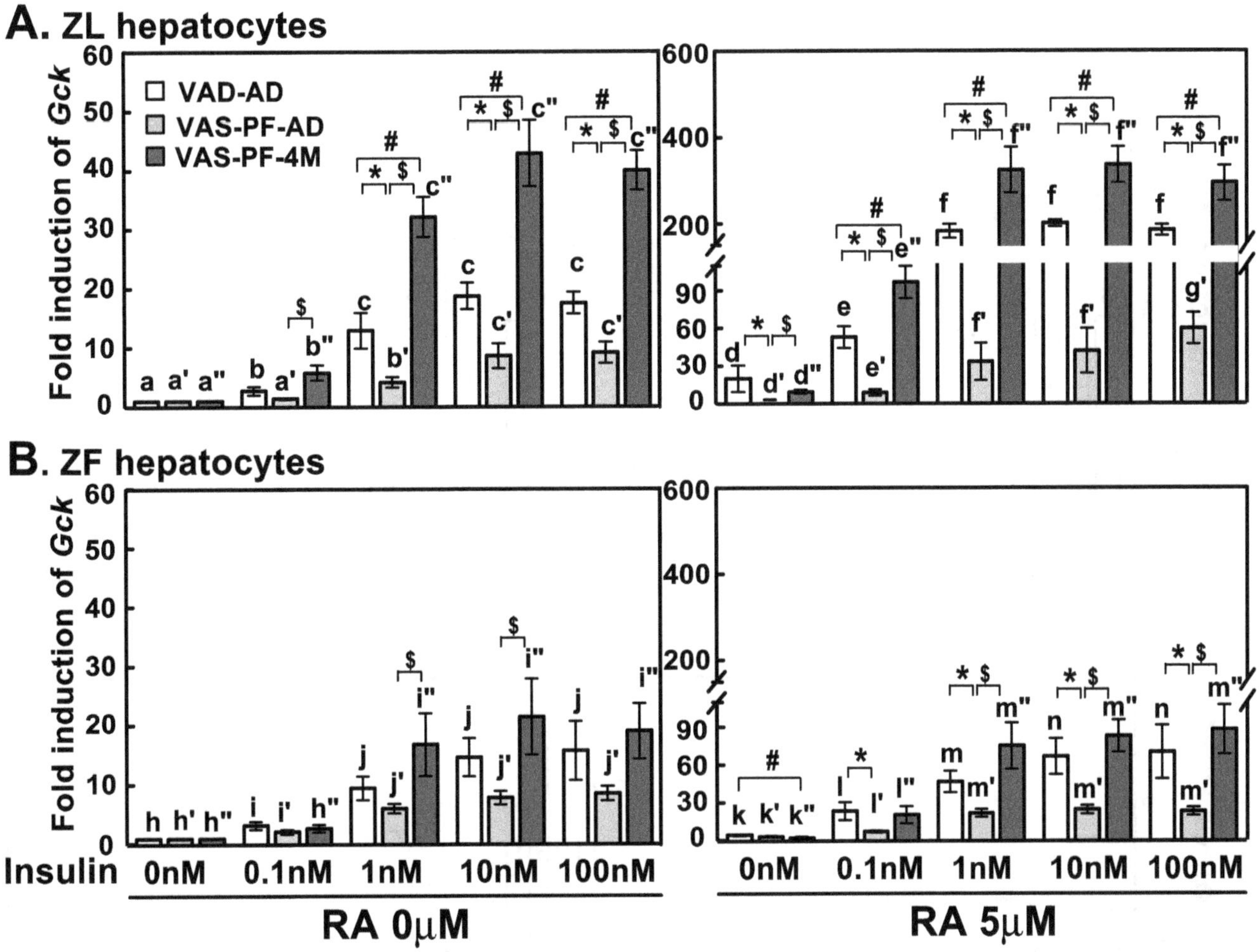

Figure 5. Insulin-induced *Gck* expression was attenuated in hepatocytes from VAS-PF-AD, but not VAS-PF-4M rats. The primary hepatocytes were treated by insulin (0 nM to 100 nM) with or without RA (5 μM) in medium A for 6 hours. The expression level of *Gck* was determined by real-time PCR analysis, and the data were expressed as fold induction. The gene transcript levels from the no treatment group (0 nM insulin, no RA) for both ZL and ZF were arbitrarily set to 1. All p<0.05; for (A), a<b<c, a′<b′<c′, a″<b″<c″, d<e<f, d′<f′/g′, e′<g′, d″<e″<f″; for (B), h<i<j, h′<i′, h″<i″<j″, k<l<m, j′<k′<l′, k″<i″<m″, using one way ANOVA. *, #, and $ for comparing the effects of dietary manipulations at any treatment using one way ANOVA.

Dietary manipulation and VA status regulated the expression levels of genes for VA metabolism in hepatocytes from ZL and ZF rats

To understand the impact of transient overeating on the hepatic VA metabolism, we analyzed the expression levels of key enzymes for VA metabolism and RA responses in all three groups of ZL and ZF hepatocytes. As shown in Figure 8A, the expression level of RBP4 receptor 2 (*Rbpr2*), a proposed liver-specific retinol transporter [17], was higher in VAD-AD hepatocytes than that in VAS-PF-AD and VAS-PF-4M hepatocytes (both ZL and ZF). RDH2 catalyzes the reversible conversion between retinol and retinal [18]. In Figure 8A, the expression level of *Rdh2* in VAD-AD ZL or ZF hepatocytes was higher than that in VAS-PF-4M ZL or ZF hepatocytes, respectively. The expression level of *Rdh2* in VAS-PF-AD ZL hepatocytes was higher than that in VAS-PF-4M, but lower than that in VAD-AD ZL hepatocytes.

Both RALDH1 (also known as ALDH1A1) and RALDH4 are involved in the irreversible conversion of retinal into RA [18]. The *Raldh1* (*Aldh1a1*) expression level in VAS-PF-AD ZL or ZF hepatocytes was significantly lower than that in VAD-AD and VAS-PF-4M ZL or ZF hepatocytes, respectively (Figure 8C). The *Raldh4* expression level in VAD-AD ZL hepatocytes was higher than that in VAS-PF-AD and VAS-PF-4M groups (Figure 8D), suggesting the alteration of VA metabolism in the liver. However, the *Raldh4* expression levels in all groups of ZF hepatocytes were similar.

Additionally, the expression level of *Cyp26a1* (Figure 8E), a RA catabolic gene [16,19], in VAD-AD ZL hepatocytes was significantly lower than that in VAS-PF-AD, but higher than that in VAS-PF-4M ZL hepatocytes. The *Cyp26a1* expression level in VAD-AD ZF hepatocyte was lower than that in VAS-PF-AD and VAS-PF-4M ZF groups. The *Rarb* expression levels were not different among VAD-AD, VAS-PF-AD, and VAS-PF-4M groups (Figure 8F).

Two-way ANOVA analysis showed that dietary manipulations accounted for the majority of overall variance observed in the expression levels of *Rbpr2* ($F = 23.04$, 61% variance explained), *Rdh2* ($F = 13.14$, 47%), *Raldh1* ($F = 23.27$, 61%), and *Raldh4* ($F = 3.56$, 22%). This suggests that dietary manipulation can potentially change the availability of RA in primary hepatocytes by changing the expression levels of VA metabolic genes. Aside

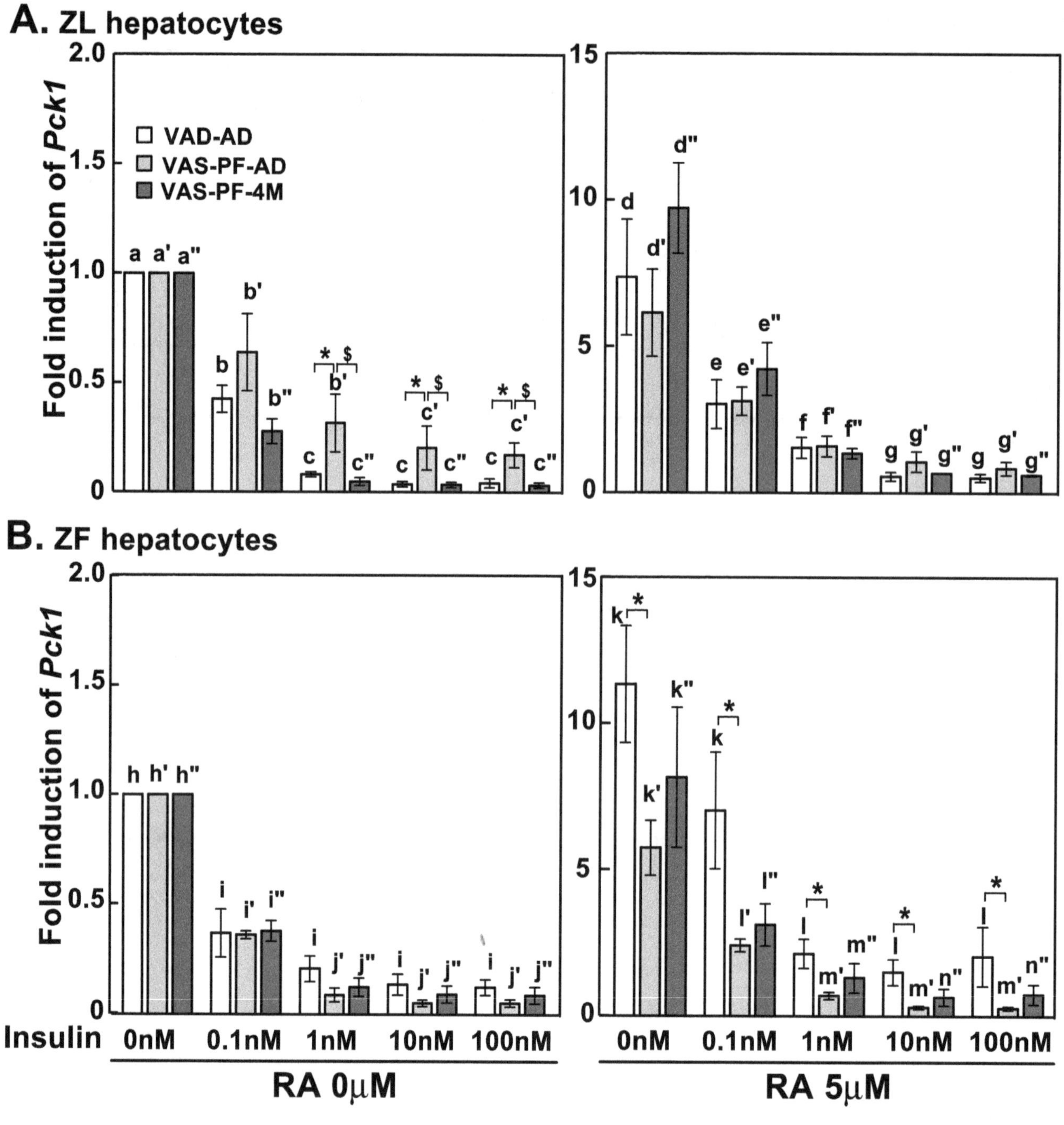

Figure 6. Transient overfeeding of the VAS diet impaired the insulin-suppressed *Pck1* expression in hepatocytes of VAS-PF-AD ZL rats. The primary hepatocytes were treated by insulin (0 nM to 100 nM) with or without RA (5 μM) in medium A for 6 hours. The expression level of *Pck1* was determined by real-time PCR analysis, and the data were expressed as fold induction. The gene transcript levels from the no treatment group (0 nM insulin, no RA) for both ZL and ZF were arbitrarily set to 1. All $p<0.05$; for (A), a>b>c, a′>c′, a″>b″>c″, d>e>g, d>f, d′>f′/g′, e′>g′, d″>e″>f″>g″; for (B), h>i, h′>i′>j′, h″>i″>j″, k>l, k′>l′>m′, k″>l″, using one way ANOVA. *, #, and $ for comparing the effects of dietary manipulations at any treatment using one way ANOVA.

from the genes described above, we also checked *Stra6*, *Rdh10*, *Raldh2* and *Raldh3*, whose transcript levels in primary hepatocytes were too low to be determined by real-time PCR analysis.

Discussion

Elucidating the molecular mechanisms resulting in hepatic insulin resistance is of great importance. It helps understand the development and progression of metabolic diseases. We investigated the effects of food intake and VA status on the insulin-regulated gene expression in primary hepatocytes of ZL and ZF rats. ZF rats, which bear a loss-of-function leptin receptor gene, develop obesity, dyslipidemia and insulin resistance due to hyperphagia [20]. We found that the insulin-regulated *Gck*, *Pck1* and *Srebp-1c* expressions were impaired in the primary hepatocytes of ZF rats fed chow diet ad libitum (Figure 1),

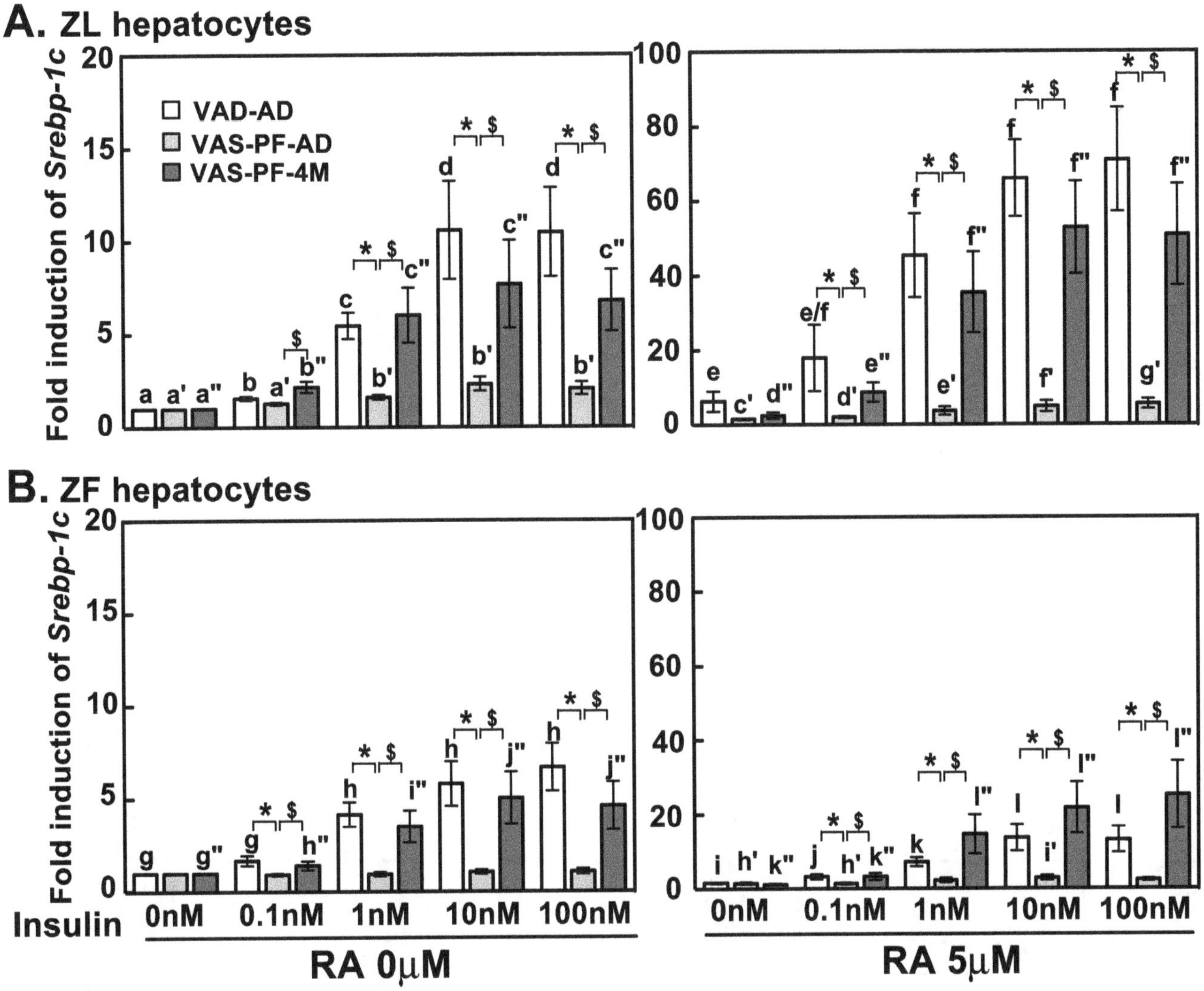

Figure 7. Transient overfeeding of VAS diet impaired insulin-induced *Srebp-1c* expression in hepatocytes of VAS-PF-AD rats. The primary hepatocytes were treated by insulin (0 nM to 100 nM) with or without RA (5 μM) in medium A for 6 hours. The expression level of *Srebp-1c* was determined by real-time PCR analysis, and the data were expressed as fold induction. The gene transcript levels from the no treatment group (0 nM insulin, no RA) for both ZL and ZF were arbitrarily set to 1. All $p<0.05$; for (A), $a<b<c<d$, $a'<b'$, $a''<b''<c''$, $e<f$, $c'<g'/f'$, $d'<f'$, $d''<e''<f''$; for (B), $g<h$, $g''<i''/j''$, $h''<j''$, $i<k/l$, $j<l$, $h'<l'$, $k''<l''$, using one way ANOVA. *, #, and $ for comparing the effects of dietary manipulations at any treatment using one way ANOVA.

confirming our previous observation [9]. VA deficiency partially corrected the impairment (Figure 2). We have reported that retinoids affect the expression levels of several insulin-regulated genes in primary hepatocytes previously. These observations are somewhat anticipated and in line with our hypothesis that both hyperinsulinemia and RA overproduction may take part in the regulation of the expression of genes for glucose and lipid metabolism, and contribute to hepatic insulin resistance at the gene expression level [1].

Compared to ZL rats, ZF rats are hyperinsulinemic [21]. Previous research showed that the insulin binding capacity of the isolated liver plasma membrane of ZF rats was not different from that of ZL rats [22]. In addition, the insulin-induced phosphorylation of AKT at Ser473 and Thr308 were similar in the primary hepatocytes of ZL and ZF rats [9]. These data indicate that the impairment of insulin-regulated gene expression in ZF hepatocytes is likely to be caused by alterations downstream of AKT activation in the insulin signaling cascade. Indeed, VA and insulin operate through separated pathways to regulate hepatic gene expression. RA, as a metabolite of VA catabolism, moves to the nucleus and activates the nuclear receptors (e.g. retinoic acid receptor, retinoid X receptor, peroxisome proliferator-activated receptor β/δ, hepatocyte nuclear factor 4α, and chicken ovalbumin up-stream transcription factor II) that are located in the promoters of the target genes [1]. How these two pathways interact with each other in normal or disease states deserves further investigation.

We also found that the degree of the impairment of *Srebp-1c* expression was more profound than that of *Gck* and *Pck1* in ZF hepatocytes (Figure 1). It suggests that branching points may exist in the downstream of insulin signaling pathway, below which the expressions of *Gck*, *Pck1* and *Srebp-1c* are differentially regulated by nutritional and hormonal stimuli. This is in accordance with other studies. For example, a bifurcation point at mTORC1 in the insulin signaling pathway separated the insulin-induced *Srebp-1c* expression and the insulin-suppressed *Pck1* expression [23]. The knockout of SREBP cleaving-activating protein gene in *ob/ob* mice

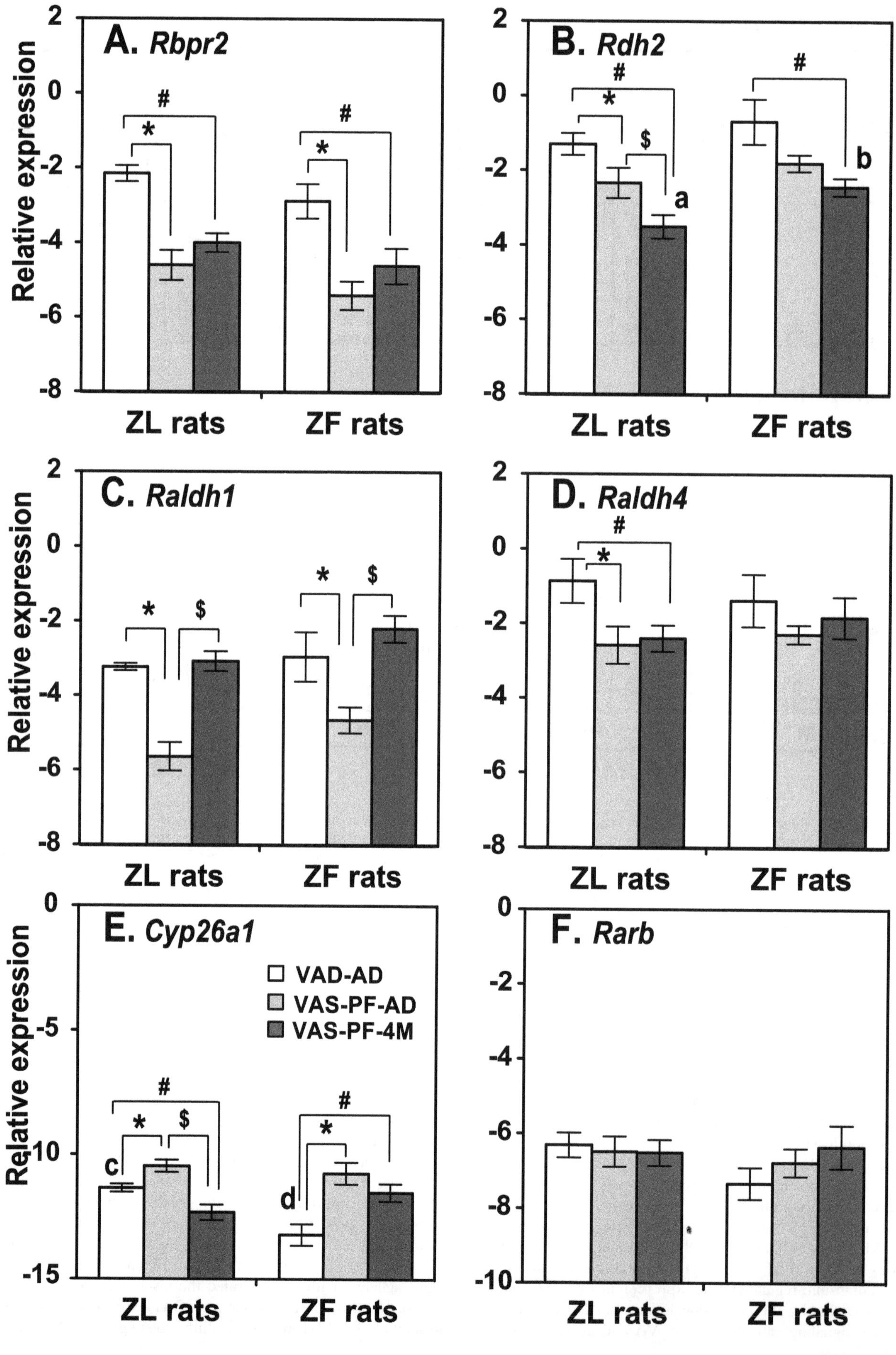
A. Rbpr2
B. Rdh2
C. Raldh1
D. Raldh4
E. Cyp26a1
F. Rarb
Relative expression
ZL rats
ZF rats
VAD-AD
VAS-PF-AD
VAS-PF-4M
#
*
$
a
b
c
d

Figure 8. Differential expression levels of vitamin A metabolic genes in ZL and ZF primary hepatocytes. The expression levels of *Rbpr2* (A), *Rdh2* (B), *Raldh1* (C), *Raldh4* (D), *Cyp26a1* (E), and *Rarb* (F) were determined by real-time PCR in the cultured primary hepatocytes receiving no treatment. The data were expressed as $-\Delta$Ct (36B4 - gene of interest). All $p<0.05$; *, #, and $ for comparing the effects of dietary manipulation variables on gene transcript levels using two-way ANOVA with Bonferroni's post-hoc test; a>b, and c>d, using Student's t-test to compare ZL with ZF with the corresponding dietary manipulation.

resulted in the amelioration of hepatic lipogenesis without the improvement of hepatic gluconeogenesis [24]. Additionally in primary rat hepatocytes treated with insulin, the *Gck* expression reached the peak level 6 hours earlier than did the *Srebp-1c* expression [10]. Further studies are needed to dissect these branching points and discover any change of regulation in insulin resistance.

The negative effects of short-term overfeeding on the hepatic insulin sensitivity have been observed in both rodents and humans with unrevealed mechanisms. The pair-feeding study indicates that the transient overeating of the VAS diet caused the impairment of insulin-regulated *Gck*, *Pck1* and *Srebp-1c* expressions in the primary hepatocytes of ZL rats (Figure 5, 6, 7). In contrast, VAS-PF-4M ZL rats showed normal insulin-regulated gene expression. This suggests that, in the liver of so called insulin-sensitive ZL rats, insulin sensitivity at gene expression level can be acutely impaired after excessive food intake, and then restored overtime. Indeed, in young human subjects, a 7-day overfeeding increased circulating adiponectin and glucagon-like peptide 1 levels, which are proposed to act against the hepatic insulin resistance [25,26]. On the other hand, transient overeating of the VAS diet caused worsened impairment of insulin-regulated *Gck* and *Srebp-1c* expressions in the primary hepatocytes of ZF rats (Figure 5, 7). ZF rats persist in overeating state due to deficient leptin signaling. This may hamper the restoration of insulin sensitivity after food intake. As a result, ZF rats fed VAS or chow ad libitum manifest the hepatic insulin resistance at the gene expression level.

Long term VA deficiency decreased the insulin-regulated expression of *Gck*, but not that of *Pck1* and *Srebp-1c*. In VAS-PF-AD ZL rats, the insulin-induced *Gck* expression was significantly lower than that in VAS-PF-4M ZL rats (Figure 5), showing that adequate VA status is instrumental to the insulin-regulated *Gck* expression in insulin-sensitive ZL primary hepatocytes. This observation demonstrates that VA status differentially affects the hepatic insulin-regulated gene expression, suggesting complex interactions of VA and insulin signaling systems.

The impairment of insulin-induced *Gck* (Figure 5) and insulin-suppressed *Pck1* expressions (Figure 6) in VAS-PF-AD hepatocytes suggests an elevation of plasma glucose level and an acute loss of insulin-sensitivity in over-feeding state. This is supported by the elevated tail tip whole blood glucose level observed in these animals (Figure 3E), and may explain the elevated hepatic glucose production in human subjects who are overfed for short terms [27,28]. The dysregulation of insulin-induced hepatic *Srebp-1c* expression after the transient overeating (Figure 7) suggests increased *de novo* lipogenesis, which may explain the increased hepatic fat content observed in short-term overfed humans [29]. More importantly, the impairment was observed in both ZL and ZF rats after transient overeating. These data suggest the existence of a mechanism that may dynamically regulate hepatic insulin sensitivity at the gene expression level in response to feeding status.

Short-term overeating provides excessive intake of not only calories but also micronutrients. We showed transient overeating for one day greatly affected the expression levels of genes involved in VA metabolism in primary hepatocytes of ZL and ZF rats (Figure 8). VAD-AD rats exhibited high hepatic levels of *Rbpr2*, *Rdh2*, *Raldh1 (Aldh1a1)* and *Raldh4* transcripts, showing compensatory upregulation of the VA metabolic genes. In contrast, VAS-PF-4M rats exhibited low hepatic transcript levels of *Rbpr2*, *Rdh2* and *Raldh4*. These suggest that the hepatic VA metabolic gene expression is greatly influenced by the availability of dietary VA.

VAS-PF-AD rats had lowered hepatic levels of *Rbpr2* and *Raldh1 (Aldh1a1)* transcripts. Indeed, the *Rbpr2* expression is inversely related to the liver retinol stores, and RA reduces the *Rbpr2* mRNA level in HepG2 cells [17]. Additionally, the elevated RA controls its biosynthesis by down-regulating RALDH1 (ALDH1A1) through the modulation of retinoic acid receptor α and CCAAT/enhancer binding protein β [30,31]. These suggest that the expression levels of VA metabolic genes are modulated in VAS-PF-AD rats to prevent the RA overproduction in response to the transient influx of the dietary VA. Despite the negative feedback regulation, excessive RA may have been produced. This is supported by the increased expression level of *Cyp26a1* [19], a RA-responsive gene, in VAS-PF-AD hepatocytes (Figure 8E). The excessive RA may affect the expression of hepatic metabolic genes, and promote the hepatic insulin resistance at the gene expression level [1]. It is interesting to note that the VA status does not seem to affect the expression levels of *Raldh1* (*Aldh1a1*) gene in primary hepatocytes as its expression levels are similar in VAD-AD and VAS-PF-4M groups. The underlying mechanism deserves further investigation.

In summary, we have demonstrated that both VA and feeding statuses affected the hepatic insulin sensitivity at the gene expression level. This finding provides insight into the development of the hepatic insulin resistance, and helps find solutions to combat metabolic diseases.

Author Contributions

Conceived and designed the experiments: WC GC. Performed the experiments: WC MLH YL RL. Analyzed the data: WC GC. Contributed reagents/materials/analysis tools: GC. Wrote the paper: WC GC.

References

1. Chen G (2013) Roles of Vitamin A Metabolism in the Development of Hepatic Insulin Resistance. ISRN Hepatology 2013: 1–21. doi:10.1016/j.cmet.2011.12.017.
2. Brown MS, Goldstein JL (2008) Selective versus total insulin resistance: a pathogenic paradox. Cell Metab 7: 95–96. doi:10.1016/j.cmet.2007.12.009.
3. Angulo P (2002) Nonalcoholic fatty liver disease. N Engl J Med 346: 1221–1231. doi:10.1056/NEJMra011775.
4. Johnson AMF, Olefsky JM (2013) The Origins and Drivers of Insulin Resistance. Cell 152: 673–684. doi:10.1016/j.cell.2013.01.041.
5. O'Brien RM, Granner DK (1996) Regulation of gene expression by insulin. Physiol Rev 76: 1109–1161.
6. Iynedjian PB (2009) Molecular physiology of mammalian glucokinase. Cell Mol Life Sci 66: 27–42. doi:10.1007/s00018-008-8322-9.

7. Brown MS, Goldstein JL (1997) The SREBP pathway: regulation of cholesterol metabolism by proteolysis of a membrane-bound transcription factor. Cell 89: 331–340.
8. Lefebvre P, Martin PJ, Flajollet S, Dedieu S, Billaut X, et al. (2005) Transcriptional activities of retinoic acid receptors. Vitam Horm 70: 199–264. doi:10.1016/S0083-6729(05)70007-8.
9. Zhang Y, Chen W, Li R, Li Y, Ge Y, et al. (2011) Insulin-regulated Srebp-1c and Pck1 mRNA expression in primary hepatocytes from zucker fatty but not lean rats is affected by feeding conditions. PLoS ONE 6: e21342. doi:10.1371/journal.pone.0021342.
10. Chen G, Zhang Y, Lu D, Li N-Q, Ross AC (2009) Retinoids synergize with insulin to induce hepatic Gck expression. Biochem J 419: 645–653. doi:10.1042/BJ20082368.
11. Li R, Chen W, Li Y, Zhang Y, Chen G (2011) Retinoids synergized with insulin to induce Srebp-1c expression and activated its promoter via the two liver X receptor binding sites that mediate insulin action. Biochem Biophys Res Commun 406: 268–272. doi:10.1016/j.bbrc.2011.02.031.
12. Zhang Y, Li R, Chen W, Li Y, Chen G (2011) Retinoids induced Pck1 expression and attenuated insulin-mediated suppression of its expression via activation of retinoic acid receptor in primary rat hepatocytes. Mol Cell Biochem 355: 1–8. doi:10.1007/s11010-011-0831-4.
13. Zhang Y, Li R, Li Y, Chen W, Zhao S, et al. (2012) Vitamin A status affects obesity development and hepatic expression of key genes for fuel metabolism in Zucker fatty rats. Biochem Cell Biol 90: 548–557. doi:10.1139/o2012-012.
14. Mayer J, Krehl WA (1948) Influence of vitamin A deficiency on the gross efficiency of growth of rats. Yale J Biol Med 20: 403–405.
15. Anzano MA, Lamb AJ, Olson JA (1979) Growth, appetite, sequence of pathological signs and survival following the induction of rapid, synchronous vitamin A deficiency in the rat. J Nutr 109: 1419–1431.
16. Li Y, Zhang Y, Li R, Chen W, Howell M, et al. (2012) The hepatic Raldh1 expression is elevated in Zucker fatty rats and its over-expression introduced the retinal-induced Srebp-1c expression in INS-1 cells. PLoS ONE 7: e45210. doi:10.1371/journal.pone.0045210.
17. Alapatt P, Guo F, Komanetsky SM, Wang S, Cai J, et al. (2013) Liver retinol transporter and receptor for serum retinol-binding protein (RBP4). Journal of Biological Chemistry 288: 1250–1265. doi:10.1074/jbc.M112.369132.
18. Napoli JL (2012) Physiological insights into all-trans-retinoic acid biosynthesis. Biochim Biophys Acta 1821: 152–167. doi:10.1016/j.bbalip.2011.05.004.
19. Wang Y, Zolfaghari R, Ross AC (2002) Cloning of rat cytochrome P450RAI (CYP26) cDNA and regulation of its gene expression by all-trans-retinoic acid in vivo. Arch Biochem Biophys 401: 235–243. doi:10.1016/S0003-9861(02)00043-7.
20. Phillips MS, Liu Q, Hammond HA, Dugan V, Hey PJ, et al. (1996) Leptin receptor missense mutation in the fatty Zucker rat. Nature Genetics 13: 18–19. doi:doi:10.1038/ng0596-18.
21. Zucker LM, Antoniades HN (1972) Insulin and obesity in the Zucker genetically obese rat "fatty". Endocrinology 90: 1320–1330.
22. Clark JB, Keen S, Clark CM (1982) Studies on the regulation of insulin binding by liver plasma membranes from Zucker fatty rats. Diabetes 31: 867–873.
23. Li S, Brown MS, Goldstein JL (2010) Bifurcation of insulin signaling pathway in rat liver: mTORC1 required for stimulation of lipogenesis, but not inhibition of gluconeogenesis. Proceedings of the National Academy of Sciences 107: 3441–3446. doi:10.1073/pnas.0914798107.
24. Moon Y-A, Liang G, Xie X, Frank-Kamenetsky M, Fitzgerald K, et al. (2012) The Scap/SREBP pathway is essential for developing diabetic fatty liver and carbohydrate-induced hypertriglyceridemia in animals. Cell Metab 15: 240–246. doi:10.1016/j.cmet.2011.12.017.
25. Cahill F, Amini P, Wadden D, Khalili S, Randell E, et al. (2013) Short-term overfeeding increases circulating adiponectin independent of obesity status. PLoS ONE 8: e74215. doi:10.1371/journal.pone.0074215.
26. Wadden D, Cahill F, Amini P, Randell E, Vasdev S, et al. (2013) Circulating glucagon-like peptide-1 increases in response to short-term overfeeding in men. Nutr Metab (Lond) 10: 33. doi:10.1186/1743-7075-10-33.
27. Heilbronn LK, Coster ACF, Campbell LV, Greenfield JR, Lange K, et al. (2013) The effect of short-term overfeeding on serum lipids in healthy humans. Obesity (Silver Spring). doi:10.1002/oby.20508.
28. Magkos F, Smith GI, Reeds DN, Okunade A, Patterson BW, et al. (2013) One day of overfeeding impairs nocturnal glucose but not fatty acid homeostasis in overweight men. Obesity (Silver Spring). doi:10.1002/oby.20562.
29. Lecoultre V, Egli L, Carrel G, Theytaz F, Kreis R, et al. (2013) Effects of fructose and glucose overfeeding on hepatic insulin sensitivity and intrahepatic lipids in healthy humans. Obesity (Silver Spring) 21: 782–785. doi:10.1002/oby.20377.
30. Elizondo G, Corchero J, Sterneck E, Gonzalez FJ (2000) Feedback inhibition of the retinaldehyde dehydrogenase gene ALDH1 by retinoic acid through retinoic acid receptor alpha and CCAAT/enhancer-binding protein beta. J Biol Chem 275: 39747–39753. doi:10.1074/jbc.M004987200.
31. Elizondo G, Medina-Díaz IM, Cruz R, Gonzalez FJ, Vega L (2009) Retinoic acid modulates retinaldehyde dehydrogenase 1 gene expression through the induction of GADD153-C/EBPbeta interaction. Biochem Pharmacol 77: 248–257. doi:10.1016/j.bcp.2008.10.011.

Markers of Tissue-Specific Insulin Resistance Predict the Worsening of Hyperglycemia, Incident Type 2 Diabetes and Cardiovascular Disease

Mária Fízel'ová[1], Henna Cederberg[2], Alena Stančáková[1], Raimo Jauhiainen[2], Jagadish Vangipurapu[1], Johanna Kuusisto[2], Markku Laakso[2]*

1 Department of Medicine, University of Eastern Finland, Kuopio, Finland, **2** Department of Medicine, University of Eastern Finland and Kuopio University Hospital, Kuopio, Finland

Abstract

We investigated the ability of surrogate markers of tissue-specific insulin resistance (IR, Matsuda IR, Adipocyte IR, Liver IR) to predict deterioration of hyperglycemia, incident type 2 diabetes and cardiovascular events in the Metabolic Syndrome in Men (METSIM) Study. The METSIM Study includes 10,197 Finnish men, aged 45–73 years, and examined in 2005–2010. A total of 558 of 8,749 non-diabetic participants at baseline were diagnosed with new-onset diabetes and 239 with a new CVD event during a 5.9-year follow-up of this cohort (2010–2013). Compared to fasting plasma insulin level, Matsuda IR (IR in skeletal muscle) and Adipocyte IR were significantly better predictors of 2-hour plasma glucose and glucose area under the curve after adjustment for confounding factors. Liver IR was the strongest predictor of both incident type 2 diabetes (hazard ratio = 1.83, 95% confidence interval: 1.68–1.98) and cardiovascular events (hazard ratio = 1.31, 95% confidence interval: 1.15–1.48). Hazard ratios for fasting insulin were 1.37 (95% confidence interval: 1.32–1.42) and 1.11 (95% confidence interval: 1.00–1.24), respectively. Tissue-specific markers of IR, Matsuda IR and Adipocyte IR, were superior to fasting plasma insulin level in predicting worsening of hyperglycemia, and Liver IR was superior to fasting insulin level in predicting incident type 2 diabetes and cardiovascular events.

Editor: Chiara Lazzeri, Azienda Ospedaliero-Universitaria Careggi, Italy

Funding: This work has been supported by the grants from the Academy of Finland, the Finnish Diabetes Research Foundation, the Finnish Cardiovascular Research Foundation, the Strategic Research Funding from the University of eastern Finland, Kuopio, Finland, and EVO Grant 5263 from the Kuopio University Hospital to M.L. The funding bodies named above had no role in the design and conduct of the study; collection management, analysis, and interpretation of the data; and preparation, review, or approval of the manuscript.

Competing Interests: The authors have declared that no competing interests exist.

* Email: markku.laakso@kuh.fi

Introduction

Insulin resistance (IR) and impaired insulin secretion are two major pathophysiological defects in type 2 diabetes [1]. Insulin resistance, typically present for several years before the manifestation of type 2 diabetes [2], is an important predictor for the development of type 2 diabetes and contributes to an elevated risk of cardiovascular disease (CVD) events [3–6]. Insulin secretion defect has been recognized as a key determinant for the progression to type 2 diabetes [7–10].

Euglycemia is maintained by a complex interaction between many tissues. In the fasting state the majority of glucose utilization takes place in the brain (~50%), splanchnic organs (~25%), and in skeletal muscle (~25%) [11]. Postprandial increase in circulating insulin promotes the uptake of glucose into insulin-sensitive tissues. Glucose is stored principally in the form of glycogen mostly in the muscle (accounting for ~60% of whole body uptake), liver (~30%) and adipose tissue (~10%) [11,12]. Hepatic IR is characterized by enhanced gluconeogenesis in the fasting state and an impaired suppression of hepatic glucose production in response to insulin in the postprandial state [13]. Insulin resistance in skeletal muscle leads to postprandial hyperglycemia [14]. Adipose tissue IR results in elevated levels of plasma free fatty acids levels [15] and overproduction of proinflammatory cytokines (interleukin, tumor necrosis factor-α, C-reactive protein) which impair insulin sensitivity. Moreover, decreased insulin-mediated glucose uptake in different tissues leads to increased plasma insulin levels to maintain normoglycemia. Elevated fasting insulin concentrations reflect IR [16] and are associated with increased risk of CVD events [5,17,18].

Insulin sensitivity can be estimated with the hyperinsulinemic euglycemic glucose clamp [19], intravenous glucose tolerance test [20] or with indices calculated on the basis of insulin and glucose levels in the fasting state or after a glucose load [19,21,22]. Many of these surrogate markers have been validated against the hyperinsulinemic euglycemic glucose clamp [23–25]. While several tissue-specific IR indices have been developed [14,26] it remains unknown whether they differentially predict the deterioration of hyperglycemia, progression to overt type 2 diabetes or incident CVD events, and whether they are better predictors of type 2 diabetes and CVD events than fasting insulin level. To address these questions, we investigated the ability of three validated tissue-specific IR indices to predict the deterioration of hyperglycemia, incident type 2 diabetes and CVD events in participants of the Metabolic Syndrome in Men (METSIM) Study, and compared their predictive power with that of fasting plasma insulin level.

Materials and Methods

Subjects and clinical measurement at the baseline study

The Metabolic Syndrome in Men (METSIM) Study was performed in 2005–2010 at the Clinical Research Unit at the University of Kuopio. It included 10,197 men, aged from 45 to 73 years, randomly selected from the population register of Kuopio, Eastern Finland (population 95,000). Each participant attended a 1-day outpatient visit to the Clinical Research Unit at the University of Kuopio, as described in detail previously [23]. An oral glucose tolerance test (OGTT, 75 g of glucose, glucose and insulin measurements at 0, 30 and 120 min) was performed, and glucose tolerance was classified according to the American Diabetes Association criteria [27]. Subjects with previously diagnosed type 1 diabetes ($n = 25$) or type 2 diabetes ($n = 763$) were excluded, and none of the participants included in statistical analyses were on anti-diabetic medication. A total of 9,398 men without diabetes or with newly diagnosed diabetes were included in the current analyses (age 57±7 years, body mass index (BMI) 27.0±4.0 kg m^{-2}, mean±SD).

Subjects and clinical measurement at the follow-up study

A follow-up started in 2010, and so far 5,419 individuals have participated. The study protocol and measurements are identical to those of the baseline study.

Diagnosis of incident type 2 diabetes and CVD events

Out of 8,749 non-diabetic participants at baseline, 558 participants developed incident type 2 diabetes and 239 participants had a CVD event between the date of the baseline METSIM Study and 31 December 2013 (5.9-year follow-up). Diagnosis of new-onset type 2 diabetes was based either on an OGTT or HbA1c≥6.5% (297 cases of new diabetes) among 4,806 non-diabetic individuals who participated in the ongoing follow-up study to date in 2010–2013, or anti-diabetic medication started between the baseline and 31 December 2013 ($n = 261$ cases of new diabetes; information obtained from the National Drug Reimbursement registry for all 8,749 non-diabetic participants). The incident CVD event was defined as myocardial infarction, coronary heart disease death, or fatal and non-fatal cerebral infarction which occurred between the baseline study and 31 December 2013. CVD events were defined according to internationally accepted criteria [28,29] and verified from the hospital records. Individuals with non-fatal myocardial infarction and stroke before the baseline were excluded from statistical analyses.

Ethics Statement. The study was approved by the Ethics Committee of the University of Eastern Finland and Kuopio University Hospital and was conducted in accordance with the Helsinki Declaration. All study participants gave written informed consent.

Measurements

Height and weight were measured to the nearest 0.5 cm and 0.1 kg, respectively. Body mass index (BMI) was calculated as weight (kg) divided by height (m) squared. Waist circumference was measured at the midpoint between the lateral iliac crest and lowest rib. Body composition was determined by bioelectrical impedance (Bioimpedance Analyzer Madel BIA 101, Akern SrL, Florence, Italy) in subjects in the supine position after a 12-h overnight fast. Smoking status was defined as current smoking (yes vs. no). Family history of diabetes (yes vs. no) was defined as the first or second-degree relative having diabetes vs. no family history of diabetes. Physical activity (physically active vs. inactive) refers to leisure time exercise (physically active, regular exercise at least 30 min 1–2 times per week vs. physically inactive, occasional exercise or no exercise). Alcohol intake was defined as total alcohol intake in grams per week. Diagnosis of hypertension was based on the use of antihypertensive medication (information obtained from the National Drug Reimbursement registry).

Laboratory measurement

Plasma glucose was measured by enzymatic hexokinase photometric assay (Konelab Systems reagents, Thermo Fisher Scientific; Vantaa, Finland). HbA1c was analyzed with a Tosoh G7 glycohemoglobin analyser (Tosoh Bioscience, Inc. San Francisco, CA, USA). Plasma insulin concentrations were measured by a luminometric immunoassay measurement (ADVIA Centaur Insulin IRI, no 02230141, Siemens Medical Solutions Diagnostics, Tarrytown, NY, USA). LDL cholesterol (LDL-C) was measured by enzymatic colorimetric test (Konelab Systems reagents, Thermo Fisher Scientific; Vantaa, Finland).

Calculations

The trapezoidal method was used to calculate glucose area under the curve (Glucose AUC) from the OGTT using samples collected at 0, 30 and 120 min. Insulin resistance was measured by surrogate indices of tissue-specific IR. Calculation of Matsuda ISI as a measure of whole body insulin sensitivity, representing mainly skeletal muscle insulin sensitivity, has been previously described [30]. For consistency with the other indices expressed as IR, Matsuda IR (calculated as 10/Matsuda ISI) was used in all statistical analyses. The Adipocyte IR index (Adipocyte IR), was defined as the product of fasting free fatty acid levels and fasting plasma insulin [24]. We used our previously validated Liver IR index [26] as a marker of hepatic IR. Insulin secretion index ($InsAUC_{0-30}/GlucAUC_{0-30}$) was calculated as reported previously [2]. The disposition index (DI) (a measure of pancreatic β-cell function) was calculated as Matsuda ISI×$InsAUC_{0-30}/GlucAUC_{0-30}$.

Statistical analysis

Statistical analyses were conducted using IBM SPSS Statistics version 19. All traits except for age were log-transformed to correct for their skewed distribution. IR indices and fasting plasma insulin levels were compared across the fasting plasma glucose (FPG) and 2-hour plasma glucose (2hPG) categories with ANOVA. ANCOVA was used to adjust for covariates (age and BMI). Linear regression model adjusted for the follow-up time was used to evaluate the ability of IR indices and fasting plasma insulin levels to predict worsening of FPG, 2hPG and Glucose AUC. Results are presented as unstandardized effect sizes (B and SE) and standardized regression coefficient beta. Fishers r-to-z transformation was performed to test the difference between the standardized beta coefficient of IR indices and fasting insulin levels. Cox regression analysis was used to evaluate the ability of IR indices and fasting insulin levels to predict incident type 2 diabetes and CVD events. Hazard ratios (HRs) are presented with the 95% confidence intervals (CI). Linear and Cox regression models were additionally adjusted for age, BMI, smoking, physical activity, alcohol consumption, family history of type 2 diabetes, DI, Glucose AUC at baseline, and linear regression model additionally for follow-up time. Cox model evaluating the risk of incident CVD

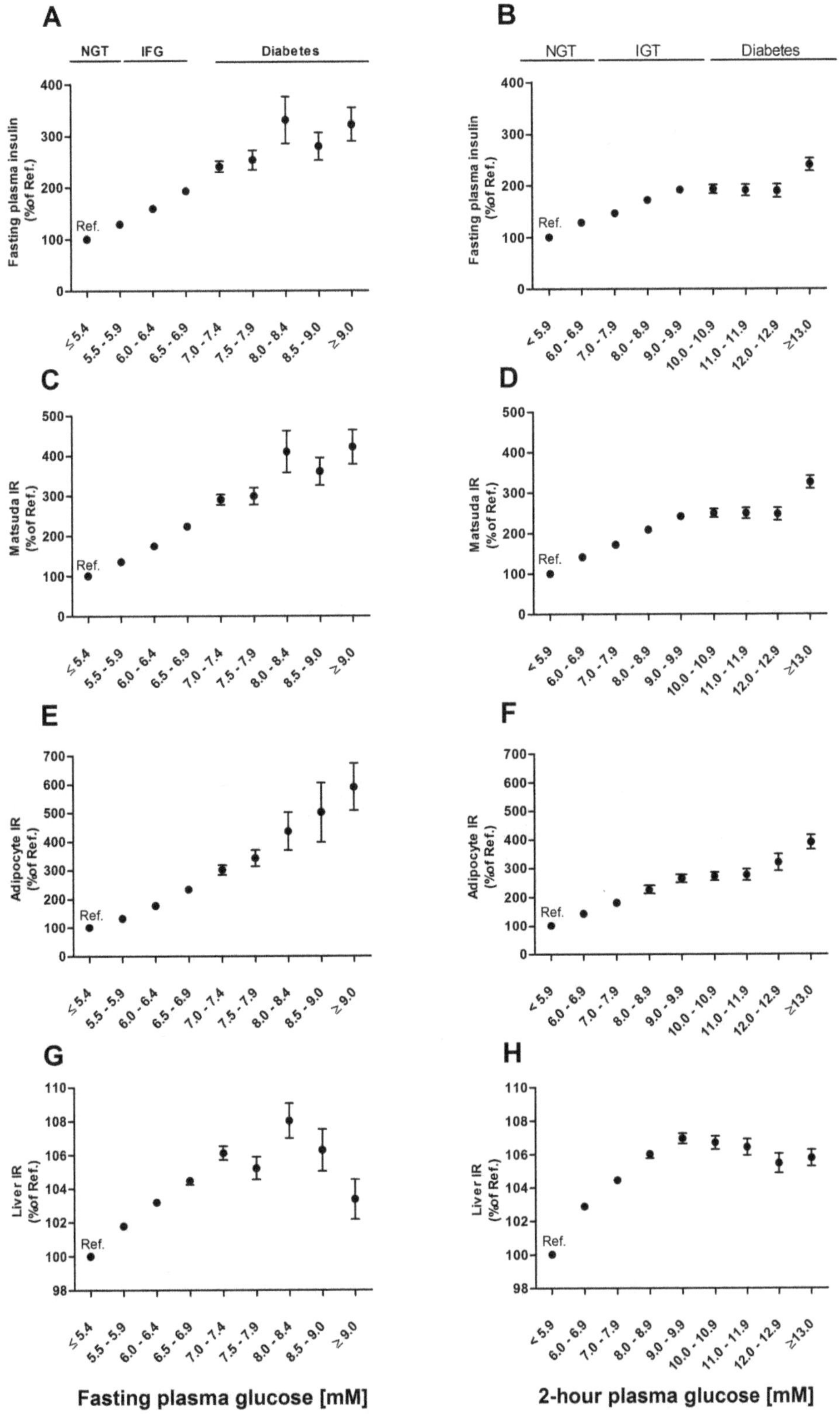

Figure 1. Mean values and standard errors of the mean (%) for tissue-specific insulin resistance (IR) indices across the fasting and 2-hour glucose categories. All indices and fasting insulin levels across the categories were significantly different from the reference category (fasting plasma glucose ≤5.4 mmol/L, 2-hour plasma glucose ≤5.9 mmol/L, $P<0.001$). *P* values for the trends, adjusted for age and BMI, were as follows: A) 4.7×10^{-181} B) 3.2×10^{-131} C) 6.5×10^{-299} D) $<6.5\times10^{-299}$ E) 1.7×10^{-204} F) $<6.5\times10^{-299}$ G) 1.3×10^{-20} H) 1.9×10^{-119}. NGT indicates normal glucose tolerance, IFG impaired fasting glucose, and IGT impaired glucose tolerance. Participants with previously diagnosed diabetes are excluded, N = 9,398. Abbreviations: IFG, impaired fasting glucose; IGT, impaired glucose tolerance; IR, insulin resistance; NGT, normal glucose tolerance; Ref, reference.

Table 1. Tissue-specific insulin resistance indices and fasting plasma insulin as predictors of hyperglyceamia at the 5.9-years METSIM follow-up study, Kuopio, Finland.

	FPG at follow-up							
Index at baseline	**B**	**SE**	**Beta**	P	P^a	P^b	P^c	P^d
Matsuda IR*	0.038	0.002	0.280	**1.5E-81**	**3.4E-39**	**3.8E-13**	**5.8E-07**	**4.3E-07**
Adipocyte IR	0.028	0.002	0.248	**9.4E-64**	**6.2E-25**	0.015	**0.001**	0.217
Liver IR	0.264	0.020	0.196	**5.2E-40**	**2.1E-06**	**8.9E-08**	0.733	**2.0E-03**
Fasting plasma insulin	0.036	0.002	0.248	**4.1E-64**	**1.3E-24**	**2.9E-04**	**1.4E-08**	**6.5E-04**
Index at baseline	**2hPG at follow-up**							
	B	**SE**	**Beta**	P	P^a	P^b	P^c	P^d
Matsuda IR*	0.150	0.007	0.312	**1.0E-101**	**1.6E-53**	**3.0E-19**	**5.6E-07**	**4.4E-07**
Adipocyte IR	0.126	0.006	0.319	**8.1E-106**	**5.5E-59**	**6.9E-16**	**1.2E-14**	**7.0E-10**
Liver IR	1.276	0.068	0.269	**3.7E-75**	**2.1E-23**	**1.4E-28**	**2.1E-06**	**1.3E-13**
Fasting plasma insulin	0.132	0.007	0.262	**2.4E-71**	**9.5E-32**	**6.5E-06**	**1.3E-09**	**2.8E-05**
Index at baseline	**Glucose AUC at follow-up**							
	B	**SE**	**Beta**	P	P^a	P^b	P^c	P^d
Matsuda IR*	0.091	0.004	0.361	**2.5E-137**	**4.0E-77**	**7.9E-28**	**7.9E-04**	**7.5E-04**
Adipocyte IR	0.073	0.003	0.356	**8.0E-133**	**1.0E-73**	**2.4E-15**	**1.2E-08**	**1.2E-05**
Liver IR	0.685	0.036	0.277	**4.3E-79**	**1.2E-21**	**2.4E-29**	0.063	**9.1E-05**
Fasting plasma insulin	0.077	0.004	0.294	**5.6E-90**	**1.5E-39**	**6.6E-05**	**3.7E-07**	**4.4E-04**

Abbreviations: B, unstandardized effect size; Beta, standardized regression coefficient; FPG, fasting plasma glucose; Glucose AUC, glucose area under the curve; 2hPG, 2-hour plasma glucose; IR, insulin resistance SE, standard error. Linear regression analysis. Values were calculated using log-transformed variables (except for age). Individuals with type 1 diabetes (N = 25), with known type 2 diabetes (N = 763), newly diagnosed type 2 diabetes at baseline (N = 649) or diagnosed with diabetes between baseline and follow-up (N = 117) were excluded, N = 4,474 for FPG and 2hPG, and 4,450 for glucose AUC. Bold font indicates statistical significance $P<0.0125$.

P, adjusted for follow-up time.

P^a, adjusted for follow-up time, age, BMI, smoking, physical activity, alcohol consumption and family history of type 2 diabetes.

P^b, adjusted for follow-up time, age, BMI, smoking, physical activity, alcohol consumption, family history of type 2 diabetes, and disposition index at baseline.

P^c, adjusted for follow-up time age, BMI, smoking, physical activity, alcohol consumption, family history of type 2 diabetes and glucose AUC at baseline.

P^d, adjusted for follow-up time, age, BMI, smoking, physical activity, alcohol consumption, family history of type 2 diabetes, disposition index and Glucose AUC at baselin.

*Matsuda IR was calculated as: 10/Matsuda ISI.

Disposition index was calculated as: Matsuda ISI $\times InsAUC_{0-30}/GluAUC_{0-30}$.

Table 2. Comparison of predictive ability of tissue-specific insulin resistance indices with fasting plasma insulin levels at baseline in predicting worsening of hyperglycemia at the 5.9-years METSIM follow-up study, Kuopio, Finland.

	FPG	
Indices at baseline	**Comparisons of Beta coefficients**	*P*
Fasting plasma insulin vs. Matsuda IR*	0.248 vs. 0.280	0.104
Fasting plasma insulin vs. Adipocyte IR	0.248 vs. 0.248	-
Fasting plasma insulin vs. Liver IR	**0.248 vs.0.196**	**0.010**
	2hPG	
Indices at baseline	**Comparisons of Beta coefficients**	*P*
Fasting plasma insulin vs. Matsuda IR*	**0.262 vs. 0.312**	**0.010**
Fasting plasma insulin vs. Adipocyte IR	**0.262 vs. 0.319**	**0.003**
Fasting plasma insulin vs. Liver IR	0.262 vs. 0.269	0.722
	Glucose AUC	
Indices at baseline	**Comparisons of Beta coefficients**	*P*
Fasting plasma insulin vs. Matsuda IR*	**0.294 vs. 0.361**	**<0.001**
Fasting plasma insulin vs. Adipocyte IR	**0.294 vs. 0.356**	**<0.001**
Fasting plasma insulin vs. Liver IR	0.294 vs. 0.277	0.383

Abbreviations: Beta, standardized regression coefficient; FPG, fasting plasma glucose; Glucose AUC, glucose area under the curve; 2hPG, 2-hour plasma glucose; IR, insulin resistance.
Beta was obtained from linear regression analysis. The difference between the standardized coefficients of IR indices and fasting insulin was tested using Fishers r-to-z transformation. Individuals with type 1 diabetes (N = 25), with known type 2 diabetes (N = 763), newly diagnosed type 2 diabetes at baseline (N = 649) or diagnosed with diabetes between baseline and follow-up (N = 117) were excluded, N = 4,474 for FPG and 2hPG, and 4,450 for glucose AUC. Bold font indicates statistical significance $P<0.0125$. *P*, unadjusted.
*Matsuda IR was calculated as: 10/Matsuda ISI.

events was additionally adjusted for age, BMI smoking, physical activity, alcohol consumption, family history of type 2 diabetes, hypertension, and LDL cholesterol at baseline. $P<0.0125$ was considered as statistically significant given the 3 IR indices and fasting insulin tested. $P<0.05$ was considered as nominally significant.

Results

Tissue specific insulin resistance indices in the categories of glucose tolerance

The association of the IR indices in non-diabetic individuals and individuals with newly diagnosed type 2 diabetes across the FPG and 2hPG categories in the cross-sectional analysis of the METSIM study cohort is shown in Figure 1. Categories of FPG≤ 5.4 mmo/l and 2hPG≤5.9 mmol/l were set as the reference categories. The fasting plasma insulin levels increased significantly ($P=4.7\times10^{-181}$ and $P=3.2\times10^{-131}$, respectively) across the range of both FPG and 2hPG categories. Matsuda IR increased significantly with increasing FPG ($P=6.5\times10^{-299}$) and 2hPG categories ($P<6.5\times10^{-299}$), adjusted for age and BMI. Compared to the reference categories, Matsuda IR increased up to +124% in the impaired fasting glucose (IFG) category and up +321% in newly diagnosed diabetes, and in the 2hPG categories up to + 150% and +226% in the impaired glucose tolerance (IGT) category and in newly diagnosed diabetes respectively. Adipocyte IR also showed a significant association with the FPG ($P=1.7\times10^{-204}$) and 2hPG ($P<6.5\times10^{-299}$) categories. Adipocyte IR increased up to +133% in individuals with IFG and up to +490% in individuals with newly diagnosed diabetes, and in the 2hPG categories up to 172% and 291% in IGT and in newly diagnosed diabetes, respectively, compared to the reference categories. Liver IR increased significantly across the entire range of FPG ($P=1.3\times10^{-20}$) and 2hPG ($P=1.9\times10^{-119}$). Across the FPG categories, Liver IR increased up to +4% in IFG and up to + 3% in individuals with newly detected diabetes as compared to the reference category. In the 2hPG categories Liver IR increased up to +7%, and +6% in IGT and in newly diagnosed diabetes, respectively.

Insulin resistance indices and fasting plasma insulin levels as predictors for the worsening of hyperglycemia

Matsuda IR, Adipocyte IR, Liver IR and fasting plasma insulin levels significantly predicted an increase in FPG, 2hPG and Glucose AUC (Table 1). Matsuda IR and Adipocyte IR were the best predictors of 2hPG and Glucose AUC. The associations were attenuated, but not abolished, after the adjustment for known risk factors of type 2 diabetes (age, BMI, smoking, physical activity, alcohol consumption and family history of type 2 diabetes). Additional adjustment for DI and Glucose AUC at baseline abolished the predictive value of Adipocyte IR and Liver IR in predicting FPG. Matsuda IR and Adipocyte IR were significantly better predictors for 2hPG and Glucose AUC than were fasting plasma insulin levels (Table 2).

Insulin resistance indices and fasting plasma insulin levels as predictors of incident diabetes and CVD events

A total of 558 of 8,749 non-diabetic men at baseline developed incident type 2 diabetes and 239 men a CVD event. In unadjusted

Table 3. Tissue-specific insulin resistance indices and fasting plasma insulin as predictors of incident type 2 diabetes in the 5.9-years METSIM prospective study, Kuopio, Finland.

	Incident type 2 diabetes								
	N								
Index at baseline	Events	Total	HR	95% CI	P	P^a	P^b	P^c	P^d
Matsuda IR*	556	8,697	1.46	1.40–1.52	**1.3E-70**	**2.2E-19**	**0.013**	0.746	0.985
Adipocyte IR	557	8,743	1.36	1.31–1.42	**1.3E-48**	**7.0E-11**	0.950	0.435	0.092
Liver IR	555	8,674	1.83	1.68–1.98	**3.8E-46**	**1.4E-08**	**1.7E-04**	0.855	0.237
Fasting plasma insulin	557	8,745	1.37	1.32–1.42	**2.3E-59**	**1.1E-10**	0.347	0.073	0.600

Abbreviations: CI, confidence interval; HR, hazard ratio; IR, insulin resistance.
HRs and their 95% CI were obtained from Cox regression analyses. HRs were calculated using standardized predictors (unit = one standard deviation). Individuals with type 1 diabetes (N = 25), type 2 diabetes (N = 763) or newly diagnosed type 2 diabetes at baseline (N = 649) were excluded. A total of 558 individuals were diagnosed with incident type 2 diabetes during the 5.9 year follow-up, 8,191 participants remained non-diabetic. Bold font indicates statistical significance $P<0.0125$.
P, unadjusted.
P^a, adjusted for age, BMI, smoking, physical activity, alcohol consumption and family history of type 2 diabetes.
P^b, adjusted for age, BMI, smoking, physical activity, alcohol consumption, family history of type 2 diabetes and disposition index at baseline.
P^c, adjusted for age, BMI, smoking, physical activity, alcohol consumption, family history of type 2 diabetes and glucose AUC at baseline.
P^d adjusted for age, BMI, smoking, physical activity, alcohol consumption, family history of type 2 diabetes, disposition index and glucose AUC at baseline.
*Matsuda IR was calculated as: 10/Matsuda ISI.
Disposition index was calculated as: Matsuda ISI×InsAUC$_{0-30}$/GluAUC$_{0-30}$.

Cox regression models all tissue-specific IR indices and fasting plasma insulin levels significantly predicted an increased risk of incident type 2 diabetes (Table 3) and incident CVD events (Table 4). Liver IR was the strongest predictor of both incident type 2 diabetes (HR = 1.83, 95% CI: 1.68–1.98, $P = 3.80 \times 10^{-46}$) and CVD events (HR = 1.31, 95% CI: 1.15–1.48, $P = 4.0 \times 10^{-5}$). Matsuda IR, Adipocyte IR and fasting plasma insulin levels had comparable ability to predict incident type 2 diabetes and CVD events.

Discussion

Insulin resistance is an important predictor for the development of type 2 diabetes and contributes to an elevated risk of CVD events [3–5,7–9,17]. None of the previous studies has investigated the association of different markers of tissue level IR with the worsening of hyperglycemia, conversion to type 2 diabetes or incident CVD events. Our study showed that Matsuda IR (representing mainly IR in the skeletal muscle), Adipocyte IR (representing IR in the adipose tissue), Liver IR (representing IR in the liver) and fasting plasma insulin levels significantly predicted the worsening of hyperglycemia and the conversion to type 2 diabetes, independently of the confounding factors (age, BMI, smoking, physical activity, alcohol consumption, family history of diabetes, insulin secretion and baseline glycemia). Importantly, Matsuda IR and Adipocyte IR were superior to fasting insulin levels in predicting 2hPG and Glucose AUC. All markers of IR significantly predicted an increased risk of CVD events in unadjusted models.

Hyperinsulinemic euglycemic clamp is the gold standard for measuring whole-body insulin sensitivity [11]. Combined with radiolabelled glucose it allows to quantify individual contribution of liver and muscle insulin resistance to impaired whole-body glucose disposal [30]. These techniques are not, however, applicable to large population-based studies. Therefore, markers of IR suitable for large-scale studies have been developed. An index of muscle insulin sensitivity developed by Abdul-Ghani et al. [4] is based on the measurement of glucose and insulin during an OGTT at 8 time points. This index had a correlation of 0.78 with the M value from the clamp [4]. Because several blood samples are needed, this measure is not possible to apply in large-scale population-based studies. Instead, we calculated Matsuda IR based on three measurements (0, 30 120 min) during an OGTT. We have previously shown that Matsuda ISI, based on five measurements (0, 30, 50, 90 and 120 min), has a correlation of 0.77 with the M value from the clamp, and that Matsuda ISI based on five and three measurements gives very similar results (correlation of 0.985) [31]. Therefore, we believe that 10/Matsuda ISI reliably measures skeletal muscle IR in insulin-stimulated state. We have developed a new index of Liver IR having a correlation of 0.65 with a product of tracer measured hepatic glucose production and fasting insulin [26]. This index was used as a surrogate marker of liver IR in our statistical analyses. Insulin resistance in adipose tissue leads to an impairment of insulin's antilipolytic effect, contributing to increased flux of free fatty acids into the circulation. We estimated Adipocyte IR with an index validated previously, calculated as the product of the fasting plasma insulin concentration and the fasting plasma FFA concentration [32].

Matsuda IR, reflecting insulin resistance mainly in the skeletal muscle, and Adipocyte IR had comparable ability to predict the worsening of hyperglycemia, measured by 2hPG and Glucose AUC in an OGTT, after adjustment for all confounding risk factors, including insulin secretion and baseline Glucose AUC.

Table 4. Tissue-specific insulin resistance indices and fasting plasma insulin as predictors of total incident CVD events in the 5.9-Years METSIM prospective study, Kuopio, Finland.

	Incident CVD events					
	N					
Index at baseline	Event	Total	HR	95%CI	P	P^a
Matsuda IR*	237	8,301	1.14	1.02–1.27	0.021	0.559
Adipocyte IR	239	8,346	1.12	1.01–1.24	0.032	0.536
Liver IR	237	8,283	1.31	1.15–1.48	**4.0E-05**	0.126
Fasting plasma insulin	239	8,348	1.11	1.00–1.24	0.049	0.599

Abbreviations: CI, confidence interval; CVD, cardiovascular disease; HR, hazard ratio; IR, insulin resistance; LDL-C low-density lipoprotein cholesterol.
Cox regression analysis. HRs were calculated using standardized predictors (unit = one standard deviation). Individuals with previously or newly diagnosed type 2 diabetes and type 1 diabetes at baseline were excluded from the analyses, as well as individuals with myocardial infarction and stroke before the baseline. Bold font indicates statistical significance $P<0.0125$. Individuals with type 1 diabetes (N = 25), type 2 diabetes (N = 763) or newly diagnosed type 2 diabetes at baseline (N = 649) were excluded.
P, unadjusted.
P^a, adjusted for age, BMI smoking, physical activity, alcohol consumption and family history of type 2 diabetes, hypertension (diagnosis was based on drug reimbursement) and LDL-C at baseline.
*Matsuda IR was calculated as: 10/Matsuda ISI.

This is not surprising since skeletal muscle is responsible for >60% of glucose disposal in insulin-stimulated states. Both indices predicted better an increase in 2hPG and Glucose AUC at follow-up than fasting plasma insulin levels. Liver IR was the strongest predictor of the conversion to type 2 diabetes (HR = 1.83, 95% CI: 1.68–1.98, $P = 3.80 \times 10^{-46}$) and incident CVD events (HR = 1.31, 95% CI: 1.15–1.48, $P = 4.0 \times 10^{-05}$) in our 5.9-year follow-up study, although Matsuda IR, Adipocyte IR and fasting plasma insulin levels also significantly predicted incident type 2 diabetes and CVD events.

The strengths of our study include the examination of a large, population-based sample of men across a broad age range and standardized assessment of diabetes with an OGTT, and the measurement of tissue-level IR with validated markers. Limitations of our study are that it included only men, and one ethnic group. Although we used validated markers for IR, direct physiological measurement of insulin sensitivity at tissue level (euglycemic clamp, radiolabelled glucose etc.) are more accurate. However, direct tissue level measurements are not possible to perform in studies of several thousand participants.

In conclusion, tissue-specific markers of IR predicted the worsening of hyperglycemia, incident type 2 diabetes and CVD events, independently of confounding risk factors. Matsuda IR and Adipocyte IR were stronger predictors of the worsening of 2hPG and Glucose AUC than fasting plasma insulin levels. Liver IR was the best predictor for incident type 2 diabetes and CVD events. Our study shows that tissue-specific markers of IR offer a new approach to evaluate the role of insulin resistance beyond and above fasting insulin level in the prediction of incident type 2 diabetes and cardiovascular disease.

Author Contributions

Conceived and designed the experiments: ML JK. Performed the experiments: MF HC AS RJ JV. Analyzed the data: MF HC AS RJ JV. Contributed reagents/materials/analysis tools: ML JK. Contributed to the writing of the manuscript: MF ML HC AS.

References

1. Defronzo RA (2009) Banting Lecture. From the triumvirate to the ominous octet: a new paradigm for the treatment of type 2 diabetes mellitus. Diabetes 58: 773–795.
2. Tripathy D, Almgren P, Tuomi T, Groop L (2004) Contribution of insulin-stimulated glucose uptake and basal hepatic insulin sensitivity to surrogate measures of insulin sensitivity. Diabetes Care 27: 2204–2210.
3. Lillioja S, Mott DM, Spraul M, Ferraro R, Foley JE, et al. (1993) Insulin resistance and insulin secretory dysfunction as precursors of non-insulin-dependent diabetes mellitus. Prospective studies of Pima Indians. N Engl J Med 329: 1988–1992.
4. Abdul-Ghani MA, Matsuda M, Balas B, DeFronzo RA (2007) Muscle and liver insulin resistance indexes derived from the oral glucose tolerance test. Diabetes Care 30: 89–94.
5. Laakso M, Sarlund H, Salonen R, Suhonen M, Pyorala K, et al. (1991) Asymptomatic atherosclerosis and insulin resistance. Arterioscler Thromb 11: 1068–1076.
6. Bressler P, Bailey SR, Matsuda M, DeFronzo RA (1996) Insulin resistance and coronary artery disease. Diabetologia 39: 1345–1350.
7. Ferrannini E, Natali A, Camastra S, Nannipieri M, Mari A, et al. (2013) Early metabolic markers of the development of dysglycemia and type 2 diabetes and their physiological significance. Diabetes 62: 1730–1737.
8. Lorenzo C, Wagenknecht LE, D'Agostino RB Jr., Rewers MJ, Karter AJ, et al. (2010) Insulin resistance, beta-cell dysfunction, and conversion to type 2 diabetes in a multiethnic population: the Insulin Resistance Atherosclerosis Study. Diabetes Care 33: 67–72.
9. Walker M, Mari A, Jayapaul MK, Bennett SM, Ferrannini E (2005) Impaired beta cell glucose sensitivity and whole-body insulin sensitivity as predictors of hyperglycaemia in non-diabetic subjects. Diabetologia 48: 2470–2476.
10. Lyssenko V, Almgren P, Anevski D, Perfekt R, Lahti K, et al. (2005) Predictors of and longitudinal changes in insulin sensitivity and secretion preceding onset of type 2 diabetes. Diabetes 54: 166–174.
11. DeFronzo RA (2004) Pathogenesis of type 2 diabetes mellitus. Medical Clinics of North America 88: 787–835.
12. Zierath JR, Kawano Y (2003) The effect of hyperglycaemia on glucose disposal and insulin signal transduction in skeletal muscle. Best Practice & Research Clinical Endocrinology & Metabolism 17: 385–398.
13. Cherrington AD (1999) Banting Lecture 1997. Control of glucose uptake and release by the liver in vivo. Diabetes 48: 1198–1214.
14. Abdul-Ghani MA, Matsuda M, DeFronzo RA (2008) Strong association between insulin resistance in liver and skeletal muscle in non-diabetic subjects. 25: 1289–1294.
15. Gastaldelli A, Natali A, Vettor R, Corradini SG (2010) Insulin resistance, adipose depots and gut: interactions and pathological implications. Dig Liver Dis 42: 310–319.
16. Laakso M (1993) How good a marker is insulin level for insulin resistance? Am J Epidemiol 137: 959–965.
17. Gast KB, Tjeerdema N, Stijnen T, Smit JW, Dekkers OM (2012) Insulin resistance and risk of incident cardiovascular events in adults without diabetes: meta-analysis. PLoS One 7: e52036.

18. Kuusisto J, Lempiainen P, Mykkanen L, Laakso M (2001) Insulin resistance syndrome predicts coronary heart disease events in elderly type 2 diabetic men. Diabetes Care 24: 1629–1633.
19. Matsuda M, DeFronzo RA (1999) Insulin sensitivity indices obtained from oral glucose tolerance testing: comparison with the euglycemic insulin clamp. Diabetes Care 22: 1462–1470.
20. Bergman RN, Ider YZ, Bowden CR, Cobelli C (1979) Quantitative estimation of insulin sensitivity. Am J Physiol 236: E667–677.
21. Stumvoll M, Mitrakou A, Pimenta W, Jenssen T, Yki-Jarvinen H, et al. (2000) Assessment of insulin secretion from the oral glucose tolerance test in white patients with type 2 diabetes. Diabetes Care 23: 1440–1441.
22. Katz A, Nambi SS, Mather K, Baron AD, Follmann DA, et al. (2000) Quantitative insulin sensitivity check index: a simple, accurate method for assessing insulin sensitivity in humans. J Clin Endocrinol Metab 85: 2402–2410.
23. Stancakova A, Javorsky M, Kuulasmaa T, Haffner SM, Kuusisto J, et al. (2009) Changes in insulin sensitivity and insulin release in relation to glycemia and glucose tolerance in 6,414 Finnish men. Diabetes 58: 1212–1221.
24. Abdul-Ghani MA, Molina-Carrion M, Jani R, Jenkinson C, Defronzo RA (2008) Adipocytes in subjects with impaired fasting glucose and impaired glucose tolerance are resistant to the anti-lipolytic effect of insulin. Acta Diabetol 45: 147–150.
25. Matthews DR, Hosker JP, Rudenski AS, Naylor BA, Treacher DF, et al. (1985) Homeostasis model assessment: insulin resistance and beta-cell function from fasting plasma glucose and insulin concentrations in man. Diabetologia 28: 412–419.
26. Vangipurapu J, Stancakova A, Kuulasmaa T, Paananen J, Kuusisto J, et al. (2011) A novel surrogate index for hepatic insulin resistance. Diabetologia 54: 540–543.
27. American Diabetes A (2006) Diagnosis and classification of diabetes mellitus. Diabetes Care 29 Suppl 1: S43–48.
28. Thygesen K, Alpert JS, Jaffe AS, Simoons ML, Chaitman BR, et al. (2012) Third universal definition of myocardial infarction. Eur Heart J 33: 2551–2567.
29. European Stroke Initiative Executive C, Committee EW, Olsen TS, Langhorne P, Diener HC, et al. (2003) European Stroke Initiative Recommendations for Stroke Management-update 2003. Cerebrovasc Dis 16: 311–337.
30. Defronzo RA, Simonson D, Ferrannini E (1982) Hepatic and Peripheral Insulin Resistance - a Common Feature of Non-Insulin-Dependent (Nidd) and Insulin-Dependent Diabetes (Idd). Clinical Research 30: A523–A523.
31. Lorenzo C, Haffner SM, Stancakova A, Laakso M (2010) Relation of Direct and Surrogate Measures of Insulin Resistance to Cardiovascular Risk Factors in Nondiabetic Finnish Offspring of Type 2 Diabetic Individuals. Journal of Clinical Endocrinology & Metabolism 95: 5082–5090.
32. Groop LC, Bonadonna RC, Delprato S, Ratheiser K, Zyck K, et al. (1989) Glucose and Free Fatty-Acid Metabolism in Non-Insulin-Dependent Diabetes-Mellitus - Evidence for Multiple Sites of Insulin Resistance Journal of Clinical Investigation 84: 205–213.

Permissions

All chapters in this book were first published in PLOS ONE, by The Public Library of Science; hereby published with permission under the Creative Commons Attribution License or equivalent. Every chapter published in this book has been scrutinized by our experts. Their significance has been extensively debated. The topics covered herein carry significant findings which will fuel the growth of the discipline. They may even be implemented as practical applications or may be referred to as a beginning point for another development.

The contributors of this book come from diverse backgrounds, making this book a truly international effort. This book will bring forth new frontiers with its revolutionizing research information and detailed analysis of the nascent developments around the world.

We would like to thank all the contributing authors for lending their expertise to make the book truly unique. They have played a crucial role in the development of this book. Without their invaluable contributions this book wouldn't have been possible. They have made vital efforts to compile up to date information on the varied aspects of this subject to make this book a valuable addition to the collection of many professionals and students.

This book was conceptualized with the vision of imparting up-to-date information and advanced data in this field. To ensure the same, a matchless editorial board was set up. Every individual on the board went through rigorous rounds of assessment to prove their worth. After which they invested a large part of their time researching and compiling the most relevant data for our readers.

The editorial board has been involved in producing this book since its inception. They have spent rigorous hours researching and exploring the diverse topics which have resulted in the successful publishing of this book. They have passed on their knowledge of decades through this book. To expedite this challenging task, the publisher supported the team at every step. A small team of assistant editors was also appointed to further simplify the editing procedure and attain best results for the readers.

Apart from the editorial board, the designing team has also invested a significant amount of their time in understanding the subject and creating the most relevant covers. They scrutinized every image to scout for the most suitable representation of the subject and create an appropriate cover for the book.

The publishing team has been an ardent support to the editorial, designing and production team. Their endless efforts to recruit the best for this project, has resulted in the accomplishment of this book. They are a veteran in the field of academics and their pool of knowledge is as vast as their experience in printing. Their expertise and guidance has proved useful at every step. Their uncompromising quality standards have made this book an exceptional effort. Their encouragement from time to time has been an inspiration for everyone.

The publisher and the editorial board hope that this book will prove to be a valuable piece of knowledge for researchers, students, practitioners and scholars across the globe.

List of Contributors

Julio Plaza-Diaz, Carolina Gomez-Llorente, Sergio Muñoz-Quezada, Angel Gil and Luis Fontana
Department of Biochemistry & Molecular Biology II, School of Pharmacy, University of Granada, Granada, Spain
Institute of Nutrition & Food Technology "José Mataix", Biomedical Research Center, University of Granada, Granada, Spain

Laura Campañ a-Martin
Institute of Nutrition & Food Technology "Jose´ Mataix", Biomedical Research Center, University of Granada, Granada, Spain

Francisco Abadia-Molina
Department of Cell Biology, School of Sciences, University of Granada, Granada, Spain,

Maria Jose Saez-Lara
Department of Biochemistry & Molecular Biology I, School of Sciences, University of Granada, Granada, Spain

Fernando Romero
Hero Global Technology Center, Hero Spain, S.A., Alcantarilla, Murcia, Spain

Juancong Dong and Shunzi Jin
School of Public Health of Jilin University, Changchun, China

Minglong Shao
School of Public Health of Jilin University, Changchun, China
Chinese-American Research Institute for Diabetic Complications, Wenzhou Medical University, Wenzhou, China
Ruian Center of Chinese-American Research Institute for Diabetic Complications, the Third Affiliated Hospital of the Wenzhou Medical University, Wenzhou, China

Xiao Xing
School of Public Health of Jilin University, Changchun, China
Changchun Institute for Food and Drug Control, Changchun, China

Chi Zhang
Chinese-American Research Institute for Diabetic Complications, Wenzhou Medical University, Wenzhou, China
Ruian Center of Chinese-American Research Institute for Diabetic Complications, the Third Affiliated Hospital of the Wenzhou Medical University, Wenzhou, China

Weitao Cong, Xiaokun Li and Litai Jin
Chinese-American Research Institute for Diabetic Complications, Wenzhou Medical University, Wenzhou, China
School of Pharmacy, Wenzhou Medical College, Wenzhou, China

Yi Tan and Lu Cai
Chinese-American Research Institute for Diabetic Complications, Wenzhou Medical University, Wenzhou, China
Kosair Children's Hospital Research Institute at the Department of Pediatrics, University of Louisville, Louisville, Kentucky, United States of America

Xuemian Lu
Ruian Center of Chinese-American Research Institute for Diabetic Complications, the Third Affiliated Hospital of the Wenzhou Medical University, Wenzhou, China

Xiaojie Wang
School of Pharmacy, Wenzhou Medical College, Wenzhou, China

Yunqian Li
Department of Neurosurgery, the First Hospital of Jilin University, Changchun, China

Jun-Yuan Huang and Lee-Young Chau
Institute of Biomedical Sciences, Academia Sinica, Taipei, Taiwan, Republic of China
Graduate Institute of Life Sciences, National Defense Medical Center, Taipei, Taiwan, Republic of China

Ming-Tsai Chiang
Graduate Institute of Life Sciences, National Defense Medical Center, Taipei, Taiwan, Republic of China

Feng Tian, Ya Jie Zhang and Ying Xie
Department of Gastroenterology, Shengjing Hospital of China Medical University, Shenyang, Liaoning Province, China

Yu Li
Department of Gastroenterology, Third People's Hospital of Dalian city, Dalian, Liaoning Province, China

Wenjuan Li, Chuanlong Wu, Yiran Lu, Xinguo Hou, Jun Song and Peng Lin
Department of Endocrinology, Qilu Hospital, Shandong University, Jinan, China

Li Chen and Lei Sun
Department of Endocrinology, Qilu Hospital, Shandong University, Jinan, China
Institute of Endocrinology and Metabolism, Shandong University, Jinan, China

Ruxing Zhao
Department of Endocrinology, Qilu Hospital, Shandong University, Jinan, China
Institute of Endocrinology and Metabolism, Shandong University, Jinan, China
Research Center for Cell Therapy, Key Laboratory of Cardiovascular Remodeling and Function Research, Qilu Hospital, Shandong University, Jinan, China

Dongqi Tang
Research Center for Cell Therapy, Key Laboratory of Cardiovascular Remodeling and Function Research, Qilu Hospital, Shandong University, Jinan, China

Shounan Yi
Centre for Transplant and Renal Research, Westmead Millennium Institute, The University of Sydney at Westmead Hospital, Westmead, New South Wales, Australia

Shun-Fa Hung
Division of Urology, Department of Surgery, Far Eastern Memorial Hospital, Ban Ciao, Taipei, Taiwan
Graduate Institute of Clinical Medicine, College of Medicine, Fu-Jen Catholic University, New Taipei, Taiwan

Chao-Yuan Huang
Department of Urology, National Taiwan University Hospital, Taipei, Taiwan
Management Office for Health Data, China Medical University Hospital, Taichung, Taiwan

Chia-Hung Kao
Graduate Institute of Clinical Medical Science and School of Medicine, College of Medicine, China Medical University, Taichung, Taiwan
Department of Nuclear Medicine and PET Center, China Medical University Hospital, Taichung, Taiwan

Melania Manco, Claudia Brufani and Rosa Luciano
Research Unit for Multi-factorial Diseases, Obesity and Diabetes, Scientific Directorate, Bambino Gesù Children Hospital, Rome, Italy

Lidia Castagneto-Gissey, Eugenio Arrighi, Annamaria Carnicelli and Geltrude Mingrone
Department of Internal Medicine, Catholic University, School of Medicine, Rome, Italy

Junji Takaya, Sohsaku Yamanouchi and Kazunari Kaneko
Department of Pediatrics, Kansai Medical University, Moriguchi, Osaka, Japan

Bernard Cudjoe Nkum, Frank Botsi Micah and Theophilus C. Ankrah
Department of Medicine, School of Medical Sciences, Kwame Nkrumah University of Science and Technology, Kumasi, Ghana

Ousman Nyan
Department of Medicine, Royal Victoria Teaching Hospital, Banjul, The Gambia

Hong Soon Kang, Grace Liao, Laura M. DeGraff and Anton M. Jetten
Cell Biology Section, National Institutes of Health, Research Triangle Park, North Carolina, United States of America

Kevin Gerrish
Microarray Group, National Institutes of Health, Research Triangle Park, North Carolina, United States of America

Carl D. Bortner
Laboratory of Signal Transduction, Division of Intramural Research, National Institute of Environmental Health Sciences, National Institutes of Health, Research Triangle Park, North Carolina, United States of America

Stavros Garantziotis
Matrix Biology Section, LRB, National Institutes of Health, Research Triangle Park, North Carolina, United States of America

Chuyan Wu, Feng Lin, Shuwei Qiu and Zhongli Jiang
Department of Rehabilitation Medicine, The First Affiliated Hospital of Nanjing Medical University, Nanjing, China

Nike Müller, Dominik M. Schulte, Susann Hillebrand, Kathrin Türk, Jochen Hampe, Mario Brosch, Rainald Zeuner, Johann O. Schröder, Marta Stelmach- Mardas, Carina Saggau, Stefan Schreiber and Matthias Laudes
Department I of Internal Medicine, University of Kiel, Kiel, Germany

Clemens Scafmhayer, Witigo von Schoönfels and Markus Ahrens
Department of General, Abdominal, Thoracic and Transplantation Surgery, University of Kiel, Kiel, Germany

Matthias Blüher
Department for Internal Medicine, Clinic for Endocrinology and Nephrology, University of Leipzig, Leipzig, Germany

Christian Gutschow
Department of General, Visceral and Cancer Surgery, University of Cologne, Cologne, Germany

Sandra Freitag-Wolf
Institute of Medical Informatics and Statistics, University of Kiel, Kiel, Germany

Qiang You
Department of Biotherapy, Second Affiliated Hospital, Nanjing Medical University, Nanjing, Jiangsu, China, Skaggs School of Pharmacy and Pharmaceutical Sciences, University of Colorado Anschutz Medical Campus, Aurora, Colorado, United States of America

Cynthia Ju
Skaggs School of Pharmacy and Pharmaceutical Sciences, University of Colorado Anschutz Medical Campus, Aurora, Colorado, United States of America

Brittany V. Martin-Murphy
Barbara Davis Center for Diabetes, University of Colorado Anschutz Medical Campus, Aurora, Colorado, United States of America

Hong Wang
Division of Endocrinology, Diabetes & Metabolism, University of Colorado Anschutz Medical Campus, Aurora, Colorado, United States of America

Becky A. De La Houssaye and Jacob E. Friedman
Department of Pediatrics, University of Colorado Anschutz Medical Campus, Aurora, Colorado, United States of America

Timothy P. Reilly
Drug Safety Evaluation, Research & Development, Bristol-Myers Squibb Company, Princeton, New Jersey, United States of America

Karsten Kristiansen
Department of Biology, University of Copenhagen, Copenhagen, Denmark

Lisa Kolden Midtbø, Lene Secher Myrmel, Ulrike Liisberg Aune and Lise Madsen
Department of Biology, University of Copenhagen, Copenhagen, Denmark
National Institute of Nutrition and Seafood Research, Bergen, Norway

Anita Røyneberg Alvheim, Nina S. Liland, Bente E. Torstensen, Bjørn Liaset and Trond Brattelid
National Institute of Nutrition and Seafood Research, Bergen, Norway

Mohammad Madani Ibrahim
National Institute of Nutrition and Seafood Research, Bergen, Norway
Institute of Biomedicine, University of Bergen, Bergen, NorwayStavanger, Norway

Seung-Hwan Lee, Hae Kyung Yang, Moo-Il Kang, Ho-Young Son and Kun- Ho Yoon
Department of Internal Medicine, College of Medicine, The Catholic University of Korea, Seoul, Korea
Division of Endocrinology and Metabolism, Department of Internal Medicine, Seoul St. Mary's Hospital, Seoul, Korea

Hyuk-Sang Kwon
Department of Internal Medicine, College of Medicine, The Catholic University of Korea, Seoul, Korea
Division of Endocrinology and Metabolism, Department of Internal Medicine, Yeouido St. Mary's Hospital, Seoul, Korea

Hee-Sung Ha and Won-Chul Lee
Department of Preventive Medicine, College of Medicine, The Catholic University of Korea, Seoul, Korea

Yong-Moon Park
Department of Preventive Medicine, College of Medicine, The Catholic University of Korea, Seoul, Korea
Department of Epidemiology and Biostatistics, Arnold School of Public Health, University of South Carolina, Columbia, South Carolina, United States of America

Hyeon-Woo Yim
Department of Preventive Medicine, College of Medicine, The Catholic University of Korea, Seoul, Korea
Clinical Research Coordinating Center, College of Medicine, The Catholic University of Korea, Seoul, Korea

Seung Hee Jeong
Clinical Research Coordinating Center, College of Medicine, The Catholic University of Korea, Seoul, Korea

Jin-Hee Lee
Catholic Institute of U-Healthcare, The Catholic University of Korea, Seoul, Korea

Lathika Mohanraj and Qing Cai
Department of Pathology, Virginia Commonwealth University, Richmond, Virginia, United States of America

Youngman Oh
Department of Pathology, Virginia Commonwealth University, Richmond, Virginia, United States of America
Biocure Pharma LLC, Richmond, Virginia, United States of America

Ho-Seong Kim, Woo Jung Lee and Jung Hyun Kim
Department of Pediatrics, Institute of Endocrinology, Yonsei University College of Medicine, Seoul, Korea

Wei Li
Biocure Pharma LLC, Richmond, Virginia, United States of America

Ki Eun Kim
Department of Pediatrics, CHA University College of Medicine, Seoul, Korea

Hye-Jung Shin
Department of Pediatrics, National Medical Center, Seoul, Korea

Yong-Jae Lee
Department of Family Medicine, Yonsei University College of Medicine, Seoul, Korea

Rachael Fletcher, Christopher Gribben, Xuiquan Ma, James G. Burchfield, Kristen C. Thomas and Daniel J. Fazakerley
Diabetes and Obesity Program, Garvan Institute of Medical Research, Sydney, New South Wales, Australia

James R. Krycer
Diabetes and Obesity Program, Garvan Institute of Medical Research, Sydney, New South Wales, Australia
School of Biotechnology and Biomolecular Sciences, The University of New South Wales, Sydney, New South Wales, Australia

David E. James
Diabetes and Obesity Program, Garvan Institute of Medical Research, Sydney, New South Wales, Australia
Charles Perkins Centre, School of Molecular Bioscience, The University of Sydney, Sydney, Australia

Nan Gu, Xiaowei Ma, Junqing Zhang, Aimei Dong, Mengmeng Jin, Nan Feng, Hong Zhang and Xiaohui Guo
Endocrinology Department, First Hospital, Peking University, Beijing, China

Nanda Gruben, Marcela Aparicio Vergara, Niels J. Kloosterhuis, Henk van der Molen, Stefan Stoelwinder, Jan Albert Kuivenhoven, Bart van de Sluis, Marten H. Hofker and Debby P. Y. Koonen
University of Groningen, University Medical Center Groningen, Department of Pediatrics, Molecular Genetics Section, Groningen, the Netherlands

Sameh Youssef and Alain de Bruin
Utrecht University, Faculty of Veterinary Medicine, Dutch Molecular Pathology Center, Utrecht, the Netherlands

Dianne J. Delsing
Merck Research Laboratories, MSD, Department of Immune Therapeutics, Oss, the Netherlands

Wei Chen, Meredith L. Howell, Yang Li, Rui Li and Guoxun Chen
Department of Nutrition, University of Tennessee at Knoxville, Knoxville, Tennessee, United States of America

Mária Fízel'ová, Alena Stančá ková and Jagadish Vangipurapu
Department of Medicine, University of Eastern Finland, Kuopio, Finland

Henna Cederberg, Raimo Jauhiainen, Johanna Kuusisto and Markku Laakso
Department of Medicine, University of Eastern Finland and Kuopio University Hospital, Kuopio, Finland

Index

N

O

P

R

S

T

V

W

www.ingramcontent.com/pod-product-compliance
Lightning Source LLC
LaVergne TN
LVHW060606210926
848485LV00005B/1377

* 9 7 8 1 6 3 2 4 2 9 5 3 7 *